ANNALS OF THE NEW YORK ACADEMY OF SCIENCES

Volume 809

COMMUNICATION WITH THE CANCER PATIENT

INFORMATION AND TRUTH

Edited by Antonella Surbone and Matjaž Zwitter

The New York Academy of Sciences
New York, New York
1997

∞ *The paper used in this publication meets the minimum requirements of American National Standard for Information Sciences—Permanence of Paper for Printed Library Materials, ANSI Z39.48-1984.*

Library of Congress Cataloging-in-Publication Data

Communication with the cancer patient : information and truth / edited by Antonella Surbone, Matjaž Zwitter .
p. -- (Annals of the New York Academy of Sciences, ISSN 0077-8923 ; v. 809)
Includes bibliographical references and index .
ISBN 0-89766-985-1 (cloth : alk. paper). -- ISBN 0-89766-986-X (pbk. : alk. paper)
1. Cancer--Patients--Congresses. 2. Physician and patient--Congresses. 3. Cancer--Psychological aspects--Congresses. I. Surbone, Antonella. II. Zwitter, Matjaž. III. Series.
[DNLM: 1. Neoplasms--psychology--congresses. 2. Truth Disclosure--congresses. 3. Cross-Cultural Comparison--congresses. 4. Physician-Patient Relations--congresses. W1 AN626YL v.809 1997 / QZ 200 C7346 1997]
[RC262]
500 s--dc21
DNLM/DLC
for Library of Congress 96-29490
CIP

CCP
Printed in the United States of America
ISBN 0-89766-985-1 (cloth)
ISBN 0-89766-986-x (paper)
ISSN 0077-8923

ANNALS OF THE NEW YORK ACADEMY OF SCIENCES

Volume 809
February 20, 1997

COMMUNICATION WITH THE CANCER PATIENT

INFORMATION AND TRUTH

Editors
ANTONELLA SURBONE AND MATJAŽ ZWITTER

CONTENTS

Part II. Africa

Part III. The Americas

Financial assistance was received from:

- CANCER ETHICS FUND
- POP TV (LJUBLJANA)

Foreword

Communication is the oldest of all our skills. It is often taken for granted and rarely included in the curricula of medical schools. Being in the shadow of the explosion of knowledge about the diagnostic and therapeutic medical disciplines, a discussion of the approach toward the patient is too often regarded as boring and of little innovative potential. Ambitions for development and cultivation of the communication process, invariably linked to a significant investment of the physicians's time, may also become an obstacle in the competitive world of references, citations, and academic achievements.

Yet communication—whether verbal or nonverbal—remains the single most important tool of the medical profession. New technologies are not replacing the need for a caring, compassionate physician. On the contrary: in the ever more alienated and sophisticated environment in our medical institutions, with the increasingly complex interventions offered to our patients, communications skills are not only desirable but indeed of crucial importance.

The origins of this project may be traced to our daily work with patients. Vivid discussions and correspondence with many friends around the globe, and the experience of practicing oncology under quite dissimilar cultural backgrounds led us to realize the close link between different cultures and the practice of communication with patients, including the fundamental question of withholding or disclosing the truth to those with a serious illness.

Dry information is not enough, and the physician's paternalistic approach is now increasingly regarded as unacceptable. But are patients and also doctors everywhere ready to cope with the demands of a distressing reality? And can reality be grasped in a single event that we call "truth"? Does truth ever exist in such a sense as to be similar to an object?

All these dilemmas are old, some of them as old as humanity. Yet, a clear discussion of these questions is urgently needed, or else the progress of medicine will be stuck in a traffic jam of mistrust and misunderstanding.

This book is an attempt to address the many aspects of truth-telling, including the cultural and the anthropological. The result is, we believe, a volume that provides the reader with an impression of the diversity of the present practices; of the somewhat less diverse views of future needs for proper communication and sincere relations; and of the very similar basic needs of all patients, regardless of their culture or education, to share the truth about the disease with their physician.

No book on such a topic may aim at universal coverage of the subject, and ours is no exception. Contributors share their personal views, as practicing physicians, rather than representing any official position of their countries. Varied personal styles of discussion reflect the preference of each contributor as well the specific aspect of the subject they chose to treat. Also, several of those invited to contribute a chapter could not do so; for this reason some parts of the world are not adequately represented, while others may appear to be overrepresented. Clearly, then, another selection of essays might lead to a very different volume. The reader is asked to kindly understand this obvious imperfection of our venture. Your critical comments, better addressed to the editors than to the authors, will be appreciated; even more welcome would be a notice about your willingness to formulate your own view—possibly a dissenting one—in a chapter for our next publication.

We are grateful to all our friends world-wide who have helped us so much in composing this unique symphony. We are indebted to Mr. Richard Stiefel for his enthusiasm and his editorial work. We are also indebted to Ms. Gladys Gonzalez for her most valuable assistance.

ANTONELLA SURBONE
MATJAŽ ZWITTER

Learning from the World

The Editors' Perspective

ANTONELLA SURBONE[a] AND MATJAŽ ZWITTER[b]

[a]*Department of Medicine*
Memorial Sloan-Kettering Cancer Center
New York, New York 10021

[b]*Institute of Oncology*
1105 Ljubljana, Slovenia

UNIVERSAL VALUES, PLURALISM, AND CULTURAL DIVERSITY

One of the most important lessons that we learned from the work of the colleagues from all over the world who have contributed to this book is that Western cultural hegemony is indeed a myth—a myth we should deny and oppose and for which we should substitute a universal cultural sensitivity. As was recently said, "ethical norms and human rights are universal not because they are recognized by certain countries or cultures, but because the human dignity in which they are grounded is universal." And "genuine respect for human dignity requires deeper understanding of the patient's values, culture, family and community."[1]

The implications are twofold: that differences exist, and that there is something universal about human dignity and therefore an ethical duty to respect it.

The first of these is what we could also refer to as pluralism. Pluralism is a de facto reality of our multiethnic societies, but also—most importantly—it is an essential principle of democracy. Pluralism does not have to lead to the intrinsic pessimism of cultural relativism, by which the ethical debate is paralyzed.[2] On the contrary, pluralism enriches ethics by fostering historical concreteness and by adding the dimension of the non-repeatibility of values,[3] which always express themselves within a precise contextual dimension. The common ethical principles that stem from the equal right of every human being to life and dignity[4] and that have led to the Universal Declaration of Human Rights[5] are real and cross-cultural in their essence. However, the modality in which they are expressed is influenced by cultural and historical differences—i.e., by their context.

The medical act is no exception, as it always takes place in a contextual dimension. Both physician and patient are bound in a network of beliefs, customs, experiences, prejudices, rules, responsibilities; and both have limited choices. This is why, for example, formalistic informed consent requirements can be possible and beneficial in certain contexts (see the prevailing Western attitude), but not in others. The different emphasis that different cultures place on autonomy versus community as basic ethical principles shapes the medical act as well as any other interaction among members of a society.

However, the issue goes beyond cultural differences, and facing some more fundamental questions will help us move from the descriptive level to the ethical. When speaking of truth-telling, we imply that we know the meaning of truth. Do we? Do we know what truth is as persons? Do we know it as doctors? It seems that the answer is no, we do not know what truth is. What we can know, though, is how we perceive truth. If we perceive truth as the mere opposite or absence of falsehood, we imply that truth is a fixed object that merely awaits description and/or verbalization.[2] In medicine, this leads to seeing information as a procedure, rather than a process. The justification for this is that there exists an objective static medical truth, and that truth equals information; hence, information suffices. But this is not the case, for truth is a relational state and develops over time and space through interactions that modify and shape truth itself. Accurate, comprehensible, continuous information remains an essential element of truth, but truth goes well beyond information alone to reach the level of communication.

This is no easy task, and it will be increasingly difficult in the face of modern medicine with its high technology, superspecialization, and economic pressure. But it is indeed now that we need to restore a human face to medicine, and one way of doing so is by practicing cultural sensitivity[6,7] and intense, systematic imaginative empathy.[8] All the contributions to this book seem to be in favor of this approach: they are not only honest reports of various ways of facing the issue of truth-telling, but they are also an incredible source of practical and theoretical suggestions for each one of us to practice imaginative empathy.

Imaginative empathy is difficult, as it requires a reappraisal of the physician's role that we will achieve only through major changes in the educational system. The education and training of doctors must aim at developing not only the scientific curriculum but also the moral character of each physician. Sooner or later we will all be patients, and we will hope to meet a doctor to trust for his or her moral character no less than for his or her expertise, because it is only on the basis of both that healing is possible.

Communication requires honesty, humility, and the complete abandonment of the doctor's more or less explicit desire for power. Imposed formalistic information,for instance, can be a means of increasing the doctor's power, rather than of giving freedom to patients. Giving such information can, as much as witholding the truth, be a way of delegating the entire burden of decisions to the patient, thus avoiding professional responsibilities.[9] Excessive medicalization of life and death, in which technology, hospitals, and health-care teams leave no place for the patient's personal system of support—family, friends, values, religious beliefs and practices—is another sign of the abuse of the doctor's power; it is dangerous, ineffective, and ethically unjustifiable. Last but not least, there are things in life that cannot—and should not—be communicated. Forcing the barriers of the incommunicable is an intrusion into the patient's privacy and intimacy—another abuse of the doctor's power.

The patient-doctor relationship is asymmetrical. For the patient disease is a personal—most often devastating—event in his or her life, with a past, a present, and a future, however short it might be. The doctor, on the other hand, must focus on the objective dimension of the disease. The patient's and the doctor's narratives are different. The patient is inevitably in a more vulnerable position. The ethics of the patient-doctor relationship must take into account this asymmetry. All the contributions to this volume show us that we must *care.* We cannot stop at the view of the autonomous moral agent, whose moral responsibility exhausts itself in relationships among peers. We need to add the dimension of trust and of respect of the patient's vulnerability: the doctor as a moral agent is called to acknowledge the asymmetry of the relationship with the patient and should consider sensitivity, including cultural sensitivity, as a fundamental ethical requirement.

CULTURAL DIVERSITY AND THE CHANGING WORLD.

When the relationship between communication in medicine and cultural diversity is analyzed, three conclusions emerge. First, cultural diversity is a reality that cannot be ignored. Second, in a rapidly changing world patients and physicians are among those who will most clearly experience the tension between the old and the new. Last but not least, justice in the availability of proper medical care is of great importance when sincere communication between patient and doctor is sought, particularly for underprivileged patients throughout the world.

Modern medicine is certainly not a folklore festival, and nice words about the rich diversity of cultures may sound idealistic when the primary objective of a physician is effective treatment for cancer. However, one of the important messages of contributors to this volume from all parts of the world is that the rich diversity of cultures is a reality. No matter how unusual some of the beliefs, rituals, and sociological patterns may be to an outsider, the physician cannot ignore the patient's cultural background and his or her support network. Human understanding of disease and death is an important part of all cultures and religions. It is closely linked to how we define the position of an individual in a society. The seeds of this understanding have been sown early in childhood, and their roots are far-reaching. Beliefs about causes and classification of diseases, assumptions about the links between the body and external and internal spiritual forces, the existence and life of the soul before birth and after physical death of the body—these are eternal questions whose answers greatly influence the ways in which patients cope with disease and suffering. The consumer-oriented approach of favoring treatment over prevention, excessive emphasis on the effectiveness of modern treatments for cancer, and the lack of efforts to integrate the acceptance of our own mortality and the demands of our life seem to be typical products of the Western world and of this century. Most modern Western cultures appear to exorcise suffering and dying and limit exposure to these events. Thus the norm becomes health and happiness, while sickness is seen as a deviation to be avoided at all cost. In more traditional cultures, on the contrary, disease, suffering, and death are not taboo, not even for children; on the contrary, they are occasions and most powerful tools for instilling and inspiring religious, spiritual, and philosophical beliefs.

In our multicultural, multiethnic societies the outer appearance and behavior of an individual human being may change with the adoption of another cultural pattern. In critical situations, however, it is the roots, not branches or leaves, that determine our responses: when facing serious disease or death we often return to the cultural values and practices to which we were first exposed in childhood. Moreover, there is an active effort to preserve cultural identity, which is not only understandable but very appropriate: in the new world of continuous stress and of global marketing (including political marketing), old cultural traditions find a new and most important role in relieving tensions, preserving local identity, and preventing the dissolution of human diversity into a pool of six billion competing individuals.

The world is changing, however; and compared to changes in the past, those of today are rapid and global. People in remote villages feel the waves of modern life with new technologies and emphasis on everyone's individual capabilities, rights, and responsibilities. The tension between the old and the new is felt worldwide, very likely to an equal extent in developing and in economically well-developed countries. We have said that patients and physicians will clearly feel tensions between the old and the new—the patients, since their health and life are at stake; and physicians, since they have to strive to achieve an often impossible balance between responsibility towards the patient, which includes establishing a sincere relationship, and the expectations of the patient's support network. Often relatives or other figures in the patient's life attempt to dominate the situation in an effort to protect the ill person from too painful a truth. In such a situation, the patient may silently sink into a passive role—and offer a nice example to those physicians who still believe that most patients do not wish to be properly informed about their disease. The physician's task is also to reveal the true, often hidden expectations, questions, fears, and misconceptions of the patient, while respecting his or her cultural and family backgrounds. This may involve lengthy, sometimes hostile argument with those who feel that they are in charge of the patient. Often the physician tries not to cross the line beyond which the family would reject him as healer, or beyond which the effort to introduce more sincerity into the interhuman relations would actually lead to their total obstruction. The goal is to break down, not to build, barriers.

JUSTICE

Justice in the availability of proper medical care, we have said, is the third aspect that illustrates the influence of a particular culture upon the process of communication with the cancer patient. There is no doubt that for many patients the possibility of a cure lies in the hands of those who decide on the allocation of resources for medical care and cancer treatment. Many of our colleagues, especially those from the developing countries, mention the critical shortage of appropriate medical institutions, equipment, drugs, and manpower. To what extent are patients informed about this? It seems that quite often physicians are reluctant to suggest a transfer of a patient to another institution, for instance, very likely at substantial financial and emotional cost, without a guarantee for a cure. Although this might be seen as a paternalistic position, it is often the most honest solution. The major impact of economic considerations on the quality of health care for patients in different socioeconomic groups and in different societies is an ethical quandary, and it also affects the issue of communication.

Specific problems of communication with women in the developing countries and with the underprivileged in some of the most developed countries, such as the United States—two groups particularly suffering from lack of proper medical care—have rarely been mentioned even in this volume written by very open, sincere, honest physicians. Discrimination against women is not only linked to certain traditions, religions, or cultures, but also extends to the so-called democratic societies. Behind almost ideal constitutional rights we still find men in dominating positions, and this is reflected in differences of access to health care and research.

The existence of grossly underprivileged populations in some affluent countries seems to be an unavoidable consequence of the Western emphasis over the last two centuries on personal achievement and success. Yet, even for a large part of the North American and European populations, reliance on complete autonomy and individual self-determination may be more illusion than reality: the underprivileged and those who are simply unlucky (perhaps because of the unexpected occurrence of a serious disease) would probably be happy to subscribe to a system of greater interdependence and solidarity. For the majority of the world population, emphasis on absolute autonomy is neither a goal nor a dream.

What are the specific aspects of communication with the cancer patient if this patient is, for instance, a single mother of two preschool children in Russia, or a man in the United States whose potentially life-saving treatment will not be covered by insurance? Clearly, many pressing questions remain unanswered.

We hope that this book will open an intense, productive discussion on all aspects of truth-telling, from its philosophical and anthropological foundations to its social and political implications.

REFERENCES

1. Gostin, L. O. 1995. Informed consent, cultural sensitivity, and respect for person. JAMA **274:** 844–845.
2. Surbone, A. 1994. Informed consent and truth in medicine. Eur. J. Cancer **30A:** 2189.
3. Bellino, F. 1993. I fondamenti della bioetica. Città Nuova. Roma.
4. Thompson, I. E. 1987. Fundamental ethical principles in health care. Br. Med. J. **295:** 1461–1465.
5. General Assembly of the United Nations. 1948. Universal Declaration of Human Rights. United Nations. Geneva
6. Blackhall, L. J, S. T. Murphy, G. Frank, V. Michel & S. Azen. 1995. Ethnicity and attitudes toward patient autonomy. JAMA **274:** 820–825.
7. Girgis, A. & R. Sanson-Fisher. 1995. Breaking bad news: Consensus guidelines for medical practitioners. J. Clin. Oncol. **13:** 2449–2456.
8. Carrese, J. A. & L. A. Rhodes. 1995. Western bioethics on the Navajo reservation. Benefit or harm? JAMA **274:** 826–829.
9. Surbone, A. 1992. Truth telling to the patient. JAMA **268**: 1661–1662.

Information, Truth, and Communication

For an Interpretation of Truth-telling Practices throughout the World

ANTONELLA SURBONE

Department of Medicine
Memorial Sloan-Kettering Cancer Center
New York, New York 10021

On se fait un idole de la verité elle meme: car la verité, hors de la charité, n'est pas Dieu; elle est son image, et un idole qu'il ne faut point aimer ni adorer.
—PASCAL

Pascal's words ("We make an idol of truth in itself. But truth, outside of love, is not God: it's simply His image, an idol that we should neither love nor adore") still represent one of the most powerful warnings against the idolatry of truth—an idolatry that is perpetuated by our limited reflection upon the many epistemic and ethical implications of truth.

Truth and epistemology: What is truth? Is truth a simple matter of coherence account? Is truth a matter of adherence? If so, to what? Does a single truth exist? If more than one truth exists, will the many truths one day reconcile in a single one? Does truth exist outside of relationships (the "love" of Pascal), outside of a connectional dimension?

Truth and subjectivity: Does truth exist outside of contexts? Are facts sufficient to determine truth?

Truth and medicine: Is the objective component of medical truth sufficient to speak of truth? Should medicine not combine cognitive and affective information to reach the truth? Is truth a unilateral concept or is it a concept shared between patient, doctor, and society? Finally, are patient and doctor simply engaged in discovering a truth that is already there, or are they creating a truth? If the latter, is it an historical or a narrative truth?

Truth and ethics: Can there be a technology of ethics? Are truth and truth-telling objects of ethical inquiry?

ETHICS IN MEDICINE

For the ancient Greeks, the sphere of ethics was not distinguished from that of esthetics; according to Aristotle courage is beautiful.[1] Exactly what, then, does ethics mean?

The word *ethics* has two different roots: *εθοσ* and *ηθοσ*. The word *εθοσ* means habit, custom. There is a dimension of ethics that has been called reactive,[2] aimed at preserving the identity of mankind. In this respect, ethics relies on a system of rules of behavior, hence on habits reflecting ethical virtues. The word *ηθοσ*, on the other hand, means home or usual place. Ethics, then, is the home of human beings, and it implies an active, continuous effort at understanding how mankind remains in this home.[3]

Ethics in medicine can be defined as the dimension in which both patient and doctor find themselves at home—a home in which they remain by acting according to ethical virtues.

TRUTH AND MEDICAL ETHICS

Truth is not merely the opposite of falsehood; rather, it is a relational state, which evolves through interactions in time. Truth can suddenly reveal itself when least expected. Truth can develop slowly, and we may be asked to wait patiently for it. Truth is a matter of now as well as of tomorrow. Can we affirm truth with certainty? Even if we think we recognize it for ourselves, can we impose it on others? Truth should above all be respected.

In the patient-doctor relationship, we need to respect the truth by the act of truth-telling, in which telling does not strictly mean using words, nor does it indicate which words; and in which truth does not equal information, but goes far beyond it.

In its action/activity implications, in its epistemological and its narrative component, truth-telling seems to be the real object of medical ethics and of our daily work as physicians.

Truth-telling is, however, only a component of a larger project, that of making truth. Truth is no longer a matter of idolatry: it is a matter of discovering as well as creating and recreating, in medicine as well as outside of medicine, in disease as well as outside of disease.

INFORMATION AND TRUTH

Clearly, information is only one component of truth. Information reflecting mere objective scientific truth does not take into account that the latter is a chimera. No knowledge is ever abstract from the context in which it was produced: knowledge is always situated knowledge, and this includes scientific knowledge. Medical truth is never value free, nor does the patient-doctor relationship ever take place in a value-neutral context.

In medicine, there is an objective dimension of truth, which can be expressed through information. The nature and likely course of disease itself, the treatment options, the possible side effects, the likely prognosis are all objective elements of medical truth. However, there are two more dimensions of truth in medicine, and they are equally important: the subjective—i.e., the patient's perception of the disease—and the contextual, which varies according to the historical, cultural, and religious backgrounds of the patient and the doctor. These three dimensions can be expressed only in the process of communication.

COMMUNICATION

Information becomes truth only in the context of communication. But what is communication? The origin of the word, from the Latin *communis*, implies sharing something in common. Hence, communication can be defined as the process by which meanings are exchanged between individuals through a common system of symbols, such as language, gestures, and signs. In the patient-doctor relationship, communication is the timely and appropriate answer to the problem of truth.

Communication is a bidirectional process. It implies information, but it goes beyond information. It is not only verbal, but also consists of a universal language of signs, gestures, objects. It develops over time. It takes into account all the variables that, by their interaction, can modify the truth in the patient-doctor relationship: the patient, the health-care team, the family, society in its entirety, the disease and its course, the medications. Communication is creative and never results from imposition. Communication respects and expresses the truth.

OBSTACLES TO COMMUNICATION

That communication is not an easy task we know from our personal lives, long before we enter our profession. In the patient-doctor relationship, many are the obstacles to communication. As in the rest of life, we face problems of language, reality and its limits, expectations and finally the presence of the incommunicable.

Language is about words, about meanings, and about imagination. Language is the major obstacle to communication, insofar as it refers not only to the linguistic property of a certain group of people, but also to the meaning that different persons attribute to the same words. "But is language the only language?" asked Ludwig Wittgenstein in his *Notebook*.[4] Later on, he wrote: "Since language stands in internal relation to the world, it and these relations determine the logical possibility of facts." Language is not merely a convention; on the contrary, it stands in a close, internal, logical relationship to the world. Language and facts are thus connected in a new dimension.

When thinking of language in the patient-doctor relationship, we might wish to think of the role of narrative in medicine. Medicine is based upon narratives—the patient's but also the doctor's. Illness narrative is a mainstay of medical practice: the stories that patients tell us are the first moment of the relationship and, indeed, shape it. Do patients' narratives depict objective experience only? Do they follow cultural models (templates, plots, literary roles)? And finally, to what extent do patients and doctors share the narrative? Because doctors have their narratives too, they work in a cultural context, they belong to multiple contexts (the general culture and also the medical culture). Doctors speak about medical knowledge as absolute, natural, universal; but is not medical knowledge also a narrative?

Reality has limitations that communication does not overcome. On the contrary, the limitations of reality can become obstacles to communication. Let us think of the following: we are not immortal, economic pressure is increasing, distributive justice needs to be considered, major therapeutic advances are not common, available therapies have severe side effects, more is not always better. Finally the medicalization of life and its quality is ineffective and dangerous. Communication about these issues is difficult, as it engages us in facing those limitations of reality against which we struggle and fight. We do not like these limitations of reality, and we tend not to talk about them. Actually, we participate in creating different expectations for us and our patients.

That expectations are often unrealistic is a fact. But who creates expectations? Society and culture first, the patient and his or her microenvironment, doctors, and medicine itself. Our goal should be to establish realistic expectations without subtracting hope. It is often an impossible task, as it involves some aspects of our lives, some webs of our thoughts that are incommunicable.

There is a threshold in the patient-doctor relationship, as in every relationship of life, that we cannot overstep. We need communication, but we also need privacy and respect. The "ponderable imponderables" (in Simone Weil's powerful expression) exist; the "ultimate concerns" of Paul Tillich cannot be communicated. There is a time when the incommunicable takes precedence.

TRUTH IN MEDICINE THROUGHOUT THE WORLD

The medical act involves a moral agent as well as values and goals. The agent, who is both the patient and the doctor, has character and virtues, responsibility and rights, a certain degree of free will and control. The agent also has memory, imagination, creativity.

The values involved in the patient-doctor relationship are attributed to the act by the agents. The values are attributed to an act before, during, and after the act takes place. The a priori attribution of values is contextual, insofar as it is learned and shared among persons in a particular context.

The *telos* of the medical act is healing. However, the goals of the medical act (and its consequences, too) might not necessarily be the same for the patient and the doctor, as they are strongly influenced by the asymmetry of the patient-doctor relationship. Think of the different meanings that a partial remission has for the patient and for the doctor where cancer is concerned, or consider the debate on quality of life and how to measure it.

Indeed, active work of communication is needed for the patient and the doctor to establish and reach a common purpose of the medical act. Unlike relationships among peers, the patient-doctor relationship cannot be described simply as a contract. There is a state of slavery induced by disease that renders the patient vulnerable; also, it makes the purpose of the medical act that of setting the patient free from the slavery of disease. We all are so familiar with our medical terminology that we probably no longer pay attention to its meaning: "disease-free," "freedom from relapse," "freedom from symptoms" are recurrent idioms in the medical, and especially the oncological, literature. Spiritual freedom, achieved by sharing the path to make truth, is also a goal of medicine.

In this book we read about the complexity of the issue of communication with a patient affected by a serious, often lethal, disease. We shall learn about different contexts, about different ways and—honestly—quite different degrees of informing patients, about different efforts to make a truth between the doctor and the patient. Also, we shall learn about different ethical frameworks and justifications of different practices of information—or noninformation—throughout the world.

FOR A POSSIBLE ETHICAL INTERPRETATION OF DIFFERENT PRACTICES THROUGHOUT THE WORLD

In reading the different chapters of this book, I first felt a strong positive feeling of breathing honesty—in itself a moral value. Then, I was fascinated by everything I learned, by the many facts and values that I had been ignoring. Finally, I tried to understand what the common ethical background behind such a tremendous variety of practices could be.

It is certainly not my intention to analyze or systematize the work of others. On the contrary, I am simply offering a review of what appear to me as the two dominant leitmotifs with respect to the ethics behind those practices: an interpretation resting on the interplay of the principles of respect for autonomy and of beneficence towards the patient on the one hand; an interpretation stemming from *phronesis,* or practical wisdom, on the other—the former emphasizing the act, the latter the agent. As a matter of fact, after reading all the chapters, the two appear to be closely intertwined.

While "what is truth" is a metaethical question, ethics is faced with the issue of truth-telling—as previously alluded to, an action-oriented problem. And we might remind ourselves of the Kantian definition of ethics as a practical philosophy.[5,6]

Quite often, the issue of truth-telling is approached from the point of view of principles of medical ethics—namely, respect for autonomy and beneficence. Many contributors have employed this terminology, or implied it in their discussion. The word "autonomy" refers to the patients' rights to be respected in their life and dignity, as well as their right to self-determination with regard to their health. The word "beneficence," on the other hand, refers to a duty of the physician—that of doing the patient's good. Implicit in the latter is the assumption that the medical knowledge of the doctor translates into a certain responsibility to determine what is best for the patient; this need not necessarily be a form of paternalism, as most of the contributors show in their chapters. There are other principles of medical ethics, such as nonmaleficence and justice, although these are not directly involved in articulating the discussion about truth-telling. Most ethical theories see truth-telling as a specification of the principle of autonomy.[7]

Kant, in his *Foundations of the Metaphysics of Morals*,[5] defined truth-telling as essential in order to respect the autonomy of each individual—the only way to treat a person as an end and never as a means. For Kant, indeed, the "sublimity" of a person comes from being morally autonomous. Kant spoke of the "autonomy of the will," which he contrasted with "heteronomy"—the former referring to acting according to the categorical imperative, the latter to acting according to motivations other than universal moral principles. Never does autonomy in Kant assume any libertarian connotation, as it does in present Western cultures and bioethics. Mill, on the contrary, regarded autonomy as necessary for each person to shape her life—a process he preferred to call "individuality."[8]

The use of principles in bioethics is derived primarily from the work of W. D. Ross,[9] to whom we owe the definition of "prima facie" duties or principles. There are many different moral obligations that present themselves in any given situation, and at times they conflict. These different moral obligations are basic, valid moral principles, but because they can conflict, it may be impossible to honor them all at the same time. In this sense, they are not absolute, and they can be "rendered wrong": moral principles for Ross are thus conditional, prima facie. In Ross's work there is no hierarchy of principles, although he tends to assume that nonmaleficence takes priority over beneficence.

The lack of a hierarchical order leads, in my opinion, to an important consequence—that any choice, even the right one, will always leave out something that we know to be of moral value, and that does not cease to be such. Hence moral life can be difficult, if not tragic: moral dilemmas exist; they are the rule rather than the exception. We do not live in Kant's world of noumenal moral duties, where "obligationes non colliduntur"; and when dilemmas arise, they do not destroy obligations as such. Moral dilemmas are a fact of life, a "misfortune of moral life."[10] They are not simply the result of imperfect understanding of the duties of the case; and Kantian theory ignores "regrets and related considerations" by eliminating "the ought that is not acted upon."[11]

There have been many lines of criticism of the use of prima facie duties, and excellent reviews of these issues have recently appeared in the literature.[12] I shall briefly summarize these criticisms for the reader who is not necessarily familiar with the subject. First, one could deny the existence of conflicts of duties when seeing conflicting duties as conditional. Second, acceptance of prima facie duties could devastate common sense morality, by hiding actual duties. The provisional character of prima facie duties with their qualifications has also been severely attacked as lacking a theory of reference and thus being inadequate in accounting for the complexity of moral life: autonomy per se, for instance, does not mean anything if we do not specify (somehow a priori with reference to a systematic moral theory) its subject and its content. Also, the use of prima facie duties has been criticized as being procedurally emphatic. Finally, it has been seen as abstracted from the real world of morality and from the sociocultural context. The latter indeed appears to be a valid criticism to me, while the previous seem to ignore the instrumental value of prima facie duties. If we consider them as being at an intermediate level between a systematic moral theory and the pluralism of different narratives, they provide us with an effective tool for a preliminary reading of the moral experience. They enable us to define the duties at stake in a particular moral experience and/or moral dilemma. They also enable us to recognize the elements necessary to formulate a moral judgment in a concrete situation.[13] Thus prima facie duties may help in the "delimitation of a range of acceptable actions"—which seems to be the purpose of an ethical code.

The use of principles in bioethics has been extremely valuable in providing instruments by which to frame moral dilemmas in medicine.[7] Truth-telling, for instance, can easily be framed in terms of autonomy and beneficence, although often our final ethical choice finds its justification outside the framework of principles alone.

This is first because autonomy and beneficence cannot be abstracted from the contextual dimension. As seen repeatedly in the discussion about truth-telling in medicine, contextual aspects can never be eliminated, as moral life does not happen in the world of ideas; it happens in a here and now, in a given society, with its cultural background, its economic and political circumstances. And the patient-doctor relationship is no exception: it is, indeed, always part of a broader patient-doctor-society relationship. Contextualism does not necessarily mean relativism, but it brings to the surface the reality of pluralism in our world: different interpretations and different expressions of moral principles in different cultures coexist with the same universal right to dignity of every human being and with the same universal duty to respect this dignity.[14,15]

It is, indeed, the aim of this book project to show in how many different ways truth-telling can occur and under which circumstances truth-telling might not occur, at least not in the Western understanding of the word. An initial explanation for these cultural differences, as we have just seen, is that the two principles of autonomy and beneficence cannot be abstracted from the contextual dimension, and, on the contrary, depend on the shared meaning of each in any given culture.[16] A second explanation is that autonomy and beneficence are interrelated principles, never existing without each other; truth-telling, then, stems from a balance between the two. That this is not a "semantic somersault"[17] is proved by the extensive literature on the subject, and certainly by the many contributions to this book.

Also, as previously alluded to, important justifications for the different ways of approaching truth-telling in the patient-doctor relationship lie outside the strict world of principles. Virtues, responsibility, and trust play equally essential roles, by emphasizing the moral agent and her character and role in solving ethical dilemmas.

Thus truth-telling becomes a matter of phronesis, of practical wisdom—which is itself a leitmotif of our book and its narratives. Phronesis —in Aristotelian terms[1]—refers to the "prudent weighing of the alternatives in situations of uncertainty and stress."[18] Its roots resting upon the integrity of the physician, upon his or her moral character, phronesis leads to the timely and appropriate way of responding to each individual patient's needs, including that of being told the truth that he or she wishes to hear.

Thus truth-telling becomes a matter of responsibility, both the doctor's and the patient's. The professional responsibility is the doctor's, whose situation in the patient-doctor relationship is that of the more knowledgeable, hence more powerful, figure. The doctor has responsibility as a healer; and we all know to what extent cultural and personal sensitivity can increase the therapeutic efficacy of the medical act. The patient's responsibility lies in his or her narrative, as well as in being honest in the relationship with the doctor. Finally, there is their mutual responsibility in sharing the process of making truth, in coauthoring a truth for the present and the future.

Thus truth-telling becomes a matter of trust.[19] The patient-doctor relationship is an asymmetry, and as such it escapes the realm of contractual relationships among peers. Kantian autonomy, based on reciprocal promises and on a moral accountability limited to autonomous equal relationships, does not cover all aspects of the patient-doctor relationship. The patient and the doctor are, indeed, equal human beings, with equal moral and social status and deserving equal respect. The patient-doctor relationship is also a form of covenant, and as such it calls for special attention to the expectations and promises of both partners. But the patient-doctor relationship is in essence a fiduciary act, based on mutual trust. Unlike most other contracts, it involves a very delicate aspect of our being human: the dependence that we all have on our body and its functioning—the basis of human life. When we put our health and life in someone else's hands, we need to trust in more than the doctor's honoring his or her part of the contract. We need to trust in the doctor's caring for us. After all, do we not all speak of medical *care*?

CONCLUSIONS

Truth-telling is only one step in the patient-doctor relationship and in the process of communication. Many other variables contribute to the cocreation by the patient and the doctor of an evolving truth: the role of society both as macro- and microenvironment, the evolution of the disease, the pharmacological component, the "unexpected" in life.

Truth-telling is an essential step, though, to care; and we should never feel relieved of our responsibility to be truthful to our patients, according to our cultures and to sensitivity to individual circumstances.

Truth-telling, finally, is not only toward our patients, but also among our professional colleagues: the honesty of each of the contributions to this volume is proof of this dimension of truth-telling. Honesty is at the core of this project, its main value. We will learn from others' experiences about different ways of making truth within the context of a highly valued patient-doctor relationship.

Can it be that one of the determining aspects of the healing process is, indeed, how much the patient and the doctor value their particular relationship? It does appear to be so, from my personal experience and, if I have correctly interpreted the contributions to this volume, from the experience of many others throughout the world.

REFERENCES

1. ARISTOTLE. Nichomachean Ethics.
2. MASULLO, A. 1995. Il Tempo e la Grazia. Donzelli ed. Roma.
3. HEIDEGGER, M. 1979. Heraklit. (1943–1944). Gesammtausgabe. Vol. 55, pp. 205 & 214. Klostermann. Frankfurt am Main.
4. WITTGENSTEIN, L. 1979. Notebooks, 1914–1916. 2nd edit. University of Chicago Press. Chicago, IL.
5. KANT, I. 1988. Fundamental Principles of the Metaphysics of Morals.

Prometheus Books. Buffalo, NY.
6. KANT, I. 1963. Lectures on Ethics. Evanston. New York, NY.
7. BEAUCHAMP, T. L. & J. F. CHILDRESS. 1994. Principles of Biomedical Ethics. 4th edit. Oxford University Press. New York, NY.
8. MILL, J. S. 1974. Utilitarianism, On Liberty, Essay on Bentham: Together with Selected Writings of Jeremy Bentham and John Austin. New American Library. Meridian.
9. ROSS, W. D. 1930. The Right and the Good. Oxford University Press. Oxford.
10. RESCHNER, N. 1987. Ethical Idealism: An Inquiry into the Nature and Function of Ideals. University of California Press. Berkeley, CA.
11. WILLIAMS, B. 1977. Ethical Consistency. *In* Problems of the Self: p. 175. Cambridge University Press. Cambridge. (Discussed and cited in N. Reschner, Ethical Idealism, p. 40.)
12. BEAUCHAMP, T. L. 1995. Principlism and Its Alleged Competitors. Kennedy Inst. Ethics J. **5**(3): 181–198.
13. CATTORINI, P. 1993. Bioetica di Fine Vita. Liviana Medicina. Napoli.
14. GOSTIN, L. O. 1995. Informed consent, cultural sensitivity and respect for person. JAMA **274:** 844–845.
15. GENERAL ASSEMBLY OF THE UNITED NATIONS. 1948. Universal Declaration of Human Rights. United Nations. Geneva.
16. PELLEGRINO, E. D. 1992. Is truth-telling to patients a cultural artifact? JAMA **268:** 1734–1735.
17. BREWIN, T. B. 1993. How much ethics is needed to make a good doctor? Lancet **341:** 161–163.
18. PELLEGRINO, E. D. 1995. Toward a virtue-based normative ethics for the health profession. Kennedy Inst. of Ethics J. **5**(3): 253–277.
19. BAIER, A. C. 1994. Moral Prejudices: Essays on Ethics. Harvard University Press. Cambridge, MA.

Cancer Patients and Medical Practice

Some Historical and Cultural Considerations

JOSEP LLUÍS BARONA

Department d'Història de la Ciència i Documentació
Universitat de València
Blasco Ibáñez, 17
46010 València, Spain

A Carmen Barona Alcalá
IN MEMORIAM

Disease is a natural phenomenon that affects human beings on many levels. Even from the purely biological point of view, for an individual disease and death include not only medical and scientific conceptions, but also a cultural background about what life and the human body are and mean. Likewise, other social, metaphysical, and even metaphorical dimensions of death and disease must be considered, inasmuch as they occupy part of the mind of humans, in their own way of understanding themselves, in every time and culture. Religious and philosophical traditions have, throughout history, constructed cultural images of death and mortal disease, of their sense and meaning, linked to beliefs on their relationship to the supernatural. Obviously, medical attitudes and theories have also had great influence on the way disease is regarded and play an important role in the complex crossroads of traditions that meet in the mind of the patient. That is why the social importance and meaning of certain diseases should not be measured only through their statistical incidence in a certain population and time. If we look at the past, it is easy to understand why some diseases such as the plague, syphilis, leprosy, and tuberculosis were endowed with a rich popular, religious, metaphorical background—a social image that determined not only personal or social reactions in the face of disease, but also scientific and political attitudes and strategies. Cancer takes the same cultural place in our modern societies as the diseases just mentioned, inasmuch as it represents for the general populace the archetype of the most unavoidable illness.

The present contribution analyzes the different aspects of the idea of cancer. It takes into account medical and individual attitudes to mortal disease, taking as a point of reference the historical construction of the medical concept of cancer, as well as the cultural implications of the disease. The paper also discusses the cultural stereotype of cancer and the most common attitudes and reactions of the patient facing his/her situation. The content and cultural considerations of this contribution are applicable mainly to a Mediterranean country such as Spain. Also considered are the hospital as a place of life, relationships, and treatment; the principal problems and strategies involved in communicating with cancer patients; and their reactions to new therapeutic procedures and their consequences. The paper refers both to general oncological service and to specific groups.

THE RELATIONSHIP BETWEEN DOCTOR AND PATIENT: SOME GENERAL CONSIDERATIONS

The clinical act is the nucleus around which medical assistance is shaped.[1,2] It is the point of encounter between the patient—a person who has lost his/her healthy condition and is seeking help to recover it—and the doctor—a person who is supposed to have the technical knowledge and ability to accomplish the patient's purpose. One of the most evident features of the doctor-patient relationship today is its organization into a ritual involving a sequence of acts. The necessity of organizing the clinical retrieval of information has brought about a perfectly structured anamnesis; examination of the patient has become a largely technical exercise. Medical decisions, with the traditional family doctor a consequence of subjective intuition based upon accumulated personal experience (clinical perspicacity and historical knowledge of the life of the patient), are now the result of a more objective, technical, impersonal clinical process.

Two of the main factors influencing the human, psychological, cultural, and historical aspects of the doctor-patient relationship are the social assessment of disease and the unavoidable inequality between health staff and patient. It is well known that illness is considered differently by each society according to its own cultural values. In our Western tradition ever since the French Revolution's Declaration of Human Rights there has been legal recognition of the right of all citizens to medical care without social or economic restriction.

The social, psychological, and personal situation of the doctor is quite different from that of the patient when they meet at the moment of the clinical act. The doctor is engaged in his/her professional activity, which means that the situation is completely normal for him/her. The entire health staff shares a professional, technical approach to disease. Doctors are carrying out their social function when they are fighting disease through their relationship with the patient. Furthermore, they obtain through this a certain social prestige and financial support for further professional training and research. On the other hand, the situation of the patient is not a normal one, but an exceptional one, without any social or professional motivation. The patient's only aim is to know what kind of illness he/she is suffering from in order to recover his/her heath.

This inequality of situation between doctor and patient is even wider when one considers it from the point of view of their respective cultures of disease. Whereas for the doctor disease is a concept full of scientific and technical content, for the patient it is something concrete, a source of personal suffering that disturbs his/her everyday life. Furthermore, the patient often has a particular way of understanding disease based on cultural values firmly rooted in folk-medical or popular thinking, including extrascientific, symbolic, and moral considerations and values. These differences between doctor and patient often generate a wide range of practical attitudes that can hinder mutual understanding between them. The psychological consequences of these differences can influence the communication process and the positive attitude in the patient that would promote his/her recovery.

There is no doubt about the clinical importance of open communication between doctor and patient, inasmuch as it is the starting point of a constructive attitude in the face of disease and a requirement for the success of therapy. The process of doctor-patient communication has varied historically in response to the changing cultural values relating to disease and the changing social organization of medical assistance. The specific mechanisms of transference between doctor and patient have shown themselves in different ways depending on the cultural framework. Obviously the codes of communication are not the same in a primitive population in central Africa as they are in a suburb of New York City or in a general hospital in southern Europe in the 16th century. One should take into account at least three aspects or levels of the doctor-patient relationship that can either help or hinder their mutual understanding: individual attitudes, the conceptualization of health and disease, and the social organization of the health system.[2]

Individual Attitudes

A positive understanding of the roles of doctor and patient involves, on the part of the patient, the desire to recover his/her health, which means being unwilling to accept the role of patient as a way of life—as a refuge from disease; and an attitude of trust and confidence in the technical ability of the doctor. The doctor, on the other hand, should understand the anamnesis and examination procedures as a way of learning about disease, not only as a method of discovering its biological signs or objectifying its symptoms. The patient should be considered a human being, not only a subject for study, research, and professional activity. These considerations imply not only the possibility of intellectual communication, but also the necessity of establishing some kind of emotional connection with the patient.

The Conceptualization of Health and Disease

Not only are the personal situations of the doctor and the patient different; also their intellectual understanding of what disease represents can be quite far from one another. Popular interpretations of disease include moral, supernatural, magical, symbolic, esthetic, and religious conceptions that remain out of the frame of the scientific perspective of disease. The relationship between disease and moral behavior—for example, the identification of disease with moral punishment for sin or moral disorder, is one of the ideas that may create a sharp division between the world of the patient and that of the doctor. Some illnesses are associated with dirtiness or depravity. Even when patients do not have such a point of view, their understanding of disease is not a scientific one. Their view of a given disease often involves a superficial, vague, or vulgarized version of scientific concepts that is very different from the exact information the doctor has about the biological changes that have taken place in the body and mind of the patient. These views of the patient are full of cultural traditions and cultural patterns that have been passed on from generation to generation. The popular ideas of what cancer, AIDS, depression, intestinal worms, or ulcers mean are often vague and sometimes do not go beyond the simple idea of gravity or curability, or beyond the feelings of fear or surprise promoted by the social stereotypes of these diseases.

This is one of the matters about which doctor-patient communication should establish links that are more solid and on a higher level: the doctor should be able to receive the story told by the patient, understand the patient's personal experience of the disease, learn from it, and promote a reinterpretation of the patient's view in his/her own language and mode of thought. This is probably one of the most difficult tasks to accomplish.

The first obstacle is language. Through many centuries Western medicine has developed a sophisticated medical terminology that aims—as does any scientific language—to be the international vehicle of communication between scientists. One of its principal attributes is a precise meaning for each term. Medical terminology is not an artificial language created for the purpose of excluding from medical knowledge and understanding those who have not been initiated. On the contrary, it was derived from the actual nature of scientific knowledge to facilitate exact international agreement on words and concepts. Nevertheless, the same instrument that serves as the main means of communication among members of the medical professions is a barrier to communication with lay people. It creates difficulties for the social diffusion of scientific concepts and, of course, for good understanding between doctor and patient, between specialist and layman, inasmuch as only one of the two people is familiar with it. In that sense medical terminology can be a great obstacle to communication that can be overcome only by a continuous effort to translate concepts into popular terms.

While respecting the privacy and personal feelings of the patient, the physician should attempt to present the scientific perspective regarding the biological and psychological aspects of the disease. This can be done only through simplified explanations. This effort of popularization need not involve an ideological defense of certain ethical or moral values regarding life and death. Although each society should establish general rules of behavior regarding these matters—often inspired by religious, moral, or other cultural values—in my opinion they should remain out of the realm of scientific discussion, belonging, rather, to the realm of personal decisions, beliefs, and freedom. For instance, doctors should inform their patients about the risks to health that smoking represents, but ultimately the option of smoking or not smoking must be left to the will and choice of the individual. It seems to me extremely important to accept this kind of distinction in order to avoid the excessive intervention and pressure of the normative impact of hygienic rules (always based on scientific laboratory criteria and not on cultural or social ones), which inevitably lead to widespread rejection of medical influence on private, personal life. It is necessary to distinguish very clearly between giving medical information and this inhuman process of medical intervention in everyday life. The latter is rejected by a large segment of the population.

The Social Organization of the Health Care System

This is the context in which the clinical act, the relationship between the doctor and the patient, takes place and hence can help or hinder it. The increasingly technological development of medical practice involves a series of difficulties that ought to be taken into account. First, one has to consider the problem of coordination involved in the hospital clinical act: many specialists often take part in examining and treating the patient, contributing their specific technical knowledge. In our health institutions the patient usually feels helpless because he lacks an advocate, a single person responsible for attending to him and returning him to health. Only careful planning of the clinical act can coordinate the necessary specialization with the overall consideration of the patient.

Second, instead of understanding illness as incapacity, as a disturbance felt on all human levels, there is a strong tendency in medicine to reduce disease to a biological problem, taking the patient's body as an object of study, a source of medical knowledge. The general attitude in contemporary medicine, relying on laboratory techniques as the main criterion of health and disease, constitutes a reductionist point of view, to the detriment of the more social, human dimension of the problem felt by the patient. He/she often feels handled by impersonal medical technicians. These considerations assume special importance in the case of cancer.

As a general conclusion one can say that a more fruitful relationship between doctor and patient should be defined as encompassing several factors, including verbal communication, positive attitudes in developing their respective roles, and exchange of information from their particular points of view regarding the disease. On the one hand it requires an effort to explain simply and clearly the achievements of medical thinking and techniques. On the other hand it requires a more inclusive conception of what disease represents for a particular human being. This holistic conception would result in a more humane conception of the clinical act, which in turn would enhance patient-doctor communication.

THE CONCEPT OF CANCER: DISEASE AND CULTURAL CONSTRUCTION

As far as we know, cancer has existed throughout human history. One can find several testimonies to its existence in the ancient texts of Asiatic cultures and in the well-known *Corpus Hippocraticum*.[3] Nevertheless, the existence of cancer patients does not mean that cancer played an important role in the societies of the past. In fact, it is possible that the transformation of cancer into the social illness par excellence is relatively recent. The increased importance of cancer is a consequence of the so-called demographic and epidemiological transition in modern Western societies. This transition—which took place in most Western countries in the course of the 19th century and the first decades of the 20th—is characterized by a decline of general and infant mortality and infectious disease and an increase in life expectancy. Once birth rates permanently overtook mortality rates, a spectacular increase in population took place, and new diseases came to the fore as primary causes of death. Chronic diseases, cardiovascular and cerebral accidents, and degenerative problems became the main health problems in the increasingly older populations.[4,5] In this context cancer took on new medical, psychological, and epidemiological meanings and importance in the same way as other diseases had in the past.

Cancer has a rich, interesting, and important symbolic meaning. Its astrological reference relates to the sign of the zodiac located in the middle of the year, the moment of transition from the zenith to the unavoidable decline. Perhaps there is also an impression of astrological fatality in the idea of cancer. The idea that something is wrong, that a destructive force has awoken inside the body, encourages the idea that cancer is unavoidable. Everybody is vulnerable to that sleeping animal inside that can wake up at any moment and eat your body. (The identification of cancer with an animal is a popular idea among Spanish people.) Cancer is considered a destructive force that acts at random, and this image of fatality, that nothing can be done against it, is extensive.

In addition, cancer today is symbolically associated with the idea of degradation, with both personal and environmental self-destruction. This image of degeneration and decay is often associated with suffering, pain, and death. This seems evident in some of the metaphorical uses of the word—for instance, when speaking of terrorism as a *cancer of society*. Cancer is seen as a process of internal destruction—for the human body or the social structure.[6] In her well-known discussion of illness as metaphor Susan Sontag emphasizes the use of military terminology, expressing the concept of cancer as invasion. Terms like *eradication of cancer*, or *war, battle, or crusade against cancer* suggest a correspondence between disease and military strategy—a comparison that has been common throughout the history of medicine.[7] These cultural constructions should make us realize that the subjective experience of disease is built not from biological, medical considerations, but from cultural images and social practices.

THE CANCER PATIENT AND THE MANY DIMENSIONS OF THE DISEASE

Cancer is a disease that, more than others, makes us conscious of the influence and coincidence of the somatic, psychological, and social aspects of disease in its onset, diagnosis, and treatment.[8] In fact, cancer patients, to a greater extent than other patients, have to challenge the idea of death and therefore become aware of the dangers represented by disease. This involves a necessary process of adaptation to new conditions of life, assuming the reality of a body attacked by disease. For the patient, cancer represents a complex disease, not only in its physical manifestations, but also in its diagnosis and treatment. It involves a type of health care that sometimes requires the participation of a number of specialists and professionals and the transfer of the patient to several medical practices or test facilities. In such circumstances it seems unavoidable that the cancer patient feel like an object of research, fragmented, reduced to consideration of a sick lung, liver, or breast. The sick part of the body assumes disproportionate importance in a reductionist process in which the human being seems to be reduced to the sick part of the body. That is why it becomes crucial that the doctor-patient relationship encompass not only human, personal consideration, but also social consideration, including personal feelings, familiar and social surroundings, professional problems—all those aspects that transform a human being into something more than merely a biological structure, whether healthy or sick. In his/her relationship with the cancer patient, the doctor should include all the aspects of human life that help people be capable of dignity, of being loved. If cancer is the only link between them, the other aspects of the patient's life will suffer.

If we take into account the possibility that the condition of a sick person might last a long time and even be permanent, it is easy to understand the specific difficulties that a long, stable relationship implies. Cancer is an uncertain illness, and often the patient perceives uncertainties in the doctor during a long, stable relationship.[9] Once the establishment of an integral program of assistance is assumed as a general aim, then it is the whole person that should take part in the relationship between doctor and patient. If this is achieved, the technical part of the treatment will be reinforced by a series of positive stimulations and attitudes. Furthermore, the patient will feel him/herself to be an integral person only if he/she is sure that the partial care received from different professionals is integrated into a holistic perspective.[10]

From the very beginning, at the very moment in which the name of the disease is communicated, some details seem to be quite important; for instance, the facial expression and mood of the doctor at that moment will be interpreted by the patient, in some cases given more weight than even the name of the disease. Obviously the patient does not have a technical, professional approach; what he/she really wants to know is the gravity of the illness, which is communicated by the physician's expression. Sometimes, after knowing his/her situation and program of treatment, a process of negotiation takes place in which the patient tries to obtain certain benefits or reductions. The answer should be carefully pondered in relation to the psychological situation of the patient. For instance, incomplete emotional development prior to the patient's knowledge of the illness could provoke uncertain behavior; often, hypochondriacal symptoms appear in patients with prior depressive tendencies. In fact, logical, rational processes are blocked by anxiety when fear appears suddenly. A mature personality always gives the patient more possibilities for better assimilating the difficult circumstances. That is why the patient's personality seems to have a great influence on the process of adaptation to disease.

At the first stage the patient receives the diagnosis of cancer and elaborates an internal answer to it: the information received shapes a new self-diagnosis, including anxieties, hopes, and pain. After that, he/she initiates a selective search for new information, willing to hear what is favorable. Then the patient usually tries to convince the health staff of his/her self-diagnosis and to obtain changes or reductions in treatment. Often patients resort to superstitious ideas or religious beliefs and wait for a miracle, especially if the prognosis is bad. At that moment the attitude of the doctor is very important: his/her response can reinforce or restrain the patient's negative impulses.[11] The doctor should counteract the negative impulses that fix the patient onto fantastic ideas or a mistaken self-diagnosis.

It is also important to consider that time is a disturbing factor. After the first manifestations of disease and the first suspicion on the part of the patient of what might happen, a wait is usually imposed until the first exploratory tests are carried out. Sometimes there is a second wait before a surgical operation; then a third, until the time of going home. All these periods of uncertainty influence the psychological disposition of the patient and should be controlled, never neglected, by the health staff. Usually the preoperative period is characterized by the patient's inability to control negative thoughts, with attacks of anxiety often accompanied by somatic manifestations such as tachycardia, acceleration of respiratory rhythm, pains, nausea, coughs, nightmares, etc. In this situation the reaction of the family seems to be very important; negative attitudes may arise from feelings of lack of control. In some cases, such as with a mother who plays a central role in the stability of the family, the patient's sickness may initiate a process of impairment of family relationships and a chain of illnesses among family members.

The relationship between doctor and patient plays a fundamental psychotherapeutic role. An important aspect of this is the perception or image of the illness that is elaborated by the patient, inasmuch as this will be the starting point of either a positive or a negative attitude. It is obvious that patients suffer a deep transformation of their representation of the world, and their position in it is translated to different coordinates. Through this adaptation process, a flexible relationship with the doctor has a pedagogic influence that helps reduce self-destructive tendencies.[12]

Moreover, the cancer patient has to take on and solve several problems involved in his new condition as chronically sick: he/she has to assume disease and its consequences, often involving pain and incapacity, as a permanent state. He/she has to get used to living in a hospital, submit to special treatments, and develop an adequate relationship with the medical staff. His/her new state implies new, adverse life circumstances. Adapting to this situation requires that the patient preserve his/her emotional stability, a positive self-image, and normal links with the family and prepare him/herself for an uncertain future.[13] The progressive development of these abilities in each patient depends on the specific characteristics of the illness, the patient's personality, and the social circumstances in which he/she is involved. In general, we can summarize the attitudes cancer patients display as follows:

1. Denial that illness constitutes a serious problem for his life and survival, as a mental mechanism of escape or as a simple way to while away the time.
2. Displacement of negative feelings (anger, frustration, etc.) to another object, often a nearby person such as the marital partner or the doctor. This displacement pushes away the fears of being invaded and destroyed by disease.
3. Finding a personal, social, or religious frame of reference in which the new situation can become integrated. This implies a recon-

struction of his/her being in the world, assuming cancer as a permanent state.

4. Preview of all the possible evolutions of the disease, which often implies discussing them or even anticipating sorrow for the death or loss of a part of the body that could happen.[10]

THE HOSPITAL AS A LIVING MILIEU FOR THE CANCER PATIENT

Modern hospitals are usually organized more for the doctors' convenience than the patients'. Often the patient feels like an intruder, who becomes an instrument of research in a great, uncontrollable display of technology. He/she enters into a space in which he loses control of his/her body and is threatened by death. That is why in hospital care subjective feelings and collective images of disease are decisive. They structure a network of support between the patient, his/her social context, and the doctor, in which uncertainty and loneliness in the face of death and misfortune are shared. In the hospital there is a clear definition between the patient—sick, defenseless, ignorant of what is happening—and the doctor—the one who knows. Sometimes this situation comes to resemble one based on religious faith: to the patient the hospital and its doctors make miracles possible—this in a supposedly secular society.[14]

The doctor, on the contrary, develops in his hospital practice a tendency to reduce the procedures that challenge disease to the level of managing its biological aspects. Insofar as hospital practice ignores the social network that surrounds the patient, the hospital becomes an inhospitable place. An autonomous social network may arise, consisting of members of the families of patients who share common attitudes and difficulties, affected by the influence of critical disease. If they develop a belief that medical practice works miracles as the only means to recovery, it is likely that they will take refuge in superstition, religious beliefs, or pure ignorance. In the context of this kind of thinking with regard to the medical profession, the supernatural appears as an instrument to allow humans to go beyond the limits of human understanding.[13] Such sentences as "Only a miracle could save him," sometimes even pronounced by the health staff, can promote this seeking of refuge in belief in the supernatural influence on disease.[10]

CANCER AND COMMUNICATION: GUIDELINES AND BOUNDARIES

When trying to solve the complex problem of telling the patient of the diagnosis of cancer—which will be a time of crisis for the patient—the doctor has to take into account several factors. One is the legal and moral right of the patient to be informed about his/her disease and the boundaries of this right. Other factors are: the extent of the responsibility of the doctor or medical unit for the treatment, the different ways of telling the truth, and the best moment for doing it.[15]

One must take all these factors into account in designing a specific strategy for each case; there does not appear to a single general rule that is suitable for all cases. The medical unit often has to fact the question of deciding if the truth should be told or not. The answer to this question will influence the patient's attitude to all that follows, particularly communication between doctor and patient. If a general rule is that patients must be told the details of their illness, their prognosis, and life expectancy, that implies that patients can and should fully assume their responsibilities; but one must investigate whether they really are prepared for that. If, on the other hand, the rule is to hide from the patient the diagnosis and consequences of cancer, that implies that the patient is not able or prepared to face the truth. Telling the truth means recognizing in the patient his/her human value and right to take part in decisions about his/her body and life—that is, to share risks. Inasmuch as the reactions of every human being are conditioned by previous experiences and everyone has his/her own way of reacting to frustrations, it is important to consider the specific features of each patient's personality and his/her ability to deal with critical situations. Telling the truth to the patient requires the establishment of a support program and mechanisms for free communication for discussing problems related to the disease, and also for channeling fears and anxieties.[16]

Obviously there are some limits to, and precautions to be taken before, communicating to the patient what is going on. First, nothing should be said before one is completely sure of the diagnosis; and once the diagnosis has been told, it is very important to explain to the patient and his/her family its meaning, prognosis, ways of treatment, and the effect of the disease on everyday life at the social, professional, family, and personal levels. It must be recognized that information about the disease is not transmitted solely through verbal expression: all attitudes, silences, smiles, and avoidances will be interpreted by the patient in one way or another through his/her "sixth sense." Therefore it is important that all these aspects of nonverbal communication be coherent with the diagnosis when it is told to the patient. Members of the patient's family play an important role inasmuch as they can help or hinder this complex process of communicating information.

In light of what has been considered above it is evident that in the process of doctor/patient communication, the clinical information given to the patient is extremely important. Nevertheless, communication is not a unidirectional process; it includes listening to the patients and learning from them. They should feel free to communicate their own understanding of disease and use this open form of communication to focus and channel their anxieties. The manifestation of fears and anxieties should not be repressed, but should be accepted by the medical team as a part of the therapeutic program that will provide better information about the situation and disposition of the patient. Obviously, time is needed for this to take place.

Finally, there are situations that arise in the course of treatment that require the communication of specific information. Oncological surgery, for instance, usually modifies the normal functioning of the body; it is important that all foreseeable repercussions be explained. When radiotherapy is used, its purpose, risks, and benefits should be clearly understood by the patient, and he/she should be prepared for the encounter with the mysterious, frightening machine. With chemotherapy, as it involves a certain degree of toxicity, the patient often feels worse during the treatment than before. This can easily lead to misunderstanding, distrust, and even leaving the doctor. That is why the patient must be fully informed about the aim of the treatment and its possible side effects. Only a full understanding by doctor and patient of what cancer means, in its physiopathological, psychological, and human dimensions, can establish the optimal conditions for a successful treatment program.

REFERENCES

1. LAIN ENTRALGO, P. 1964. La relación médico enfermo. Historia y Teoría. Guadarrama. Madrid.
2. BARONA, J. LL. 1993. Communication obstacles in the doctor/patient relations. *In* International Workshop on History, Anthropology and Epistemology of Medicine. Società Italiana di Storia delle Scienze Biomediche. Senigallia.
3. GRMEK, M. D. 1983. Les maladies à l'aube de la civilisation occidentale. Payot. Paris.
4. LIVI BACCI, M. 1991. Modelos regionales de transición demográfica en España y Portugal. J. Gil Albert/Seminari d'Estudis sobre la Població. Alacant.
5. BERNABEU MESTRE, J. 1995. Enfermedad y Población. Seminari d'Estudis sobre la Ciència. València.
6. SONTAG, S. 1978. Illness as Metaphor. Farrar Straus & Giroux. New York, NY.
7. BARONA, J. LL. 1993. Social order and human body in Renaissance medical thought. Hist. Philos. Life Sci. **15**(2): 165–180.
8. KAUFMANN, A. E., Ed. 1984. Cáncer y sociedad, un enfoque integral. Ed. Mezquita. Madrid.
9. STRAUSS, A. L. & B. GLASER. 1975. Chronic Illness and the Quality of Life. The Mosby Co. St. Louis, MO.
10. CAMPOS, H. 1984. La asistencia integral al paciente oncológico. *In* Cáncer y sociedad, un enfoque integral. A. E. Kaufmann, Ed. Ed. Mezquita. Madrid.
11. CARBONELL RODRIGO, J. M. Psicología aplicada a la conducta intrahospitalaria. Doctoral thesis. University of València.
12. BARD, M. & R. B. DYK. 1956. The psychodynamic significance of belief regarding the cause of serious illness. Psychoanal. Rev.

13. MOSS, R. H. & V. DAVIS TSU. 1977. Coping with physical illness. *In* The Crisis of Physical Illness: An Overview. Plenum. New York, NY.
14. COMELLES, J. M. 1995. La sacralización de la práctica hospitalaria. Del despliegue tecnológico a la institucionalización del milagro. *In* Malaltia i Cultura. J. Ll. Barona, Ed. Seminari d'Estudis sobre la Ciència. València.
15. ALLUE, M. 1982. La gestión del morir: Para una antropología del enfermo terminal en la sociedad actual. Primeres Jornades d'Antropol. Med. **2**(1): 4–34.
16. GOOD, M. J. *et al.* 1990. American oncology and the discourse on hope. Cult. Med. Psychiatry **14:** 59–81.

A Discourse Ethics Approach to Quality of Life Measurement[a]

ANDREW EDGAR

Centre for Applied Ethics
School of English Studies, Communication and Philosophy
University of Wales Cardiff
Cardiff CF1 3XB, Wales, United Kingdom

The purpose of this essay is to explore the role that quality of life measures may have in enhancing communication between patients and members of the medical profession. I am not therefore concerned as such with the communication that occurs between the individual patient and the individual doctor, or between the patient and his or her family, but rather with the cultural preconditions of that communication, and thus with the part that quality of life measures might play in highlighting those factors that inhibit such communication.

The measurement of health-related quality of life has become increasingly important in the understanding and planning of health care provision over the last two decades. While numerous measures have now been developed, they may be classified according to two broad criteria. Quality of life measures are either indexes or profiles. Indexes reduce the patient's quality of life to a single index number (typically with 1 representing good health and 0 representing a state equivalent to death). Various health states, defined according to more or less complex parameters, may then each be given a value. Profiles differ insofar as the various dimensions of the health states are considered separately, although each dimension may have several components. The quality of life of the patient cannot then be reduced to a single number. Rather, each dimension has its own number, so that a more complex picture of the patient's health is given. Quality of life measures may also be either disease specific or global. A global measure is designed to be applicable to patients suffering any disease. Disease-specific measures, in contrast, are designed to be applicable only to certain ranges of disease.

Ethical debates about quality of life measurement have tended to focus on the use of non–disease-specific indexes, and in particular the Quality Adjusted Life Year (QALY), to influence resource allocation across

[a]An earlier version of this essay was presented at the 1995 OECI Conference on Cancer and Quality of Life, held at Bled, Slovenia.

a health care system.[1,2] Such measures are criticized for justifying the removal of health care resources from patients (or patient groups) that have some prima facie entitlement to them. Profiles, such as the Sickness Impact Profile or the Nottingham Health Profile, and disease-specific indexes, such as those typically intended for use with cancer patients, are less directly concerned with such resource allocation decisions. While they remain relevant to allocation—for example, by providing tools for medical technology assessment—they may typically be seen as justifying the movement of health care resources towards patients, insofar as they indicate either the type of health care that is most appropriate for the patient, or the complexities of the patient's health state and thus the patient's need for care. Such measures have in consequence received far less attention from moral philosophers.

Reflection on the use of disease-specific quality of life measures, and upon profiles rather than indexes, shifts the philosopher's attention away from the pressing problems of resource allocation, towards what are more fundamental concerns. I will suggest that at the foundation of quality of life measurement are presuppositions about the way in which the medical profession, patients, and lay people talk about and understand disease and illness. To use a quality of life measure to allocate resources, or to assess technology or a patient's progress, entails an articulation of our understanding of disease and health, and thus a confrontation with our ability to communicate that understanding to others and to ourselves. My interest is then with the potential that quality of life measures have for unraveling the confusions, fears, and prejudices that beset the lay person's thinking about cancer, and that may inhibit communication between the medical staff, the patient, and the patient's family and friends.

DISCOURSE ETHICS

The approach that grounds these reflections is derived from discourse ethics.[3,4] At the core of any such analysis is the view of human beings as social creatures, continually involved in understanding their (physical and cultural) environment, communicating that understanding to others, and being capable of defending that understanding (more or less well) in open discussion. Any statement that an agent utters can, in principle, be challenged on a number of grounds. Upon saying "QALYs are used in health care allocation," I might be challenged as to what I mean (by, for example, someone who is unaware of the concept of "the QALY"), or as to whether the statement is true or not (by, for example, someone who doubts that QALYs have ever been used by a government or health authority), or even as to whether or not I have any right to make such a statement (as I am, after all, only a philosopher, and not, say, a health economist). In each case I can defend myself, by explaining what QALYs are, by giving an example of the use of QALYs, and by pointing out that, philosopher that I am, I have spent a good deal of time studying health policy and health economics. Of course, my replies may not satisfy my interrogator, in which case our discussion must continue (so that I may discover that my example of QALYs being used is actually fictitious, and that my study of health policy is not as satisfactory as I thought it was).

Discourse ethics may thereby be seen to focus upon communication as that process by which human beings articulate their factual understanding and evaluation of the world to themselves and to others. To communicate successfully to another human being is to provide information that makes sense, that is true, and that does not violate any moral principles that the respondent may hold dear. The doctor who thus uses technical language that a patient cannot understand, or the doctor who lies about the potential success or outcome of the treatment, or the doctor who forces the patient to accept a form of treatment—such as, for example, an abortion or blood transfusion—that is not permissible according to the patient's personal morality, has violated certain fundamental principles that ground and make possible communication. In principle, if not in practice, the patient may challenge the doctor to use nontechnical language, to provide evidence for his or her estimations of outcomes, and to justify the enforcement of an unacceptable treatment.

From this simple model of human understanding and interaction, a significant and possibly unexpected consequence can be derived. What human beings understand as truth and goodness are products of a consensus. Any statement that expresses a truth, be it a mundane fact of everyday life or a complex scientific theory, does so because those people to whom it matters accept it to be so. More precisely, a true statement is such that no one can offer a generally accepted challenge to it. Similarly, a statement expresses a desirable moral value because those affected by it accept it as such, and are unable to mount a successful challenge to it.

This account must be qualified. As it stands, it appears to be counterintuitive on a number of grounds. First, it appears to divorce truth claims from the way the world actually is. A statement could seemingly be true, or at least be regarded as true, despite its failure to correspond to reality. Superficially, discourse ethics seems to be suggesting that my statement to the effect that "the cat is sitting on the mat" will be true if everyone accepts that it is true, despite that fact that the cat is not sitting on the mat. This problem is resolved when it is recognized that truth depends upon the ability of those who profess the truth to defend their belief. One of the most powerful defences will be the appeal to empirical evidence. There is a consensus not merely on what is true, but also on the most appropriate means of establishing truth. Within the scientific community, repeatable, controlled experiments and peer review of research enshrine ideals of open, well-informed, rational debate.) Second, with respect to morality, the consensus theory seems to lead to relativism. The term "moral relativism" refers to the theory that moral values and norms will be grounded in particular cultures. Members of different cultures will accept different values and norms (or at least different combinations of values and norms) as being morally binding upon them. That which is morally good will thus be relative to the beliefs of a particular community. If a particular community holds that murder is acceptable, then, at least within that community, murder is indeed acceptable. More problematic, people from another culture cannot coherently condemn the murderous acts, for in so doing they merely impose their values on the other culture. Moral relativism thus challenges the possibility that there are any universal moral values.

This raises, for discourse ethics, more profound questions about the way in which consensus (about moral and factual issues) is achieved. Ideally, consensus is a product of open, well-informed, rational debate. Anyone who perceives him- or herself as being unfairly harmed by, for example, a moral principle, should be entitled to object, and to have his or her objection acted upon, or to be given a reasoned reply. This ideal is implicit in the idea of communication itself. In practice, consensus is brought about by more questionable means. Crucially, it may be suggested that any consensus actually achieved (be it over morality or truth) is at best provisional, because the process of reaching consensus inevitably falls short of the ideal. Three mechanisms that distort the process of debate may be recognized. First, participants may be ill-informed. For example, the theory or technology necessary to recognize or to resolve key problems in currently accepted scientific knowledge may not yet be available. Conversely, prejudices and superstitions, widely accepted within a culture, may not yet have been rigorously challenged. Second, rhetoric may hold greater sway than well-informed, reasonable argument. Excessively emotive language may thus, paradoxically, inhibit communication, not least because it blurs the grounds upon which one might reasonably challenge the information or ideas conveyed. Third, potential participants in a discussion may be silenced or otherwise excluded from the debate due to imbalances in social power. Someone may thus be afraid to challenge what a superior says, perhaps because of the consequences that such a challenge might have in terms of physical harm or career prospects. More significantly, the powerless may not even realize that they have any right to challenge the statements and commands of the powerful.

Discourse ethics thereby suggests that any existing consensus—be it in everyday life, in science, medical research and practice, or in morality—is provisional, and open to further critical examination. Knowledge may be improved, superstitions and prejudices challenged, and the powerless given a voice. The task of the philosopher is to facilitate such critical examination. In ethics, the philosopher does not resolve moral dilemmas, but struggles to ensure that the lay processes that lead to any such resolutions are rational and, as far as possible, well informed. The political philosopher and the social scientist have the additional responsibility of ensuring that debate is genuinely open. While inherently desirable, the ideal of open consensus is impossibly demanding, and can never be achieved. Precisely because of this, any existing consensus is always open to question.

This overview of the key ideas of discourse ethics, crude as it necessarily is, may begin to stimulate reflection upon communication about health. Doctors have more power than most of their patients. This power may be rationally grounded in their expert knowledge, and may therefore be used in what are perceived to be the patients' best interests. This power may, however, be abused, so that the doctor may, innocently or otherwise, assume that he or she knows best what is in the patients' interests, without presuming to consult them. This raises questions, not merely about the need for openness, and thus for communication, and about the way in which knowledge is communicated, but also about the superstitions and prejudices that may hamper communication. Fears and misinformation among lay people about disease, its cause and transmission, may lead them to enter into discussion about health and illness only on the basis of presuppositions that actually serve to disrupt the possibility of open, well-informed debate and communication. Again, my concern is therefore with the failure of communication about cancer, and thus with the absence of the conditions that would facilitate open, well-informed debate.

QUALITY OF LIFE MEASUREMENT

The interest in quality of life measurement that has developed over the last few decades has, to a significant degree, been grounded in an antipaternalistic ethos.[5] Implicitly, quality of life measures serve to question the legitimacy of the preponderant role that medical professionals took in decision making. Quality of life measures serve to give the patient and the general public a new, more sophisticated voice in the allocation of health care resources, in the determination of priorities and objectives for health care, and in the evaluation of that care. As such, quality of life measures may be seen to empower lay participants in debates about health care provision. The mechanisms of this empowerment are twofold. On the one hand, patients and the general public (as appropriate) may be consulted about the relevant dimensions of health, and thus the parameters that would occur in any particular measure. Typically, the statements that describe health states—for example, in such instruments as the Nottingham Health Profile or the Sickness Impact Profile—are derived from what lay people say about their own health. The profile or index thereby comes to reflect what is important to the lay person (rather than to the doctor) about the experience of being ill or healthy. On the other hand, the weightings of these health states, and thus the relative importance that they have with respect to each other and to some putative state of good health, may be generated through surveys of patients or the public. Again, the quality of life measures thereby come to reflect the evaluations of lay people. Some of the implications that these mechanisms have for the recognition and development of a dialogue between patient and medical professional may be rehearsed.

While it is a common complaint that there is no clear or agreed-upon definition of "quality of life," and there are thus a plurality of measures, each operationalizing the concept in a distinctive manner, "quality of life" clearly goes beyond the physically quantifiable symptoms of an illness, in order to embrace "psychosocial well-being."[6] By responding to the statements elicited from patients (and possibly their carers and other members of the public) about illness, disease and health, the crude biomedical model of health (that implicitly legitimates the dominant role of the physician in all health-related decision making) is challenged. The health of a patient is seen, variously, to impact on and in turn be affected by, his or her psychological state; his or her ability to function in the family and community, and in political and working environments; and the cultural resources that allow sense to be made of the illness and its consequences. It may be suggested that the biomedical model rapidly gives way to a humanistic model of health, where "health" depends less on the physical well-being of the patient than on the patient's ability to cope with his or her illness.[7]

The weighting of health states within an index matrix or within the individual parameters of a profile further allows the collective or aggregate opinions of patients (or the public) to find expression in the assessment of health care. Here further discrepancies between lay and professional judgments may be noted. Indexes are typically designed to allow the respondent to express a trade-off between years of survival and quality of life, and thus to determine the objectives of a treatment program. Selby points to the role that quality of life measures may play in focusing a patient's decision on the balance between the efficacy and toxicity of a cancer treatment. Western patients may express a willingness to suffer surprisingly high levels of toxicity for relatively little chance of an effective cure.[6,8] Conversely, from outside Western culture, Segun Gbadegesin has offered the example of a Yoruba woman who refused a mastectomy, knowing that this was the only treatment available that would save her life, on the grounds that the social stigma associated with the resultant deformity would make her life valueless.[9] If it is assumed that such a preference is representative of the Yoruba culture as a whole, then it may pose a fundamental challenge to medical presuppositions of the appropriate treatment for breast cancer—and indeed to the relationship between Western and non-Western understandings of health and illness.

If quality of life measures serve to highlight disagreements between patients, the public, and physicians (and, indeed, variations between societies or cultures), either over the definition of health or over priorities and weightings, then they thereby serve to highlight those points at which communication has broken down—and, possibly more pertinently, points at which the breakdown is not otherwise acknowledged or recognized. The antipaternalism inherent in quality of life measures cannot be so construed as to suppress the physician's voice altogether. A physician will have reasons for employing a restricted, biomedical model of health, and for using the technical language that goes along with that model and its knowledge base. Those reasons may be perfectly defensible in many situations. Similarly, as Selby points out, the patient's willingness to tolerate highly toxic treatments may represent the patient "clutching at straws." Such reasons may well be ultimately indefensible, insofar as they reflect the patient's inability to cope with his or her own mortality. In this case, the fault lies not with the patient as such, or at least not with the patient understood as an isolated individual, but rather with the inability of the patient's culture to provide him or her with the resources to make sense of mortality, which is to say to communicate with herself about mortality. Similarly, while the Yoruba woman's fears about being stigmatized must be respected, there is also a case for challenging the roots of that stigma in the culture as a whole, for example, through health education.

In summary, disagreement is a lack of consensus and indeed marks the potential breakdown of communication; and if consensus is desirable, then further means need to be found to allow the disputants to explore and to understand each others' positions, and indeed to understand their own. Quality of life measures may serve to expose the discrepancies that exist between doctor and lay person (and possibly the healthy and the ill) in understandings and evaluations of health. The process of debate that should result from this recognition may serve to reveal the distortions that contribute to mutual misunderstanding, and thus inhibit mutual understanding. Unjustifiable fears about mortality, social isolation, and dysfunctioning may inhibit the respondent's ability to give a reasonable, well-informed opinion on health states. Equally, a failure to recognize the impact that such fears have upon a patient's quality of life may lead to patients being directed into unnecessarily demanding or distressing forms of treatment.

QUALITY OF LIFE AND CANCER

A problem of certain approaches to quality of life measures has been to assume that measuring instruments, including such methodologies as the time trade-off or standard gamble, elicit the respondents' preexisting subjective attitudes to health and health states. Such attitudes are seen as basic data, which cannot further be challenged. In reply it may be suggested that typically respondents can give reasons, or should be expected to give reasons, for ranking states as they do, or for understanding "health" in the way that they do. The emphasis upon communication, and the inherent possibility of challenging any given statement, could thus be imposed upon the process of deriving quality of life matrices and weightings.[10] Certain reasons may not be defensible in open discussion, and as such should not be used in the construction of quality of life measures, or as straightforward guides to health policy and treatment. To give a particular health state a low ranking may reflect not the simple experience of that state, but rather the stigmas and prejudices that surround such conditions or the people who suffer from them. For example, people with physical disabilities frequently express disquiet over the use of quality of life measures, precisely because of the ill-informed judgments of the able-bodied, as to the experience and degree of dignity of those with disabilities, which may be encoded into the quality of life matrices.

A response to this problem may be to exclude those who have not suffered from a relevant disease state from the process of weighting. While this may be acceptable on some counts, from the discourse ethics perspective it misses a crucial opportunity. It prevents the comparison of the evaluations and understandings of different groups, and possibly serves further to isolate those who suffer illness and disease from dialogue with the healthy community. To recognize the discrepancy between the evaluations elicited from different groups serves to initiate the process of challenging and defending those evaluations, and thus the process of explicating the sorts of cultural assumptions that underpin them. This is to suggest that weighting may be affected by the sort of cultural factors that inhibit open, rational discussion of disease, and thus communication with sufferers. Thus, while in the preceding section I emphasized the potential that quality of life measures have for exposing the prejudicial assumptions and blind spots that inhibit communication about disease, it is important also to note that the uncritical use of quality of life matrices may perpetuate those very blind spots. The difficulty in discussing cancer—and in communicating the fears, aspirations, and experiences of the cancer patient, the doctors, and the patient's relatives and friends—may be suggested to rest precisely upon the paucity of cultural resources available to communicate such material, and the associated stigma and misunderstanding of cancer and its sufferers.

The rhetoric that surrounds any discussion of cancer is almost uniquely significant insofar as it at once inhibits and enables debate and expression. On the one hand, 'cancer' itself provides a key metaphor in expressing our distaste at much that is evil and threatening in society. This metaphorical use of the term is at once grounded in, but thereby serves to reinforce, public attitudes to the disease itself. As Selby points out, the perceived evil of cancer serves to isolate the patient from the rest of society, disrupting work and family life.[6] On the other hand, the patient's fear of his or her own illness is typically mitigated by dealing with cancer in terms of metaphorical narratives—for example, of the patient's struggle or battle with the illness.[11] Metaphors thereby allow the patient to construct an understanding of the disease and of his or her relationship to it. A doctor who reports, "You have to give people something to wake up for in the morning, otherwise they might as well take some cyanide"[11] highlights the role that such metaphorical narratives have in sustaining any quality of life at all in the patient. The wish for suicide is indicative of no quality of life, or of the QALY score that is less than zero.

The tension between these two uses of metaphor is indicative of the breadth required in the understanding, and consequent treatment, of the disease. Quality of life studies, by involving patients and the general public in the definition and evaluation of disease, reveal that cancer, and indeed any other disease, is a phenomenon not merely of the body, but of culture. A public's fear that cancer patients are infectious may be unfounded. Yet such irrational fears have real consequences for patients, and treatment of the disease may therefore require health education programs that can challenge such misinformation, and thereby serve to reintegrate the cancer patient into the overarching dialogue of social life itself. Quality of life measures are, on the one hand, crucial in indicating the dimensions of everyday life that the disease impinges upon, and also in raising questions as to the most appropriate ways of dealing with that loss of quality. On the other hand, they may serve to indicate the fears that the healthy have about cancer, and the difficulty with which such fears are articulated. The patient's fears of his or her own cancer, and the threat that it poses to life, are real; but they may also be indicative of a culture that is fundamentally unable to deal with, and talk about, its own mortality. The metaphors that sustain the patient, and that allow patient and doctor to discuss treatment regimes, are enabling, but possibly only to a point. A number of studies suggest that, paradoxically, even terminal cancer may have its positive side.[12] Imminent death puts one's life into perspective, and the burdens and stresses that occupy so much of the time and energy of the healthy, may be revealed as trivial. Inappropriate, albeit well-meaning, metaphors of "struggle" and "hope" may underestimate the quality of life found through stoicism. They may enable one form of dialogue at the cost of another, potentially richer dialogue.

In conclusion, the application of quality of life measurement within cancer treatment has been presented as giving the patient, and the public, a new voice in debates over treatment and policy. It may begin by highlighting those points at which there is no real dialogue. The understanding of what is entailed in cancer is thus expanded, and the cultural context of cancer and the cancer patient becomes a pressing concern. The eliciting of patient and public opinion about cancer care does not end a debate, but rather begins it. Quality of life measures must be understood as much to be indicators of public and patient ignorance and fear as they were initially understood to be indicators of physicians' ignorance and insensitivity.

REFERENCES

1. HARRIS, J. 1987. QALYfying the value of life. J. Med. Ethics **13:** 117–123.
2. BELL, J. M. & S. MENDUS, EDS. 1988. Philosophy and Medical Welfare. Oxford University Press. Oxford.
3. HABERMAS, J. 1990. Discourse ethics: Notes on a program of philosophical justification. *In* Moral Consciousness and Communicative Action. Polity Press. Cambridge.
4. OAKESHOTT, M. 1975. On Human Conduct. Clarendon Press. Oxford.
5. HUNT, S. M., J. MCEWEN & S. P. MCKENNA, Eds. 1986. Measuring Health Status: 1–19. Croom Helm. London.
6. SELBY, P. 1993. Measuring the quality of life of patients with cancer. *In* Quality of Life Assessment: Key Issues in the 1990s. R. Walker & R. Rosser, Eds.: 235–265. Kluwer. Dordrecht.
7. SEEDHOUSE, D. 1986. Health: The Foundations of Achievement. John Wiley. London.
8. SLEVIN, M. *et al.* 1990. Attitudes to chemotherapy: Comparing views of patients with cancer with those of doctors, nurses and general public. Br. J. Med. **300:** 1458–1460.
9. GBADEGSIN, S. 1994. Presentation to the Second World Congress of the International Association of Bioethics, Buenos Aires, October 1994.
10. EDGAR, A. 1995. Weighting health states and strong evalution. Bioethics **9:** 240–251.
11. VECCHIO GOOD, M. *et al.* 1995. Oncology and narrative time. Soc. Sci. Med. **38**(6): 855–862.
12. KAGAWA-SINGER, M. 1993. Redefining health: Living with cancer. Soc. Sci. Med. **37**(3): 295–304.

Truth, Disease, and Prognosis

An Historical-Anthropological Analysis

OLIVIO GALEAZZI[a]

Department of the History of Medicine
University of Bologna
Bologna, Italy

Discourse on the truth between the doctor and the cancer patient can be based on applied research and experimentation (clinical, psychological, legal, bioethical, etc.), or it can be based on humanistic methodologies: historical, anthropological, epistemological, the so-called medical humanities.

I will approach the daily problems—often harrowing—of the doctor's thinking, decision making, and medical actions from the humanistic point of view. I will shed light on three crucial elements in this complicated (delicate) task of communicating the truth about cancer: the meaning of truth, the meaning of illness, and the meaning of prognosis.

THE MEANING OF TRUTH

Communication between doctor and patient is mainly verbal (oral and/or written): words link the doctor and the patient primarily, the act of saying in its full anthropological complexity (biophysical, semiotic and linguistic, psychological).

The doctor must decide whether, how, and when to reveal the truth to the cancer patient. He must reflect on saying and truth, interconnected and always essential in a doctor's work, even in its most routine aspects.

We must consider the meaning of truth, which has been the main focus of philosophy and theology. Truth does not mean reality. What is real is not necessarily true. What does reality need to have to be considered true? Reality and truth are obviously very close to each other. Reality has to be presented in a certain way in order to be considered truth. This particular presentation consists in the act of saying. Reality becomes truth only when it is said.[1]

Indeed, truth has no autonomous existence; it is a relationship between a portion of reality and its statement. In other words, an unex-

[a]Tutte le mie gratitudine alla Signora Snežana Stiefel per il complesso e riuscitinicero lavoro di traduzione in inglese.

pressed truth cannot exist. When this relationship does not exist, we can talk about falsehood. Falsehood is the opposite of truth the way nonreality is the opposite of reality. Therefore, the absence of truth (the relationship that verifies an aspect of reality) does not allow us to deny the reality, no matter how bizarre or difficult it may be to accept it as true.

Reality cannot be considered truth until the very moment it is stated. Even before it is stated, we must admit that the human mind can perceive it, but this is not sufficient to consider it true. Reality becomes truth only when it is said, named, defined, stated—in short, communicated.[2]

These considerations, applied to a delicate relationship between doctor, patient, truth, and cancer, assume a new meaning: the truth can only be communicated, the heart of clinical truth lies in the act of telling between doctor and patient. Clinical reality certainly exists, discovered by scientific medicine (clinical and technical), but this reality is different from the truth, and it exists as objective fact separate from the act of communicating. When a doctor talks to a cancer patient, the truth that emerges from his words should also contain the clinical and technical evidence, but it should not and cannot be limited to it.[3]

The truth comes after and within the act of communicating, not the other way around; it lives and gains meaning in the words, not the other way around. The words come before the truth; they precede, illuminate, and give meaning to the truth; they make the truth true.

Is it possible to state some practical consequences of these eminently philosophical arguments? The doctor has two options. First, the great bioethical accomplishment of the autonomy of the patient[4] need not make us forget that the efficacy of therapy depends on the recognition of the relationship between the illness and medicine, and on the degree to which the doctor recognizes, accepts, and masters the inevitable presence of profound emotions in the patient as well as in himself in every moment of their daily rapport: to reject that medical staff should be unfeeling does not mean to be less professional or scientific; it means to be more professional and more scientific.[5] The mutual involvement in the fateful rendezvous between patient and doctor expands the doctor's theoretical and practical horizons, and induces in him a behavior that needs to be controlled.

Second, to tell the truth about cancer means that the doctor has to make true an unpleasant portion of reality.[6] He must start from the clinical-technical reality but must be aware that his words will make the truth sprout, will give it form, meaning, and fulfillment. The doctor needs to pass the illness through his own judging and telling subjectivity in order to communicate it to the patient as truth.

This complicated passage is the very essence of medicine at any time and place: reality observed by the doctor becomes knowledge and science in the same way as in any other scientific discipline, in every area of human knowledge. Up to this point, the method of medicine is essentially identical to that of all other sciences, particularly the sciences that study life and man.

The difference arises at the moment when the doctor must act as a mirror and convey to the patient (the natural source of his knowledge) the conclusions of his observations, in a sort of short circuit between the observer and the observed, a process in which the whole person of the doctor (his thoughts, his gestures, even his very body) is engaged.

All the sciences are based on communication (within the community of researchers and between it and society at large), but only in the practice of medicine is full, constant, mutual communication required between the subject—the observer—and the object—the observed, for the simple reason that both of them are human, with the same fears, the same pain, and the same hopes.

The final product of this complicated epistemological short circuit is the truth. As unpleasant and discouraging as it may be, this truth is always new, always different, always individual—a far cry from the dry, useless statistics of survival and from the enumeration of different hypothetical "slalom paths" that the patient has to run before he arrives at the final goal of death.

The clinical condition of the cancer patient (his reality, his cancer) is not the truth; they become the truth only in the hard-to-utter spoken word (always new and always the same) through which the doctor finds the strength to communicate with the patient.

THE MEANING OF ILLNESS

> If illness, like climatic variations, the search for food, and competition among species, is a constant element of our existence as living animals, illness, or the channel through which the phenomenon of illness becomes a variable in human history, is one of the typical results of the creative capacity with which man modifies his surroundings.[8]

This quotation introduces and emphasizes the distinction between two polarities: on the one hand, illness understood as a natural constant that exercises a selective and undifferentiated pressure, and, on the other hand, illness as a variable that is historically determined and subordinated to the modifications of the habitat by man's creativity.

This main distinction brings a second one, of equal theoretical importance: that between illness as a possible reality (an object of the natural world, a circumscribed episode of life), and illness as a relational reality, a formidable experience of communication.[9]

It is evident that the two elements of the phenomenon of illness— personal suffering and the impulse to communicate—are inseparable.

In the case of the human animal, the greatest part of what we consider the environment consists of nature and man-made nature, the net of interrelations between man and culture. The greatest part of the habitat of civilized man (in contrast to that of other species) is created by his own civilization, by his material and nonmaterial parameters, by his achievements and his symbols.[10]

There are manifold reasons that justify the permanent historical and interpretative need always to shed light on the relationship between medicine and communication. Any attempt to connect the concept of illness with the concept of communication (speaking in metaphors for illness) should inevitably depart from the definition of illness as a condition of "more onerous citizenship."[11]

This definition leads back to a very precise historical and ideological concept. This definition could be defined as historical, as it establishes a cultural criterion that surpasses the culture in which it was formulated.[12]

Since we stated that illness defines the limits (narrow and distressing) of a "more onerous citizenship," we need a second proposition to fullfill two logical purposes:

(l) to ascertain the existence of a common, typical behavior of that "population" that in different ways experiences the conditions of a "burdensome citizenship" (minorities forced into social subordination, groups in objective situations of suffering from lack of resources, cultures that by ideological choice submit to very harsh living conditions);

(2) to ascertain whether such typical behavior can be found in a "group of burdensome citizenship" consisting of a vast and always changing population of sick human beings.

As a working hypothesis, we can identify the cultural "marker" (specific to all human population subordinated in different ways) with a radical semiotic intention: all the conditions of impairment and hardship (and above all those that derive from illness) seem to inflict a behavioral automatism, an irrepressible compulsion to communicate that impairment and that hardship, to make "others" in some way involved in that impairment and in that hardship.[13]

We are faced with an archaic "vis semiotica" with a tendency to translate into a sign (howl, weeping, song, metaphor) the hardship inherent in the illness.[14]

The patient's production of signs corresponds naturally to the healer's production of signs; this is the way the primordial exchange of messages takes place, from which the illness as such gains form and substance; and this is how we (patients and doctors) identify it: as an inseparable mixture of subjective and corporal moments and of objective moments (taxonomic and ideological) with the coexistence in both worlds (from which it suffers and by which it heals) of immediate, "volcanic" elements or of strongly controlled elements on the level of a culture.[15]

Literature and poetry are important sources for medical humanistic research. As a matter of fact, the paradigm of communication between the world of suffering and the world of help is rendered, in its dramatic perfection, in one of the key passages of the dialogue between Achilles and his mother in what we can consider the first real product of world literature—Homer's *Iliad:*

> Eyes wet with tears,
> he spoke, and her ladyship his mother heard him
> in green deeps where she lolled near her old father.
> Gliding she rose and broke like mist from the inshore
> grey sea face, to sit down softly before him,
> her son in tears; and fondling him she said:
> "Child, why do you weep? What grief is this?
> Out with it, tell me, both of us should know."
> Akhilleus, fast in battle as a lion,
> groaned and said: "Why tell you what you know?"[16]

In this archaic example of therapeutic drama (the first one in the history of our culture) all the phases of communication are present in a foreseeable and logical way. They are aroused always and everywhere by physical and emotional suffering, which is described by Homer with absolute precision and expressive economy:

(1) request for help ("Eyes wet with tears he spoke");
(2) hearing the request ("and her ladyship his mother heard him,""Gliding she rose and broke like mist from the inshore grey sea face");
(3) the activation of nonverbal forms of therapeutic communication ("to sit down softly before him," "fondling him");
(4) request to tell a story ("'why do you weep?'" "'What grief is this?'")[17];
(5) the difficulty of complaining and the therapeutic function of sharing the suffering ("'Out with it, tell me, both of us should know.'");
(6) the existence in the consoling goddess as well as in all the other help givers of an operative, taxonomic "previous knowledge," a specific knowledge of what is being cured; it is assumed that the help giver knows all the possible causes, forms, and cures of the specific illness and suffering ("'Why tell you what you know?'").[18]

Besides the more obvious aspects of the communicative encounter between the doctor and the patient, such as, for example, the inherent cathartic function of expressing one's suffering, or the sublimating function of representation (magical, dramatic, figurative, etc.) of the medical impairment, there are other subtle aspects.[19]

The manner in which this communication is rendered—originated by the patient, as in all the subjugated cultures—is typical of a group that is temporarily in a subordinate position, and therefore hermetic, exclusive, and ad hoc.

Paradoxically, communication about pathology between patients and doctors, doctors and doctors, and, above all, patients and patients is exclusive and coded. Especially among patients, but even in the slang of doctors and paramedics, an enigmatic world of cryptic verbal and non-verbal signs is evoked or accepted to assuage fear, to exclude "strangers," to use special and unusual resources. What interests patients and doctors is not the universal clarity and intelligibility of their communication, but creation of a parallel, conventional universe of symbols, signs, and even of enigmas and cryptograms built on pain and the communication of pain.[20]

In anthropological terms, the invisible danger, the most serious trap inherent in illness is that it, like a solid rock, appears in front of the us and blocks our capacity to reason, to act, to change, by robbing us of "soul," courage, and hope.

Both medicine and popular knowledge have aimed not so much to cure as to overcome this radical, annihilating danger—to remove the obstacle of illness, and to give illness the capacity to move, evolve, to give it the meaning and dynamics of change that would help the patient recover his or her potential resources.[21]

Illness can "function," can progress (toward improvement or deterioration) only if it is duly restrained in a linguistic and metaphoric net. This net is the most potent and most essential remedy that humanity has distilled over the millennia to confront disease.[22]

Medicine and the symbolic-linguistic universe go hand in hand; they are interconnected and influence each other. The clinician must be fully aware of this fact and must act in such a way as to use the vision of illness (operating in the culture and in the sick person) as an everyday "working tool," especially in the crucial moment in which he must communicate to the patient an unpleasant truth.

The pathological, therapeutic insight, the result of the metaphoric rendering of the illness, should be used by the doctor as a resource, not as a limiting or conditioning element—a resource that for the purpose of diagnosis and therapy avails itself of the entire philosophical, psychological, religious, and ethnic background of the patient and his culture, which may vary from culture to culture, from person to person, and even within a single individual.

Every generation has elaborated, with meticulous accuracy, a complicated body of beliefs, practices, and symbols relating to illness that acts as a semiotic silencer of bodily and mental suffering. This elaboration, specific to each culture, of a cultural paradigm of illness has been paralleled by, and very interactive with, the theoretical evolution of official medicine (prescientific or scientific), which was working on the elaboration of a scientific paradigm of illness.

If the patient, when he addresses the doctor, moves, with more or less awareness, on the basis of this enormous symbolic patrimony, the doctor, meanwhile, needs to become familiar with and to recognize that patrimony and to know how to use and manipulate it in the interest of the patient, according to the principle of beneficence—above all in the communication of unpleasant truth.

THE MEANING OF PROGNOSIS

Since the most unwelcome moment in the communication between doctor and cancer patient is that in which the future outcome is discussed, it is important to dwell briefly on the meaning of the subtle intellectual operation that is called prognosis.

What does the patient ask of the doctor? The patient turns to the doctor for the immediate relief of suffering (tactic) and the prognosis of the cure (strategy)—and also, always, for coparticipation in knowledge (gnosis). To know the name of the illness (and its hypothetical tale, with the probable stages of a future story, always the same and always different) is no less important to the patient than the cure.

As strange as it may seem to a utilitarian mentality, this hunger for knowledge, more or less conscious, more or less articulated, always intervenes in the therapeutic relationship, unavoidably and almost automatically; this is so essential to the stabilization of the relationship, that we cannot even conceive this doctor-patient relationship (in a transcultural milieu) if it does not also contain this (more or less conscious) request for knowledge.

The name of the illness corresponds, in a prelogical and symbolizing vision of the events of reality, to the very essence of illness. It contains the forms and the fate of the illness. The name is the illness, its real being, its intimate soul.[23] To know the name of the illness means to know its secret. It means to unmask it, to uncover its real and specific character. It means to nail it down to its very essence, to divest it of all fluidity, of all vagueness and indeterminateness, that are characteristics of a blind and anonymous suffering.

To name an illness (or anything, animate or inanimate) allows one to place it in the context of its evolution, in its own perspective of change and (if possible) of cure. The sick person does not know the name of the disease. Those who do know the name of illnesses and can name them are usually socially designated as ad hoc experts, recognized as a culturally homogeneous group (doctors or medicine men); it is from them that the sick person learns the name of his or her illness and becomes, by means of this initial communication, an adept, a limited participant in a higher, mysterious knowledge.

This is a primordial, universal way (nominalistic mentalization) in which the human mind conquers "scientifically" the world, for the purpose not only of cataloging reality, but also of enabling the transmission of knowledge (nosological and therapeutic) either vertically (through successive generations of healers and patients) or horizontally (among doctors and patients who are contemporaries).

This "nosography" (naming illnesses) is eternally problematic and is, by definition, never definitive. It is always deeply felt, always unsatisfying work in medicine of all ages and cultures. Every phase of the history of medicine reinvents tirelessly, radically, the whole nosographic terminology, in order to adapt it to the permanent evolution of theories and falsifications, in the very way in which ethnic medicine diversifies the names of illnesses in order to adapt them to changeable mythologies and rituals.

Some contemporary societies[25] avoid mentioning the word cancer. The reason for this caution, with origins in magic, is simply that the name of the illness automatically contains the prognosis of the illness—not the scientific prognosis, but the common-sense prognosis. A mixture of foretelling and predestination confusedly persists in the mind, inexorably dark and inauspicious, because of the symbolic and extraordinary emotional charge of the name of the illness—cancer.

The moment of the prognosis is fundamental in all the encounters between doctor and patient, from the most fleeting and banal to the most fateful and dramatic. Since the communication of the prognosis to the patient is what needs to be done and what is so difficult to do, especially in the case of cancer, it is important to focus on the concept of this key moment in the relationship of doctor and patient.

We have seen that two different levels of the prognosis of cancer (but not solely of cancer) exist in the mind: the scientific prognosis of the doctor, which, through wisdom, slowly improves over time, and the emotional prognosis of the patient, which continues to carry the historical burden of endless suffering and death, recent and long past.

Medical-historical reflection explains the complexity of the concept of prognosis: the basic systematic definition is still, after 25 centuries, that articulated by Hippocrates and his school. Hippocratic prognosis is the center, the pillar of the whole edifice of medicine. To practice medicine, according to Hippocrates, is to make prognosis. Hippocratic prognosis is, however, fundamentally different from what we doctors of today mean by the term. To understand this difference is to grasp the essence of the dilemma of information and truth in relation to the cancer patient.

By the Greek term *prognosis,* the School of Cos did not mean what is understood in modern medical practice—namely, foretelling the future development of the illness to the patient. Our kind of prognosis was, in the Hippocratic cultural milieu, designated by the restrictive term *prog-*

nosticon, in which the prefix "pro" assumes the chronological connotation of "before." Therefore, it is a knowledge of a future evolution of the illness of a certain patient, a present knowledge, before such future even started.

The prognosis of Hippocrates was something different.[26] The prefix "pro" did not indicate simple chronological antecedence, but suggested, on one hand, philosophical antecedence—the doctor and the expert must possess a preknowledge of the illness, a code for pigeonholing all possible events, even the rarest, most unpredictable and inexplicable. On the other hand, for Hippocrates this prefix had what has been defined as an "extensive-intensive value." This value of the preposition "pro" gave to the term knowledge *(gnosis)* not so much the meaning of "knowledge before the time," "knowledge of the future,"as the meaning of deep, advanced knowledge, more advanced than everyday knowledge—the paradox of a "rational clairvoyance" that is exercised for the purpose of giving relief to (*pro*) the sick person. And this, in my opinion, is the extensive-extensive semantic meaning of Hippocratic prognosis.[27]

Prognosis is, therefore, always a form of knowledge of illness with the following characteristics:

1. It is knowledge that is present in the doctor even before a concrete case of illness appears.
2. It is complex knowledge of the whole of the illness (in its abstract and concrete aspects), of its past *(anamnesis)*, its present (*diagnosis*) and its future *(prognostikon).*
3. A part of such knowledge (*prognostikon* according to Hippocrates, prognosis in the modern sense) concerns the probable future fate of the illness and the patient (survival or death, duration of relapse-free survival, relapse rates, cure rates).
4. It is knowledge that the doctor projects toward and for the purpose of helping the patient (another accepted meaning of the prefix "pro"), transforming it into plain, rational verbal communication. The term *gnosis* is never, in the mind of antiquity, mute and closed in the mind of the knower. Knowledge automatically leads to expression *(logos).* It does not exist as, and is inconceivable as, unexpressed awareness. Like the truth, knowledge can be called such only when it takes on meaning with the human word. Prognosis exists only as a central focus of the communication (verbal, but not only verbal) between doctor and patient.

Anamnesis, diagnosis, and prognosis (*prognostikon*), integral parts of Hippocratic prognosis in a wider sense, thus consist of the act of saying—of these three crucial moments in which "the force of the words that express the reflection, the act of the spirit" is exercised professionally.[28]

The word is the instrument that allows human intelligence to explore the unknown by formulating tentative logical conclusions, by searching out hypothetical solutions, by constructing simulated realities, in an art of combining inexhaustible potentialities.

Verbal communication between doctor and patient assumes the importance that it merits. "I maintain that it is a truly positive fact that a doctor foretells the future. If he is capable of knowing the past, the present, and the future of a patient without his help and of filling in the gaps in the patient's account, he will be considered capable of handling different cases, and people will entrust him with their treatment with confidence."[29]

The importance, in the history of ethics and of the medical profession, of the eternal question of trust in the relationship between doctor and patient is a logical consequence of the prognosis that the patient demands from the doctor and that the doctor cannot avoid giving the patient.

Mutual trust between doctor and patient is at the basis of the correct information and truth that needs to be given to the cancer patient. If the patient does not have trust in his doctor, no information, no truth about the illness will have any meaning, and it will seem provisional, weak, and doubtful. If the doctor does not have trust in his patient, in his ability to change, to collaborate, even to be a protagonist in his own cure, the doctor will probably give him a generic, perfunctory, dryly statistical, anguish-causing, unproductive prognosis that will not lead to a cure.[30]

"To be useful, or at least, not to harm" the patient: the principal of prima facie beneficence is, in conclusion, confirmed as being equal in importance to that of autonomy, not only concerning the bioethical, philosophical, and medico-legal level, but also on the humanistic level (historical, philological and anthropological). Beneficence and autonomy coexist with equal dignity, above all else, because both are rooted in the word (communicating, confiding, healing) that tirelessly connects doctor and patient. Everything that can happen to them and between them can be articulated in words. No reality, no matter how tragic or irreversible, can be considered a priori excluded from words (or from the knowing silence that represents their vital echo). It is precisely such words that the doctor has to find every day, words that are always the same and always new.

NOTES AND REFERENCES

1. "The use of true and false is a bit misleading, because it refers to the idea of 'agreement' or 'correspondence' with the facts (or with reality), which is anything but easy to explain . . . . On the basis of this agreement it is assumed that a statement is true if it agrees with the facts or with reality." (Gaetano Calabró. 1981. Vero/Falso. In Enciclopedia Einaudi, Vol. 14, p. 1035. Einaudi. Turin.) It is assumed, though, that truth (or falsehood) is something that concerns the statement of reality, and not the reality stated. Reality will never be true or false—only the statement about reality.
2. The spoken word and its intrinsic power of truth, as the power of relation-

ship, has relevance in the Western classical and Christian traditions, with smaller and less diverse relevance in other traditions. ". . . I assert that God does not know because He is, but that He exists because He knows; because God is intellect and knowledge and His knowledge is the very essence of His being." Then John 1.1 says: "In the beginning was the Word, and the Word was with God, and the Word was God." The Evangelist did not say: In the beginning there was being, and God was being. The Word refers totally to the intellect, as the act of telling and as the spoken word that holds within itself being and nonbeing. That is why the Savior says in John 16.6, 'I am the truth.' Reality watches over the intellect. This relationship receives its whole being from the soul . . . ." (Meister Eckhart. 1953. La nascita eterna. *In* Antologia sistematica delle opere latine e tedesche. G. Faggin, Ed.: 5. Sansoni. Florence. Quaestio "Utrum in Deo sit idem esse et intelligere," 1302–1304).

What assures the existence of a bond between language and the world? The act of naming or baptizing things in the world is always a conventional act, but it always establishes a relatively stable reference between a name and the thing that it indicates; the act of showing that a certain thing has been baptized with a certain name is the basic causal mechanism that stabilizes the relationship between the signifier and the signified. Cf. Thomas Kuhn, 1985, La metafora della scienza—Il riferimento dei termini scientifici e il cambiamento delle teorie., Pegaso **1**(1): 46.

3. It should be remembered that the act of saying that makes reality true is always an act of selective saying, which sees and underlines only the essential part of reality. Only this part of reality is seen and expressed; only it matters. The truth or the idea that we have about what the truth is is such only when it presents a particular element, a signature, a sign of reality. It is obvious that a complex reality requires, in order to be identified, a complex variety of signs. The same is true in the case of the truth about cancer as for the identification of every level of truth. There are strong analogies with anatomical-clinical iconography: " . . . we are not so much dealing with a single mark of truth in anatomical illustration, but with complex varieties of truths which carry the marks or imprints of a wide range of factors—intellectual, visual and social . . . ." (Martin Kemp. 1993. The mark of truth: Looking and learning in some anatomical illustrations from the Renaissance and the eighteenth century. *In* Medicine and the Five Senses. W. F. Bynum & Roy Porter, Eds.: 121. Cambridge University Press. Cambridge.)
4. Cf. Antonella Surbone, 1993, Dire la verità ai pazienti, JAMA Ital. edit. **5**(1): 33–35; Edmund D. Pellegrino, 1993, Dire la verità al paziente è un artefatto culturale? JAMA Ital. edit. **5**(1): 36–37; Howard D. Silverman, L'arte di comunicare cattive notizie, *in* Medico e Paziente (Trad. da Senior Patient), McGraw-Hill, New York, NY; Antonella Surbone, 1993, Which truth to the patient? *in* International Workshop on the History, Anthropology, and Epistemology of Medicine, Third Stage, Senigallia, Italy, November 27–28, 1993 (i.p.).
5. Therapy becomes effective only if the doctor gets profoundly and intensely, although maybe unconsciously, involved in his relationship with his patient. An involvement that could only lead to change is essential to all healing dynamics. (Girgio Bert & Silvana Quadrino. 1993. Il medico e il counseling. Il Pensiero Scientifico Ed. Rome.) A relationship of reciprocal availability between both poles of the therapeutic dyad (doctor and patient)

could be delineated from the model formulated in T. S. Szasz & M. H. Hollender, 1956, A contribution to the philosophy of medicine: The basic models of doctor-patient relationship, Arch. Intern. Med. **97:** 585 (cited in Costantino Jandolo, 1985, Il malato inosservante, p. 60, Armando, Rome). To the three models—parent-child ("activity/passivity"), parent-adolescent ("guidance/cooperation"), adult-adult ("mutual participation")—should be added a fourth: child-child, which exists at the moment of change or growth that is essential in all types of healing dynamics. See also Rosaria Conte & Mauro de Angelis, 1984, Scopi e conflitti di ruolo del medico nel rapporto col paziente, *in* Esplorare la vita quotidiano, Carlo Gerbaldo, Ed., p. 237, CNR-Il Pensiero Scientifico Ed, Rome. In the history of the professions, and especially of the medical profession, two opposing tensions coexist: the capacity to remain objective in the exercise of a role (T. Parsons, 1939, The professions and social structure, *in* Essays in Sociological Theory, Pure and Applied, T. Parsons, Ed., The Free Press, Glencoe, IL) and the availability for intimate involvement in the therapeutic relationship (Olivio Galeazzi, 1992, Rapporto terapeutico e antropologia della sessualità, *in* Atti 34 Congr. Naz. Storia Med., Messina, November 27–29, 1989, pp. 583–603.) It is not by chance that the element of secrecy is of the essence of the development of the very concept of profession, though in some cases the secret is activated in the opposite direction. "It should be observed that under the guise of the affirmation of truth and the professional secret, the position of a doctor is clearly different from that of a lawyer. The client confides to the lawyer a secret that he himself (the client) knows, while the patient confides to the doctor a secret concerning the condition of his health that he himself does not know and that he wishes to learn about from the doctor . . . ." (Francesco Carelli, 1993, Verità o bugie al malato? Meditime **25**(11): 16.)

6. Cf. C. Melodia & C. de Beretolini, 1990, L'immagine del cancro: Dalla morte alla rinascita, Psichiatria e medicina, October: 22–24.
7. "How much a patient should know depends on his desire and on his character, on the wishes of his family, on the state of his affairs, and maybe on his religious convictions . . ."; ". . . one thing is sure, it is not your job to put on a black hood and assume the role of a judge who pronounces a death sentence, to dash all hope of the patient . . . hope that counts so much for all of us (William Osler) . . . ." (1975–1976. Harrison's Principi di medicina interna e terapia, various authors, vol. 1, p. 12, Vallardi, Milan.) Even though all these elements—the desire of the patient, his/her character, the wishes of the family, the state of affairs, religious convictions, keeping hope alive, etc.—are facts of reality that should enter into the clinical evaluation, they are also clinical facts essential in the communication of reality. The Oslerian concept of judge and sentence evidently evolved in the last century. A judge should show wisdom in passing a sentence the way a doctor should show wisdom in forming and communicating a diagnosis. See Maria Giovanna della Vecchia, 1993, Verità vo cercando, Tempo Medico, **11**(12): 11.
8. Aurelio Mauri Paolini. 1987. Evoluzione tecnico-scientifica. Costi sanitari crescenti. Ritardi culturali nelle strutture amministrative-decisionali del S. S. N. attuale. *In* International Workshop on the History, Anthropology and Epistemology of Medicine, Senigallia, Italy, November 27–28, 1987 (Abstr.).
9. Cf. in Tito Pignedoli, n.d., Fede e malattia, in "Doctor": ". . . only human consciousness has been the cause of the fact that suffering itself has not become

isolated and ignored by the community. On the contrary, this very consciousness of the existence of suffering has caused the development of studies and research, the development of medication and countermeasures to prevent it. This has happened because the sick have made the healthy conscious that pain exists, even though the healthy do not have it at the moment." To give meaning to suffering by means of converting it into a universal, communal, shared hope—in other words, a cultural hope—is a primary historical requirement of sick humanity.

10. About the social and cultural (and specifically urban) origin of the entire modern pandemic of chronic degenerative diseases (cardiovascular, neoplastic, psychopathological, etc.) see Sandro Spinsanti, 1993, Il peso della dimensione sociale nel determinarsi della malattia, *in* Il Medico d'Italia **42:** 8; and Olivio Galeazzi, 1994, Ethnopathology in urban contexts: Anthropologtical and historical notes, *in* Actas 32 Congr. Intern. Historia Medicina, J. L. Carillo & G. Olague de Ros, Eds., pp. 543-551, Seville.
11. The hypothesis that illness is a message of the invisible exists in every historical and cultural context. It could represent divine or diabolical punishment or revenge, caused by a spell, a prophecy come true, the eruption into everyday reality of deep yearnings, not necessarily negative but endowed by a creative potency, unexpressible any other way, of the individual or collective unconscious (cancer as "symbolic pregnancy," ethnic and "paranormal" pathologies, etc.). Cf. Alessandra dal Ri, .n.d., Voglio guarire, quindi guarisco, in "Doctor": ". . . All emotion that is not lived is lived by the body. This is a very old idea. For ancient Egyptians illnesses are 'confessions' of the soul. In renaissance medicine Paracelsus says: 'The invisible becomes visible through analogy.' About illness as creativity, i.e., as an "esthetic moment," see Arnaldo Cherubini & Francesca Vannozzi, 1993, Note bibliografiche sull'uso (e l'abuso) del patologico nel Romanticismo, *in* Healing—Storia e strategie del guarire, Olivio Galeazzi, Ed, pp. 75–92, Olschki, Florence. On the capacity of illness to reveal a level of the invisible and otherwise inaccessible "other" reality, see Renato di Michele, 1993, Il corpo ammalato come emittante di segni, *in* Healing (op. cit.), pp. 65–73.

    Illness is something that should be harnessed, tamed, and translated into a different language; suffering requires an interpretation. See Marc Augé, 1982, Simbolo, Funzione, Storia, Liguori, Naples.
12. "Illness is the night-side of life, a more onerous citizenship. Everyone who is born holds dual citizenship, in the kingdom of the well and in the kingdom of the sick." (Susan Sontag. 1978. Illness as Metaphor. Farrar, Straus and Giroux. New York, NY.)
13. A hermeneutic of illness cannot exist without anthropological categories, because just as anthropology is a science of "elsewhere" (of others different from oneself, of the other that is in us), in the same way illness, in its very presence, requires the existence of "others" and of an "elsewhere," where the suffering can find the cause as well as its alleviation. See Ferdinando de Marco & Anselmo Palma, 1993, Condividere il disturbo è una terapia? Comunicazione ed espressione del disagio nella dimensione della antropologia quotidiana, *in* International Workshop on the History, Anthropology, and Epistemology of Medicine, Third Stage, Senigallia, Italy, November 27–28, 1993 (i.p.).
14. Illness is perhaps the most tellable and most memorable event of human existence. There are structural analogies between the story of illness and the

other types of stories present in the different literary genres. In all of them the tension escalates until the climax, in which all the moments of narration lead toward the final resolution. In such stories every passage gradually prepares us for the final catastrophe, of which the audience is aware, yet without knowing until the very end the actual outcome of the story. War stories, travel stories (a kind of story of homecoming), comic stories (jokes and gags), and, above all, detective stories: How will it end? Who will recognize the killer? Who will win the war? What will be the outcome of the illness? How will the joke end? These genres of story finds their meaning only at the end. Cf. Walter J. Ong, 1986, Oralité e scrittura—Le tecnologie della parola, Il Mulino, Bologna.

15. There exists a rhetorical hypertrophy in medicine, caused by the great linguistic intensity that characterizes the relationship between doctor and patient. The need to resolve a semiotic and emotional block has always made the therapeutic encounter relatively rigid and constrained. The encounter with the doctor is always changeable, yet stable and with a rigid protocol, like a repetitive ritual. However, in scientific medicine, a standard encounter with the doctor combines the maximum of methodological rigidity with the maximum of flexibility, of expressive spontaneity. In an optimal doctor's visit, a doctor should know how to be spontaneous (to go beyond the pure protocol), while the patient should know how to be rigorous (in order to conform to the rigor of clinical work). See Olivio Galeazzi & Gianni Jacovelli, 1986, Medicina come linguaggio e linguaggio degli strumenti clinici, *in* Medicina e Storia, O. Galeazzi, Ed., Il Lavoro Edit., Ancona; Josep Lluis Barona, Communication obstacles in the doctor-patient relation, *in* International Workshop on the History, Anthropology, and Epistemology of Medicine, Third Stage, Senigallia, Italy, November 27–28, 1993 (i.p.). The concept of "volcanic eruption" is applicable to the primal, physiological stage of basic emotions and behavior, which only in the second stage acquires a certain cultural transformation, as happens with mourning, sexuality, nourishment and help-seeking, etc. See Wulf Shiefenhovel, 1985, Sterben und Tod bei den Eipo im Hochland von West-Neuguinea, Curare **4**: 191–208.

16. Homer, Iliad, 1: 357–365, translated by Robert Fitzgerald, 1974, Doubleday, Garden City, NY. The goddess, who is a mother and a healer, appears under the guise of fog. This means that the one who is helping needs above all to be a presence. The forms, techniques, and good manners of the doctor mean very little if his presence is weak, or if the sick person does not perceive at the outset the inexpressible healing effectiveness inherent in the presence of the doctor.

17. Cf. D. Mechanic, 1976, Illness, illness behavior and help-seeking. Implications for increasing the responsiveness of health services, *in* The Growth of Bureaucratic Medicine, D. Mechanic,Ed., Wiley, New York, NY.

18. "Have you seen a case like mine before?" A primary and unconscious desire of the patient for the doctor to have seen a case like his before, a hundred, a thousand cases like his (preknowledge of the doctor). This releases his suffering from the chaos of the unknown and anchors it onto the medical (and magical) knowledge that gives meaning to the pain and resolves it. (J. N. Blau. 1993. Behaviour during a cluster headache. Lancet **342:** 723–725.)

19. It should be remembered that communication has a primitive, "vulcanic" worth that cannot be reduced to a purely utilitarian vision. Healing, like

sexuality, proceeds originally from a language. See Francesco Voltaggio, 1993, Eidos: Paradigma nosologico e prescrizione del farmaco, *in* Healing (op. cit.), pp. 241–267.

20. In all cultures there is a need to construct a philosophy of illness and healing capable of making suffering a model, a scheme, a syndrome. Cf. Francesco Voltaggio (op. cit.); La malattia e i suoi modelli, Convegno del Ministero dell'Università e della ricerca scientifica e tecnologica, Forlí, Italia, January 26-28, 1995; Filosofia della medicina, Corsi di medicina e scienze umane dell'Istituto Scientifico H. San Raffaele, Milano, 1988-1989/1989-1990.
21. A series of translations is embedded in illness—a naturalistic, pathological manifestation sets off a series of translations. It becomes translated into a precultural, primordial scream for help, which, in turn, is tranlated into a prefolkloric, prescientific common language. This is then translated into the language of the ethnomedical knowledge of illness and healing (prescientific folklore); and this is then finally translated by official medicine into scientific language (learned lore).

    This cascade of translations leads to the knowledge of illness and allows it to complete its course, to have a life as an "object" to be studied and to be tellable—which means treatable in its time outside of time.
22. Francesco Voltaggio, (op. cit.): "My research has led me to evidence that the School of Cos (fifth century B.C.) has elaborated a peculiar concept of illness in which every illness (*nosos*) is an *eidos*.
23. Mirko D. Ormek, 1985, Le malattie all'alba della civiltà occidentale, Il Mulino, Bologna, which cites the momumental J. E. Hebebstreit, 1751, Exegesis nominum graecorum quae morbos definiunt, Lankisch, Leipzig. On this theme see the text of a Babylonian tablet, "The people do not know the names of illnesses"; and the Bambara proverb "Illness is a thing that is searching for a buyer"—i.e., is seeking to be called by its name. (From the lectures of V. De Micco & M. A. Coccanari, respectively, *in* International Workshop on the History, Anthropology, and Epistemology of Medicine, Third Stage, Senigallia, Italy, November 27–28, 1993 (i.p.). On the "baptizing" of things refer to the quotation from Kuhn in Note 2.
24. All cured patients become followers and propagandists of a particular cure, of a particular doctor, of a particular hospital in the field of either official medicine or folk medicine. This phenomen is at the root of the modern health pilgrimage, of the so-called voyages of hope—an unavoidable element of the popular experience of illness. See Olivio Galeazzi, 1988, Ethnoiatrical operators in central Italy, Proc. 30 Intern. Congr. Hist. Medicine, Dusseldorf, 31-8/5-9/1986, Leverkusen, Vicom KG, pp. 701-713.
25. Olivio Galeazzi, 1991, Linguaggio folklorico e malattia in una popolazione ambulatoriale: Funzioni rituali e ascendenze culte, in Atti Conv. Psichiatria Magia Medicina popolare, Ferentino, November 14–16, 1991; Storia e Medicina Popolare **9**–2,3(1991): 98–109; Lido Valdré, 1988, Medicina scientifica e Linguaggio del senso comune, *in* Nuova Civiltà delle Macchine," VI-**24:** 50-55 (monograph edited by O. Galeazzi: Strategie del quarire).

26 "Prognosis is composed of pro- (before) and -gnosis (knowledge)—foreknowledge, foresight. In the Hippocratic language it has a slightly different meaning: it designates the totality of an illness, past, present, and future, because the prefix pro- assumes an extensive-intensive meaning. Knowledge of the future was expressed by the word prognostikon, as part of the prognosis . . . ." (Enrico Marcovecchio. 1993. Dizionario etimologico

storico dei termini medici. Festina Lende Ed. Impruneta, Italy.) See also Innocenzo Mazzini, 1989, Introduzione alla terminologia medica, Patron, Bologna.

27. On the illustrious topic of the use of intuition (rational clairvoyance) in medicine, see the following: Mauro Di Giandomenico, L'occhio clinico tra teoria e storia; Giovanni Federspil, L'occhio clinico: Occhio magico o occhio logico? Cesare Scandellari, L'occhio clinico: Occhio magico o occhio logico? Emanuele Riverso, Strategie dell'occhio clinico; Enrico Garulli, Occhio clinico: Arte o scienza? All are *in* Epistemologia, metodologia clinica e storia della scienza medica, various authors, pp. 129–172.
28. Storia della medicina, della farmacia, dell'odontoiatria e della veterinaria, various authors, Vol. 1, p. 335, Walk Over, Bergamo, 1982.
29. See Albert S. Lyons & Joseph R. Petrucelli II, 1992, La storia della medicina, Vol. 2, p. 218, Momento Medico, Salerno.
30. "It is not important what is said or how it is said, but to whom it is said. Before establishing what to say and before talking, it is important to foresee the psychological response of the patient to the news. Difficult!" Carelli, op. cit. See also Maurizio Imperiali, 1991, Negli ambulatori non si sa che dire, Tempo medico **15**(5): 11.
31. See 1990, La relazione medico-paziente: I seminario sulla comunicazione, various authors, Snamid, Milan; Constantino Iandolo, 1984, Parlare col malato: Tecnica, arte ed errori della comunicazione, Armano, Rome; Franca Laudi, 1978, Il dire implicato, Il polso, January 15, 1978; Majla Paci, 1985, La comunicazione della diagnosi, Medico e bambino **7:** 539–542.

Truth in the Relationship between Cancer Patient and Physician

JOHANN G. KLOCKER,[a,b] URSULA KLOCKER-KAISER,[c] AND MARKUS SCHWANINGER[d]

[a]*Oncological Institute,*
1st Medical Department and
[c]*Center for Mental Health*
General Hospital
A-9026 Klagenfurt, Austria

[d]*University of St. Gallen*
CH-9008 St. Gallen, Switzerland

HONESTY TOWARD CANCER PATIENTS: PAST AND PRESENT

Hardly a quarter of a century has elapsed since the time physicians were educated to tell compassionate and merciful lies to cancer patients. The words of Christoph Wilhelm Hufeland (1762-1836, a physician in Jena and Berlin) at the beginning of the 19th century, "to prophesy death is to cause it," have had lasting effect. It is remarkable that concealment of diagnosis and falsification of medical findings appeared suitable, especially in the case of cancer patients. Greater openness was practiced toward patients suffering from other illnesses with a comparable prognosis (myocardial infarct, cerebral insult, kidney and liver diseases). This must surely have something to do with the word "cancer," which has become a metaphor for agonizing pain, invalidity, and death.[1]

In an age when illness, invalidity, and death had been banned from the daily life of society and delegated to institutions, it was inevitable that diagnosis of such a disease must have caused anxiety and terror. In a culture that refused to face illness and death, it was understandable that a patient was told merciful lies in order to protect him/her and to avoid anything that might worsen the course of disease. The attending physicians were only too happy to evade any involved conversation with the cancer patient, the patient's room was shunned, and the absence of the patient from his room during the physician's rounds was quite welcome.[2]

[b]Corresponding author.

In the first instance, it was the relatives of the patient who were informed about the condition, and they were then left alone with the patient and the terrible truth.

With the growing emancipation of patients wanting to take their destiny in their own hands and with increasing success in the healing of cancer, discussions regarding honesty towards cancer patients have become more frequent.[3] At the same time, *suffering* and *death* have become acceptable words in polite society and are topics that it is permissible to discuss in the drawing room. Literature and films containing descriptions of suffering have become bestsellers. "In an emotionally drained form, the taboo surrounding dying and death has been lifted," says Wolfram Eberbach, a forensic lawyer.[4,5] Descriptions of death appear in all news media, and various discussions about euthanasia fill the evening programs on television.

It is not surprising that it has become the highest duty of a physician to provide true information to the patient; according to law, the patient must be informed of the truth, with the small proviso that the patient shall suffer no harm thereby. However, the duty to tell the truth on the one hand, and the injunction that the patient be unharmed by information on the other, puts the practicing oncologist in a difficult situation. Even though suffering and death have come to be accepted as normal components of the life cycle, contact and discussion with severely ill people, especially with cancer patients and their relatives, take place in a border region where all those concerned are not only emotionally deeply involved but are also forced to search for meaning in life.[6]

There is no doubt that the patient must be met with openness and honesty. "All men by nature desire to know" (Aristotle). The belief that it may be acceptable to tell lies in a difficult situation such as that of having to deal with severely ill people often arises from an overwhelming arrogance on the part of the physician who thinks too highly of himself/herself. In such a situation, it is not simply the spoken words that are important, but rather the confrontation between the whole being of the physician and the whole being of the patient; a lie creates a fundamental imbalance between the two and is therefore unsuitable as a means of communication with a severely ill person.[7]

The Greeks called truth *aletheia*. In Greek mythology Lethe is the river of forgetting. Aletheia then means to stand firm against the river of forgetfulness, it means not to forget, it means not to evade the truth, not to deny it. The continuous struggle for truth can be understood in the context of this concept of aletheia. The ever-flowing river of forgetfulness stands against the constant striving after truth. Perhaps this is the picture from which the concept of truth as a process originates.[8] Attention must be drawn to this aspect of truth, to its being a process in the interaction of the physician with the severely ill.

The question that needs to be answered is not whether truth has a place in communication with severely ill people, but rather how truth is to be placed in this context, how truth is relevant to the patient at the given moment. While it is not difficult for the physician to force the objective truth upon the patient, it is easy to forget that the patient needs to be rescued from his subjective distress. The existence of these two opposing poles of the "objective" truth of the physician and the subjective situation of the patient should be understood as a sort of warning. The physician talks of cytology and histology, but the patient wants to know about the role and value of illness; the physician means by objective truth the progress of the disease, but the patient is interested in the why of the disease, the exogenous and endogenous causes. The patient is seldom interested in the diagnosis; what interests him/her is the prognosis. Thus, the subjective condition of the patient may be more truthful than the objective findings.[9]

The discussion of four problematic polarities in the following should help highlight the difficulties of communication with patients and their relatives about the true nature of the illness. This should enable us to see better how truth as a means of healing can be introduced into a dialogue with the cancer patient.

FOUR PROBLEMATIC POLARITIES

Protection of the Patient versus Self-Protection of the Physician

Concealment of truth in order to protect the patient is a widespread approach to communication with cancer patients. To put it bluntly, this means that lies are conceived as a humanitarian act towards the patient. It is not always clear whether lies are intended to protect the patient or whether they serve rather to protect the physician. In the past few years there has been an increasing demand for openness toward patients and their relatives. This has put the physician under pressure to communicate truth as quickly and as comprehensively as possible, without taking into consideration whether the patient and his/her relatives have the emotional strength to bear it and whether the physician himself/herself is in a strong enough condition emotionally to communicate the truth at that given point of time. Under conditions when neither the patient and his/her relatives nor the physician is emotionally equipped to face the reality of illness, there should be no consulting session. It is necessary that the physician clarify for himself/herself the issue of whether open disclosure and discussion about the disease is at all possible at the given time, and how much of as well as which aspects of the truth can be brought into the conversation.[10] The physician must be able to assess his/her own emotional strength as well as that of the patient. This means that only a physician who is capable of reflecting upon existential questions regarding his/her own finiteness and that of others and who has come to terms with his/her own mortality can assume the task of exchanging frank information about the disease with the patient. A certain modesty on the part of the physician is necessary, as are also a recognition of the limits of his/her own strength and a readiness to accept these limitations. On the other hand, as physicians we also often experience the emotional limits of the patient, especially when existential issues are discussed. A physician must be sympathetic, sensitive, and understanding in order to be able to respect and accept the limits of the patient's capacity and willingness to face the truth; he/she must be ready to expose the patients and their relatives to the truth in stages—if necessary, in small doses. Thus, disclosure of truth to patients is a balancing act between a justified wish for openness on the part of the patient and concealment on the part of the physician for the protection of the patient. A physician who can accept his own feelings will be better able to understand the actual emotional situation of the patient.

Quality of Life of the Patient versus the Physician's Struggle for Success

As before, survival curves and rates of remissions remain the objective criteria of success in oncology on the basis of which a physician is judged. They also represent to a large extent the relevant criteria for scientific research.[9] The assessment of the quality of life of the patient is rather of secondary importance. The primary reason for this is the difficulty of scientifically capturing and measuring the quality of life,[11,12] because of which these tasks are delegated to other disciplines, such as psychology. We consider this withdrawal of the physician and clinical research from the area of quality of life of the patient as a questionable standpoint and suggest, rather, that precisely this has to be a main concern of the physician. This demands a highly differentiated sensitivity towards the patient. Questions such as, what does the patient mean by quality of life? and, how is his quality of life to be improved? require greater attention.

If the concept of quality of life of the patient is excluded from the physician's concern, then an important area of physician-patient relationship—namely, emotional contact, is prevented. In order to comprehend the quality of life of a patient, it is necessary for the physician to be highly sensitive to the patient's situation; this enables him/her to become aware of further dimensions of truth affecting the patient—namely, the emotional-social-familial dimensions. However, this demands a certain competence in interaction. There may, however, be occasions and situations when a physician does not have confidence in his/her own capacity for this kind of interaction. In such cases, he/she may require some support.

Even if no immediate "official" success follows concern with the quality of life of a patient, we still believe that it is useful to focus on this area in the interest of an open, honest relationship: what helps the patient must be carried out.

Therapeutic Abstinence versus the Physician's Involvement

Therapeutic abstinence as far as emotional involvement is concerned is still regarded as the ideal approach of the physician towards his/her professional activities: only thus can a physician help the patient in difficult situations; only thus is it possible for him/her to have a correct overview and to make a realistic assessment of the situation. This is true to some extent, since too great an emotional closeness to the patient may make the physician blind to negative findings, and may cause great anxiety, impairing his/her space of action. On the other hand, in dealing with severely ill patients faced with threatening existential questions, only an emotional involvement of the physician is credible. A competent technique of discussion with a patient cannot simply be learned; it demands from the physician a readiness to realize and bear with his/her own finiteness and mortality as well as with that of the patient. A physician who is armed with technical knowledge but has failed to confront existential anxiety in himself/herself is likely to be experienced by the patient and his/her relatives as being emotionally cold. The loneliness of a severely ill or dying person whose care is centered primarily on fighting the disease with every weapon made available by the whole machinery of medicine and hospital, but whose emotional and mental needs are ignored, is one of the most terrible situations a human being can experience.

Dominance of the Physician versus Partnership with an Emancipated Patient

In critical situations demanding quick decisions and the employment of radical therapeutic measures to save the life of a patient, dominant behavior on the part of the physician can be both useful and meaningful. But as soon as the crisis has been overcome, the same dominating behavior can become a disturbing element in the interaction between the physician and the patient, who may have to take responsibility for the therapy, be it about the way he/she wants to lead his/her further life or about his/her willingness to accept supporting measures and, in the final instance, about the whole quality of his/her life. In all of these points, the patient must be regarded as the physician's partner; the physician is dependent upon the patient's feedback even for his/her decisions concerning therapy and diagnosis. As far as the emotional aspects are concerned, in order to establish a therapeutic relationship with a patient, the communication between physician and patient must be open, honest, and on a partnership basis. Only thus can the patient feel himself/herself cared for and supported comprehensively within the therapy regimen.

TRUTH CAN BE A VIRTUOUS DRUG

Whatever the sociocultural and legal pressures on the physician to communicate truth to the patient might be, it must be recognized that truth is a very powerful drug in the context of contact with severely ill persons, and one must be careful how one goes about using it. On the one hand, the therapeutic value of truth is very limited; and on the other, its use must be learned just as the use of cytostatics must be learned. Before truth can be administered, there needs to be clarity on the following questions: to whom is it to be administered, by whom, and in what doses?

In principle, the question regarding who should be told the truth can be answered. The communication partner will always be the patient himself/herself, but he/she must be allowed to have the opportunity of drawing support from his/her relatives. From a system-theoretical point of view, an illness touches the system in its entirety, especially the family, but also the professional world. Communication can be most valuable when the patient can get his family members to participate in a consulting session. A discussion of the illness with the relatives in the presence of the patient presupposes a climate of trust and confidence not only among the members of the family of the patient, but also between the physician and the relatives. What must be avoided at all costs is private communication with the family, since this inevitably leads to isolation of the patient. When patients remain uninformed but the family is in possession of "the truth," the basis for communication within the family is totally lost. It must be pointed out that this is a highly problematic issue also from the legal point of view. A difficult situation arises when relatives do not wish the truth regarding the illness to be communicated to the patient. The family may he afraid that the patient would not be able to bear facing the truth. Unfortunately, there are no ready-made solutions to deal with such situations. Although it is certainly easy for the physician to fall back upon the legal duty to provide information, it is perhaps not the most human and reasonable way to deal with the situation. It has been found useful to meet the family under the supervision of a family therapist in order to gently convince the relatives of the meaningfulness of shared truth. Very often the desire of relatives not to inform the patient of his illness is an indication of a severe disturbance in intrafamilial communication.

Who should be the one to inform the patient and his/her relatives?

The immediate response to the question will usually be the attending physician. From what has been described above, the key role is played by the physician providing information. It is he/she who has the great responsibility to communicate the truth adequately. The primary prerequisite is that he/she be competent in his/her field. Over and beyond that, the human and emotional competence of the physician plays a decisive role.

On the basis of C. R. Rogers's work, we describe three attitudes on the part of the information-providing physician as a precondition for a productive, open talk with a severely ill person:[13]

1. A physician should have a sensitive, sympathetic, and precise understanding of the patient.
2. The physician should accept the patient completely.
3. There should be authenticity and congruity on the part of the therapist.

A sympathetic and sensitive physician with an attitude of complete understanding toward the patient is able to judge how much of the truth is to be communicated to the patient, and whether at a given time it is at all possible to communicate truth. This attitude should regulate the talk between the physician and the patient, in which questions of when and how much can be clarified.

The complete acceptance of the patient in all his fears, needs, and wishes is a further essential attitude. The patient must also have the right to deny the situation he/she currently finds himself/herself in. It may be the only correct or possible attitude for him/her at that point of time. It is highly relevant to keep in mind here the nature of truth as a process, and this should help answer the questions of how and when. It is the patient who determines in the first instance both the time and the amount of information he/she is to be given.

Authenticity and congruity of the therapist are behavioral patterns that determine the atmosphere in which communication with a severely ill person takes place. We have already pointed out that the communication of truth is directly dependent on the way the information-providing physician feels and thinks. It is imperative that the physician has himself/herself confronted the emotional and philosophical aspects of illness, invalidity, and death. Only a physician who can be emotionally moved, who questions, and who is humble can find his/her way to authenticity and congruity; the smooth, untouchable, all-knowing physician cannot. The physician who is open, congruent, and well-balanced within himself/herself has the ability to communicate truth to the patient and also the readiness to accept the responsibility that such communication involves. It has to be pointed out that when truth about the illness comes out into the open, a new dimension develops in the relationship between the patient and the physician. Truth is a link that strongly unites the two; they become allies, working together in the struggle to conquer the disease.

CONCLUSION

The question is not whether or not to communicate truth to a severely ill person. It is rather a question of the timing and the proper measure of truth to be communicated. This presupposes a high degree of sensitivity and readiness to reflect on the part of the physician. A few heuristic principles of how to deal with truth in the relationship between physician and the cancer patient are formulated below.

Assessment of the Patient's Ability to Understand

A patient can only be provided with truth that he/she is capable of understanding. In the process of providing information and explanation, the physician must be keenly aware of exactly how much truth should be communicated to the patient, avoiding too much and also too little. As Rolf Verres said, "Es kann auch inhuman sein einem Menschen das Wissen um seinen Tod gleichsam aufzuzwingen und ihn dadurch in ein Stadium von Hoffhungslosigkeit zu versetzen." ("It can also be inhuman to force upon a person knowledge of his death and thus place him in a situation of hopelessness.")[14]

Focus on Relevant Truth

Today, a widespread epistemological and ontological point of view is the concept of truth as being in principle relative. We find this questionable. At the same time we object to the views of those physicians who, in the belief that they are in possession of the objective truth, make prognoses to their patients about how much time they still have to live. Misled by a mechanistic worldview, they have the hubris to claim to know what human beings cannot know. A more productive concept appears to be that of relevant truth. The dialogue with the patient must be directed in such a way that those aspects are discussed that are relevant for his/her recovery and also for planning how to lead his/her life further. Relevant in this context is whatever helps patients find new strength and mobilizes their powers of self-healing. These aspects can be recognized only in an intensive encounter with the patient or with the patient and his/her family. Relevant truth is thus a dynamic concept.

Holistic Approach

Restricting therapy to physical aspects must remain reductionistic. Behind such an approach seems to be the maxim of curing for the sake of curing; in this process, the question of the meaning of life tends to get excluded. Truth demands that the physician be ready and willing to deal with the emotional, mental, and spiritual aspects of his/her patient. He/she must not desert the patient when it comes to the so-called ultimate questions.

Help the Patient Bear His/Her Suffering

The highest-ranking duty of a physician is to alleviate the suffering of the patient. Next in importance is his/her duty to help the patient bear suffering. No one has put it more clearly than Viktor E. Frankl: "Es gilt, das Leiden anzunehmen, das Schicksal zu bejahen, sich zu stellen. Auf diesem Weg allein kommen wir an die Wahrheit heran, kommen wir ihr nahe, auf diesem Weg allein, nicht auf den Wegen der Flucht und Furcht vor dem Leiden." ("The issue is to accept suffering, to approve of destiny, to be ready to face it. Only along this way can we approach truth, come close to it—along this way alone, and not along the way of escape and fear of suffering.")[15]

Suggestions Based on Practical Experience

From what has been said above, it is clear that high demands are placed on a physician dealing with oncological cases. In order to be able to meet these demands, we would like to present some suggestions:

- Work in the area of oncology presupposes availability of adequate staff and optimal space.
- Continuous further training and education are indispensable if physicians are to remain competent in their field.
- A stable basis for work in this area is provided by building an interdisciplinary team consisting of all those employed in the oncological field—namely, nurses, nursing aides, social workers, psychotherapists and physicians. Regular exchange of information in consulting sessions of the team, with and without psychotherapeutic supervision, makes it easier to master the demanding situations.
- A physician engaged in the oncological area should acquire psychotherapeutic abilities and under individual supervision reflect upon his/her work.

REFERENCES

1. SONTAG, S. 1987. Illness as Metaphor. Anchor and Doubleday. London.
2. SENN, H. J. 1992. Wahrhaftigkeit am Krankenbett bei Tumorpatienten. *In* Onkologie für Krankenpflegeberufe. A. Glaus, W. F. Jungl & H. J. Senn, Eds. Thieme. Stuttgart.
3. WANAGAT, L., Ed. 1991. Wandel der Krebskrankheit, Ethische Probleme. 3. Bad Mergentheimer Onkologisches Gespräch. Thieme. Stuttgart.
4. EBERBACH, W. H. 1984. Die Aufklärung des Patienten vor dem Hintergrund der Einstellung zum Tode. Medizinrecht **6**.
5. POTTHOF, P. 1980. Der Tod im medizinischen Denken. Thieme. Stuttgart.
6. KÖNIG, W. 1993. Umgang mit Extremsituationen. *In* Jahrbuch der Psychoonkologie. Springer Verlag. Vienna.
7. WATZLAWICK, P., J. H. BEAVIN & D. D. JACKSON. 1967. The Pragmatics of Human Communication. Norton. New York, NY.
8. BLOCH, E. 1995. Principle of Hope. Vol. 2. MIT Press. Cambridge, MA.
9. RICHTER, H. E. & M. W. WIRSCHING, Eds. 1991. Neues Denken in der Psychosomatik. Fischer. Frankfurt am Main.
10. BRÄUTIGAM, W. & F. MEHRWEIN, Eds. 1985. Das therapeutische Gespräch mit Krebskranken, Fortschritte der Psychoonkologie. Hans Huber. Bern.
11. AULBERT, E. & N. NIEDERLE, Eds. 1990. Die Lebensqualität des chronisch Kranken. Thieme. Stuttgart.
12. TÜCHLER, H. & T. LUTZ, Eds. 199 l. Lebensqualität und Krankheit—Auf dem Wege zu einem medizinischen Kriterium Lebensqualität. Deutscher Ärzteverlag. Cologne.
13. ROGERS, C. R. 1951. Client Centered Therapy. Houghton Mifflin. Boston.
14. VERRES, R. 1994. Die Kunst zu Leben. Krebsrisiko und Psyche. Piper. Munich.
15. FRANKL, V. E. 1975. Anthropologische Grundlagen der Psychotherapie. Huber. Bern.

Truth, Science, and the Oncologist

LARRY NORTON

Breast Cancer Medicine Service
Memorial Sloan-Kettering Cancer Center
1275 York Avenue
New York, New York 10021

I vividly recall two lessons about truth that I was taught as a medical student. The first was by an imposing professor who interrupted my attempt to explain a physical finding, which I began with the phrase "I think," with the reprimand: "A physician is expected to know, not 'think.'" His comment was provocative on many levels: The interruption, the arrogance, the incorrect assumption that I was using the phrase "I think" to mean "I guess" rather than "I reason." My reactions to this episode were tempered shortly thereafter when I was told, by another eminent professor, that as a judge is an advocate of justice and a philosopher an advocate of truth, so is a physician an advocate of health. I recall pondering the meanings of knowledge, justice, truth, and health,! and wondering about their linkage beyond the bond of simple virtue. Was not justice the victory of truth over duplicity? Was not knowledge truth? Was not health a result of justly applied knowledge?

What brought these lessons recently to mind was an event this past summer: I heard my mother admonish my nine-year-old daughter to dry her ears thoroughly upon emerging from a swimming pool. The history of this seemingly innocent remark, a staple of my own childhood, is as follows. In the mid-1920s, my mother's pubescent brother developed an otitis media that progressed to a fatal bacterial meningitis. The treating physician—let us call him Dr. Past—carefully explained that the etiology was the boy's failure to dry his ears thoroughly after swimming at school. This pronouncement effectively transferred the fault for the death away from the true villain, the lack of antibiotics, to the patient's misbehavior or his teachers' or parents' misguidance. Instantly, the tragedy of a young death was compounded by the imposition of parental guilt, propagated to an entire extended family. The result was not only much profound, acute sorrow but even unfounded apprehension and compulsive behavior more than seventy years later.

What was Dr. Past's motivation? We must discount the possibility of an intentional misrepresentation as being unconscionably iniquitous. The greater likelihood is that Dr. Past sincerely believed in the connection between wet ears and otitis media. Perhaps he intended his instruction as constructive, aimed to thwart future transgressions! The critical point, however, is not an understanding of his motivation, but rather the recognition that Dr. Past never expressed, and probably never regarded, his own ignorance as central to the unfolding of events. How could he, after all, foresee medical advances that would soon focus on the cure of bacterial infections rather than the avoidance of a dubious etiology?

We assume, therefore, that Dr. Past thought he was speaking the truth: he was stating a fact that he believed was true. Many physicians and laypersons of his time and generation would probably have agreed with him, so that by the criterion of conceptual validation, what he said was true. Yet even if he did not plan his statement as self-exculpation, it had been useful for this purpose. So who was served? Not the health of the dead patient, nor justice for the bereaved family, nor knowledge, for discovery starts with an acknowledgment of ignorance. Only the physician's narcissism benefited, at a huge cost in the pain of others. Is this the value of truth in medicine?

Before we wrestle with this central question, let us reexamine Dr. Past's statement. As modern oncologists we are not unfamiliar with the temptation to transfer blame. Does a man die of lung cancer because he smoked tobacco? Partially, yes, but also because of our inability to eradicate his cancer cells with any available therapy. Our patients "know" this, because of their sometimes unrealistic expectations of our resources; but we do, too, because we now expect future medical advances to empower us as they have formerly. This is an important distinction between an enlightened modern view and that of Dr. Past: we can no longer seek exoneration in ignorance, because we are conditioned to believe in the transience of ignorance. Or at least we should be. When I was an undergraduate student, all children with leukemia died By the time I was a medical student, most of these children were being cured, but all patients with Hodgkin's disease were still dying. When I started my oncology fellowship, most patients with Hodgkin's disease were being cured, but all men with testicular carcinoma continued to die, and now most of these are being cured as well. Before each of these advances there were many who said that it could not happen, and all the pessimistic voices were wrong. So it is rational to be optimistic about the future. Yet to the patient suffering now, and to ourselves presiding over what will someday be preventable pain and loss, our long-range optimism is bitterly ironic.

There is another difference between Dr. Past's worldview and our own, one that concerns an issue of even more direct relevance to truth in medicine than the issue of culpability. The issue is the source of knowledge. Dr. Past used his knowledge—wet ears cause otitis media, which in turn can lead to lethal complications—as a barrier between himself and his responsibility. However, what was the origin of his knowledge? Was it based on observation? On intuition? On inference from previously established facts? On rigorous, controlled experiments? On guessing? On folklore? In fact, Dr. Past's beliefs were not founded on solid experimental science. How much pain could have been avoided had my mother's family asked Dr. Past how he knew that wet ears cause fatal meningitis, and had they been able to correctly interpret the validity of his allegation!

The modern dictum is that opinion without knowledge is suspect, if not outrightly absurd. Knowledge itself—tempered by experience, certainly, and explicated by deduction—is now largely derived from formal scientific inquiry. Oncologists in particular now insist on randomized, prospective clinical trials whenever possible. In some cases, prospective trials are not possible. Here, knowledge can be based on observation, followed by hypothesis generation, then confirmatory observation, in multiple iterations until a stable system of beliefs is achieved. I was once told (and I suppose that this qualifies as a third lesson about truth) that a true scientist should respond to the question "Do you believe in spirits?" with the answer "I have no evidence in favor nor against, so I have no opinion on this subject!" The question of the existence of spirits is clearly not one that is subject to prospective, randomized trials. However, when a topic is amenable to properly designed prospective studies, such experiments are by far the most reliable method of accumulating knowledge. I assert that it is unethical not to perform randomized, prospective trials when they are needed, lest we promulgate the destructive ignorance epitomized in Dr. Past's remark.

I will defend this latter view using an example from my own field of inquiry, the management of breast cancer. For most of this century the standard treatment for invasive cancers was surgical, the radical mastectomy. This practice was based on a theory of the biology of metastases: cells from the tumor in the breast could reach the systemic circulation only by invading lymphatic channels and then by breaking through the filter of the axillary lymph nodes. This theory was based on observations Patients with axillary metastases developed distant metastases at a much higher rate than those with clean axillary nodes. Motivated by this theory, surgeons became adept at the en bloc resection of the cancer along with the whole breast, the muscles of the chest wall, the axillary contents, and sometimes even more local tissue. The results of this radical, very mutilating procedure were truly momentous, with perhaps a third of patients being cured; all of these patients would otherwise have gone on to extensive local invasion and life-threatening systemic metastases.

The development of the radical mastectomy can be considered a prototype of the nonexperirnental approach to acquiring knowledge: observation led to a theory that led to a manipulation producing results consistent with the theory. So compelling was the knowledge so gained that the radical mastectomy became fixed in the armamentarium of oncology—so fixed, indeed, that it has taken us almost a century to successfully challenge the theory and practice. Prospective randomized trials have conclusively demonstrated that modified radical mastectomy, sparing the muscles of the chest wall, and now breast-conserving surgery plus radiation therapy to the remaining breast tissue, are equivalent to radical mastectomy in terms of survival. Even more counter to the prevailing wisdom is the observation, again from a randomized trial, that inadequate local control—as by intentionally not irradiating residual breast tissue postlumpectomy—does not dramatically impair survival in spite of a very high rate of recurrence in the ipsilateral breast. The notion evidently supported by these observations, a notion popularized by the work of Bernard Fisher, is that, in most cases, if metastatogenic cancer cells would ever colonize distant sites, they would have already done so by the time of initial presentation. Hence, many practitioners have concluded, local control is not a prerequisite to systemic control. To really increase the rate of cure—that is, decrease the rate of systemic recurrence—we would have to kill cells already metastatic at the time of initial presentation. This cannot be accomplished with local treatments like surgery or radiation therapy. This task would depend on the action of such systemic therapies as chemotherapy and hormonal therapy. Indeed, adjuvant systemic therapy—such as drug therapy or surgical oophorectomy—do decrease the risks of systemic and local recurrence, and improve the odds of survival in nearly all categories of primary disease. This has been shown by dozens of randomized trials, and has been confirmed by overview analyses conducted over two decades.

Although we must acknowledge that recent information is now qualifying Fisher's view, its fundamental tenets remain intact. Postmastectomy radiation therapy does decrease, very slightly, the systemic recurrence rate as well as the local recurrence rate. Whether or not to use this information in the clinic would depend on the relative balance of cost and benefit in the individual case, for radiation therapy does have some negative effects and does increase the monetary cost of care. Nevertheless, the biological implication, which is pivotal, is that local cancer cells residual after mastectomy can be a further source of metastatic cells after the time of initial presentation. In addition to its theoretical significance, this concept may turn out to be important regarding clinical practice. Nevertheless, we must recognize that quantitatively most of the metastases will still have occurred prior to mastectomy. Hence, Fisher's fundamental concept remains valid, and we owe this concept entirely to the victory of randomized, prospective trials that challenged the ideas prevalent in the day the trials were initiated.

Most oncologists now believe in the value of breast-conserving treatment and adjuvant drug therapy, and most of us believe that our beliefs are based on solid knowledge. We believe this because our knowledge originates from prospective, randomized clinical trials, which we assume are a pathway to truth. Furthermore, we believe that this latter assumption is well founded, because the knowledge gained from prospective trials has proved durable, verifiable, and useful. Certainly, a true statement does not have to be based on scientific evidence, for even random thoughts are sometimes valid by chance alone. However, experience has shown that the conduct of science does increase the likelihood of a belief deriving from the conduct's being true.

I dwell on this ostensibly unnecessary defense of science because we are living in an age of great paradox in the public perception of the relevance of science to daily life. The same people who will depend on technology to convey them in modern automobiles on modern roads, or inform their lives by television or Internet, will turn to unproved, untested, inexplicable remedies for serious illness. The same people who will check safety records carefully before boarding an airplane will ingest unspecified, unpurified plant products to regain or assure health. Dr. Past's ignorance is multiplied by orders of magnitude in every "health food" store in the nation, every business day. There are thousands of practitioners who feed on such senseless behavior, leading to untold suffering because of the denial of effective treatments, and countless economic loss as well. Is there fault in this? Certainly, unscrupulous practitioners and merchants bear a significant burden. The hapless victim who refuses to be educated bears some as well. But modern physicians and scientists are not blameless, because by failing in our educational duty we set the stage on which these travesties are played out.

We have, therefore, found three problems with Dr. Past's remark. The first is that his knowledge was incomplete: even if wet ears do cause meningitis, medical ignorance regarding effective treatment was at least partially to blame in my uncle's death. The second is that his knowledge was faulty. The third is that he failed to understand why his knowledge was incomplete and faulty, and thereby spread falsehood by speaking the truth as he saw it. In fact, his truth was incomplete. Contrast his statement with others he might have used: "I believe that your son's going out into the cold with wet ears contributed to the development of his ear infection, but I have no proof of this"; "I have seen other people with severe ear infections who did not give a history of wet ears"; "I'm sorry that we do not yet have drugs to treat infections like your son has."

If we define truth as the honest transmission of knowledge, I contend that truth is not enough to do justice to the health of our patients. We need a broader definition of truth, one that includes our uncertainties, our human qualities. Part of this uncertainty is intrinsic to the philosophy of science: the concept of knowledge as unchanging fact obscures the process of acquiring knowledge by inquiry, judgment, and reasoning. In this regard I contend—in contrast to my neurosurgical professor—that it is more important for the physician to think than to know. We are not authorities because of what we know, we are authorities because of what we can learn.

Recently, I was interviewed by an infamous television reporter who charged that my colleagues and I were preventing effective anticancer therapies from being developed by refusing to accept the claims of various practitioners of "alternative" medicine. My argument—that we test hundreds of new compounds and new approaches per year, finding most not useful but some highly promising, such as paclitaxel, a derivative of tree bark—fell on deaf ears. He could perceive only that we defended one set of treatments, while the alternative doctors defended another: authority vs. authority. Why could this journalist not see that the practitioners of untested approaches were the closed-minded ones, not providing data for objective, independent scrutiny or subjecting their hypotheses to the bright light of the scientific method?

In the world of conventional medicine, we often make the same error, although cloaked in more subtle garb. The reason I avoid writing editorials in journals is that once you express an opinion on a controversial topic, you are expected to defend that opinion forever. To change one's view would be considered "waffling." Nothing could be more destructive to scientific progress than to deny change. The bedrock of our professional lives is not truth as hard fact, but the intellectual progression toward information that is ever more useful.

Practical value, after all, is the heart of the matter. The physician is not just the advocate of health; the physician is the advocate of the patient, health being an important part of the package. We exist as professionals to serve that advocacy. What we do, and what we say, should make a positive impact on our patients' lives.

Dr. Past spoke truth, and did harm. We must be different: we must accept our responsibilities to heal and to comfort. When we do not heal because medical knowledge is lacking, we cannot deny our accountability. Not to try to comfort is an unforgivable transgression. But an equally great failure is not to take part in improving the state of affairs, not to be involved in the process by which real advances are accomplished.

We also fail when we are arrogant. One of the tools we use to help people is knowledge of biology. But knowledge, even if it is based on science, is not automatically truth any more than the ruling of a judge, even if it is based on jurisprudence, is always justice. In honest circumstances, however, both knowledge and judgment are approximations to those ideals. We must teach that the scientific method is our best way of achieving reliable knowledge, but it is not infallible, its findings are not immutable, and its applications are not incontrovertible. To do less is to invite the authoritarianism that defeats our best intentions.

We must also accept our human limitations, even use them to advantage. Although we are experts in medicine, only our patients are experts in the structure of their lives. We physicians can access research data, can interpret technical information, can exercise our personal diagnostic and therapeutic experience, can apply our formally taught and informally learned interpersonal skills. But only the patient can tell us what they need, and can constructively implement what we can provide. Truth, justice, health, and humanity: perhaps, in the final analysis, the bond of simple virtue is the one bond that unites us all.

Truth-telling, Risk, and Hope

ANTONELLA SURBONE

Department of Medicine
Memorial Sloan-Kettering Cancer Center
1275 York Avenue
New York, New York 10021

Reason transforms the tears of time into the smile of grace. Grace, by freeing hope and responsibility, without words calls us to the responsibility towards our hope.[1]

If truth-telling is difficult in the face of the established reality of a disease, it becomes a real quandary when dealing with risk. Yet, in medicine we often face risks more than certainties, and to present them to and discuss them with our patients pose tremendous problems. In many cultures and societies, risks are seldom discussed. In the name of beneficence, doctors most often evaluate risks without involving the patient, and then act according to what appears to be in the patient's best interest, for the patient's good.

In most Western countries, however, the patient as an autonomous agent, responsible for decisions regarding his or her health, is entitled to full disclosure of the risks involved in any medical or surgical procedure, as well as in any therapeutic measure. Moreover, both patients and healthy individuals should be able to gather information on the risks involved in certain lifestyles (the subject of preventive medicine). Finally, it seems that now all persons should be entitled to inquire about their genetic risks.

Far from aiming at a philosophical discussion of risk and hope, I shall offer some elements of consideration that are drawn from my practice and thus quite limited to a Western reality. I am well aware that genetic predisposition, for instance, exists for all human kind, but not all have the luxury of living in a society in which genetic research is available and feasible. What constitutes risk and hope might be quite different in different contexts.

TRUTH-TELLING AND RISK

The intricacy of the issue of truth-telling with regard to risk increases as we go from the first aspect mentioned, risks associated with therapies, to the others, risk associated with lifestyle and genetic risk. Inherent in the discussion of risk is the uncertainty both in the prediction of events and in the impact that such prediction might have on different people. The information provided, as well as its relevance and meaning, can easily be manipulated—not necessarily intentionally, but as a consequence of the imbalance of power created by the different degrees of knowledge between the two interlocutors. Often information does not immediately translate into wisdom for the patient, and providing information can remain a unilateral imposition onto the patient. Unless it is done in a context that allows for a true exchange between doctor and patient, giving information can reproduce all the characteristics of a more or less paternalistic form of dominance.[2] This is particularly evident when discussing risk.

Emphasizing or deemphasizing a piece of information while providing it is almost inevitable. Also, much of what is retained by the patient depends on factors other than the information per se: the patient, exposed to overwhelming, often traumatic information, generally relies on the tone of voice, gestures, and expression of the physician and on those words that accompany the raw information. Consider the different effects of telling a woman with node-negative breast cancer that she has a 25% risk of recurrence in 10 years versus telling her that 1 woman in 4 in her situation will have a recurrence of breast cancer in 10 years; the latter is a less abstract, much more graphic way of representing the risk, and can have quite a different impact on the patient.

RISKS ASSOCIATED WITH THERAPIES

Medicine almost invariably entails an estimate of the so-called risk/benefit ratio, and, indeed, one of the reasons for seeking medical advice is to consult an expert who will help us deciding when a therapeutic measure is necessary and worthwhile. The time when a woman would enter the operating room for a breast biopsy and wake up to find herself with a mastectomy scar (it happened in my family in Italy not very long ago) should be over. Whether or not modified radical mastectomy was the appropriate surgical choice is not the issue; the patient has to participate in such a choice.

Not all cases are so clearcut, though; and even in countries, such as the United States, where the emphasis is on patients' right to self-determination (autonomy), there is still a lack of uniformity of opinions and practices with respect to informing patients about risk.

In cancer research, for instance, written informed consents provide an exhaustive list of all possible risks, including immediate and delayed side-effects, mortality rates, long-term sequelae, and possible unexpected outcomes. However, detailed informed consents are not generally used for "standard therapies," where the extent of risk discussion is left to the discretion of the treating physician. Also, written information guarantees the legal aspects of the duty to inform, more than it does the real comprehension of the information provided.[3]

Many cancer therapies have a very low probability of success. This is the case of phase I and phase I-II trials and of many of our recommended therapies for patients with advanced cancer. When we administer third- or fourth-line chemotherapy to a patient with a solid tumor, we know that the expected benefit is quite marginal. The risk here is of no therapeutic benefit. How do we present such risk to patients? Can or should the patient entering a phase I trial knowing that all standard therapies have already failed be deprived of the hope of success, no matter how unrealistic? Almost all oncologists would agree that it should be explained to the patient in a phase I trial that the purpose of the trial is to explore the pharmacology and toxicology of a new compound. And patients almost everywhere in the world actually sign informed consents where those words clearly appear. However, it seems that rarely does a patient enter a trial for altruistic reasons only; most patients hope to benefit personally from the therapy.

At first glance the issue seems to be whether we should take away hope from our patients and not let them believe that a particular drug might, indeed, help them personally. And, more important, what right would anyone have to do so? After all, pharmacokinetics is not likely to change under the effect of some hope or to be influenced by a placebo effect. What justification would we have, then, for denying our patients the right to hope? For hope is a right to be acknowledged and respected as much as other rights. Furthemore, we, as doctors, also live with hope, for ourselves and our patients. In our specialty in particular, much of what we do belongs to the sphere of hope, and it is remarkable how little we know about such an essential ingredient.

However, more important than the question of whether we should or should not take away hope is that we acknowledge that we all have a responsibility towards hope. As doctors, we have a responsibility not to deceive our patients. The patient should not be given false hope of a cure; the doctor should encourage the patient to positively and realistically assess and reassess his or her situation. The doctor has the responsibility to help the patient in the advanced stages of disease see that the goals of therapy have changed and that there is still room for hope, although the object of hope is no longer cure.

Hope plays a delicate and essential role in discussing risk. Any evaluation of risk implies precise knowledge of the present situation, an accurate estimate of the future outcomes, and finally an evaluation (prediction). Any choice based on estimate of risk inevitably ignores some of the other variables in life, while it might, indeed, happen that these ignored variables determine the final outcome. Therefore, in making a decision based on risk, factors other than rational calculation come into play—among these, fear and hope. That similar risks can assume quite different proportions and meanings for different individuals, depending on their hopes, is a matter of simple observation. Patients come to disease with their own personal histories and cultural backgrounds, and they go through disease in absolutely unique ways. The fears of cancer patients are clearly related to their individual pasts and presents as well as to the realities of their disease.[4] Here are examples from one day in a clinic attended only by women with breast cancer.

> A. has an aggressive tumor. She is very young but has a history of severe infections, and avoiding neutropenia is essential. I tell her proudly that the use of cytokines nowadays allows us to prevent neutropenia, but she immediately asks about the possible stimulatory effect of cytokines on the bone marrow. A very bright and well-informed woman, she wonders about possible future development of hematologic malignancies due to hyperstimulation of the bone marrow. Although I tell her that the issue has been addressed and that no data support such a fear, she agonizes over her decision. A. has been sick before, and she is now. The remote risk of again having to face a major unknown disease is more important to her than the actual risk of leaving her breast cancer untreated now.
>
> B. appears totally overwhelmed by her "altered body image." She is a beautiful 36-year-old woman with node-positive breast cancer, treated with conservative surgery and radiation therapy. Her scar is barely noticeable, and cosmesis by physicians' standards is optimal. Yet the scar is a metaphor, and it appears to mean so much to B. that she believes "no man will ever touch her again." B. wishes to have children, and her fears are far from being simply cosmetic. She tells me that "if she can no longer have children, why should she bother living." The risk for her is not recurrence, but sterility.
>
> C. has gone through bone marrow transplantation for metastatic breast cancer and is now in remission. She tells me that she has to accept that she is a "terminal patient." I believe she has a misconception of her prognosis and is overestimating her immediate risk. But then I learn that she has invested all her hopes in being able to take care of a severely handicapped child throughout his life, without ever institutionalizing him. It is the risk to her son that is haunting her, not her personal risk: by "terminal" she means "it will be the end for my son, too."

What is unique about cancer, mostly because of its metaphorical implications, is that, once diagnosed, a person knows that her life span is limited. The knowledge that the time remaining to you is to be counted in months or years is a devastating one, profoundly different from the awareness that we all have—and should have—of being mortal. This, in turn, has a profound effect on hope, and on how patients perceive their risks and then act upon them. Any discussion about future risks, whether of complications of treatment, recurrence, or death, should take into account the particular vulnerability of the patient: she is overwhelmed by the reality of the present disease, and finds herself asked to make a decision based on the evaluation of future risks. It is easy to see how difficult this might be for any patient, and how easily the patient can be manipulated at this stage. A choice based on risks implies a frame of mind that the patient rarely has; to calculate and weigh the pros and cons of a choice is far more difficult in a time of crisis. Yet, it is just at this time that the patient's autonomy is most in need of protection, rather than being bypassed in a paternalistic effort. It is at this point that we should accompany our patients, sharing with them what we know about their future risks, without imposing our values on them. While this certainly takes more time than simply acting in the patient's best interest, it is the only way to fully respect the patient's dignity.

However, this can be a quandary at times, for we also have, as human beings and as doctors, our own perception of risk, as well as our own standards of what level of risk we deem acceptable for us and for our patients.

> One of our patients, a 43-year-old woman, was admitted for rapidly progressing metastatic breast cancer, with brain involvement. The patient came to us for observation and was not previously known by us. She could barely communicate with us. It was unclear whether she understood her situation and could make decisions for herself. After she had progressed through chemotherapy and radiation therapy, we had several long discussions among us and with her relatives. As a result, the patient was transferred to a hospice facility for palliative care. I have no doubt that this was the best medical decision, since continuing with active treatment would have had no chance of success, but, on the contrary, could have negatively affected her already-poor quality of life. The risk of toxicity was far greater than the expected benefit. Moreover, the decision was thoroughly and repeatedly discussed also with her family, and was finally made after several days of pondering the alternatives. Yet I felt uncomfortable and extremely sad when the patient left for the hospice. In discussing my feelings afterwards, I learned that I was not alone: every member of the staff had felt uncomfortable. We tried to understand why, since we all had agreed on this being best for the patient: it was because we could never hear a yes from her, nor could we ever know whether she agreed within herself, what she wished to do, how she wanted to live her last few weeks, what she hoped for.
>
> A year ago, on the contrary, a patient requested to be treated on a high-dose regimen after her doctors, including myself, had estimated that the risk of toxicity would have been too great in her case. Unlike the previous patient, she clearly expressed her wishes, but there was genuine disagreement among us. The patient was eventually successfully treated, but a long process of education was necessary before we could safely give her the therapy. While I am happy to see the patient in remission, I cannot

help thinking that the risk was exceedingly high for her. I would not have given her that treatment if she had been my primary patient.

The balance between the autonomy of the patient and beneficence is a very delicate one; rarely is it so delicate as in the estimate of risks.

RISKS ASSOCIATED WITH LIFESTYLES

Preventive medicine aims at eliminating or reducing those risk factors that play a role in the development of diseases, such as cancer. This effort often involves active control of the environment as a major social and political enterprise. Prevention also often involves more specific intervention, aimed at controlling or modifying certain lifestyles or behaviors that increase risk;[5] such interventions raise special ethical concerns.

The risk of developing cancer later on in life is not necessarily perceived by everyone with equal concern, and it is legitimate to wonder to what extreme public intervention should go in the attempt to change certain risk-incurring lifestyles. The perception of risk, here, is strictly intertwined with the right of individuals to self-determination. Whether autonomy can or should be allowed to take precedence over all other ethical principles is, in itself, a matter of debate. In preventive medicine, the issue is, in essence, whether the knowledge that smoking, for instance, is detrimental to a person's health is sufficient to limit this person's freedom out of beneficence. Even the most thorough understanding of risk does not necessarily translate into the choice of actively preventing it: how many oncologists continue to smoke and would not accept limitation of their freedom? Moreover, there is another factor to consider—the good of society as a whole. Preventive medicine is not only concerned with the good of individuals; its main concern is the good of society, the public health. Beneficence towards the patient and society has to be balanced against the autonomy of the individual. Justice becomes a leading principle, and the role of truth-telling assumes different connotations and proportions. We can learn from preventive medicine some important lessons about truth-telling and risk, as well as about the interplay of autonomy and beneficence when the good of society is the main consideration.

GENETIC RISK

The enormous, rapid progress in human genetics is charged with profound ethical implications. The major issues are informed consent; privacy and confidentiality; the right to be tested or not to be tested; the right of access, or nonaccess, to genetic information; possible discrimination in health insurance, at the workplace, or in the process of adoption; consequences of the use of genetic information in prenatal diagnosis; and, finally, its possible use for the purpose of eugenics.[6] One equally important, yet more subtle, ethical implication of human genetics is the concept of genetic risk itself. What exactly is genetic risk? How does it differ, if at all, from other risks? Is there any particular caution we should have with respect to genetic risk?

Genetic risk appears (but only appears) to be different from other risks. There is something about the power and the mystery of genes that makes us perceive genetic risk as something more real, more true, more fundamental, and more immediate than other risks. So genetic risk may, indeed, influence our decisions more than any other risk.

> While I was obtaining informed consent from a young breast cancer patient who participated in a genetic testing program, she told me that if she had known in advance that she would develop breast cancer, she would never have divorced her husband—a decision that was, she said, one of the best of her life.

Somehow I could easily relate to such a remark and imagine myself making different decisions about my life if I were told that I would soon develop breast cancer. Soon afterwards, though, I started thinking about her and my reactions. We were both thinking of genetic risk as a "worse risk." Yet there are many risks in our lives that are not inscribed in our genome, but no less real or scary; and we face them all the time. Hence, what is "wrong" with genes? Why is genetic risk immediately perceived as an irrevocable sentence? First, genetics is still a new field, and discoveries in this field are not easily apprehended, even by members of the medical profession. There is tremendous confusion about the terminology, and we are far from doing everything possible at present to make our genetic jargon clear. Also, as a consequence of poor understanding, genetic predisposition is becoming a new metaphor for death, after TB, cancer, and AIDS.

Indeed, there are many ways of dying; being paralyzed by risk could be one of them. Yet, the medical community may be overconcerned about the possible negative consequences of genetic information. Maybe the perception of genetic risk in the lay public is more accurate than we expect. For instance, reacting to a paternalistic article in the press suggesting that women might not be ready to deal with BRCA1, a young patient of mine stated that the medical community is underestimating the intelligence of women and that "women are not likely to jump onto an operating table" because of a gene mutation.

Certainly the perception of genetic risk is greatly influenced by our culture and society. Now that we are faced with knowing our genome, it is up to us as a society to properly understand genetic diversity and to prevent it from changing our belief in human equality.[7] At the same time, it behooves us as a society and as individuals to accept genetic risk as another kind of information, to be dealt with on an individual basis, without unduly expanding its meaning.

Although diseases always result from the interaction of genetic and environmental factors, genetic predisposition is seen by some as a major limitation of our freedom, an expression of determinism. For others, awareness of genetic risk can foster a more active effort at prevention, an expression of increased control over life. Certainly, the very delicate subjective balance between risk and hope is deeply challenged by genetics.

CONCLUDING REMARKS

"Hoping against all hope," reads the Bible; and many of our patients do this. Hope is a response to the risks of life, a legitimate positive response. Hope is difficult to define, although we all can grasp its meaning. Hope is an attitude towards life—and for many towards death, too—and it does not need to have "cure" as its object. Whether we are patients or not, we have hopes, and our hopes are different. Based on our hopes, we then take and face risks.

"Those who do not hope in the unexpected will never find it," wrote Heraclitus. At times, we can hope for something totally unexpected. At times, we feel there is nothing left to hope for. At all times, we have to approach hope with a deep sense of responsibility.

REFERENCES

1. MASULLO, A. 1995. Il Tempo e la Grazia. Donzelli Ed. Rome.
2. PRESIDENZA DEL CONSIGLIO DEI MINISTRI DIPARTIMENTO PER L'INFORMAZAIONE E L'EDITORIA. 1992 Societa ed Istituzioni. Informazione e consenso all' atto medico. Comitatio Nazionale per la Bioetica. Rome
3. AARONSON, N. K, E. VISSER-POL, G. H. M. W. LEENHOUTS *ET AL.* 1996. Telephone-based nursing intervention improves the effectiveness of the informed consent process in cancer clinical trials. J. Clin Oncol. **14:** 984–996.
4. SURBONE, A. 1995. The patient-doctor-family relationship: At the core of medical ethics. *In* Cancer and the Family. L. Baider, C. L. Copper & A. Kaplan De-Nour, Eds. John Wiley & Sons. West Sussex.
5. VINGERHOETS, A. J. J. M. & F. H. G. MARCELLISSEN. 1988. Stress research: Its present status and issues for future developments. Soc. Sci. Med. **26:** 279–291.
6. SURBONE, A. 1995. The ethical issues in genetic testing. Memorial Sloan-Kettering Cancer Center and the European School of Oncology. Breast Cancer. Postgraduate Course. June 1995.
7. REILLY, P. 1992. ASHG statement on genetics and privacy: Testimony to United States Congress. Am. J. Hum. Genet. **50:** 640–642.

On the Spirituality of the Doctor-Patient Relationship

BOŽIDAR VOLJČ

Ministry of Health
Republic of Slovenia
Štefanova 5
61000 Ljubljana, Slovenia

Throughout human history, disease has had an influential role in developments of the human mind, fostering biological and cultural changes in the individual and in human society as a whole. On the personal level, a serious disease, with its effects on the patient and his close family circle, may reveal the profound riches of the human mind.

From a personal viewpoint, disease and health are as hard to define as happiness and human life. Each individual experiences them differently, in accordance with his inner self. Disease and health are interrelated; they cannot be considered as two extreme values on a health measuring scale. Some people, though terminally ill, may in certain circumstances feel well and happy. In an individual's life experience there is no clear-cut line between health and disease. In everyday life, people rarely speak of their health or disease; rather, they discuss their physical condition, which is either good or bad. Hence, health and disease are estimated concurrently.

BUILDING THE RELATIONSHIP BETWEEN PATIENT AND DOCTOR

Treatment of chronic disease has always been associated with frequent contact between patient and doctor. The relationship between the two is therefore different from the short-term relationship that is established between a doctor and a patient with a minor health problem. A general practitioner who cares for a patient and follows his health problems is sooner or later aware of the fact that the quality of health care depends to a great extent on their building a long-term, partnership-like, bidirectional relationship based on mutual understanding and equality.

The patient's relationship with his doctor follows the same principles that apply in everyday communication. We know that relationships among people in general can be bad or good. From their experience, doctors can tell that patients are not all alike: with some it is easy to become close and immediately win their confidence; with others it takes years and a lot of effort; with certain patients it is impossible to establish an intimate relationship.

During a conversation between two persons, and in particular between a patient and his doctor, their inner thoughts are revealed and exchanged; this process is a clue to their further mutual understanding. Every human being, having his own thoughts and personal experiences, creates his own microcosm, through which he is able to communicate with the outer world even without using words. Every human creature is unique, and so is his inner microcosm. A discussion on a given topic between two individuals never develops in the same way as it would between two other individuals, even though they all would be speaking on the same subject. A patient explains his health problems differently to different doctors. A doctor who has the capacity to penetrate into a patient's innermost microcosm through his own will do a lot for the patient and will also get a lot from him. A doctor's work is far from only giving; it is also receiving—an invaluable privilege of this profession; because of the uniqueness of individual patients, a doctor never stops benefiting from his relationships with them

HARVESTING THE FRUITS OF THE RELATIONSHIP

When a patient learns that he is incurably ill and that his days are numbered, he assigns entirely new values to time and life. A day counts more, and life is more intense. He is ready to listen to his doctor and is grateful to him for the understanding, appreciation, and respect that the doctor is conveying to him through nonverbal communication. A terminal disease therefore facilitates the approach to a patient's mind. The richness of a patient's mind does not depend upon his physical condition, but, rather, vice versa. The family, friends, and medical team who care for the patient during the difficult period of his illness are often taken by surprise at recognizing how rich a seriously ill patient's soul can be; he may be a precious gift to any community. As long as the disease does not affect consciousness, the human mind will grow and develop.

Terminal disease is most often associated with death. However, human beings experience the imminence of dying in various ways. Many of those who are already lying at the death's door are not quite prepared to enter it. The idea of the inevitability of death impels them to discomfort and fear. No matter how the patient confronts his dying—with anger, resignation, or despair—he poses himself questions about his departure, sense of life, responsibility, and consciousness. More subtle patients wonder what will happen to their soul when death transfers it to another place and time, where questions and answers arise no more. While searching deep inside himself in an attempt to answer these questions, a terminally ill patient recognizes the immensity of his mind, from which he is able to draw the willpower to prepare himself for the inevitable departure, fully reconciled with himself, instead of awaiting it in restlessness and fear.

When active treatment is no longer indicated and doctors and nurses stop using military terms in talking about the disease, the language of the mind comes to the fore. These are not technical terms, used for specifying medical examinations, tests, and equipment, but the language of those who are capable of listening, understanding, and generous consideration.

The common feature of all chronic diseases is their incurability. A treatment that leads to physical remission of the disease may be insufficient for a successful recovery. When it comes to terminal disease, the most a doctor can do for the patient is help him become reconciled with the disease and stimulate him to follow the experts' advice. The patient will thus be better able to cope with the disease and will live a more dynamic life. The doctor should strive toward mutual understanding between his own and his patient's mind, so that throughout the rest of his life the barriers and distresses of the disease may be alleviated. By doing this, the doctor is also further improving his own human qualities, and he may then come to regard his profession as a holy assignment—one that also helps him overcome his personal difficulties.

Communicatin with the Patient in Clinical Research

MATJAŽ ZWITTER

Institute of Oncology
1105 Ljubljana, Slovenia

INTRODUCTION

A discussion of communication with the patient in clinical research is often reduced to the practice and contents of informed consent. This is an unbearable oversimplification. There is no way to separate such a discussion from a more general discussion on the relations between a doctor and a patient. The patient in clinical research is still, and first of all, a patient. Similarly, a commitment to clinical research should not influence the physician's primary role as a physician. As far as their communication is concerned, the fact that the physician is proposing a clinical trial should not influence his relation to the patient. A discussion of communication in clinical research is therefore just one chapter of a general discussion of communication between physician and patient.

Starting any treatment is technically possible without much explanation. The danger of treating an uninformed patient can be compared to that of administering chemotherapy without checking blood counts and providing adequate support measures. Instead of tailoring the treatment to the individual, average tolerance is presumed, and average doses of drugs are given. The result may be a suboptimal effect on the tumor; in addition, unforeseen complications may arise that further intervention cannot alleviate. The same is true for the treatment of an uninformed patient: after a while, both doctor and patient may realize that the results of the treatment are different from what was anticipated and may find their relationship blocked in an atmosphere of mistrust.

The dangers and shortsightedness of concealing the proper information during routine treatment increases to become an unsurmountable obstacle when clinical research is concerned. Few of us doubt the benefits of clinical research not only for future patients but also for the actual patient enrolled in an exactly specified prospective trial and thence subjected to most rigorous quality assurance and control.[1] Nevertheless, the potential benefits of clinical research do not justify manipulating the patient for the purpose of obtaining his or her consent: no patient should ever enter a prospective trial without clear, thorough information, first on the disease and its implications, and then on the proposed research trial. Without much exaggeration, the practice of not informing the patient in a trial about the diagnosis, and thence about the purpose, logic, and potential consequences of the procedures to which he or she is to be exposed, may easily be compared to experiments on laboratory animals, or to the sad experience with human experimentation in the not-too-distant past.[2,3]

After such a clear position regarding the necessity that a patient in clinical research be fully informed, what issues remain to be discussed? I have deliberately omitted some of the more frequently discussed questions on the ethics of clinical research or on the individual physician's preference versus collective equipoise[4,5] and have instead devoted more attention to those questions that profoundly influence communication. We will present the stage first, then the actors, and finally the play itself. The first section therefore presents the three phases of trials in clinical oncology, with special consideration of the issues of importance for the communication process. The second section presents the pressing dilemmas that the physician and the patient face when confronted with a research protocol. In the last section, an attempt will be made to describe the form and content of the communication process itself.

THE STAGE: THREE PHASES OF CLINICAL RESEARCH IN ONCOLOGY

Phase I Trials

A key moment when introducing a novel drug into clinical use is its very first application to humans. This is a phase I trial, which aims at establishing the pharmacokinetic parameters of the drug, its main side effects, safe dose range, and an acceptable—though not yet necessarily optimal—application schedule.

For most drugs, the research subjects in a phase I trial are healthy volunteers. The initial doses of the drug are only a percentage of the effective dose,[6] as predicted on the basis of animal testing. If no untoward side effects are noted, the dose is then gradually increased. However, anticancer drugs are invariably linked to severe acute side effects and potential late consequences such as carcinogenicity and organ dysfunction, and so research subjects in phase I trials of anticancer drugs are not healthy volunteers but patients with cancer that is not amenable to standard curative treatment.

If noted, an antitumor effect is recorded, but this is not among the main objectives of a phase I trial. Due to uncertain effectiveness of the drug, and especially due to the dose escalation schedule, which starts with extremely small doses, an objective tumor response is seen in less than 5% of patients in a phase I trial.[7,8] The subjects in a phase I trial appear to be used not for their own benefit, but predominantly for the benefit of medical knowledge and of other, future patients; phase I trials may thus be regarded as ethically the most problematic type of clinical research in oncology.[9]

Phase II Trials

The aim of phase II trials is to identify tumor types for which the treatment appears promising. A phase II trial usually enrolls patients with a measurable tumor and in fair general condition for whom no effective anticancer treatment is known. The new drug is first tested as a single-agent therapy and later, if it is considered at least moderately effective, in combinations with other effective drugs.

Phase III Trials

After an innovative treatment has been tested in a phase II trial, a comparison with the best standard treatment is needed. To minimize the risk of a bias, random choice of the treatments to be compared is the rule for phase III trials.

The ethical issues linked to clinical trials with a random choice of treatment have not yet been resolved. For some, randomized phase III trials are a proof that clinical research—previously often a mixture of observations, unproved postulates, and wishful thinking—has become a true science. Other authors have expressed deep concern regarding this particular type of clinical research.[2,10] Utilitarian arguments about important past or future advances in medical knowledge as a contribution of randomized trials do not justify manipulating the individual patient with regard to his or her true interests and consent—a topic that will be discussed later. In addition, proper attention to the physician's personal preferences seem justified, and the methodology of other types of clinical research should also be further developed.[10,11]

THE ACTORS: THE PHYSICIAN AND THE PATIENT

Dilemmas of the Physician

Am I Primarily a Physician, or a Researcher?

Although it is frequently discussed,[11,12] this dilemma seems to me somehow artificial. After the physician has come to the end of questions about his readiness and competence to participate in the trial, and about the appropriateness of inviting the particular patient into the trial, then he clearly has to accept both roles simultaneously. It would be bad science if coercion were used in order to rigidly follow the research protocol, with little respect for the patient's interests: the reader of such a report would underestimate the side effects of the treatment that is being advocated. It is in the interest of the physician and of the researcher—of the medical profession and of medical science—to produce a sincere report, including the difficulties in following the predetermined research protocol.

A good clinical investigator should always also be an excellent physician. Clinical competence and devotion to the physical and emotional needs of a patient, honest sharing of experiences with colleagues, and seeking their advice when needed are among those personal characteristics that are equally essential for the performance of good medical practice and of medical research.

Every rule has its exceptions. Our opinion that the physician and the clinical investigator should best be one and the same person is easy to defend for phase I and phase II trials, which represent the majority of clinical research; however, in some randomized trials, splitting the roles of the clinical investigator and the physician participating in the trial may be warranted. For statistical reasons, randomized trials will frequently enroll several hundred or even several thousand patients. When dealing with a trial of such dimensions, the organizational and statistical tasks become very complex and demand specific skills and experience that most physicians do not possess. The other reason for separating their roles is the physicians' preference for one of the treatment options. It is desirable that a randomized trial address an important dilemma; yet, in such instances, many physicians will have a clear preference for one treatment option or the other. In such a situation, splitting the roles of the clinical investigator and the physician participating in the trial may, indeed, be desirable: after full informed consent and after randomization, the patient would be treated by the physician with a preference for that particular treatment option. Not only would the technical performance of the treatment be higher, but also communication with the patient would be much easier if a physician who believes in adjuvant chemotherapy for non–small-cell lung cancer treats patients with chemotherapy, and a nonbeliever just gives good supportive treatment.

Yes or No for Participation in a Trial

When a research protocol is being prepared and circulated among potential collaborators, the really important question is whether to join a research group and promise to encourage patients to enter a specific trial. This question should not be reduced to just the scientific validity of the question formulated in the protocol, to the physician's competence and technical experience with the proposed treatments, or to a feeling of a strong personal preference for one of the treatment options—questions that are beyond the scope of the present discussion and that have been extensively discussed.[13,14] If the answers to all these questions go in favor of joining the trial, further questions arise, and these further questions are linked to communication with the patient.

Unfortunately, it seems that the doctor's decision to join a research team is often taken very lightly. As a consequence, many, if not the majority, of trial protocols overestimate by far the expected dynamics of patient accrual. Of more than 1300 active clinical trials for cancer listed with the Physician Data Query service at the National Cancer Institute, it is most likely that the majority may never accumulate enough patients to allow a meaningful interpretation of the results and reach publication.[1].

The physician should know that a decision to participate in a trial means considerable additional time for explaining to the patients the purpose of the trial with appropriate and comprehendible explanations of the technical details, the expected outcome(s), and the alternatives. Although leaflets prepared in advance can be helpful, no written word can replace personal, customized, repeated explanation—and that is very time-consuming.

I have no experience in programs specifically designed to improve communication skills for the medical profession. However, two decades of observing my colleagues and their behavior with patients permits me to conclude that some physicians are simply unable to respond to the basic requirements for proper communication with a patient in a clinical trial. The ability to adjust to the level of understanding of each particular patient, the ability to present the current dilemmas and the need for continuous research, a proper balance between the two unacceptable extremes—coercion on one side and "it is totally your choice" on the other—accessibility for and patience with the patient's frequent additional questions, and compassion are among those personal characteristics that everyone discussing a trial with a patient should possess. Whether in research or not, the patient depends on the physician and cannot be considered as absolutely autonomous;[16] thence, he needs not only information but also help and friendly advice.

To Propose or Not Propose Entry into a Trial to a Particular Patient

The criteria for eligibility of the patient for a trial include parameters such as age, diagnosis and stage of the disease, performance status, or kidney function. After these criteria are met and after a thorough general discussion of the disease and its perspectives with the patient, the physician should realistically assess whether the particular patient will be able to understand the dilemmas that are to be resolved by the trial, together with his own role in medical research. It is neither a favor to the patient nor a pleasant task for the physician to start a lengthy, embarrassing, and possibly even hostile discussion if the chances for a relatively smooth resolution of these questions are slim. An experienced physician will anticipate such an outcome and will not start a discussion about a trial, but rather propose the best available standard treatment. Therefore, not only the criteria of eligibility listed previously, but also the physician's assessment of the patient's capacity to accept his role in medical research should be considered before the proposal is formally presented to the patient and his consent is granted or refused.

Dilemmas of the Patient

For the purpose of this discussion, we will suppose that the patient has been properly informed about the diagnosis, natural history of the disease, and perspectives of the best available standard treatment. As we said above, no sincere discussion about the patient's participation in a clinical trial may start before these basic questions have been approached. Still, the scenario of the communication between doctor and patient is never written in advance: the patient will often come back to questions already discussed and seemingly resolved long ago—another reminder of the shortsightedness of the practice of concealing the truth.

Am I a Patient or a Research Subject?

This question is rarely clearly formulated, yet it lies behind the patient's dilemmas and hesitation in consenting to enter a trial. However altruistic some patients may be and no matter how they respect medical science and the need for clear and scientifically valid answers to the dilemmas of modern medicine, the patient is always still the patient, with his or her unique individuality and interests. The patient then may be expected to consent to a trial only if he is convinced that this offers him better chances, or at least no worse a chance than choosing one of the standard treatment options.

THE PROCESS OF COMMUNICATION

Thornton wrote that after the operation on her breast, she received a text prepared to explain her diagnosis, together with an invitation to enter a randomized trial of postoperative radiotherapy.[17] This report best illus trates what the communication process with the patient should not look like. Communication is a bidirectional process, is continuous rather than once-and-for-all, and is based primarily on personal contact.

A message concerning a description of a health problem and the options for its management is never a simple process. The more complicated the problem is, the greater is the need for building close relations based on mutual respect and confidence. After the initial, introductory discussion, the patient will certainly need additional explanations and will try to adapt the information to his personal understanding of the role that a disease, with its consequences, may play in his life.

The patient's dilemmas will occasionally culminate in a crisis of adaptation to his or her changing position in relation to the social environment, and in relation to his or her ideal self-image. The physician should help the patient understand and overcome this often predictable, yet always unique, episodes.

All that has been said so far on the process of communication applies to an even greater extent to a patient in research. Apart from his normal demands as a patient, he has accepted participation in a clinical trial, with all the additional dilemmas that that may involve. It is more than just, then, that the patient in clinical research is treated as a partner to the medical profession. The practical implications of such a statement will be presented in the next section, in particular when discussing the patient's right to be informed about preliminary results of a study in which he is invited to participate.

Informed Consent

According to McKenna,[18] the elements of informed consent include:

- Adequate information about risks and benefits;
- An on-going process of communication between the doctor and the patient, rather than a one-time event;
- Comprehension by the patient of detailed explanations provided in appropriate language and reading level;
- Voluntary and uncoerced consent;
- Adequate documentation of the process used to obtain consent.

The process of informed consent should not only be specified in a research protocol, but should also be adhered to in clinical practice. A marked divergence between the declared policy and its practical implementation, as revealed in our recent study,[19] is a reason for serious concern and deserves more attention.

Oral or Written Information

Talking with the patient has always been the basis of our communication, and should remain so. Nothing can replace the physician's duty to repeatedly discuss with the patient the current knowledge about his or her disease, and future treatment options. A conversation can be only supplemented, never replaced, by written information such as leaflets describing a specific situation. I strongly believe that this is true not only for a patient in routine clinical practice, but also for a patient in clinical research: he also has the right to, and the need for, a caring physician with whom he can share his doubts, his fears, and his hopes.

It seems, then, that the difference between oral and written communication is somehow artificial. While some differences between the patient in clinical practice and the patient in research cannot be denied, the basic process of informing the patient and of obtaining his consent is very similar.[20] Fair, open, repeated conversation with the patient is always the basis of our communication. Written information, which is becoming indispensable in clinical research, is the supplement to oral communication.

The Patient's Signature

Should the patient sign his approval to enter a prospective clinical trial? Before we answer this question, two circumstances need to be mentioned. The first is that the consent always includes a statement that at any time the patient may withdraw from the trial. The second is that the responsibility for all elements of clinical research, from planning a trial to its practical implementation, always remains with the physician. In a randomized trial, it is the personal responsibility of the principal researcher that the trial really compare treatment options considered optimal for the entire time, until the last patient enters the trial. In the same way, it is also the personal responsibility of each participating physician that the treatment be delivered according to the highest standards of quality of patient care. Even if the patient lends his signature, he will never share the responsibility for the trial with the principal investigator or with his physician.

All this implies that signing a consent form is not to be compared to signing a contract between equal parties. The need for the patient's signature depends on cultural and legal circumstances, which may vary considerably from one country to another, and indeed even within the same community when patients with quite different educational and spiritual backgrounds are involved. The meaning of the signature can be only that he or she was informed about the research and does not disagree to participate in it. Never can the patient's signature be used against him or her and interpreted as the patient's sharing the responsibility for eventual untoward events.

Detailed or Basic Information?

Should the written information really include a terrifying list of potential complications? My personal opinion is that the information should include all complications that are normally expected, but not those seen only exceptionally. Whatever happens, the legal and moral responsibility remains with the physician. If a consent form is more than one page of simple text and if it includes a lot of medical terminology, then it has been written for the protection not of the patient, but of the doctor or the sponsor of the research.

The Meaning of Words

We said that the researcher should do his best to prepare a text comprehensible to a lay person. In spite of all efforts, however, there may be a great gap between the understanding of the words, and the actual experience. No words can bring the experience of a disease to a healthy person. Likewise, a patient may not fully understand the real meaning of "febrile neutropenia." There is no remedy to this inadequate capacity of words, other than our responsibility to propose trials of true scientific value and to provide continuous psychological support to our patients, regardless of whether they do or do not participate in research.

Specific Aspects of Phase I, Phase II, and Phase III Trials

Phase I Trials

At first glance, there seems to be no conflict of interest between a clinical researcher and a patient consenting to participate in a phase I trial of a novel anticancer drug. After a thorough, compassionate presentation of their situation, patients with advanced cancer will usually consent to be included in the trial of a new drug: for most patients, uncertainty and hope linked to the new drug is preferable to the definitively grim prognosis that may be offered by supportive treatment alone. However, it is precisely this line of reasoning of a patient with advanced cancer that may offer an opportunity to manipulate the patient in order to obtain his consent: patients included in phase I trials rarely realize that the main objective of the trial is not to test the efficacy of the new drug, but to study its pharmacokinetics, preferred application schedule, and toxicity.[21] Consent to participate in a phase I trial and to all the associated additional investigations, frequent visits to the clinic, and eventual side effects often stems from false hopes that the patient has a chance for a positive response—when this chance is really less than five percent.

It seems that a phase I trial would be much more acceptable to patients if the dose escalation schedule would permit a quicker, albeit admittedly more risky, testing of the drug in its anticipated effective dose range. When a patient consents to the trial, he should have some chance of winning. This would allow the clinical investigator to communicate with the patient with open cards, instead of hiding his real objective of testing the pharmacology and toxicity of the drug behind an unrealistic promise of therapeutic improvement.

Phase II Trials

From the ethical point of view, phase II trials are the least problematic type of clinical research in oncology. The interests of the researcher are very close to those of a well-informed, consenting patient.

Randomized Phase III Trials

Inherent in the performance of phase III trials are conflicting interests, possibilities for manipulation of patients' consent, and pressures for distortion of physicians' ethical principles.

From the patient's perspective, randomized clinical trials can be grouped under three categories:

- Trials comparing two treatments of approximately equal anticipated effectiveness and similar comorbidity. Numerous trials comparing different chemotherapy regimens fall into this category.
- Trials comparing radical treatment with a more conservative approach, stemming from a hypothesis that the less aggressive treatment is not less effective. Trials of radical versus organ-preserving surgery, of routine postoperative radiotherapy versus surgery alone, or of long-term adjuvant chemotherapy versus short-term perioperative chemotherapy may be mentioned in this category of randomized trials.
- Trials comparing the standard treatment of known low potential to influence the downhill course of the disease against an innovative treatment.

The patient should have relatively few problems in consenting to a trial of the first type. The patient's dilemmas with trials of the second and third types stem from their misunderstanding of the difference between a hypothesis and the real role of a particular treatment that is still to be established.[22] Furthermore, patients also have their preferences regarding choice of treatment. The patients' preferences may be related not only to treatment of the cancer itself, as the most common end point to be evaluated in a study, but also to the acute and late side effects, long-term morbidity, and the expected interference with the patient's normal life. It is quite natural that patients look at the problem through their own eyes, not through the eyes of a scientist. When experts hide their opinion under "collective equipoise," patients' preferences should be considered.[23,24] Thus, Mrs. Thornton wrote that she would refuse postoperative irradiation if so many doctors feel that it is unnecessary and may be even harmful. Why should she offer her body to scientifically prove something that is very likely to be true?[17] Similar is the dilemma of that patient with inoperable pancreatic cancer who believes that someday an effective treatment for his condition will be found. As he has not much to lose, why should he consent to a randomized trial (and, thence, to a 50% chance of getting only supportive treatment) and not ask for some kind of innovative treatment right away?

Finally, months or years after entering the trial and completing the treatment, the patient's disease may progress. As a patient is often inclined to seek an explanation for his or her condition in the outer world, so also eventual progression of the disease may appear to be linked to the particular treatment option to which he or she had been assigned by random choice. The patient may feel that his well-being had been sacrificed for the sake of the progress of medical science. Whether expressed openly or in a more discrete mode, the patient will have even more grounds for such a statement in case he had actually been assigned to a treatment option that proved to be inferior in subsequent analysis. Therefore, the roles of the clinical investigator and of the physician do not end after the results of the trial have been made known to the scientific and lay community. Responsibility for the patient continues. The ground for potential conflict diminishes if the relationship has been based on sincere, humane mutual understanding rather than on hierarchy and the physician's professional superiority.

Has the patient the right to know the preliminary results of a study in which he was invited to participate? This question is particularly pressing in randomized clinical trials, in which patient accrual is usually protracted over several years and in which new patients are still entering the trial while the events (remissions, complications, or survival) from earlier patients have already been recorded. The present practice is that the cancer patient is not entitled to know the preliminary experience and the interim results. Indeed, some authors state that even the physicians participating in the study should not be told about the preliminary results. The reason for this is clear: when the interim results show an advantage of one of the treatment arms, the uncertainty principle may be seriously compromised and neither doctors nor patients will accept further randomization.

Beyond the scope of this presentation are the practical implications of the idea that the patient has the right to be informed about the preliminary results of the trial he is about to enter. Here, I will say only that trials with a long patient accrual period very often become unethical. Many years of slow recruitment of patients into a trial will frequently lead to a situation with an obvious but statistically still unconvincing advantage of one treatment over the other. In such a situation, accrual of new patients cannot proceed without ignoring their right to be informed about the preliminary results. Completion of a trial in a short time is therefore highly recommended, not only for scientific but also for ethical reasons.

DISCUSSION AND CONCLUSIONS

Dissecting and analyzing the communication process may be both dangerous and artificial: such an attempt is not far from discussing what we mean by "love" through a detailed analysis of the motivations and actions of those involved. Being aware of the limitations of such an approach, I nevertheless have found no other way to present my personal view of the various general problems linked to communication with the patient, and in particular with the patient in clinical research.

In everyday communication, words can be an adequate medium only for very simple messages. Whenever emotions are involved—and this is the case in every decisive moment of our lives—movements and gestures, physical contact, silence, and the mere feeling of spiritual proximity are among the invaluable means for conveying messages.

Everyone responsible for another person is also responsible for his spiritual adaptation. Our roles are changing constantly: the physician of today may be a patient at the same time, or will certainly be a patient in the future. When it comes to clinical research, it is unacceptable that physicians involve patients in trials in which they themselves would not be willing to participate.[25–27] This is a clear sign of the erosion of moral principles among the medical community. The situation may be worse than just a predominance of utilitarian ethics over Kantian ethics, according to which a human being can never become a means. Professional ambitions linked to the fruits of clinical research, or even financial reimbursement offered as compensation for involving one's patients in research may have wider and more profound influences on the behavior of our profession than we would even wish to think.

The resolution of these dilemmas may be sought in true partnership with patients.[28] Some principles and practices of clinical research should probably change. Nobody should be forced to perform clinical research.

A physician should join a clinical research team only after all the implications of such a decision have been considered; sincere motivation for continuous communication with the patients in clinical research is not among the least important of these implications.

REFERENCES

1. STILLER, C. A. 1989. Survival of patients with cancer. Those included in clinical trials do better. Br. Med. J. **299:** 1058-1059.
2. HELLMAN, S. & D. S. HELLMAN. 1991. Of mice but not men. Problems of the randomized clinical trial. N. Engl. J. Med. **324:** 1585-1589.
3. BEECHER, H. E. 1966. Ethics and clinical reesearch. N. Engl. J. Med. **274:** 1354-1360.
4. FREEDMAN, B. 1987. Equipoise and the ethics of clinical research. N. Engl. J. Med. **317:** 141-145.
5. BERRY, D. A. 1989. Comment: Ethics and ECMO. Stat. Sci. **4:** 306-310.
6. EORTC PHARMACOKINETICS AND METABOLISM GROUP. 1987. Pharmacokinetically guided dose escalation in phase I clinical trials. Commentary and proposed guidelines. Eur. J. Cancer Clin. Oncol. **23:** 1083-1087.
7. ESTEY, E., D. HOTH, R. SIMON, S. MARSONI, B. LEYLAND-JONES & R. WITTES. 1986. Therapeutic response in phase I trials of antineoplastic agents. Cancer Treat. Rep. **70:** 1105-1115.
8. DECOSTER, G., G. STEIN & E. E. HOLDENER. 1990. Responses and toxic deaths in phase I clinical trials. Ann. Oncol. **1:** 175-181.
9. EMANUEL, E. J. 1995. A phase I trial on the ethics of phase I trials. J. Clin. Oncol. **13:** 1049-1051.
10. BERRY, D. A. 1993. A case for Bayesianism in clinical trials. Stat. Med. **12:** 1377-1393.
11. MUELLER, B. C. 1995. Breast cancer trials on trial. A case of conflicting ethical interests. Cancer **75:** 2403-2406.
12. LAWRENCE, W. & H. D. BEAR. 1995. Is there really an ethical conflict in clinical trials? Cancer **75:** 2407-2409
13. LIBERATI, A., W. B. PATTERSON, L. BIENER & B. J. MCNEIL. 1987. Determinants of physicians' preferences for alternative treatments in women with early breast cancer Tumori **73:** 601-609.
14. KORN, E. L. & S. BAUMRIND. 1991. Randomised clinical trials with clinician-preferred treatment. Lancet **337:** 149-152.
15. NEWCOMER, L. N. 1991. Randomized clinical trials. N. Engl. J. Med. **325:** 1513.
16. O'NEIL, O. 1984. Paternalism and partial autonomy. J. Med. Ethics **10:** 173-178.
17. THORNTON, H. M. 1992. Breast cancer trials: A patient's viewpoint. Lancet **339:** 44-45.
18. MCKENNA, R. J., J. LASZIO, J. DURANT, J. F. HERMANN, C. HUGULEY, B. LEVENTHAL, E. ROACH & M. SIEGLER. 1990. Ethical considerations. Cancer **65:** 2407-2408.
19. WILLIAMS, C. J. & M. ZWITTER. 1994. Informed consent in European multicentre randomised clinical trials—Are patients really informed? Eur. J. Cancer **30:** 907-910.
20. LEVINE, R. J. 1983. Informed consent in research and practice: Similarities and

differences. Arch. Intern. Med. **143:** 1229-1231.

21. DAUGHERTY, C., M. J. RATAIN, E. GROCHOWSKI, C. STOCKING, E. KODISH, R. MICK & M. SIEGLER. 1995. Perceptions of cancer patients and their physicians involved in phase I trials. J. Clin. Oncol. **13:** 1062-1072.
22. FETTING, J. H., L .A SIMINOFF, S. PIANTADOSI, M. D. ABELOFF, D. J. DAMRON & A. M. SARSFIELD. 1990. Effect of patients' expectations of benefit with standard breast cancer adjuvant chemotherapy on participation in a randomized clinical trial: A clinical vignette study. J. Clin. Oncol. **8:** 1476-1482.
23. ANGELL, M. 1984. Patients' preferences in randomized clinical trials. N. Engl. J. Med. **310:** 1385-1387.
24. BREWIN, C. R. & C. BRADLEY. 1989. Patient preferences in randomised clinical trials. Br. Med. J. **299:** 313-315.
25. MACKILLOP, W. J., G. K. WARD & B. O'SULLIVAN. 1986. The use of expert surrogates to evaluate clinical trials in non-small cell lung cancer. Br. J. Cancer **54:** 661-667.
26. MOORE, M. J., B. O'SULLIVAN & I. F. TANNOCK. 1988. How expert physicians would wish to be treated if they had genitourinary cancer. J. Clin. Oncol. **6:** 1736-1745.
27. MOORE, M. J., B. O'SULLIVAN & I. F. TANNOCK. 1990. Are treatment strategies of urologic oncologists influenced by the opinions of their colleagues? Br. J. Cancer **62:** 988-991.
28. MERIGAN, T. C. 1990. You can teach an old dog new tricks—How AIDS trials are pioneering new strategies. N. Engl. J. Med. **323:** 1341-1343.

Is It Wise to Tell the Truth, the Whole Truth, and Nothing but the Truth to a Cancer Patient?

SAWSAN EL-GHAZALI

Behavioral Medicine Unit
Department of Community, Environmental, and Occupational Medicine
Ain Shams University
Cairo, Egypt

INTRODUCTION

The physician-scientist, particularly as a member of a clinical cancer research institution, faces many ethically troublesome situations.[1] Those working on scientific and medical frontiers should be specifically trained to identify, analyze, and resolve ethical dilemmas. However, the question addressed—what should patients know?—is a very difficult one.[2]

Caring must be considered a major part of the management of patients suffering from cancer. Complicity-based caring is characterized by verbal and nonverbal behavior of patients sharing a common experience. This type of caring is better conducted through a third party—i.e., medical staff—who bring patients together with similar experiences. Action-oriented caring consists of interacting with other patients as an antidote for one's own fear, panic, or anguish. Solidarity-based caring helps patients find and maintain their own identity, pride, and dignity. Cooperative caring can be observed in group settings such as support groups or vegetarian cooking classes for cancer patients. Self-centered caring refers to the various forms of concern one has for oneself.[3]

Difficult moral concerns and choices are a characteristic of palliative cancer therapy. Patient information, palliative chemotherapy, treatment with unconventional remedies, and chemical drug development involve important issues.[1] Experts contend that biotechnology therapies will shift the site of cancer treatment from external systemic treatments, such as radiation and chemotherapy, to targeted tumor-specific drugs that boost the immune system. That change alone holds many implications for oncology management.[4]

The physician who treats cancer patients is particularly exposed to ethical problems in his daily routine. These ethical dilemmas occur at almost every stage of the cancer patient's treatment from diagnosis through treatment to the final stages of his or her illness, such as disclosure of the diagnosis of cancer and the place of mutilative surgery and other aggressive modalitities in cancer treatment. Only awareness of these problems and open discussion will help the oncologist to treat his or her patient in the best possible way.[5]

Some researchers have investigated the information given to their patients according to the stage of their cancer.[6] Others have identified issues that are central in the treatment of dying children and their families, assuming that management of the terminal phase of illness has a dramatic effect on the psychosocial recovery of the family.[7] It can be argued that the "bearable truth" has to be supplied to the patient; however, the application of this concept needs time and dedication to the patient.[8]

In a study of 50 patients with lung cancer,[9] 2 patients would have preferred not to have been told the diagnosis. In Chinese culture, a study was conducted of 50 Chinese families dealing with childhood cancer. All identified cancer as the most frightening disease.[10]

Another aspect of truth-telling is providing patients with the "whole truth" about treatment—e.g., its side effects and toxicity—and whether informed consent should be requested before starting treatment. The issue is what information should be revealed to the patient. In order to totally satisfy the patient's "rights," informed consent forms should be encyclopedic, providing the "whole truth" to the patients. However, this would not meet the moral goal of shared decision making, because few patients would be able to make sense of such data.[11]

Delays in seeking diagnosis and care for cancer are as prominent now as they were 50 years ago. These delays may be seen as attempts to resolve or postpone the crisis brought on an individual by the suspicion of terminal illness.[12]

Ditto *et al.*[13] and Lau and Hartman[14] have shown that typically people's thoughts about common illnesses have five components: (1) a label or name for the illness; (2) a list of consequences; (3) a time course; (4) a cause; and (5) a cure. The mental representation of an illness is called a folk belief system.[15]

This chapter will focus on patient-doctor communication and truth-telling and will include interviews with two patients from the Egyptian community who have breast cancer.

SUBJECTS AND METHODS

This study is composed of two parts. The first considers doctors' opinions on telling the truth to their patients who suffer from cancer. A questionnaire of 23 items designed by the author was distributed to male surgeons (female surgeons are very scarce in Egypt) in the field of general surgery working as staff members in a university hospital in Cairo. The

TABLE 1. Telling Patients about Their Condition

	Surgeons with > 20 y Experience (n = 50)			Surgeons with < 10 y Experience (n = 50)		
	1st Visit	Later Visit		1st Visit	Later Visit	
a. When is the patient informed about his condition?						
As 1st opinion	35 (70%)	15 (30%)		5 (10%)	45 (90%)[a]	
As 2nd opinion	41 (82%)	9 (18%)		11 (22%)	39 (78%)[a]	
Terminal stage	50 (100%)	0		50 (100%)	0	
	Yes	No		Yes	No	
b. Does the type of cancer determine the time of truth-telling?	5 (10%)	45 (90%)		18 (36%)	32 (64%)[a]	
c. Is breast cancer an exception?	35 (70%)	15 (30%)		45 (90%)	5 (10%)[b]	
d. Does the sex or age of the patient determine the time of truth-telling?	3 (6%)	47 (94%)		24 (48%)	26 (52%)[a]	
	Patient	Spouse	Relatives	Patient	Spouse	Relatives
e. Whom do you prefer to inform about the diagnosis first?	3[c] (6%)	18 (36%)	29 (58%)	0	32 (64%)	18 (36%)[a]

[a] $p < 0.001$.
[b] $p < 0.02$.
[c] Depends on the situation.

total sample consisted of 100 surgeons, who were divided into two groups for comparison, according to their length of professional practice in their specific fields of surgery. The first group had more than 20 years' experience, and the second group had less than 10 years' experience. The questionnaire requested information in six categories.

TABLE 2. Timing and Amount of Truth-Telling

	Surgeons with > 20 Years' Experience (n = 50)			Surgeons with < 10 Years' Experience (n = 50)		
	1st Visit	Later Visit		1st Visit	Later Visit	
a. When is it more traumatizing for the patient to be told the truth?	45 (90%)	5 (10%)		48 (96%)	2 (4%)[a]	
	Yes	No		Yes	No	
b. If the patient is informed at the first visit, is there a decline in mood in later visits?	5 (10%)	45 (90%)		30 (60%)	20 (40%)[b]	
	All	Some	Little	All	Some	Little
c. How much information do you prefer to disclose about the patient's condition?	15 (30%)	30 (60%)	5 (10%)	2 (4%)	28 (56%)	20 (40%)[b]

[a] $p > 0.05$.
[b] $p < 0.001$.

Category I (7 questions) included a group of questions concerning telling the patient about his condition as regarding (a) first or later visits; (b) stage of cancer; (c) type of cancer; (d) age or sex of the patient; (e) who is to be informed of the diagnosis first.

Category II (3 questions) includes a group of questions concerning the traumatizing effect of when the patient is told his diagnosis and the depth of information the patient should know.

Category III (2 questions) includes a group of questions concerning the length of time the doctor spent with his patients and whether or not it was influenced by the type of cancer or not.

Category IV (3 questions) includes a group of questions concerning the patients' acceptance of their condition; whether or not they come back to the doctor.

Category V (4 questions) includes a group of questions concerning the giving or taking away of hope.

Category VI (4 questions) includes a group of questions concerning management procedures.

TABLE 3. Length of Time Spent with Cancer Patients

	Surgeons with > 20 Years' Experience ($n = 50$)			Surgeons with < 10 Years' Experience ($n = 50$)		
	Yes		No	Yes		No
a. Do you think the type of cancer determines the amount of time spent with a cancer patient?	44 (88%)		6 (12%)	45 (90%)		5 (10%)
	15 min	20 min	30 min	15 min	20 min	30 min
b. How much time do you spend with each patient?	10 (20%)	35 (70%)	5 (10%)	18 (36%)	31 (62%)	1 (2%)

NOTE: For a and b, $p > 0.05$.

Statistical analysis was done using the chi-square test.

The second part of this study is a comparative scenario with two female patients with breast cancer, from different social classes and with different personalities. Each patient was interviewed by the author on two separate occasions, each lasting two hours. One of the cases was presented at the First International Conference of Behavioral Medicine held in Cairo, Egypt, in November 1994.

RESULTS AND DISCUSSION

Human behavior is the product of two domains. The first domain is the person, who is composed, according to the writer's point of view, of three integrated circles: body, spirit, and mind. The second domain is the person's environment, which serves as a matrix in which he/she is embedded. Cancer in our community is called the "insidious," "wicked," "cruel," or the "very bad" disease. In our community the word "cancer" is very traumatizing, as cancer and death have so often been synonymous in the minds of so many.

Many researchers have tried to measure or define the quality of life. Jenkins summarized it as three F's, feelings, function, and future.[16] To my mind this could be functionally translated into three H's, happiness, health, and hope. "Doctor" originally meant "teacher." What is the role of this teacher when facing a patient with cancer? What is the role of

TABLE 4. Acceptibility to Patient of Knowledge of Condition

	Surgeons with > 20 Years' Experience (n = 50)			Surgeons with < 10 Years' Experience (n = 50)		
		Yes	No		Yes	No
a. Do some patients wish they had never been told their diagnosis?		10 (20%)	40 (80%)		15 (30%)	35 (70%)[a]
		Return	Leave		Return	Leave
b. What percentage of patients who are told their diagnosis return to the physician, and what percentage leave?		75%	25%		5	95%[b]
	Fear	To Seek Second Opinion	Referred by Another Physician	Fear	To Seek Second Opinion	Referred by Another Physician
c. Why do you think those who leave do so?	50%	40%	10%	5%	45%	50%[b]

[a] $p > 0.05$.
[b] $p < 0.001$.

experience in handling such a problem? This study shows that the length of experience in handling patients with such an insidious disease is of great importance.

Regarding the timing of giving the diagnosis (TABLE 1a), we can observe that this was done during the first visit to the doctor (experience over 20 years) in 70% and in 82% as first and second opinions, respectively; compared to 10% and 22% among surgeons with 10 years' experience or less; the difference proved to be statistically highly significant ($p < 0.001$). This observation held for all types of cancer except breast cancer. Senior surgeons explained that they were afraid they may lose the case, that the patient may be reluctant to return for further procedures; in order to avoid that, they resorted to increasing the awareness of their patients or their relatives so that they would approach the condition with the utmost seriousness. On the other hand, the junior staff preferred to confirm the diagnosis and to gain the trust of the patient first. Also, the type of cancer and the gender or age of the patient had no effect on the

TABLE 5. Giving Hope to Cancer Patients and Their Relatives

	Surgeons with > 20 Years' Experience ($n = 50$)		Surgeons with < 10 Years' Experience ($n = 50$)	
	Yes	No	Yes	No
a. Is the patient diagnosed as terminal told there may be hope?	50 (100%)	0	50 (100%)	0
b. Are relatives of the terminal patient told there may be hope?	7 (14%)	43 (86%)	38 (76%)	12 (24%)
c. Have you ever told a patient there is no hope?	0	50 (100%)	0	50 (100%)
d. Have you ever told a relative there is no hope?	45 (90%)	5 (10%)	10 (20%)	40 (80%)

NOTE: $p < 0.001$.

mode of thinking of the senior surgeons (TABLE 1b–d). As regards who is informed first about the diagnosis, both groups preferred to face the spouse or relatives with the diagnosis rather than the patient (TABLE 1e).

The two groups agreed that giving the diagnosis on the patient's first visit is more traumatizing to the patient, as shown in TABLE 2a and b. With regard to how much information to give the patient, the two groups of physicians disagreed, with 30% of the more experienced doctors preferring to fully disclose the patient's condition, as opposed to 4% of the less-experienced group ($p < 0.001$; TABLE 2c).

TABLE 3 shows that the type of cancer affects the amount of time the doctor spends with the patient in both groups; however, as regards the actual time spent, the average time was between 20 and 30 minutes. Less experienced surgeons spent less time with their patients, presumably due to their lack of communication and comforting skills, which are more developed among the more experienced surgeons.

The acceptability of the patient's knowledge of his/her condition is revealed in TABLE 4a, which shows similar results with both investigated groups. However, the rate of patients leaving the doctor's care was greater among those physicians with less than 10 years' experience; the reason for leaving was to seek another opinion or referral to a more experienced doctor. Surgeons of more than 20 years' experience said that fear was the reason for leaving in 50% of cases (TABLE 4c).

TABLE 6. Management Procedures

	Surgeons with > 20 Years' Experience (n = 50)		Surgeons with < 10 Years' Experience (n = 50)	
	Yes	No	Yes	No
a. Do you request consent before radical treatment?	50 (100%)	0	50 (100%)	0
	Patient	Relative/ Spouse	Patient	Relative/ Spouse
b. If yes, from whom?	50 (100%)	0	45 (90%)	5 (10%)
	Yes	No	Yes	No
c. Do you think psychological therapy should be implemented as an adjunct to cancer therapy?	50 (100%)	0	50 (100%)	0
d. Do you think surgeons should undergo special training in order to deal better with cancer patients?	7 (14%)	43 (86%)	38 (76%)	12 (24%)[a]

[a] $p < 0.001$.

TABLE 5 shows physicians' practices regarding the giving and taking away of hope. In terminal cases, no one in the included sample was able to say "There is no hope" to a patient. However, with relatives surgeons with longer experience (90%) were straightforward in telling them "There is no hope," compared to 20% among the junior staff.

The last category of the first part of the study focused on the ethical procedure for consent request (TABLE 6a–c). There was no difference between both groups; however, there was greater flexibility among the junior staff (10%) to obtain consent from the spouse or relatives. The junior staff was in favor of special training in dealing better with their patients (76%), while only 14% among the more experienced surgeons was in favor of such training (TABLE 6d).

The second part of the study was an interview of two women with breast cancer (see TABLE 7). The first woman was 50 years old, married, had no children, worked as a secretary, and was of middle social class.

TABLE 7. Interviews with Two Breast Cancer Patients

Question	Response	
	Patient No. 1	Patient No. 2
What was your first reaction when you suspected you had cancer?	I felt afraid.	I couldn't believe it.
What was your reaction after the diagnosis was confirmed?	I accepted my fate.	I was severely depressed and felt devastated.
What was the message, and who told you?	You have something in your right breast, and it should be operated on My sister and a close friend.	You have an abscess in your breast and should have a biopsy taken. My mother and brother.
Did you sign a consent before your operation?	Yes.	Yes.
Did you know exactly what was written on it?	Not exactly, but I understood that a radical procedure would be done if necessary.	Not exactly, and I denied to myself that a radical procedure would be done.
Do you think you condition could be some sort of punishment?	No, I did not harm anybody; it is a test from God.	I asked myself is it a punishment? But why?
Who supported you in your crisis?	My spouse, family members, friends, and colleagues. I realized how much they love me.	My family, although I am depressed because some friends did not ask, although they knew.
What was your complaint after radiation and chemotherapy?	Gastrointestinal trouble, and I felt sad for my hair loss.	I was depressed because of my hair loss; that made me very sad.
Do you feel some difference in your coping abilities after having suffered the condition than before?	Yes, I became more sensitive than before. I couldn't bear feelings of apprehension.	I don't like feeling pitied by others. I prefer to be alone for meditation.

TABLE 7. *Continued*

Question	Response	
	Patient No. 1	Patient No. 2
What is your evaluation of this experience?	First I felt afraid. Then, in time I realized how much my family, friends, and peers love me. Thank God!	I still do not believe what happened to me. It is like a nightmare.
What do you want to say about cancer to other women?	It is fate. I never complained. Everything happened within one week.	It is surpising, but although I heard about it, I never imagined I would be a victim of cancer. It is the end.
What was the role of the doctor in your experience?	It was positive. I trusted him, and he reassured me.	It was positive, but I felt that it was my own problem.
When and how did the doctor inform you about your condition?	In my first visit he assured me and asked for investigation. In my second visit he was worried and said that I had a tumor (he never said "cancer").	He did not tell me I had something serious. Later I knew that my family had asked him not to tell me.
What was the most critical time during the whole experience?	Before and after the operation.	Before and after the operation, and now because of my hair loss.
What do you feel now?	I thank God.	I don't exactly know, but I feel that I will never be as before.

The second woman was 51 years old, particularly beautiful, married, had one married daughter and one son in final stage of his university studies, did not work, and was of high social class.

Answers given by the first woman showed acceptance of her condition. Those of the second woman showed refusal to accept her situation; she felt that what she had contracted was a sort of punishment ("I don't believe it, it's like a nightmare," etc.); also, her family played a role in asking the doctor not to tell her about her condition.

What is interesting is that neither woman knew exactly what was going to be done during her operation. The most critical time for them was immediately before and after the operation, which draws our attention to the importance of social support during that period in particular. The side effects of radiation and chemotherapy were very distressing for both of them. Loss of hair, the crown of beauty, was very depressing, particularly for the second woman, perhaps because of her social rank and beauty. Also, her comment that "cancer is the end" reflected how gloomy she felt. The first woman coped with her condition by accepting the disease as "fate" and by thanking God, while the second woman could not hide her feelings of agony and sadness, although she was also a believer. A similar story was told by a Slovenian lady whom I happened to meet during a conference.[17] This suggests that women's agony when facing breast cancer is universal.

It is interesting in this regard to refer to a study about mammography screening among a group of Egyptian females of different social backgrounds over 35 years of age.[18] This study showed that even among the group of Egyptian female medical staff, 79% did not consider having this screening, because of the fear of discovering breast cancer.

In conclusion, this study reveals that the doctor's experience plays a role in communication and truth-telling. Relatives and spouse as social supports are the recipients of this truth-telling. In the Egyptian community it is very rare to find a patient, particularly one with rural roots, visiting a doctor alone; he/she usually is accompanied by two or three relatives. While senior surgeons depend on their communication skills, junior surgeons prefer to underdo training in that field.

Finally, we should learn how to cope with cancer, how to live with it, how to make it part of our lives and not be afraid of or fight it. We should learn to be courageous and face the situation rather than trying to escape from it. Our efforts should be directed toward learning how to cope with bad news and to realize that it is part of our life.

ACKNOWLEDGMENT

The author thanks Dr. Youssef Sorour for his contribution.

REFERENCES

1. NAGEL, G. A. 1992. Ethics versus ethos: Current ethical problems in palliative oncology. Schweiz. Rundsch. Med. Prax. **81**(44): 1332–1338.
2. BOK, S. 1993. Impaired physicians: What should patients know? Camb. Q. Health Ethics **2**(3): 331–340.
3. LETTRE, L. 1992. Patients and solicitude. Can. Nurse **88**(7): 45–47.
4. LUMSDON, K. & H. J. ANDERSON. 1992. Cancer at the crossroads. Hospitals **66**(23): 22–30.
5. PFEFFER, M. R. 1993. Ethics and the oncologist. Med. Law **12**(3–5): 235–240.

6. ESPINOSA, E., M. GONZALEZ-BARON, J. POVEDA, A. ORDONEZ & P. ZAMORA. 1993. The information given to the terminal patient with cancer. Eur. J. Cancer **29A**(12): 1795–1796.
7. WHITTAM, E. H. 1993. Terminal care of the dying child. Psychosocial implications of care. Cancer **71**(Suppl. 10): 3450–3462.
8. ESPINOSA, E., M. GONZALEZ-BARON, J. POVEDA & I. DE-LA GANDARA. 1993. Bearable truth as the crux of information for the cancer patient. Ann. Med. Interne **10**(3): 147–149.
9. SELL, L., B. DELVIN, S. J. BOURKE, N. C. MUNRO, P. A. CORRIS & G. J. GIBSON. 1993. Communicating the diagnosis of lung cancer. Respir. Med. **87**(1): 61–63.
10. MARTINSON, I. M., SU-XIAO-YIN & Y. H. LIANG. 1993. The impact of childhood cancer on 50 Chinese families. J. Ped. Oncol. Nurs. **10**(1): 13–18.
11. LANTOS, J. 1993. Informed consent. The whole truth for patients. Cancer **72**(Suppl. 9): 2811–2815.
12. ZERVAS, I. M., A. AUGUSTINE & G. L. FRICCHIONE. 1993. Patient delay in cancer. A view from the crisis model. Gen. Hosp. Psychiatry **15**(1): 9–13
13. DITTO, P. H., J. B. JEMMOTT & J. M. DARLEY. 1988. Appraising the threat of illness: A mental representational approach. Health Psychol. **7**(2): 183–201.
14. LAU, R. R. & K. A. HARTMAN. 1983. Common sense representations of common illnesses. Health Psychol. **2**(2): 167–185.
15. SNOW, L. F. 1974. Folk medical beliefs and their implications for care of cancer patients: A review based on studies among Black-Americans. Ann. Intern. Med. **81:** 82–96.
16. JENKINS, C. D. 1992. Assessment of outcomes of health intervention. Soc. Sci. Med. **35**(4): 367–375.
17. OECI Conference on Cancer and Quality of Life, Bled, Slovenia, May 12–14, 1995.
18. EL-GHAZALI, S., H. I. FAHIM & A. KHELLA. 1994 "Prochaska Model" and Mammography. 1st International Conference of Behavioral Medicine, Cairo, Egypt, November 15–19, 1994.

Communication with the Cancer Patient in Nigeria

Information and Truth

TORIOLA F. SOLANKE

National Headquarters of Cancer Registries in Nigeria
University College Hospital
Ibadan, Nigeria

Nigeria is the most populated country in Africa, with 85 million people (1993) and an area of 356,699 square miles (923,773 square kilometers). It has a tropical climate, with wet and dry seasons. Three climatic patterns are distinguished: (1) tropical wet climate in the southeast, with uniformly high temperature and heavy rainfall distribution throughout the year; (2) tropical wet and dry, or savanna, climates in the north and west; and (3) the dry, or steppe, climate in the far north.

The great diversity of peoples and cultures in Nigeria is largely a result of the location of the country at the meeting point of transcontinental migration routes from north to south, west to east, and southeast to northwest. There are over 200 ethnic groups, each of which has its own customs, traditions, and languages. The major groups are the Yorubas, Hausas, Fulanis, and Igbos. In addition to the major languages, there are many dialects. The religions practiced in Nigeria are Christianity, Islam, and traditional forms of worship. The main Christian groups are Roman Catholic, Methodist, Anglican, and American Baptist. Some of these churches, as well as some Muslim sects, own their own hospitals throughout the country, where orthodox medical practice is undertaken. There are in addition traditional and alternate forms of medical practice.

The delivery of conventional health care services in Nigeria is done at three levels: the primary (local government), secondary (state government), and tertiary (federal government) health-care levels. Funding of health services in the country is provided by these tiers of government. The allocation of funds for health-care services is minimal and for cancer programs infinitesimal. The treatment modalities for cancer patients are surgery, radiotherapy, chemotherapy, immunotherapy, and combinations of these. In Nigeria most tertiary institutions can cope with the surgical aspect of cancer management, but at the moment only two moderately equipped radiotherapy centers, located in Lagos and Ibadan, are operating. These centers have only two megavoltage (cobalt-60) units. Chemotherapy is expensive and cannot be afforded by the average Nigerian cancer patient. On the whole, facilities for cancer management in Nigeria are rudimentary.

CANCER IN NIGERIA

Cancer is rising in the health agenda throughout the world, in developing as well as in developed countries. Developing countries not only experience their own forms of cancer now, but they also appear to be undergoing a cancer epidemic curve, similar to that of the developed countries. These changes are happening because many communicable diseases are coming under control; hence, more people are living into the later years of life, when cancer is relatively more frequent.[1]

Cancer has been known from time immemorial in Nigeria. One of the local names for cancer is "that condition which cannot be cured." The Yorubas refer to cancer as *Jejere*, that which devours the body. Every year cancer affects at least nine million people and kills five million globally. Its economic as well health consequences make the disease a substantial and increasing problem. In Nigeria about 100,000 new cases occur every year, and it is expected that by the turn of the century about 500,000 cases will occur annually.[2]

The common malignant tumors in Ibadan, Nigeria, as recorded in the Ibadan Cancer Registry, which collects information about cancer patients at University College Hospital, Ibadan and other hospitals within a circumscribed area, are those of the (1) breast, (2) cervix, (3) liver, (4) skin, (5) lymphoid tissue, (6) prostate, (7) connective and soft tissues, (8) Burkitts, (9) stomach, and (10) chorion and hydatidiform mole. Breast cancer is by far the most commonly encountered cancer in females (29.7%) in Ibadan. Carcinoma of the cervix is second in prevalence, followed by cancers of the chorion, ovary, and liver. In males, primary cancer of the liver is the most frequent cancer (9.5%), followed by cancer of prostate, lymphoid tissue, connective and soft tissue, and stomach (TABLES 1–3).

Cancer is regarded in Nigeria as a deadly and dreadful disease. Most people regard the diagnosis of cancer as a death sentence, even though one-third of cancers can be prevented and another third are curable, provided they are diagnosed early; and in the majority of incurable patients, quality of life can be improved by palliative care. The attitude of most Nigerians to death is influenced by religious beliefs. Death, even death from cancer, is regarded by many as an act of God that cannot be changed.

Most Nigerian patients prefer to consult traditional healers first. Although these healers do not understand the scientific basis of cancer management, they communicate effectively with their patients and instill in them some measure of hope. These patients utilize the existing facilities in conventional hospitals as a last resort. This practice causes delay in presentation at the hospital; consequently, a large proportion of cancer patients is seen in the advanced stages of the disease.

Cancer patients in Nigeria can be divided into the following groups regarding their attitude toward death and information about their condition:

TABLE 1. Ten Common Cancers in Ibadan (Male and Female)[a]

	Age in Years												
Cancer Type	0–9	10–19	20–29	30–39	40–49	50–59	60–69	70–79	80–89	90–99	Age Unknown	Total	RRF[b]
Breast	-	-	10	60	86	46	29	8	1	-	8	248	18.5%
Cervix	-	-	3	41	47	40	38	14	1	-	5	189	14.1%
Liver	-	1	6	10	19	10	12	7	2	-	2	69	4.5%
Other malignant neoplasm of lymphoid tissue	2	8	10	8	10	11	6	2	-	-	4	61	4.5%
Prostate	-	-	-	-	4	6	15	12	5	1	4	47	3.5%
Connective and soft tissues	7	9	9	5	5	2	4	-	-	-	-	41	3.1%
Other malignant neoplasm of skin	1	4	2	6	10	5	7	1	1	-	2	39	2.9%
Burkitt's tumor	15	16	4	-	-	-	-	-	-	-	-	35	2.6%
Stomach	-	-	-	4	4	6	13	6	1	-	1	35	2.6%
Chorion and hydatidiform mole	-	-	14	11	2	-	-	-	-	-	6	34	2.5%

[a]Based on Ibadan Cancer Registry, 1991 data, all cancers (1342: female, 814; male, 528).
[b]RRF = relative ratio frequency.

TABLE 2. Ten Common Cancers in Ibadan (Female)[a]

Cancer Type	Age in Years 0–9	10–19	20–29	30–39	40–49	50–59	60–69	70–79	80–89	90–99	Age Unknown	Total	RRF[b]
Breast	-	-	10	60	86	44	25	8	1	-	8	242	29.7%
Cervix	-	-	3	41	47	40	38	14	1	-	5	189	23.2%
Chorion and hydatidiform mole	-	1	14	11	2	-	-	-	-	-	6	34	4.2%
Ovary	-	1	7	1	7	7	4	1	-	-	1	29	3.6%
Liver	-	1	2	1	5	3	4	4	-	-	-	19	2.3%
Connective and soft tissues	2	3	3	4	4	1	1	-	-	-	-	18	2.2%
Burkitt's tumor	8	6	3	-	-	-	-	-	-	-	-	17	2.1%
Other malignant neoplasm of lymphoid tissue	1	1	3	2	3	2	3	1	-	-	-	17	2.1%
Other malignant neoplasm of skin	-	1	1	4	2	4	3	-	1	-	-	16	2.0%
Other malignant neoplasm of uturus	-	-	-	3	3	2	6	1	-	-	1	16	2.0%

[a]Based on Ibadan Cancer Registry, 1991 data, 814 females.
[b]RRF = relative ratio frequency.

TABLE 3. Ten Common Cancers in Ibadan (Male)[a]

	Age in Years												
Cancer Type	0–9	10–19	20–29	30–39	40–49	50–59	60–69	70–79	80–89	90–99	Age Unknown	Total	RRF[b]
Liver	-	-	4	9	14	7	8	4	2	-	2	50	9.5%
Prostate	-	-	-	-	4	6	15	12	5	1	4	47	8.9%
Other malignant neoplasm of lymphoid tissue	1	7	7	6	7	9	3	1	-	-	3	44	8.3%
Connective and soft tissue	5	6	6	1	1	1	3	-	-	-	-	23	4.4%
Other malignant neoplasm of skin	1	3	1	2	8	1	4	1	-	-	2	23	4.4%
Brain	4	7	2	3	1	2	1	-	-	-	-	20	3.8%
Nasopharynx	-	1	3	3	7	3	1	2	-	-	-	20	3.8%
Trachea, bronchus, lungs	-	-	-	2	1	4	8	4	-	-	-	19	3.6%
Burkitt's tumor	7	10	1	-	-	-	-	-	-	-	-	18	3.4%

[a]Based on Ibadan Cancer Registry, 1991 data, 528 males.
[b]RRF = relative ratio frequency.

Group A: those who take the outlook that destiny determines the path of one's life and that death is the inevitable end;

Group B: those who appreciate the efficacy of hospital treatment but still believe in traditional medical practice and are prepared to combine the traditional and orthodox forms. The pattern employed in giving information to these patients is for the doctor to solicit the help of relatives, especially the older ones in the family and/or a minister of the patient's religion, who will sift out the information to give to the patient; and

Group C: the informed group, which has faith in and is conversant with orthodox medical practice. These patients can afford the cost of medical treatment.

Members of group A usually consult traditional healers, who give varied causes (including intervention of supernatural forces) for any disease process, including cancer. These patients eventually revert to the hospital form of treatment in the very late stages of their illness. Of course, on arrival in hospital they are in the terminal stages. Information about the cause of their illness is usually not given to them; however, relatives are informed about the impending demise of the patients. Relatives and patients continue to believe and hope that by divine intervention a cure may be effected. Terminal cancer patients are not normally admitted into hospitals; and, of course, they do not come back!

Members of group B by and large prefer to be informed of their illness if the outlook is bright. Every patient has to be assessed carefully before revealing to the patient the extent of the illness. Sometimes it is necessary to get relatives or ministers of religion who are closely related to the patient to act as intermediaries in the disclosure of information about cancer to the patient or the relatives. This has a moderating affect on the patient. It has to be pointed out that counseling cancer patients in Nigeria is usually not done by trained personnel. The amount of information revealed about the extent of the disease is determined by the assessment of the patient and the situation, either by the relatives or a minister of religion because of the fear and confusion that blunt information might cause, disturbing the tranquility within the family setting. Sometimes, in order to maintain equilibrium, some facts are deliberately withheld.

Group C consists of people who have knowledge about cancer—e.g., doctors, nurses, lawyers, and teachers. It is difficult to conceal the hard facts from this group because the patient can read about their condition and appreciate the prognosis. This group experiences a lot of emotional disturbance, which requires counseling. Although these patients function adequately in many areas of their lives, they volunteer the information that cancer and its treatment have an effect on their energy, physical and recreational activities, communication with spouse, sexual and emotional functioning, occupational issues, and treatment-related situations—e.g., alopecia following chemotherapy and gynecomastia consequent on hormone therapy in males. Younger patients have more psychological, sexual, and treatment-related problems than the older ones. Some patients within this group, even though they are conversant with their grave condition, prefer not to be told the bare facts at the follow-up clinic; they prefer not to know.

COMMENTS

Diagnosis of cancer places considerable stress on Nigerian patients and requires them to make major adjustments in many areas of their lives. As a consequence, considerable demands are placed on health-care providers to satisfy the complex needs of cancer patients.[3]

Cancer patients need information to promote the understanding of events throughout the illness and support to mobilize coping strategies when they consider that the demands of the situation exceed their personal resources. It has been shown, however, that a communication barrier exists and that information does not always reach the target.[4] Although there is considerable controversy about what information regarding the diagnosis of cancer is most helpful to patients in meeting their psychological and medical needs, little research has been done on what patients are told about their diagnosis and treatment.[5] It is suggested that research in this area in Nigeria is necessary and imperative, bearing in mind the psychological and medical needs of the patient.

The literature suggests that doctors' and nurses' openness about communication with the terminally ill and their families has increased in the past two or three decades, influenced partly by the hospice movement.[6] Gaps in information given to the patients—not being told enough about what is wrong with them, not being told about the reasons for decisions about treatment, and not giving information to relatives about how to care for the patient—must be bridged. This is of particular relevance in the Nigerian setting.

Giving information to cancer patients and their family members regarding the disease, the treatment procedures, and the adaptation process for living with the uncertainty that is inherent in the diagnosis of cancer is often not effective due to people's failure to understand. The impact of emotional stress usually creates communication difficulties. Information that does not take account of the assessed learning needs and individual differences as to learning works against proper understanding.[7]

Informing the cancer patient about the illness is a difficult problem. Physicians are urged to evaluate patients, keeping in mind that most patients want information. In fact, studies show that giving patients adequate information usually impacts positively on their psychological and physical well-being.[8]

It is necessary, once the diagnosis of cancer has been established, to encourage the patient to have a positive attitude towards the illness. Hope is an essential aspect of the therapeutic relationship between cancer patients and their caregivers. Realistic hope provides considerable support, whereas unrealistic hope can be destructive by impairing the ability to make appropriate decisions about treatments and future plans and to be assured of one's personal importance.

Realistic hope exists for cancer patients at all stages of the illness. Provision of realistic hope facilitates the process of breaking bad news. Appropriate hopes are identified from the time of prediagnostic workup through the phase of definitive treatment and into the transition to palliative and supportive care. This is well exemplified by the practice of the Nigerian traditional healers, whose communication and listening skills underscore the importance of providing time and gradual adjustments in hope as the disease progresses.[9]

Traditional healers are primarily of two types—namely, "herbalists" and "diviners." The herbalists are practitioners of an indigenous system of empirical medicine with a vast pharmacopoeia, mainly of herbs and roots. The diviners base their practice on the thought system according to which there are malevolent and benevolent spirits. The traditional healers and their clients believe that when individuals or a group of people offend the malevolent gods by their acts or deeds, the gods can cause illness; and that enemies or detractors can, by magical means, cause diseases, including cancer. Traditional healers are believed to have a means of communicating with the gods. On behalf of their clients they appeal by divination and sacrifice to the benevolent gods for pardon.[10]

The patients (especially those of groups A and B) and the traditional healers in their interaction are from the beginning on the same wavelength. The rapport between them lowers the tension usually encountered at the first patient-doctor meeting, making communication easy.[11] The orthodox medical practitioner needs to borrow a leaf from the traditional healers in the creation and maintenance of rapport.

Information about the practices of these traditional healers is based on interviews grudgingly given, or observation during their treatment sessions. Traditional healers do not normally document their treatment procedures. Traditional healers exercise a lot of patience and spend much time (days or weeks) trying to understand the problem as the cancer patient sees and understands it. They accommodate varied statements of the patients that the orthodox medical doctor may consider outlandish. Orthodox medical practitioners, because of their heavy load of clinical work, have limited time to unravel the deep-seated, complex problems of the cancer patient.

It is obvious, therefore, that there is a need for closer collaboration between orthodox medical practitioners and traditional healers. The federal government of Nigeria has over the years accorded the traditional healers greater recognition and given financial support to some of their institutions. However, most doctors trained under the Western system are very uncomfortable with the claims and methods of traditional healers, while the latter fear that they may be put out of business if they reveal their healing techniques; hence, their resistance to divulging information about their techniques. It is hoped that with time the two systems will collaborate more for the benefit of the patient.

The communication and listening skills incorporated in the cancer management protocol of the Nigerian traditional healers are worthy of further intensive study and of emulation by orthodox conventional medical practitioners. There is a need to modify the current curricula for training nurses, medical students, and postgraduate medical students to include training in oncology with emphasis on listening and communicating skills as they relate to cancer patients.

For advanced cases palliative care needs to include both the patient and the family, because the needs of the family exceed those of the patient.[12] Support teams, doctors, and nurses must perceive the needs of dying patients, and this can be accomplished only through better education and organization of services. The provision of a structured patient education program, to complement the information currently given by hospital staff members, based on assessed needs and planned to meet individual differences in learning readiness and capabilities, is appropriate.

"Telling the whole truth and nothing but the truth" to the patient may have an adverse effect on the cancer patient when the "true" statement appears to be incorrect. There have been many occasions when patients with advanced disease have been informed of a prognosis of about six months to a year and the patients survived five to ten years or more. Such patients tend to doubt their physicians. The physicians, on the other hand, may be disappointed because of their inability to forecast accurately, having relied on the best information available to them at the time of informing their patients. Apparent "untruths" often cause barriers between patients and their caregivers that can lead to psychological isolation of the patients.

Information to the cancer patient must be given on an individual basis, taking into consideration environmental factors, religious beliefs, and attitudes toward death. The cancer patient's great fear and anxiety about his/her condition usually can be decreased by understanding derived from free, frank, kind discussion with the physician and caregivers. This will lead to confidence in dealing with any disability that may result from therapy and preparation for the inevitable outcome. The Oath of Hippocrates, an eternal challenge to generations of physicians, which states, inter alia, "with purity and with holiness I will pass my life and practice my art" should continue to be the guiding principle when giving basic, truthful information to the patient.

REFERENCES

1. MILLER, A. B. &. J. STJERNSWARD, Eds. 1992. National Cancer Control Programme. Policies and Managerial Guidelines. A Handbook Produced by the World Health Organization Global Programme for Cancer Control. World Health Organization Publication WHO/CAN/92.1. Geneva.
2. 1992. Report of the Workshop on "National Cancer Control Programme for Nigeria." Sponsored by the World Health Organization, Geneva; the Federal Ministry of Health, Lagos; and the National Headquarters of Cancer Registries in Nigeria, University College Hospital, Ibadan; and AGIP. Lagos.
3. WIGGERS, J. H., K. O. DONOVAN, S. REDMAN & R. W. SANSOM-FISHER. 1990. Cancer patient satisfaction with care. Cancer **66**(3): 610–616.
4. GRAHN, G. 1993. Learning to cope—An intervention in cancer care. Support. Care Cancer **1**(5): 266–271.
5. MOSCONI, R., B. E. MEYEROWITZ, M. C. LIBERATI & A. LIBERATI. 1991. Disclosure of breast cancer diagnosis: Patient and physician reports. GIVIO (Inderdisciplinary Group for Cancer Evaluation). Ann. Oncol. **2**(4): 273–280.
6. SEALE, C. 1991. Communication and awareness about death: A study of a random sample of dying experience. Soc. Sci. Med. **32**(8): 943–952.
7. GRAHN, G. & J. JOHNSON. 1990. Learning to cope and living with cancer. Learning needs assessment in cancer patient education. Scand. J. Caring Sci. **4**(4): 173–181.
8. SIMINOFF, L. A. 1992. Improving communication with cancer patients. Oncology **6**(10): 83–89.
9. LINKS, M. & J. KRAMER. 1994. Breaking bad news: Realistic versus unrealistic hopes. Support. Care Cancer **2**(2): 91–93.
10. ODEJIDE, A. O., A. O. SANDA, M. O. OLATAWURA & A. O. OYENEYE. 1978. Some socio-psychiatric attributes of patients utilizing the facilities of the traditional healers in the city of Ibadan. Trop. Geogr. Med. **30:** 115–119.
11. OLATAWURA, M. O. 1995. Personal communication.
12. HIGGINSON, I., A. WADE & N. MCCARTHY. 1990. Palliative care: View of patients and their families. Br. Med. J. **301**(6746): 277–281.

Transcultural and Language Problems in Communicating with Cancer Patients in Southern Africa

W. R. BEZWODA,[a] H. COLVIN, AND J. LEHOKA

Division of Clinical Hematology and Medical Oncology
Department of Medicine
University of Witwatersrand Medical School
7 York Road
Parktown 2193
Johannesburg, South Africa

INTRODUCTION

Patterns of Cancer in Southern Africa

South Africa is a multiethnic, multicultural, and multilingual society[1] (TABLE 1 and FIG. 1) with elements of both developed country and third world country health problems. There has sometimes been the perception in Africa that cancer is a disease of affluence and of "Westernization," but cancer registry data hardly bears out this view. While age-standardized incidence rates (ASIRs) as reported by the National Cancer Registry of South Africa[2] (TABLE 2) do appear to show a lower cancer risk in the black population as compared to Caucasians, it should be remembered that this is a pathology-based registry and as such considerably underestimates cancer incidence in less developed and rural populations. Both World Bank and World Health Organization estimates point to the increasing likelihood of cancer overtaking infectious disease as a cause of death in developing countries, including Africa, during the next decade.

Since cancer risks are largely environmentally determined, it is perhaps not surprising that the relative frequency of cancer types differs in different population groups. The five most frequent pathologically diagnosed cancers (excluding basal and squamous cell skin cancers) in various ethnic groups in South Africa are shown in TABLE 3. The available data do, however, indicate that cancer mortality patterns are already changing in South Africa. These changes include an increasing incidence of breast

[a]Corresponding author.

TABLE 1. South African Population Groups in the Nine South African Regions

	KwaZulu-Natal	Gauteng	W. Cape	E. Cape	N. Cape	N. TVL	North-west	E. TVL	Free State
Asian	770,320	147,611	28,514	14,624	1,717	4,334	7,950	10,739	990
Hindi	4,891	475	40	32	0	15	13	75	1
Tamil	4,223	146	27	13	0	0	0	9	0
Black	6,481,914	3,969,007	559,384	5,438,081	220,214	4,551,684	2,845,141	2,387,410	2,161,770
Xhosa	93,533	397,827	522,875	5,162,636	44,635	8,645	195,592	42,947	244,185
Zulu	6,308,717	1,190,743	2,648	46,070	1,926	35,537	88,603	653,761	133,406
N. Sotho	2,963	543,310	1,506	1,306	800	2,633,424	159,755	254,825	20,972
S. Sotho	16,235	696,245	6,655	130,405	3,604	11,507	138,075	44,842	1,383,273
Tswana	1,034	466,727	2,483	1,107	126,774	70,321	1,879,841	49,935	170,075
Colored	106,356	262,516	1,991,437	413,191	377,714	6,548	36,563	15,731	70,596
Afrikaans	9,505	185,159	1,679,473	379,428	365,584	4,082	30,135	10,947	63,364
White	596,935	2,079,199	838,340	369,340	121,329	138,243	263,413	289,981	365,067
English	435,318	836,277	369,951	189,105	10,476	16,447	23,620	41,590	38,040
Afrikaans	138,808	1,137,697	441,356	173,091	109,678	118,083	233,803	297,797	319,622

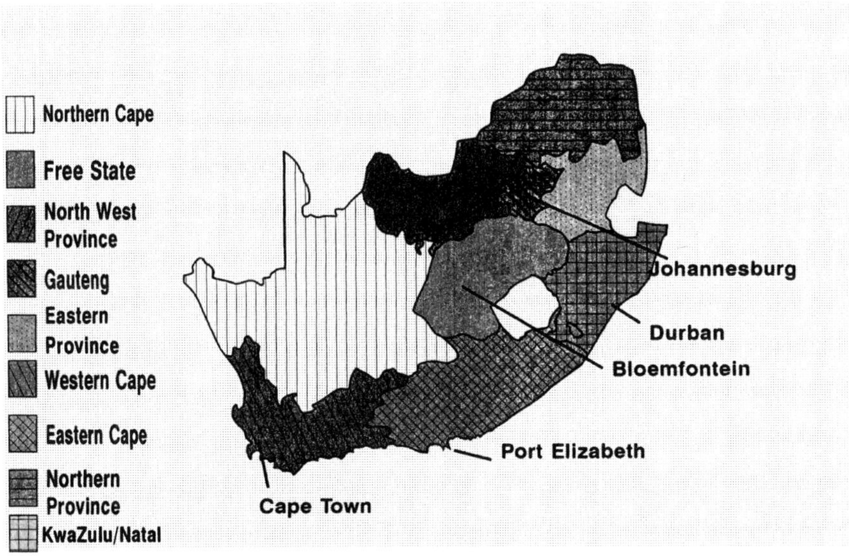

FIGURE 1. Schematic map of the nine provinces of South Africa.

cancer among black females,[3] in line with the experience in "Westernizing" populations.

A notable difference between cancers in the various population groups is the predominance of advanced stages of disease at the time of diagnosis among black patients.[4–6] While there is no clear evidence for an ethnic

TABLE 2. Crude, Age-Standardized Incidence Rates (per 100,000) and Lifetime Risk of Developing Cancer (Excluding Basal and Squamous Cell Skin Cancers) in South Africa

	Crude	ASIR	Risk
Asian			
Female	101.0	142.2	1:6.7
Male	67.4	130.1	1:6.5
Black			
Female	68.6	105.4	1:8.8
Male	64.7	116.8	1:7.8
Colored			
Female	105.6	150.5	1:6.6
Male	107.0	187.7	1:5.1
White			
Female	254.6	212.4	1:6.4
Male	263.5	217.5	1:5.1

TABLE 3. Distribution of the Five Most Frequent Cancers (Excluding Basal and Squamous Cell Skin Cancers) in South African Population Groups

	Female				Male			
	Type	Crude	Percent	ASIR	Type	Crude	Percent	ASIR
Asian								
	Breast	142	23.74	29.76	Lung	52	14.3	19.7
	Cervix	47	9.51	9.58	Prostate	27	7.34	14.3
	PSU[a]	33	6.68	6.92	PSU	36	9.78	14.24
	Endometrium	30	6.07	6.29	Stomach	29	7.88	11.22
Black								
	Cervix	3,446	35.74	40.08	Esophagus	1,806	19.47	25.34
	Breast	1,103	11.44	13.19	Lung	1,008	10.87	14.36
	Esophagus	823	8.54	10.37	PSU	978	10.54	13.58
	PSU	704	7.30	8.29	Prostate	762	8.21	13.0
	Endometrium	357	3.70	4.55	Liver	490	5.28	6.36
Colored								
	Cervix	399	22.43	34.53	Lung	211	12.09	25.23
	Breast	367	20.63	33.56	Prostate	166	9.51	22.72
	PSU	155	8.71	14.39	PSU	188	10.77	21.28
	Stomach	80	4.50	7.78	Stomach	156	8.94	18.24
	Lung	72	4.05	6.65	Esophagus	132	7.56	15.78
White								
	Breast	1,841	18.13	64.42	Prostate	1,028	8.26	43.26
	Melanoma	454	4.47	15.43	Bladder	744	5.98	30.84
	PSU	447	4.40	15.10	Lung	635	5.10	26.49
	Lung	351	3.46	12.12	PSU	450	3.61	18.78
	Colon	378	3.72	11.91	Melanoma	442	3.55	17.39

[a]PSU = primary site unknown.

difference in cancer prognosis per se,[5] late presentation is obviously a factor that influences overall disease outcome. Reasons for such late presentations are likely to reside, among other factors, in access to medical care as well as in patient perceptions of disease. Although the relationship between patient knowledge and compliance is by no means clear,[7–10] there can be no doubt that cultural perspectives (as outlined below) do influence the stage of disease at presentation. Another factor accounting for the apparently poorer treatment outcome in black patients may well be the dire economic consequences of illness experienced by patients who have little economic or job security. The effects of some of these factors on treatment compliance among patients with Hodgkin's disease have previously been documented.[11] While some of these economic consequences may well be amenable to legislative intervention, patients' perception of disease and acceptance of treatment will depend largely on the development of more effective communication systems and skills.

Traditional Beliefs Regarding Illness and Cancer

There has been little systematic study of traditional beliefs about illness and more particularly of perceptions about cancer in the black population. Gelfand,[12] writing in 1944 from a rather patronizing and heavily"Western" perspective, characterized the African population as falling into two groups with respect to lifestyle and outlook. These were the (1) "more or less sophisticated" urban dwellers, whose lifestyle and diet approximate those of the Western population; and (2) "unsophisticated" or rural Africans, whose beliefs remain largely traditional. He considered the typical "African" outlook as fatalistic about illness, with a belief system that emphasizes the primacy of "spiritual" influences on physical health. In particular, beliefs regarding the direct intervention of ancestors or other spirits on life and material welfare, the influence of the witch-doctor (*nganga*), and the malign influence of the wizard or witch were considered important components of traditional beliefs.

While there is no doubt that lifestyle patterns throughout the world have undergone considerable shifts, most frequently in direction of adoption of Western modes, it should be pointed out that this is a phenomenon not specific to Africa.

A more recent study[13] of the beliefs of black women regarding breast cancer (TABLE 4) showed that apparently only a minority (approximately 8%) thought that the illness was the result of witchcraft. This study was done as a structured interview by a trained nursing speaking the patient's own language, and included 100 patients at first presentation with breast cancer. Almost half the patient population belived that the primary lesion in the breast was an abscess. Approximately one-third of patients were not unduly alarmed by the presence of a mass in the breast and did not,

TABLE 4. Attitudes of Black Women to Breast Lumps That Later Proved To Be Breast Cancer

Believed Cause of Primary Breast Tumor	Number	Percent
Abscess	44	44
Not normal	34	34
Witch craft	8	8
Baby burping at breast	7	7
Money kept in brassiere rubbing against breast	6	6
Contraceptive use	1	1

in fact, regard a palpable mass, in the absence of other symptoms, as evidence of illness. The rest related the breast mass either to injury, the consequence of babies burping at the breast, or the consequence of rubbing from money secreted in brassieres (a popular carrying place). Only one patient, a nurse, related the breast mass to the effects of an oral contraceptive she had been using.

While it is possible that there may have been underreporting regarding belief in witchcraft, out of fear that mention of traditional healers may anger "Western" doctors. it should be pointed out that the study was performed by an experienced nurse belonging to the patient's own ethnic and language group. The low percentage who believed in witchcraft appears to be borne out by the finding that when help was sought, only 10% of patients consulted traditonal healers, while fully 81% had their initial consultation in a conventional medical setting. These settings included rural clinics (20%) and regional hospitals (61%). Despite this, the majority of patients (65%) were found to have advanced disease (stage Ill or IV) at the time of referral to an oncology service. Nine percent of patients initially sought advice from various Christian sects (among which the Zion Christian Church is the most powerful in South Africa) regarding breast masses. Many of these sects emphasize spiritual healing as part of their ministry. Patients who had undergone "healing" were often found to present with advanced disease.

It is of interest to compare these findings with the results of a survey of attitudes to breast cancer in a rural United States population, among whom 30% of those diagnosed as suffering from breast cancer were black women.[14] While no significant differences were found in regard to access to medical care by ethnic group, this study similarly found that black women were more likely to present with advanced disease. Another striking similarity to the findings in the South African study was the observation that a significant proportion of these women appeared to find the concept of breast cancer to be fairly new. "Although they were familiar with much of the popular discussion on breast cancer, many reported not having heard of it until recently and not having known anyone who died of it."

If such perceptions can exist in a community with a single predominant language (English) in which the term "cancer" would appear to have passed into common usage, how much more understandable is the situation in South Africa, where among the nine ethnic black languages only three (including Zulu, Swazi, and Xhosa; the Nguni group) have a word for cancer (*Umdlavuza, Umdlopha,* and *Umlaza,* respectively). Although these words are in some senses much more apt than the term "cancer" (crab), it should be noted that the reactions of patients to these words do not include any concept of a disease that may spread to other sites of the body or that requires any special measures to effect cure. While the Western term "cancer" is linguistically meaningless, the concept appears, at least in a greater proportion of Western patients, to trigger the response of seeking medical advice at an earlier stage of the illness.

Health Education and Knowledge about Cancer

Recently there has been a major shift, at least at the level of state health policy, towards emphasizing primary prevention of cancer rather than treatment. While by no means denying the desirability of preventing rather that attempting to cure disease, we do point to some paradoxical effects of health information campaigns in regard to patient perceptions of cancer. In South Africa media campaigns have emphasized sun exposure, smoking, and alchohol (in relation to esophageal cancer) as causes of cancer, as well as the value of healthy eating and exercise as keys to longevity. How relevant the first factor is in a country where the majority of the population is darkly pigmented is a moot point. While the benefits of health promotion campaigns appear self-evident, patients with cancer are often puzzled as to why they should be suffering from this illness despite having no exposure to these generalized risk factors. Indeed, where these public health campaigns have had an impact among the black population, the attitude, when when faced with a diagnosis of cancer, is often disbelief. The power of the media to persuade appears often to be related to a simplified presentation of what is in reality a complex problem.

Such problems may be more general given the nature of primary health education materials. A recent study regarding the utilization of public cancer information materials by Dutch general practitioners[15] found that at least half the respondents had negative attitudes towards the materials supplied, mostly on the basis that generalized information may needlessly provoke anxiety without supplying the context for specific questions about health problems. A proper balance needs to be sought between resource utilization for public health and public education, and that devoted to direct medical care. What the appropriate levels of spending for these various needs are is beyond the scope of this article.

AVAILABILITY AND ACCESS TO CANCER INFORMATION IN SOUTH AFRICA

No comprehensive, publicly funded cancer information service similar to the United States Cancer Information Service (CIS)[16] exists in South Africa, or, indeed, to our knowledge, anywhere on the African continent. A variety of nongovernmental organizations (NGOs) have attempted to fill this need. These include: (1) the Information Service of CANSA (Cancer Association of South Africa); (2) the Cancer Information and Support Services (CISS) Trust; and (3) oncology units at academic and private hospitals in South Africa.

The Cancer Association of South Africa is a charitably funded national organization that undertakes the tasks of cancer education, information, and funding of research and also has some direct involvement with patient care (mostly at the level of providing shelter for out-of-town patients undergoing cancer treatment at hospital facilities as well as home nursing support). For these latter two services, some state funds are made available. The Cancer Association is divided into a national and six regional offices. The major information campaigns of the national office are aimed at primary prevention and also at the promotion of the CANSA slogan "Cancer can be beaten." Two of the regional offices—namely, the Southern Transvaal regional office (Johannesburg) and the Western Cape regional office (Cape Town)—have patient and media centers that provide access to books, videos, audiotapes, and journal articles as well as booklets dealing with various cancers and the treatment modalities and psychosocial aspects of the disease. Verbal information is provided by a coordinator (usually a social worker). Additional information is provided by a panel of physicians who are on call and who are prepared to provide additional, specifically medical information to the coordinator. While some of the material is available in vernacular languages, the vast majority is in English and presupposes a "Western" understanding of disease.

The CISS Trust is an independent charitable trust that was initiated by a patient who felt that there was a need for an organization specifically geared to supplying cancer patients with educational information about specific cancers and their treatments. The CISS trust is based in Johannesburg but is moving towards a regional office structure. The CISS trust has negotiated with various cancer information bodies in other countries to be able to use their materials without royalty charges and in some instances to have the right, subject to suitable acknowledgment, to have the materials translated into various African languages. This process of translation a still in its infancy but will, it is hoped, help to meet the ideal of providing cancer information to all who seek it, in their own language. The problem of whether direct translation is a suitable method of providing information for people of different cultural backgrounds will still, however, have to be faced.

Oncology Units: Specialized oncology units, either radiation oncology or medical oncology based (or both) exist in six main population centers (Johannesburg, Pretoria, Cape Town, Durban, Bloemfontein, and Port Elizabeth). The first five of these cities also have academic training hospitals. A number of these treatment centers and academic units have developed their own patient information system and programs. While many of these centers cooperate, there is no national registry of materials available; and this lack leads to considerable duplication. These oncology centers are also linked mainly to either English- or Afrikaans-speaking universities and have had only limited success, if any, in providing information in the vernacular.

Patient Needs

Most of the surveys of patient information needs have been carried out among the English- and Afrikaans-speaking segments of the population.[17] Since these are Western populations, the responses, not surprisingly, have been similar to those determined in other surveys elsewhere. In this population, as elsewhere, the main information need, as expressed by patients, is the desire to obtain maximum information about their disease.[18] Priorities relate to information about possible effects (including side effects) and success rates of treatments, with more than 80% of respondents indicating a strong desire for as much information as possible about outcome as well as information regarding possible avenues for second opinions. Fewer respondents (around 70%) wanted more information about the physical nature of cancer itself. More emphasis on information resources and self-help/support groups was desired by approximately 50%, while information about "alternative" methods of therapy was wanted by only 40%. It should be remembered, however, that these results may reflect a particular cultural bias.

COMMUNICATION WITH THE CANCER PATIENT

Doctor-Patient Communication

Medical attitudes to disclosure of information about illness are still undergoing changes. The Hippocratic admonition to physicians to perform their duties

> . . . calmly and adroitly, concealing most things from the patient while you are attending him. Give necessary orders with cheerfulness and sincerity, turning his attention away from what is being done to him, sometimes reprove sharply and emphatically, and sometimes comfort with solicitude and attention, revealing nothing of the patient's future or present condition . . .

is yielding, (at least in regard to the disclosure of the diagnosis) to patients' stated desire for more information. A major impetus to formalizing doctors' positions in regard to the provision of information was taken with the publication of the American Hospital's Association's *A Patient's Bill of Rights.* Even in polities where this ethical statement lacks the quasi-legal status that it enjoys in the United States, there can be few physicians who now seriously dispute the patient's right to know. In practice, however, the situation, although improving, is still not ideal. In a survey carried out in the Division of Medical Oncology of the University of the Witwatersrand in 1991, approximately 35% of patients still claimed not to be aware that they had cancer at the time of referral. While this was substantially different from the 65% of patients from 10 years previously who did not know the diagnosis at referral (W. R. Bezwoda, unpublished observations), it still represents less than full disclosure. The ostensible reasons, when they could be established, as to why patients were not told the diagnosis were either to save the patient unnecessary distress and/or pressure from families who did not wish their relative to know the diagnosis.

A more recent study performed among patients attending the hematology/oncology unit of the University of the Witwatersrand (TABLE 5) still shows substantial differences in approach to the provision of health information to patients of different ethnic groups. The results of this study, based on a comprehensive survey of 100 patients (36 black, 11 colored and Asian, and 53 white), showed that black patients were significantly less likely to have information about their cancer provided by a doctor, or in their own language, or to be provided with reading material regarding the disease—this despite substantial efforts in this department to improve patient communication. Black patients were also significantly more likely to have consulted traditional healers or alternative practition-

TABLE 5. Provision of Information in a Multiethnic, Multilingual Oncology Unit

	Percentage Responses			
	Black	Colored and Asian	White	*p* Value
Knew diagnosis at referral	50	55	66	NS[a]
Information given by				
Doctor	61	100	86	<0.05
Nursing sister	30	0	14	
Information given in own language	61	81	86	<0.05
Claimed to have understood information	63	91	72	NS
Were offered reading material	50	73	78	<0.05
Consulted traditional healer or practitioner	36	18	10	<0.02

ers (in this instance mostly traditional healers). Indeed, in this regard this study appears to show considerably more use being made of traditional healers than did the earlier study. The reasons for this difference is probably that the more recent study was carried out among patients who had become "acclimatized" to the clinic and had grown to trust the staff.

While such failures to communicate adequately or to provide understandable information are not unique to the South African situation,[19,20] the difficulties are compounded by language and cultural differences. When communication is attempted either through the medium of a second language (either on the part of the doctor or of the patient) or through a translator, the possibility of failing to communicate adequately increases immeasurably. While it is unrealistic to suppose that these problems can ever be wholly resolved in a multiethnic and multilingual society, at the very least the doctor must be aware of and respect the cultural values of his or her patient. Factors that the Western-trained doctor often finds frustrating in dealing with patients from more traditional societies are the prolonged nature of and wider family involvement in the decision-making process, the resort to traditional healers, and the role of the husband as the absolute arbiter of decisions about his spouse's health.

While each of these processes do occasion situations in which the Western-trained doctor feels that therapy options have been adversely curtailed, the first situation, at least, should be seen as a challenge where, with time, patience, and skill, a treatment program both suitable for and acceptable to the patient can be evolved. The issue of the husband's marital power needs to be addressed by overall sociopolitical changes that improve the status of women and allow them control over their own bodies.

It should also be pointed out that while there are constraints, the doctor-patient relationship in Africa is much less adversarial than it often is in other parts of the world. Patients have an immense trust in the medical profession and in their doctors in particular. Requests for a second opinion are extremely rare, and hospitals are still perceived as places of healing This trust must not be abused.

The Patient-Liaison Nurse

Nurses are seen in virtually all societies as more patient oriented and less threatening caregivers than doctors. In the black community, in particular, the nurse is a higly respected figure and is looked up to as a confidant and guide/leader. The nurse is thus placed in the ideal position to facilitate communication with the cancer patient.

Few institutional positions have been provided in Southern Africa for a specific patient-liaison nurse. By fortunate chance and the good offices of individual chief matrons, a few units—among those the Johannesburg Hospital—have a nursing post dedicated to patient information and communication. This has had a major impact on communication, and a process of evolving a patient education program with emphasis on the needs of black patients is underway. Although group approaches such as the structured "I Can Cope" programs have proved popular among Caucasian patients, social norms and usage dictate a more individual approach in the black population. Personal health problems are discussed only after a process of getting to know each other as individuals; and although teaching materials will provide some assistance, they will not replace the individual approach.

CONCLUSIONS

It is somewhat ironic that the generations of physicians who practiced according to Hippocrates's advice are often looked back upon as providing the most human and caring medical contact, as opposed to mere technical expertise, for their patients. Information alone is obviously not sufficient for adequate communication. Form and content do interact at this level of human activity. Without two-way communication and knowledge of the cultural context, doctors will be tempted to see their role purely in terms of beneficence, regarding the decisions that they make as always in the best interest of the patient, while they may, in truth, be a manifestation of a paternalistic attitude. This temptation is particularly prominent when the "Western"-trained doctor has the weight of scientific truth, as opposed to patient "superstitions,"to back him up. These different perceptions of the meaning of disease do create tension. While it is not the doctor's role to change the entire belief system of the patient, he must in all honesty present and explain cancer and its treatment in scientifically acceptable, cell function–based terms. To do otherwise would be dishonest. When such concepts are unfamiliar to the patients, particular skill and tact need to be exercised to make the information comprehensible. Over and above content, feelings for cultural nuance and style of presentation are required. Personal contact and adequate time are required to foster a good therapeutic relationship. In these relationships the role of the oncologist trained as mediator and reinforcer of the information and education process has been found to be crucial.

REFERENCES

1. 1994. Provincial Statistics Reports 00-90-01 to 00-90-09 Population Census, 1991. South Africa.
2. SITAS, F. & R. PACELLA. 1992. Cancer in South Africa. National Cancer Registry of South Africa Annual Statistical Report for 1989: Incidence and Geographic Distribution of Histologically Diagnosed Cancer in South Africa, 1989. South African Institute for Medical Research. Johannesburg.
3. WYNDHAM, C. H. 1986. A comparison of mortality values for cancer in black adults: 1970 vs. 1980. S. Afr. Med. J. **70:** 469–471.
4. WALKER, A. R. P., B. F. WALKER, B. N. TSHABALALA, C. ISAACSON & I. SEGAL. 1984. Low survival of South African black women with breast cancer. Br. J. Cancer **49:** 241–244.
5. DANSEY, R. D., P. HESSEL, M. BROWDE, M. LANGE, D. DERMAN, M. NISSENBAUM & W. R. BEZWODA. 1988. Lack of a significant independent effect of race on breast cancer survival. Cancer **61:** 1908–1922.
6. PEGORARO, P., V. KARNAN, D. NIRMAL & S. JOUBERT. 1986. Estrogen and progesterone receptor among women of different racial groups. Cancer Res. **46:** 2117–2120.
7. COHEN, S. J. 1970. New Directions in Patients' Compliance. Lexington Books. New York, NY.
8. HAYNES, R. B. 1976. A critical review of the "determinants" of patient compliance with therapeutic regimens. *In* Compliance with Therapeutic Regimens. D. L. Sackett & R. B. Hayes, Eds.: 26–39. Johns Hopkins University Press. Baltimore, MD.
9. MCKINLEY, J. 1972. Who is really ignorant—physician or patients? J. Health Soc. Behav. **16:** 3–9.
10. PODELL, R. N. 1975. Physicians' Guide to Compliance in Hypertension. Merck. West Point, PA.
11. BEZWODA, W. R. Treatment of Hodgkin's disease in Southern Africa. In press.
12. GELFAND, J. 1944. The Sick African. Post Graduate Medical Press. Cape Town.
13. LEHOKA, J. 1988. Cultural Perspectives of Breast Cancer. 5th International Conference on Cancer Nursing, London.
14. MATHEWS, H. F., D. R. LANNIN & J. P. MITCHELL. 1994. Coming to terms with advanced breast cancer: Black women's narratives from eastern North Carolina. Soc. Sci. Med. **38:** 789–800.
15. VISSER, A., I. ALKEMA & K. VAN KOPPEN. 1994. Public cancer information by GP's: Evaluation of a Dutch campaign. Patient Educ. Counseling **24:**

117–125.
16. FREIMATH, V. S. 1989. Searching for Health Information. The Cancer Information Service Model. University of Pennsylvania Press. Philadelphia, PA.
17. MCLOUGHLIN, H. A. 1984. The Information Needs of Cancer Patients in the Republic of South Africa. Dissertation, Faculty of Arts, Rand Afrikaans Univeristy.
18. LEHOKA, J., H. COLVIN, S. MASHISHI, S. BELL & W. R. BEZWODA. Patient information about cancer in different ethnic groups. In press.
19. DERDIARIAN, A. K. 1978. Informational needs of newly diagnosed cancer patients. Part 1. Cancer Nurs. **10:** 107–115.
20. DERDIARIAN, A. K. 1986. Informational needs of recently diagnosed cancer patients. Nurs. Res. **35**: 27–35.

Communication with the Cancer Patient in Zimbabwe

L. M. LEVY[a]

Department of Medicine
Medical School
University of Zimbabwe
Harare, Zimbabwe

INTRODUCTION

A high level of communication between patient and doctor is obviously desirable but may be difficult to achieve, particularly in the filed of oncology. The word "communication" encompasses may aspects of the patient-doctor relationship, including the provision of information and support by the doctor and freedom to ask questions, make decisions, and discuss concerns and problems throughout the illness by the patient.

Telling patients the diagnosis and discussing all aspects and implications of the disorder is an obligation that must be met by doctors or, in some instances, other health workers. That the patient has a right to know is indisputable, yet there is much debate about how much to tell, and when and how to tell it.[1–3] All are agreed that bad news needs to be broached in a positive way that the patient can accept and understand. It is important to preserve hope, as the devastated patent will be extremely distressed and quite unable to make rational decisions on medical or personal issues.

Many cancer patients are critical about the information they receive from doctors and the manner in which the diagnosis is given and in which diagnostic procedures and treatment options are discussed.[4,5] Furthermore, research has shown that doctors generally underestimate both the amount and type of information their patients want, which increases uncertainty, anxiety, distress, and dissatisfaction on the part of the patient.[5,6]

Why are so many doctors unable to impart bad news in an acceptable manner? There are numerous reasons, but essentially they are reluctant to cause distress, unable to cope with the range of emotional reaction that may follow, and often uncertain about how much the patient wishes to

[a]Address for correspondence: Department of Medicine, Parirenyatwa Hospital, P.O. Box A 178, Avondale, Harare, Zimbabwe.

know. Little, if any, training in delivering bad news is given in most medical schools, yet there are many sources of helpful advice.[7–15]

It is equally important for the doctor to develop good listening skills and the ability to establish rapport with the patient.[16] This will increase the patient's confidence and trust so that he/she will be more easily able to communicate concerns.

Communication difficulties occur throughout the world and are confronted in different ways in different countries.[2,3,17] Health attitudes, beliefs, and behavior are products of culture, and are particularly important considerations when dealing with people from cultures different from one's own.[8] Furthermore, if doctor and patient have different first languages, meaningful communication may be limited. In Zimbabwe communication is greatly influenced by traditional medical beliefs, cultural mores, and social factors. The discussion below reflects my personal experience in working with cancer patients in Zimbabwe.

BACKGROUND INFORMATION ON ZIMBABWE

Zimbabwe is a land-locked country in Central Africa, with a population of 10 million. The vast majority of people are black and of either the Shona tribe living in the northeastern part of the country or the Ndebele tribe living in the southwestern areas. The population is predominantly rural based, with 70–80% of people living in communal and commercial farming areas. For patients in rural areas, travel to the main cities is difficult and expensive. The most usual means of transport is by bus, and there is fairly comprehensive service along main roads. Off the major highways service is much more limited, and patients may have to walk long distances to the nearest bus stop.

According to a study carried out in the mid-1980s, almost all Zimbabwean patients had received some primary education with only 14% receiving any secondary- or tertiary-level teaching. Since then educational opportunities have increased, so educational status varies with age, with younger people achieving a higher level of schooling.

Approximately one-third of adults are in salaried employment, most of the remainder being subsistence farmers. On a socioeconomic ranking of six groups specifically designed for use in Zimbabwe,[19] some 60% of people fall into the lowest group. Most people living in rural areas have traditional-style houses made of poles plastered with mud and thatched roofing. There is no piped water or waterborne sanitation. In high-density urban areas the houses are constructed of brick, with iron or asbestos roofing. Piped water and waterborne sanitation are usually present. Such accommodation is in short supply and often overcrowded. Urban squatter camps with no amenities are numerous.

The Shona tribe comprises a people on whom traditional beliefs exert a very strong influence. The concept of original home is vital in this regard. Wherever a person may be staying, it is rural home that provides the spiritual and emotional identity. In this place there is a sense of permanence and continuity in terms of ancestral links and ownership of land, buildings, and cattle. It is here that most people return for holidays and retirement, and also where advice will be sought in times of crisis, even if the person has been living and working in town for many years.

Closely related to this strong bond with the rural home is the belief that deceased relatives control family affairs. These beliefs greatly affect attitudes towards illness. It is not uncommon for a specific illness to be attributed to an expression of displeasure by an ancestral spirit, and the remedy will be seen to lie in acts of appeasement. Another cause of illness is believed to be the casting of spells by grudge-bearing individuals.

Faith in traditional healers is deeply engrained in Shona culture. It is believed that the traditional healer will determine the cause of illness and decide what must be done to propitiate the offended spirit.[20] In most instances traditional healers will treat patients with scarification and/or herbal remedies, but some concentrate on the spiritual approach. Occasionally a healer may recommend that the patient consult a doctor; others advise against any approach to the formal health centers.

Medical centers to serve this population include four central hospitals with specialist facilities, plus a larger number of peripheral hospitals and clinics. Over the past few decades in Zimbabwe attention has centered on the development of primary health care and preventive medicine. Curative services have been largely involved with infectious and nutritional disorders. More recently attention has turned to chronic disease, of which cancer forms a large part. Over 5,000 new cancer patients are recorded by the Cancer Registry each year; but this is a gross underestimate, with the true figure thought to be in the region of 15,000.

There are two main oncology centers where facilities such as radiotherapy equipment, cytotoxic drugs and trained personnel are concentrated. These centers are in Harare (the northeastern region) and Bulawayo (the southwastern region). The majority of cancer patients are referred to these units for investigation, treatment, and follow-up.

BREAKING BAD NEWS (DIAGNOSIS)

Informing the patient that he has a malignant condition is an early first step in communication. Every patient has the right to know his diagnosis, and although study results vary, research shows that most patients do want to have this information.[3,21,22] In some countries—e. g., the United States, Canada, and the United Kingdom—it is usual to tell the patient the diagnosis, though there may be exceptions to this rule.[17,23,24] In other countries the diagnosis is often withheld from the patient, though relatives may be informed.[3,17,25,26]

In developed countries most people have some understanding of the word "cancer," though it may mean different things to patient and doctor.[24,27] To many it is a single entity that is painful and fatal and obviously generates a mixed emotional reaction of which fear is a major component.

In Zimbabwe the situation is quite different, as most Shona patients have little or no concept of cancer. There is no word in the Shona vocabulary for cancer. Words meaning a mole burrowing in the ground or parasitic mistletoe are used by a few people, showing some understanding of the nature of the disease. On being told the diagnosis, most patients here do not respond with the range of emotional reactions described elsewhere but usually ask "What is that?' or (anxiously) "Is it AIDS?" These questions are closed followed by "What has caused it?" While there may be advantages in having patients with no preconceived misconceptions, it is difficult to answer these questions briefly and simply in what is often the first consultation. The most satisfactory approach seems to be a brief explanation of the nature of cancer in general, at a level compatible with the patient's educational background, with the promise of a fuller discussion the following day. Here, as elsewhere, patients are able to absorb only small amounts of information at any one time.

The causation of cancer poses a very difficult problem, and virtually every patient asks about this. Explanations of uncontrolled growth or predisposing causes (such as hepatitis B or bilharzia) are met with blank stares of total incomprehension. Many patients firmly believe they have displeased an ancestral spirit or that a spell has been cast on them.

At the second discussion the nature of the illness is described in greater detail, as are the necessary investigations. Treatment options and possible outcomes are introduced in broad outline only at this stage. The following day patients are asked what they understand of their illness and if they found the discussions helpful. The responses range from good understanding and satisfaction through to denial that any discussion took place. Repeated explanations and discussion follow.

TREATMENT SELECTION

In many countries prognosis seems to be the next issue discussed, but in Zimbabwe once the diagnosis has been explained the patient usually asks what can be done about it. Although the aims of treatment—i.e., cure, disease control, symptom control, or terminal care—are defined, more detailed discussion of prognosis is usually deferred.

An attempt is made to discuss possible side-effects and toxicity in such a way that the patient will not be terrified. This area is fraught with difficulty in some cases. If, for example, infertility is a possible result of treatment in a young woman, the social and cultural implications for her are enormous.

Problems relating to inappropriately intensive regimens in terminally ill patients do not often arise in Zimbabwe. Because of the limited resources, national cancer treatment policy dictates that intensive, expensive programs are offered only to those patients with prospects of a good outcome.

Following discussion of the treatment options, a few patients decline therapy and request discharge. Most are not seen again, some will present at a later date with even more advanced disease, and strangely, a few continue to attend the clinic, willing to accept treatment for infections, etc., but no anticancer therapy.

Most patients are, however, willing to undergo treatment. Unlike their counterparts in many countries,[28] they seldom express a preference for a particular modality or regimen. "Its up to you, doctor" is the common response. The concept of clinical trials is readily understood by most patients, and they are willing to participate, provided they are assured that no particular treatment is known to be superior.

The use of statistical life-expectancy data in consideration of treatment options and prognosis has become controversial in some countries.[21] These strategies are generally inappropriate for Zimbabwe and are used only occasionally at the patient's request.

In Zimbabwe the traditional healer holds an extremely important place in society. In past years it was unusual for any patient to approach the health services without having consulted a traditional healer first. This is slowly changing, but for many patients there is still conflict. Alternating between the two is common, and some patients feel the safest option is to employ both methods simultaneously. It is essential that Western-trained doctors acknowledge and respect these beliefs. Ridicule and scepticism immediately destroy rapport between patient and medical personnel. With two very different forms of medical care, it is understandable that the patient may first avail himself of the one that is both readily available and an inherent part of the culture.

PROGNOSIS

Discussing prognosis with a patient who has an early stage of a malignancy that is highly amenable to treatment poses few problems for doctors. Unfortunately, in Zimbabwe most patients present with advanced disease.

Informing a patient of a poor prognosis is a most difficult and unpleasant task and appears to be even more controversial than breaking the news about diagnosis. In theory many agree that the debate should center not on whether to tell the patient with incurable disease the prognosis, but on how to do so.[1] In practice, however, the situation is often different, and the information provided differs from doctor to doctor, patient to patient, and country to country. In Japan and parts of Europe for example most doctors will withhold the truth from terminally ill patients;[7,25,29] and in Spain the concept of "bearable truth" is used, with limited information being given.[3] Even in countries where litigation may follow, the full prognosis may not be disclosed.[21]

How and when to tell the patient about the expected outcome are also very important considerations. We feel it is preferable in most cases to provide small amounts of information over a period of time, being guided by the patient as to how fast to proceed and whether a family member should be present. In Zimbabwe it appears that patients are more comfortable, particularly in the early stages of the patient-doctor relationship, discussing what will happen to the tumor rather than what will happen to the person. Telling the patient that the tumor cannot be eradicated but that treatment should prevent it from growing for a time, or that the tumor will continue to grow but problems such as pain or bleeding will be treated promptly wherever possible, seems to be a method of providing information that is well received.

No Shona patient has ever asked me how long he or she has to live. Efforts to encourage patients to express fears and anxieties about dying are often unsuccessful, particularly in the early stages of the relationship. But with patience and empathy a time comes when the patient reveals that the concept of impending death has been accepted. For example, a patient may request that a letter be written to his place of work seeking confirmation that his pension will continue after death, or may state that a teenage relative has come to live with the family to help with care of the children "afterwards."

At this point the majority of Shona patients appear to face death with serenity and/or resignation. This may be because death is seen as part of a natural cycle and there is a strong cultural belief in an afterlife. Alternatively it may be that the patients are unwilling or unable to express their concerns and fears on this issue. Most terminally ill patients express a wish to return to the ancestral home.

CONTINUATION OF COMMUNICATION

Continuation of two-way communication throughout the course of the illness is vital. It has been documented that doctors are not good at recognizing psychological and other distress in patients.[30,31] Regrettably this is often the case in Zimbabwe. New patients are usually admitted to the relative calm of the ward for investigations and initiation of treatment, and in this environment meaningful communication is possible.

Subsequent consultations and treatments take place in a busy outpatient department, where it is easy to overlook the patient's needs. Attention of the workers may be further diverted by organizational matters such as locating the latest drug consignment, finding out when the radiotherapy machines will be functional again, or why there has been yet another protocol violation in a particular study. Yet it is imperative that time and space be found to allow patients to discuss their problems. When psychological stress is recognized, it appears that meaningful intervention is the exception rather than the rule.[32] Even with the best will in the world, this often pertains here. Because of the pressure of work, access to psychiatrists and psychologists is limited, and counseling falls largely on members of the basic oncology team.

Medical workers tend to assume that all anxieties will be directly related to the disease process, treatment, or prognosis; yet in Zimbabwe this is frequently not the case. Sympathetic questioning will often reveal a host of other worries to do with transport to the hospital; length of time away from home, work or school; care of the children; or financial concerns. In view of the socioeconomic background of most patients, these issues need to be addressed and resolved as far as possible. They form an integral part of quality of life, a concept that has only relatively recently been recognized perhaps as the most important outcome of patient care. Social workers are in short supply, so most of this work will fall on the doctors or nurses in the oncology unit. Patients greatly appreciate help with these social problems.

The Cancer Association and Island Hospice have branches in several areas in Zimbabwe. They perform excellent work in counseling and both psychological and practical support. Their assistance is sought whenever appropriate.

Compliance is an issue greatly affected by the level of communication between patient and doctor/medical team. The greater the understanding of all aspects of the disease and treatment, the more likely the patient is to comply with treatment. When patients fail to attend the clinic, efforts are made to trace them. Reasons for dropout are numerous, but the most common are "No money," "I was so well I did not think I needed any more treatment," and "I was too ill to come." The latter may be rather puzzling until one considers the arduous journey many patients have to undertake.

Group discussion sessions have had considerable success in improving communication in Zimbabwe. People with similar conditions but at different stages of treatment are invited to attend one (or more) sessions. These meetings provide patients with an opportunity to talk about problems and anxieties in a relaxed atmosphere and have proved popular. "Old timers" are of great assistance in encouraging new patients.

CONCLUSIONS

Communication with cancer patients, both in terms of providing information about the disease and in encouraging patients to express their views and fears, is beset with problems common throughout the world. In addition to these common issues, communication between patient and doctor in Zimbabwe is greatly affected by traditional beliefs. Social factors are also important. Lack of a conceptual model for malignancy is an important factor limiting the understanding by patients of the disease process and the aims of treatment. Furthermore, traditional views about the origin and treatment of disease and the presence of two very different treatment options (traditional and conventional) lead to considerable confusion in some patients. The importance of understanding these cultural aspects is vital in the establishment of good communication between patient and doctor.

REFERENCES

1. HOLCOMBE, R. F. 1994. Informed consent, cancer and truth in prognosis (letter). N. Engl. J. Med **331**(12): 811.
2. SURBONE, A. 1993. The information to the cancer patient: Psychosocial and spiritual implications. Supportive Care in Cancer **1**(2): 89–91.
3. ESPINOSA, E, P. ZAMORA & M. GONZALEZ BARON. 1994. Informed consent, cancer and truth in prognosis. N. Engl. J. Med **331**(12): 811.
4. AUDIT COMMISSION. 1993. What seems to be the matter? Communication between hospitals and patients. NHS Report 1993; No. 12. HM Stationery Office. London.
5. FALLOWFIELD, L. J, S. FORD & S. LEWIS. 1994. Information preferences of patients with cancer. Lancet **344:** 1576.
6. FALLOWFIELD, L. J. 1993. Giving sad and bad news. Lancet **341:** 476–478.
7. FAULKNER, A, P. MAGUIRE & C. REGNARD. 1994. Breaking bad news—A flow diagram. Palliative Med. **8**(2): 145–151.
8. NELSON-JONES, R. & W. CONSOLO. 1994. How to assess thinking skills in cancer patients. Palliative Med. **8**(2): 115–121.
9. FAWZY, F. I & N. W. FAWZY. 1994. A structural psychoeducational intervention for cancer patients. Gen. Hosp. Psychiatry **16**(3): 149–192.
10. FAULKNER, A, P. MAGUIRE & C. REGNARD. 1994. Dealing with anger in a patient or relative: A flow diagram. Palliative Med. **8**(1): 51–57.
11. LINKS, M, J. KRAMER. 1994. Breaking bad news: Realistic versus unrealistic hopes. Supportive Care in Cancer **2**(2): 91–93.
12. WIST,E. 1993. Teaching communication with cancer patients and terminally ill patients to medical students. J. Cancer Educ. **8**(2)119–122.
13. FREEDMAN, B. 1993. Offering truth. One ethical approach to the uninformed cancer patient. Arch. Intern. Med. **153**(5): 572–576.
14. SARDELL, A. N. & S. J. TRIERWEILER. 1993. Disclosing the cancer-diagnosis. Procedures that influence patient hopefulness. Cancer **72**(11): 3355–3365.
15. CREAGAN, E. T. 1994. How to break bad news—And not devastate the patient. Mayo Clin. Proc **69**(10): 1015–1017.
16. ROSENBLUM, D. 1994. Listening to people with cancer. Semin. Oncol. **21**(6):

701–704.
17. MUJAJI, N. T. 1994. Informed consent, cancer and truth prognosis. N. Engl. J. Med. **331**(12): 810.
18. OLWENY, C. 1994. The ethics and conduct of cross-cultural research in developing countries. Psycho-oncology **3:** 11–20
19. CASTLE, W. M. 1978. Measurement of socio-economic status in an urban African community. Trop. Doct. **8:** 44–48.
20. GELFAND, M. 1971. The principles and practice of the n'anga. Centr. Afr. J. Med. **17:** 67–78.
21. ANNAS, G. J. 1994. Informed consent, cancer and truth in prognosis. N. Engl. J. Med. **330:** 223–225.
22. CENTENO-CORTES, C. & J. M. NUÑEZ-OLARTE. 1994. Questioning diagnosis disclosure in terminal cancer patients: A prospective study evaluating patients' responses. Palliative Med. **8**(1): 39–44.
23. MURRAY, J. A. 1994. Telling the truth (letter). Lancet **344**(8916): 196.
24. BREWIN, T. B. 1994. Telling the truth (letter). Lancet **343**(8911): 1512.
25. SANTOS, Z. M, G. SANTOS & P. ABRANTES. 1994. Physician-patient communication in oncology (Portuguese). Acta Med. Portuguese **7**(6): 361–365.
26. TAN, T. K, F. C. TEO, K. WONG & H. L. LIM. 1993. Cancer: To tell or not to tell. Singapore Med. J. **34**(3): 202–203.
27. GILBERT, J. 1994. Telling the truth (letter). Lancet **344**(8916): 196.
28. MAZUR, D. J & D. H. HICKAM. 1994. The effect of physician's explanations on patients' treatment preferences: Five year survival data. Med. Decision Making **14**(3): 255–258.
29. THOMSEN, O. O, H. R. WULFF, A. MARTIN & P. A. SINGER. 1993. What do gastroenterologists in Europe tell cancer patients? Lancet **341**(8843): 473–476.
30. FORD, S, L. J. FALLOWFIELD & S. LEWIS. 1994. Can oncologists detect distress in outpatients and how satisfied are they with their performance during bad news consultations? Br. J. Cancer **70:** 767–770.
31. JONES, R. V & B. GREENWOOD. 1994. Breast cancer: Causes of patients' distress identified by qualitative analysis. Br. J. Gen. Practice **44**(385): 370–371.
32. RUCKDESCHEL, J. C, C. G. BLANCHARD & T. ALBRECHT. 1994. Psychosocial oncology research. Where we have been, where we are going and why we will not get there. Cancer **74**(4 Suppl.): 1458–1463.

Talking to a Child with Cancer

A Valuable Experience

BLANCA DIEZ,[a] EULALIA LASCAR, AND
ANGELICA ALIZADE

Buenos Aires, Argentina

INTRODUCTION

Pediatricians and health professionals who care for children know very well that talking with children and mothers is a challenging aspect of their day-by-day work. We need to talk with them in many different situations. Talking to the child is a very important part of their care and of the treatment of his/her disease. Sometimes we wish to prepare and put the child at ease before a physical examination or an invasive procedure. This is a very common aspect of our work and is appreciated by our patients and their families. We do know that timely explanations can greatly diminish stress and fears. Talking with children, particularly those with terminal illness, allows us to know whether there are any factors in the environment that can cause unexpected symptoms, and of course this knowledge helps us manage these symptoms, giving importance to the details. Children need to know what is wrong and like to discuss diagnosis and treatment. To explain how we communicate with our children with cancer and their families, we would like to describe some features of our country and its people that are quite different from those of most other countries in South America.

Argentina is a very large country, with a continental area of 2,776,888 km^2. (France has an area of 543,988 km^2.) The distribution of the population is very unbalanced. The average population density for the country as a whole is only 10.1 inhabitants/km^2. Yet in the Federal District there are 14,660.8 inhabitants/km^2, and in the province of Santa Cruz barely 0.5 inhabitants/km^2 (FIG. 1). Most of the people live in cities (83%).[1,2]

The ethnic predominance is Caucasian (mostly Spanish and Italian), with some mixture of aborigines and Caucasians, and a minority of pure aborigines (FIG. 2). It is, indeed, exceptional to find anyone of black African descent.[3]

We do not have reliable data about the general incidence of childhood cancer in Argentina. We do know that in the Federal District cancer in children and adolescents (1–19 years) is by far the most frequent medical

[a]Address for correspondence: Billinghurst 2135 9/B, (1425) Buenos Aires, Argentina.

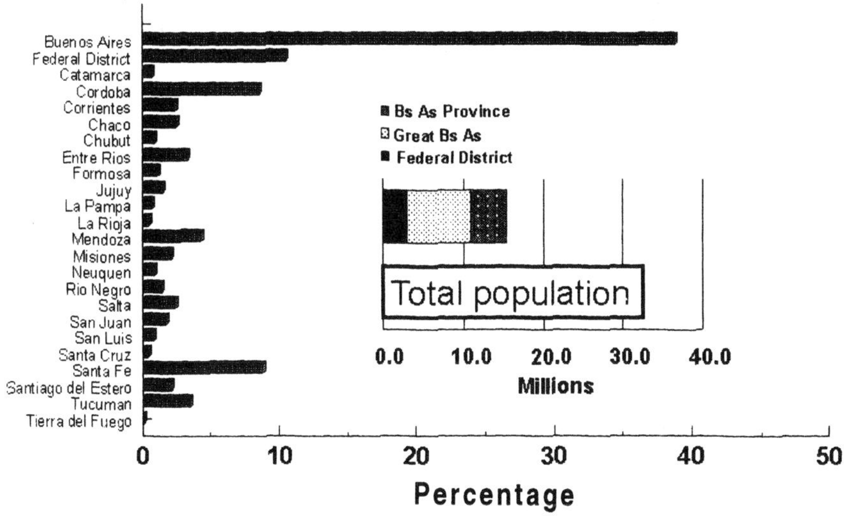

FIGURE 1. Distribution of the population of Argentina.

cause of death (FIG. 3).[4] This is also true for the country as a whole between ages 5 and 19 (FIG. 4).[5–7]

INFORMATION GIVEN AT DIAGNOSIS AND DURING CURATIVE TREATMENT

Talking about cancer in Argentina is arduous. The word "cancer" is still synonymous with death. The knowledge of the population at large about childhood cancer is at best very poor. The possibility that a child might have such an illness and the possibility of a cure are unknown by the majority. Because of this it is very difficult at diagnosis to talk with the child or the parents about the existence of cancer.

An important point is privacy; this is always essential. In our country it is often very difficult to find privacy. Hospitals (even private ones) are very noisy, and doctors in general do not consider privacy important. Frequently there are no separate conference rooms in which to meet the child and his family, and thus we suffer many interruptions when we are talking about the illness, the treatment, or the prognosis. It is very difficult to find a place with closed doors.

There are a number of important issues in communicating with children and adolescents. The first thing is to be honest. The truth carefully put is always more helpful than a distortion or an evasion, which could cause a feeling of isolation. We speak about the disease without using the word "cancer." Children learn very quickly about difficult words such as

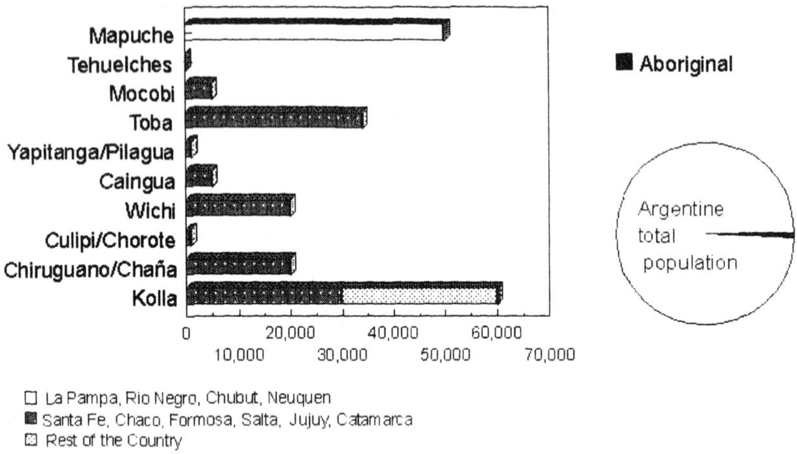

FIGURE 2. Proportion of aboriginal population in Argentina.

rhabdomyosarcoma or neuroblastoma, and use them when they explain to their pals about the disease they have. The child most often learns that a rhabdomyosarcoma is cancer, making the association that his/her treatment is similar to that of an adult known to have cancer. The child frequently comments on television movies about cancer.

In religion our population is primarily Christian (predominantly Catholic), with Jewish being in a distant second place.[8] A minority of the population profess other religions or are agnostic. Most Argentines are not actively religious; but when a serious illness such as cancer is present, religious beliefs become stronger in the family of the child and among the extended family, neighbors, friends, schoolmates, and teachers. We seriously need to take into account, when we talk with these families and the child him-/herself, their beliefs and also the beliefs of the social group to which they belong. In our country, the family characteristics very much determine our approach to the ill child and to truth-telling about the disease.

If the aim of the meeting is explanation of the treatment, it is appropriate for both parents to be present, but the doctor has to be sure that the child is properly included in the discussion. In certain circumstances the child is seen alone, particularly if a teenager. Individual interviews are used to explore private matters, fears, doubts. The child must have the opprotunity to ask questions that they are afraid or ashamed to ask in the parents' presence.

Taking into account and respecting the family and child's beliefs, we try to teach the parents the truth about the characteristics of the disease,

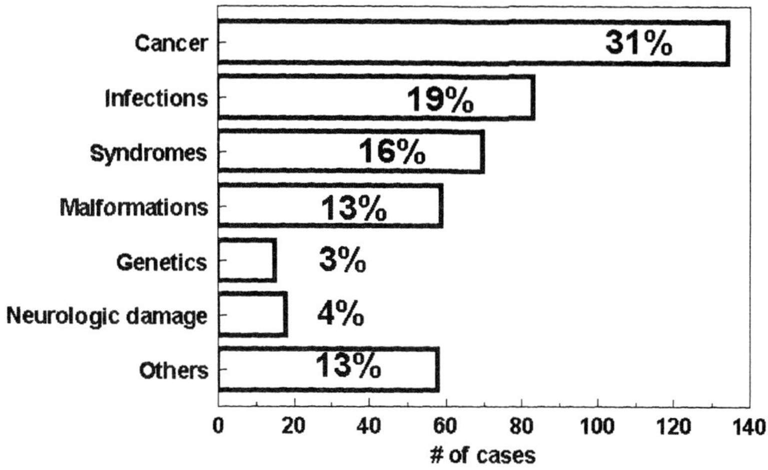

FIGURE 3. Distribution of medical causes of death of persons aged 1–19 years in the Federal District.

the treatment, and the prognosis. We are particularly flexible about who gives the information to the child, trying to meet the needs of each particular case. If the parents give the information, we plan a follow-up meeting with the child to check that he/she actually understood what was said about the illness and the treatment. In this follow-up meeting, the family can be present or not, as they wish and according to the age of the child. Children older than 10 years are very grateful if they can meet a health-care team member without their parents being present.

> Mariana, nine years old, had a local relapse of an osteosarcoma after an "en bloc" resection. Blanca talked with her parents about the amputation. The father asked, very firmly, that he be the one to tell his daughter about the surgical decision. After Mariana talked with her father at home, she had a meeting with Blanca and the orthopedic surgeon to clarify medical issues involving the surgery and the rehabilitation. She had an uneventful surgery with good, quick recovery

Adolescents have a remarkable capacity for denial. We need to learn ways of helping them and getting them to share their worries. A clear memory of one's own adolescence may be helpful during such difficult conversations.

> Juan, 18 years old, had a testicular tumor. Two years later, in a psychotherapeutic session, he came out with, "Almost without any informa-

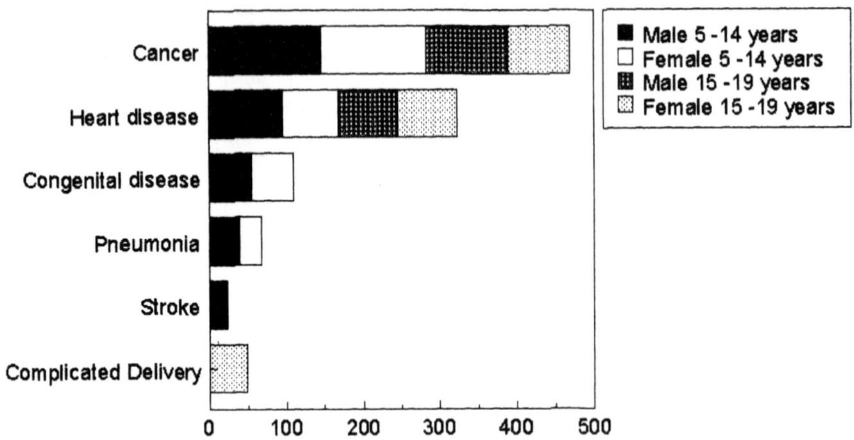

FIGURE 4. Distribution of medical causes of death of persons aged 5–19 years in Argentina.

tion I had an orchiectomy. When I woke up, I had a prosthesis instead of my own testicle. Nobody told me about the diagnosis. I thought that with the operation I would be cured. I felt very embarrassed to talk about the operation and the prosthesis with my mother or my girlfriend. I was discharged from the hospital with a letter for another doctor, who knew about the illness I had. The other doctor was a female doctor. She examined me and looked at the CT and the other reports the surgeon sent her. I was very anxious. I very eagerly awaited what the new doctor was going to say: "Is everything all right?" "Well . . . yes, but the disease you have is a tumor called germinal tumor. The CT also shows that you have a node in the abdomen, and this blood test shows that the node has the same tumor that was in the testicle." "For the first time I learned what I had. I am very grateful that the first time I saw my doctor she only explained what I had without using the word *cancer.* She told me the truth, but slowly. If she had told me that I had cancer that day, I think I would have died."

On very infrequent occasions we have the opportunity to treat a patient with very different cultural or religious beliefs from our own. This happened when we cared for an aboriginal child:

José, 12 years old, is a "Toba" Indian who lives in a reservation in the Province of Formosa (1400 km north of Buenos Aires). He was brought by his father to the Federal District because of a huge tumor in his leg. After admission to a hospital he was diagnosed as having an osteosarcoma

> without metastasis. Blanca gave the father the diagnosis and explained that the only chance for a cure was amputation followed by medication. José's father refused the amputation. "It is better that he die." He forbade Blanca to talk with José about this. Blanca asked for the help of a social worker who knew more about the Toba culture. "Perhaps we can ask the permission of a judge to talk with José and explain the situation to him. He is old enough to decide about his own life." The social worker told Blanca that in this case it would be unwise to do this. The Toba culture believes very strongly in reincarnation. José could not be reincarnated if he had an amputation. His soul would wander forever. If we forced treatment by means of the law and against the father's will, upon his return home the child would become a pariah in his own village. José went back home with only analgesics and died seven months later. It was very hard for us to endure this. The social worker told us afterwards that José talked with her, enthusiastically, about the new, healthy body he would have when he came back to earth again.

Truth-telling in childhood cancer is slowly changing in Argentina, for the better.

> María had a diagnosis of acute lymphoblastic leukemia in 1981 at the age of 10 years. She was told she had "anemia." In 1993 she came back with back pain and paraparesis. She was very upset about the symptoms and about the possibility that the "anemia" could relapse. All the workup was normal. Talking with her about the diagnosis she really had in 1981 was very useful. For the first time she could ask about the illness. She could also speak about the cancer she suspected she had and her fears about death. After these conversations all the symptoms disappeared. Today she enjoys perfect health. She is married and is the mother of a healthy girl.

PALLIATIVE CARE

Talking with the child is always a two-way process, and this is particularly true with the very ill child. Listening is the most important part. This is a dark point in our culture. We are used to talking all the time without listening to each other. We are very afraid of silence, of body communication. Listening involves not only hearing what the child says, but also noticing how it is said (tone of voice, body posture, eye contact, and facial expression). Children choose a favorite person to talk with, and it may be a parent, a doctor, or a nurse.

We try to start the discussion with a neutral, nonthreatening topic, such as the child's toys, clothes, or favorite soccer team, rather than the common "How are we today?" Using cognizance of the child's responses, imagination, and creativity, it is relatively easy to complete a good physical examination or to find out private themes that require additional exploration or discussion. Teamwork and empathy with the child make communication easier. Children communicate verbally and nonverbally, and both forms are equally important. Play can reveal much about the child that may otherwise remain unspoken: "It should be noted that children at play are not playing about; their games should be seen as their most serious activity" (Montaigne, 1588). Drawings and paintings are significant, not for what the doctor might read into them (which is pure conjecture) but for what the children say about them.

> Fernando, aged four years, had a metastatic neuroblastoma. He was treated with chemotherapy and, after he obtained complete remission, had a bone marrow transplant. He loves to draw and paint. Every time he came to the clinic he gave Blanca a painting full of colors as a present. He was very proud of this. At age six he relapsed in the CNS and became paraplegic. His drawings started to lose their colors more and more. He painted all blue or black. Blanca asked Fernando about this: "Do you have no other crayons than blue or black ones?" "Yes, I have , but I do not like them any more."

Unless parents do not want us to, we always tell children the truth they wish to know. If they can ask, they are prepared to receive the proper answer. They will know how far they can go in the discussion. Very frequently the parents do not allow us to talk with the child about the nature of the disease or the prognosis. Even if we cannot say the whole truth, we can always avoid lying. We always use age-appropriate language. Our children can talk and ask if parents allow them to. Many times we have seen that children (even smaller ones) know everything about their disease and status. They do not talk, because that is what they have learned from their parents.

> Tomás, a boy aged 12, had a brain tumor. During the last two years of his life Eulalia cared for him at home. In one of her visits Eulalia found him very sad and crying. Eulalia and Tomás began to talk about his feelings. His mother, standing behind him, asked Eulalia very desperately with body gestures not to tell the truth about his declining health and possibility of death. When this happened Eulalia felt very puzzled; she changed the subject of the conversation, not knowing what to say. Eulalia wanted to respect Tomás' decision knowmore about his condition, and she was afraid of Tomás's isolation.
>
> Eulalia spoke with Tomás's mother, who really did not want her to tell him the truth. Eulalia shared this difficult case with the team, and the decision was to respect the parents' desire as the best way of caring. After one year Tomás started to feel sicker and sicker. The side effects of the

steroids were difficult to control, and his incapacity was very significant. He did not want to go out or see his friends. He spent most of the time with his family, particularly his mother.

A day arrived when he felt very sick, and he told his mother, "If I have to live like this I would prefer to die. I know that you and Dad will be very sad." His mother answered him: "Yes, it is so, but don't worry about us. All we want is that you feel fine. The next day he said that he was afraid of Heaven. His mother asked him, "Why? It is a pleasant and quiet place." The last two days he could speak freely. These moments were very important, for himself and for his family. Tomás died the next day, peacefully, surrounded by his family and embraced by his mother. He bore his illness with the most remarkable courage and dignity. His family had a healing bereavement.

Sometimes the religious beliefs of the family make communication difficult.

Martín, 13 years old, had a bone marrow transplant because of chronic myeloid leukemia. Six months after the transplant, he developed severe, chronic graft-versus-host disease. The family were practicing Catholics. The father and mother knew the whole appalling truth about the illness, but wanted to protect their daughters (Martín's sisters) from it. They let the days go by without telling them that Martín would most probably die. Martín's room became a sanctuary full of icons of saints. "There is no need to tell the sisters. Martín can be cured by a miracle."

Angélica visited Martín two or three times a week. She worked with Martín's feelings through open-ended story books (choose your story). In the last interviews Martín chose "To Die: The Mission Had Failed."

At this point Angélica asked permission from Martín's parents to talk with his sisters. The mother approved of this meeting, in spite of her feelings. She had a good relationship with Angélica from the beginning of Martín's illness. The sisters could ask with amazement and dismay, "Is Martín really going to die?" They could cry. For the mother it was very difficult to share these feelings with her daughters. With pain she reaffirmed the family beliefs: "Martín is in the Lord's hands; we will endure His will with resignation." This meeting allowed Martín's sisters to say good-bye to him. Martín died three days later. Angélica attended the funeral and is still in contact with Martín's mother.

Sometimes we are wrong in our understanding of what the child and the family need to know about the disease. Each family has different ways of being and different needs. We cannot presume to know them; we can only suggest or hope. The final decision should be made by the family. Parents are the main caretakers, after all. If we provoke a gap between them and us, we are not providing proper help.

Felipe, a boy aged 15, had a late relapse of an abdominal neuroblastoma that had been diagnosed at age seven. His mother did not want Eulalia to tell him the truth about the disease. Felipe asked if he could be cured, and the answer was, "That is not possible." The following day he and his mother came to the clinic. Felipe was very depressed and his mother very angry. She wanted to speak to Eulalia alone. She shouted at Eulalia that Felipe could not sleep and was very sad. Eulalia tried to explain to her that those emotions were normal in the given circumstances; if he could speak them out, he would feel better. After that time Felipe was brought by his parents less frequently and only when the symptoms became unmanageable. The mother never allowed Eulalia to speak with him alone. He did not speak or ask again about his illness. Felipe died at home with some symptoms not completely controlled.

It is frequent, in our experience, that children actually try to protect their parents. They try to alleviate the burden the illness imposes upon them.

A bone marrow transplant was the last chance of curative treatment for Victor, 13 years old. His mother, divorced, was very unstable emotionally; she was under psychiatric care. She did not tolerate the presence of Victor's father. In spite of these difficulties, we tried an evaluation and family consent conference for the transplant team. The mother expressed her panic about the procedure. She cried, blaming the father for his insubstantial commitment towards Victor's illness. She also expressed her rancor about the whole situation—all this in the presence of Victor, who listened but did not speak. The climax was so terrible that Victor was asked to wait outside and talk alone with one of us. He said to Angélica very clearly that he wanted the transplant but he could not go through with it without his mother's approval and support, or if the procedure would upset her too much. He said this very calmly and firmly. Victor was not transplanted. He died at home six months later of progressive disease.

Working with a real team and being involved with the child make truly worthwhile communication much easier. "It is our responsibility to remember that medicine is not only science, but also the art of letting our own individuality interact with the individuality of the patient" (Albert Schweitzer). Working with the truth in every aspect has enabled us to learn a great deal from the families we cared for. They displayed a sincere heart, and we could see that they were true to it. A father, crying while his little girl, aged five, was dying, told Eulalia, "Now, I just know how much I have to enjoy every minute of life."

ACKNOWLEDGMENT

We wish to acknowledge with much gratitude the very much we have learned from talking with children, from our patients, and from their families.

REFERENCES

1. INSTITUTO NACIONAL DE ESTADISTICA Y CENSOS (INDEC). 1990. Hacia el censo de poblacion y vivienda.
2. INSTITUTO NACIONAL DE ESTADISTICA Y CENSOS (INDEC). 1991. Censo Nacional de poblacion y vivienda.
3. 1982. Atlas demografico de la Republica Argentina. Centro Editor de America Latina S.A.
4. SARASQUETA, P., P. BILISKY, H. MARTIN, M. NASTRI & H. SPINELLI. 1991. Mortalidad de niños y adolescentes en la ciudad de Buenos Aires en 1988. Arch. Argent. Pediatr. **89:** 303–318.
5. MINISTERIO DE SALUD Y ACCION SOCIAL REPUBLICA ARGENTINA. 1990. Programa Nacional de estadisticas de la salud, Serie 5 No. 34.
6. YUNES, J. 1993. Mortalidad y morbilidad de adolescentes en la region de las Americas. Arch. Argent. Pediatr. **91:** 303–318.
7. MINISTERIO DE SALUD Y ACCION SOCIAL REPUBLICA ARGENTINA. 1985. La Juventud en la Argentina.
8. FEIERSTEIN, R. 1993. Historia de los Judios Argentinos. Ed. Planeta. Buenos Aires.

Argentina

Telling the Truth to Cancer Patients in a Multicultural Society

M. I. DE GONZALEZ VICTORICA,[a] L. BERTOLINO, AND S. PAVLOVSKY

Fundaleu
J. E. Uriburu 1450
Capital Federal (1114)
Buenos Aires, Argentina

The following study took place in a hospitalization center for oncohematological diseases. The method used here is to describe examples of the bedside skills needed to handle the situation of truth-telling in this special relationship between the physician and the cancer patient. The age range of the population was from toddlers to elderly people. We have placed truth in a cultural context in order to try to answer the question of whether communication of the truth in cancer is culturally related or conditioned.

As in other countries, in Argentina the disclosure of truthful information to cancer patients is related to sociocultural and ethnic origins.[1–6] However, nowadays the focus is on how these ethnic groups find their intellectual level in the actual society.

We consider it a real challenge to be truthful in medicine in Argentina, taking into account that in many other aspects our country is striving to live more realistically and in confrontation with truth—social truth, the truth of its education, the truth of its economy, and the truth of its past and origins. It was not until very recently that legal action has begun to be applied in medicine; in this regard the fact of informing truthfully has become a really important issue, but more for legal reasons than for the proper spirit of truth.

At this time in our country the type and quality of information given to cancer patients concerning diagnosis, life expectancy, the prognosis of cure, as well as morbidity and mortality caused by the treatment vary tremendously among treatment centers.

[a]Corresponding author.

ARGENTINA: CULTURAL BACKGROUND AND HISTORY

We work in Argentina, a country that was formed by wide immigration currents, especially by Italians and Spanish, to whom this land offered possibilities for quick economic growth in return for labor for the local landowners. At the beginning of this century, wars, persecutions, and other situations caused a new wave of immigration to our country from eastern and central Europe, which joined the earlier settlers.

During this time, Argentina was one of the 10 richest countries in the world; this was a result of economic growth caused by an important development in cattle and agricultural production. This situation was very tempting for those wishing to start a new life abroad. They came from the poorer regions of their countries, being mainly farmers with little education and no job opportunities in their native countries; many of them were fleeing from religious persecution such as the progroms. Popular culture, especially in Buenos Aires, did not pay much respect to the original inhabitants, but instead looked up to the various foreign cultural groups. Even today, these groups still maintain their own schools, religions, meeting places, and clubs, where they keep up their language, traditions, and bonds with other communities as well.

Historically, immigration has produced a socially advanced impact on the traditional basis of a landowner society, whose national identity is determined by foreign culture. These foreigners either went back to their countries or stayed in the capital; it is in the interior of the country where the original colonization group has remained most intact. Buenos Aires, a cosmopolitan port, was considered a cultural frontier of Europe in America.

A large number of well-educated professionals, especially from the United Kingdom, Germany, France, and Belgium, came to Argentina to work in foreign companies such as the railroad, meat markets, etc. The major achievement of the immigrant generations was the massive establishment of literacy in the population; as people became culturally nourished, they wanted more information and knowledge. Most of the population, mainly from the middle classes, became integrated fairly quickly with the immigrants. This great social and cultural mobility created a new identity, which approached the 20th century in need of great change, mainly intellectual.

In recent decades there was another wave of immigration from some of Argentina's neighboring countries such as Uruguay, Paraguay, Bolivia, and Chile. These people belonged, in the great majority, to uneducated groups and were living and working in an illegal status, without any health insurance. This last group did not join the first groups of immigrants in trying to improve the reality offered by their host country.

THE ESTABLISHEMENT OF HOSPITALS AND THE EVOLUTION OF MEDICINE IN ARGENTINA

In this century, the professional workers who came from abroad to work in the companies that had been established in Argentina required medical attention. This need contributed to the establishment of hospitals devoted to patients of their community (Italian, Spanish, British, German, French, Jewish, etc.). These hospitals were set up according to the model of those in their countries of origin.

Public hospitals were built in the largest cities of our country at the beginning of the century. Similar to those in France, they had several isolated pavillions to prevent the spread of epidemic illness to the rest of the hospital. For a symbolic salary most doctors spent all morning in the government-run hospitals. All teaching and postgraduate training was done there as well. Most of the patients who received medical care in the public hospitals were indigent. The majority of the increasing number of middle- and upper-class patients were treated by the same doctors in their private consultation practices in the afternoon.

Until 1950 the greatest influence on local medicine was from Europe, especially France and Germany. The main European languages were in common use among members of the medical society, who traveled abroad for training and attended congresses. Most medical books and journals came from that continent. Our universities developed in the area of medicine and joined those in more advanced countries, reaching such important achievements as the Nobel Prize won by an Argentine doctor in 1947; to date, two other Argentine doctors have obtained this award. During this time, too, outstanding young doctors began choosing the United States as a place for training and attending specialization courses in the university hospitals where Nobel Prize winners were doing their research. When these well-specialized doctors came back and settled down in Argentina, they became pioneers and later leaders in their specific fields of medicine. The American model modified the doctors' training. Doctors have gradually incorporated the practice of informing patients of the truth and the increasing importance given to the doctor-patient relationship in the rest of the advanced countries.[7]

During the past 30 years, many changes have occurred in social medicine in our country. Workers or employees who belong to the low or lower-middle classes are now able to have health insurance provided by their employers. Also, the higher ranking employees, executives, independent professionals, and shop owners are able to have private health insurance. But there are still people without access to this kind of medical security, and they are referred to public hospitals for medical attention.

Along with changes in physicians' and popular knowledge of medical issues, there have been changes in attitudes toward disclosing information to patients about their diagnosis and prognosis. Although the quality of information given patients has evolved in the last decades, there are still doctors who provide scarcely any or no information concerning procedures, diagnosis, treatment options, and prognosis. Fear of the patient's emotional reaction is the most frequent reason for not giving patients full information. Other doctors do provide patients with more information and considerably more attention. These doctors believe that knowledge of the truth generally has a positive effect on the doctor-patient relationship. Still, the words "cancer" and "incurable or fatal diseases" are not mentioned directly to many patients.

OUR PERSONAL EXPERIENCE AND SITUATION

We work in a small cancer center, a nonprofit organization run by Fundaleu (Foundation Against Leukemia). Most of the patients treated here suffer from hematological malignancies (see TABLE 1). We have a very active autologous progenitor cell transplant program and are enrolled in several national and international clinical research protocols. Fundaleu has established an institutional review board, and all the therapeutic protocols have received approval. All the patients provide written and oral informed consent according to the requirements of the protocol.

Our population lives according to certain cultural patterns that should be taken into account when treating such a broad and deep subject as the significance of life and death. Why death? The fact that we face when working with cancer patients is the anguish produced by the word "cancer" and its relation to death. It is like the presence of death itself, suspended in time, and the fear of prolonged agony. This is the common understanding that patients have when they first hear their diagnosis, and it is because of this that many physicians face the decision of telling or not telling the truth, of communicating the diagnosis or not.

The first symptoms of the diseases we treat are not alarming, they are

TABLE 1. Patients Treated by Fundaleu

	Age		
Diagnosis	0–21	>21	Total
Leukemias	86	142	228
Lymphomas	67	298	365
Myelomas	-	72	72
Breast cancer	-	9	9
Solid tumors and others	40	81	121
Total	193	602	795

not known to be prolegomena of so serious a disease as cancer, and they are not evidence that would cause one to accept the reality of an illness. The diagnosis, on the other hand, is a laboratory fact, confirmed by the clinic. Therefore, the patient should believe what he is told; it is here where the first bond of truth starts. Forcing the truth by providing more information than the patient needs is often cruel because it removes hope. To do so is generally considered more a way of preventing legal problems in case of a lawsuit for malpractice.than a way of achieving trust and cooperation between patient and doctor.

Our policy is *truth with hope.* We believe that full disclosure of the diagnosis of cancer to competent individuals (including children) is morally, ethically, legally, and therapeutically the appropriate policy. We believe that giving patients adequate information usually has a positive impact on their psychological and physical well-being.[16]

After performing all the studies that lead to confirmation of the diagnosis, the medical team holds a meeting with the patient and close relatives, who often are the main source of emotional support and are far more available and knowledgeable about the patient than is the doctor. In this meeting, we try not to limit the time for questions and answers; all aspects of the diagnosis, side effects, prognosis, hospitalization time, and financial or health insurance coverage are discussed.

Often the patients and relatives are shocked upon hearing the initial diagnosis and ask few questions. In this first conversation we try not to saturate them with too much technical information about response to cure, percentage of response, median duration of response, survival, etc., because, since they are so disturbed by the diagnosis, they are not able to follow and understand these terms properly. Instead, we discuss the immediate steps that they have to go through during the days to come. We encourage them to meet with us again and assure them that every member of the medical team will be ready to offer support and to answer any question. Many parents and relatives are reluctant to ask for further clarification of the information, primarily because they do not want to hear more bad news.

Patients, including children, are informed when new procedures, such as bone marrow or spinal fluid studies, will be done. They are informed of the results of these studies, of blood tests and bone marrow or CAT scan reports, and of any evolution of the treatment. The patients have confidence in what the therapy team is doing. If they become refractory to therapy and, therefore, terminal, the team always tries to support them and give them the truth with hope. To provide truth and hopeful information to persuade the patient to cooperate in his cure is the first maxim governing the therapeutic relationship. There is an instant in this relationship when the patient realizes with intuitive knowledge that his doc tor is truthful and honest, and that everything that is said and done after that instant will be true and coherent with this genuine information.

DIALOGUE WITH THE PATIENT: EVOLUTION AND EXAMPLES

Dealing with oncohematological diseases is fairly new terrain internationally; only since the 1960s has oncohematology been firmly established as a field of specialization demanding a broad understanding of the whole range of medical science. In our cancer center, whose medical director has 30 years of experience at the bedside of hundreds of neoplastic patients, the communication of truth regarding diagnosis and prognosis has evolved considerably. When in 1970 we started delivering radiotherapy to the cranium to prevent central nervous system (CNS) leukemia, most patients were reluctant to receive radiotherapy for fear of losing their hair; usually those patients did not know their diagnosis or the risk of CNS relapses. This shows how something that was really important lay hidden under something much less important, the fear of losing one's hair.[9–13] After receiving news of the diagnosis, usually there is an awkward situation in the family, sometimes lasting for several days, where everybody is aware of the diagnosis but no one is able to talk about it. This kind of situation taught us the importance of giving the diagnosis to both patient and close relatives at the same time.

In general, hematologists who treat potentially curable diseases such as Hodgkin's disease, lymphomas, and acute leukemia, as well as diseases with a long survival time such as chronic leukemia, multiple myeloma, and myelodisplastic syndromes, tell the truth about the diagnosis, treatment, and general approach to prognosis to their patients. In most cases the truth of the diagnosis was softened with false hopes. This happened, for example, to the parents of a child with acute lymphoblastic leukemia. They were told that the disease was a highly curable one, but they were not given much information about the death rate due to treatment, failure of the primary treatment, or relapse. In many cases, parents try not to ask many questions, especially the most difficult. This lack of information leads to misunderstandings; if anything should go wrong during the treatment, the parents become angry with the treatment team in which they had placed so much hope.

There are four patterns of awareness: *open awareness,* in which staff members, family, and patient are aware of the diagnosis, treatment, and prognosis of the illness; *mutual pretense awareness,* in which those same persons know but pretend not to know; *suspected awareness,* in which everyone knows except the patient, who suspects the truth; and *closed awareness,* in which everyone except the patient knows.[14]

We understand that it is not the same thing to give information about diagnosis, treatment, and prognosis. At Fundaleu we always give information about diagnosis and treatment right away. The prognosis is not communicated in statistical-numerical terms. With incurable but chronic diseases such as chronic myelocytic leukemia, in most instances the patients know the diagnosis but believe that with treatment they can live forever.

A different situation exists with solid tumors: the diagnosis comes after surgery, and the main physician is the surgeon. To this day surgeons in such cases do not tell the truth about the diagnosis and prognosis. Instead, three specialists act as physicians and communicators. Here begins a false and common story. The surgeon tells the patient that the tumor was "only a premalignant disease" and that it was "totally resected." They later send the patient to the radiotherapist "just in case any tumor cells still remain and to ensure the cure." If the treatment fails, the oncologist communicates the truth about the failure of the treatment and the imminence of death only to the close relatives, very rarely to the patient. When this happens, the family, which was not properly prepared to accept the reality of the situation, usually refuses to accept it and instead searches for a magical cure, placing their hopes in alternative cures, often in quackery. When the truth is not told to patients early on, they, along with their relatives, seek cancer quackery. This is due to lack of confidence in their own physician.

When patients learn that they have cancer, their psychological reactions include fear of death, abandonment, loss of independence, disruption of relationships, and financial loss. This is why a common reaction of patients and relatives is to give in to the temptation of not facing or denying the truth of the diagnosis. We have a large referral of patients for autotransplantation. Most of them arrive at Fundaleu with little information about their diagnosis, less about their prognosis, and practically none at all about the morbidity and mortality of the transplant procedure.

Information about Palliative Care

For the medical staff, palliation should be an active process in which they are fully involved, with no hint of withdrawal or abandonment. In this stage alternative therapies are an option. Most of the providers of alternative therapies offer "nontoxic" or "natural" cancer treatments. At present, these therapies are biological and are said to improve the natural immunity against tumor cells; they also recommend a change of lifestyle in such matters as diet, vitamins, and avoidance of stress and impurities. These alternative therapies are respected and taken into account, but they should not interfere with the treatment strategy planned by our center.

TRUTH AND COMMUNICATION

"If we deliberately say *is* when we think *is not* or say *is not* when we think *is*, we are lying. The false opinion is that form of opinion which thinks the opposite of the truth."[15] When we referred to the transmission of the truth as a process, we noted that it is done in the context of a therapeutic relationship and at a given moment. What to communicate, how, and when must be known. The communication itself may be accomplished verbally and nonverbally. It has been successful when he who receives the information captures the intention of him who gives it—when there is coordination between the verbal and the nonverbal.

COMMUNICATION

It must be remembered that the patient has the right to know the diagnosis of his disease, its evolution, and its prognosis. It is necessary to communicate everything that is going on, even though he already knows intuitively that something is wrong and has an internal perception of the illness. Transmitting the truth is not merely an act of communication, it is a process in which two persons are involved, the patient and the physician.

There are three levels of communication: an intrapsychic level, in which messages are decoded according to a very personal point of view depending on one's background; an interpersonal level, where empathy and the ability to establish contact are key factors; and a social level, where the messages that are handled are part of the cultural background of the two persons in communication. The physician, in his role as communicator, should be skilled on all three levels. He should be able to decode the anguish produced in himself by the transmission of information about the diagnosis, evolution, and prognosis of illness. He should be able to carry out interpersonal communication, to engage in a dialogue with the patient and motivate him toward his cure; he should avoid giving information in a very technical manner, which would be incomprehensible and would not allow the patient's feedback. He should be a social communicator to demystify the illnesses that he treats and to forgo the omnipotence that appears when the other person is not knowledgeable about the subject being discussed. The doctor must develop a broad variety of disciplines to be able to fulfill all these steps—to understand what is going on in the process of communication and have a clear understanding of his own feelings about the situation in which he is a key participant. Medical practice involves more than specific knowledge of medicine; it also involves knowing how to communicate.

Discussions of the latest revisions of health plans in the most advanced countries refer to the necessity of providing physicians with a forum for the discussion of some of the new sociopolitical forces that affect medical action, but this is nothing new. Hippocrates pointed out that there are intellectual as well as moral conditions to be fulfilled by those who would dedicate themselves to the service of health. It is therefore very important for a doctor to know the patient's diagnosis with certainty so as to be able to establish a proper therapeutic relationship. Plato contrasts the right and wrong relation between doctor and patient by comparing the practice of the physicians who treated slaves to those who treated free men[15]: "The slave-doctor," he says,

> prescribes what mere experience suggests as if he had the knowledge, and when he has given his orders, like a tyrant, he rushes off with equal assurance to some other servant who is ill . . . . But the other doctor, who is a free man, attends and practices upon free men; he carries his inquiries far back, and goes into the nature of the disorder; he enters into discourse with the patient and with his friends and is at once getting information from the sick man and also instructing him as far as he is able; he will not prescribe for him until he has brought the patient more and more under his persuasive influence and sent him on the road to health; he attempts to affect a cure.

Hippocrates recommended that the physician cultivate prognosis not only for the guidance of his own actions but also for the sake of the patient. "By foreseeing and foretelling in the presence of the sick the present, the past, and the future and explaining the omissions that patients have been guilty of, he will be the more readily believed to be acquainted with the circumstances of the sick; so that men will have the confidence to entrust themselves to such a physician."

According to modern concepts of medicine, an overall approach to disease is necessary. External (ecological, infections, cultural, environmental) and internal (emotional, genetic, somatic, constitutional) factors and history are important and should be studied by multiple investigators working in the frames of reference in which they have been trained. This calls for a greatly expanded sharing of responsibilities among various professionals.[14]

Specifically in cancer—where improved treatments have changed an incurable disease associated with death to a frequently chronic, often curable disease—the psychological aspects of cancer, the reaction to the diagnosis and treatments, are of increasing importance. Truth-telling is an important means of obtaining the desired response to the medical treatment; it is part of the dialogue that leads to a comprehensive analysis of the patient's response to illness, his psychological and social resources, his coping style, and his psychiatric illness, if any. If the professional views disease from such a multicausal point of view, every disease can be more fully understood. A patient's presenting complaint is usually physical; patients rarely complain about their anxieties, depressions, or tension. The doctor is and should remain the one who handles the complaints, overseeing the patient's response to medical treatment.

CONCLUSION

The communication of information has been evolving simultaneously with changes in inquiries from the patient's side and in the training of medical professionals. These changes are not occurring and are not being applied in the same way throughout the country. The type and quality of information given to the patient may vary according to the patient's own knowledge and information regarding his illness. The quality of the information available to people who live near urban areas is very different from that available to people who live in more remote areas. When people have access to good information, they become more aware of the scientific basis of the illness and the limits of modern science. On the other hand, people who have little or no access to information have a different concept of the illness, its treatment, diagnosis, and prognosis.

In our country these differences are very strong. Therefore, the physician must be able to communicate with truthfulness while taking into account the readiness of the patient to receive the necessary information in a proper manner. We inform truthfully because we believe that the patient with information cooperates with his own curing process and establishes a better relationship with the physician; and this communication, in turn, helps the doctor cope with the anguish that the possibility of losing that patient generates.

REFERENCES

1. Estape, J., H. Palombo, E. Hernandez, M. Daniels, T. Estape, J. J. Grau, N. Vinolas & J. M. Mane. 1992. Cancer diagnosis disclosure in a Spanish hospital. Ann. Oncol. **3**(6): 451–454.
2. Gjerse, P., O. O. Thomsen, J. H. Larsen, H. A. Holmsgaard, K. M. Linborg & H. R. Wulff. 1995. Attitude of Danish patients and physicians to information on cancer. A questionnaire study. Ugeskr. Laeg. **157**(1): 46–48.
3. Lavrentiadis, G., N. Manos, J. Christakis & C. Semoglou. 1988. The Greek cancer patient's knowledge and attitudes towards his diagnosis and prognosis. Psychother. Psychosom. **49**(3-4): 171–178.
4. Mizushima, Y., T. Kashii, K. Hoshino, T. Morikage, A. Takashima, H. Hirata, A. Kawasaki, K. Konishi & S. Yano. 1990. A survey regarding the disclosure of the diagnosis of cancer in Toyama Prefecture, Japan. Jpn. J. Med. **29**(2): 146–155.
5. Tanida, N. 1994. Japanese attitudes towards truth disclosure in cancer. Scand. J. Soc. Med. **22**(1): 50–57.

6. THOMSEN, O., H. WULFF, A. MARTIN & P. A. SINGER. 1993. What do gastroenterologists in Europe tell cancer patients? Lancet **341**(8843): 473–476.
7. NEWALL, D. J., E. M. GADD & T. J. PRIESTMAN. 1987. Presentation of information to cancer patients: A comparison of two centres in the UK and USA. Br. J. Med. Psychol. **60**(Pt 2): 127–131.
8. SURBONE, A. 1993. The information to the cancer patient: Psychological and spiritual implications. Support Care Cancer **1**(2): 89–91.
9. LLUESMA-GONALONS, M., S. PAVLOVSKY, M. T. SANTARELLI, M. EPPINGER-HELF, E. DORTICOS BAVEA, C. CORRADO & J. CARNOT. 1991. Improved results of an intensified therapy in adult acute lymphocytic leukemia. Ann. Oncol. **2**(1): 33–39.
10. PAVLOVSKY, S., M. MASCHIO, M. T. SANTARELLI, F. S. MURIEL, C. CORRADO, Y. GARCIA, L. SCHWARTZ, C. MONTERO, F. L. SANAHUJA, O. MAGNASCO *et al.* 1988. Randomized trial of chemotherapy versus chemotherapy plus radiotherapy for Stage I-II Hodgkin's disease. J. Natl. Cancer Inst. **80**(18): 1466–1473.
11. PAVLOVSKY, S., G. MILONE, N. SOMOZA, C. CORRADO, H. MAGNASCO, Y. CERUTTI, J. SASLAVSKY, I. FERNANDEZ & S. BRUNO. 1993. Comparative study of 1st generation versus 2nd generation (CAVPE) combinations in intermediate and high-grade lymphomas. Sangre (Barcelona) **38**(1): 17–23.
12. PAVLOVSKY, S., F. SACKMANN MURIEL, M. T. SANTARELLI, E. SVARCH, E. JIMENEZ, R. KOHAN & A. ROSSO. 1992. An update of the results of intensive therapy in children with acute lymphoblastic leukemia. Leukemia **6**(Suppl. 2): 167–170.
13. CORRADO, C., M. T. SANTARELLI, S. PAVLOVSKY & M. PIZZOLATO. 1989. Prognostic factors in multiple myeloma: Definition of risk groups in 410 previously untreated patients: A "Grupo Argentino de Tratamiento de la Leucemia Aguda" Study. J. Clin. Oncol. **7**(12): 1839–1844.
14. KAPLAN, H. I., B. J. SADOCK & J. GREBB. 1994. Synopsis of Psychiatry. 7th edit. Williams & Wilkins. Baltimore, MD.
15. 1980. Truth. *In* Great Books of the Western World. Encyclopaedia Britannica. Chicago, IL.

SUPPLEMENTARY BIBLIOGRAPHY

ARIÉS, P. 1983. El Hombre ante la Muerte. Taurus Edit. Madrid.
BACHELARD, G. 1980. La Intuición del Instante. Siglo Veinte Edit. Buenos Aires.
FLORIA, C. & C. GARCÍA BELSUNCE. 1971. Historia de los Argentinos. Kapelusz Edit. Buenos Aires.
LUNA, F. 1995. Breve historia de los Argentinos. Planeta Edit. Buenos Aires.
MORGAN, J. D. 1991. Young People and Death. John D. Morgan Edit.
SENDRAIL, M. 1983. Historia Cultural de la Enfermedad. Espasa-Calpe Edit. Madrid.

Communication with the Cancer Patient

Information and Truth in Brazil

SÉRGIO L. FARIA[a] AND LUIS SOUHAMI[b]

[a]*Department of Radiation Oncology*
Universidade Católica de Campinas
Campinas, São Paulo, Brazil

[b]*Department of Oncology*
Division of Radiation Oncology
McGill University
Montréal, Québec, Canada

BRAZIL: WHERE, HOW MANY, WHO?

Brazil is the largest country in Latin America and the fifth largest in the world. It is larger than the continental United States and makes up about one-half of South America. The population of Brazil is approximately 150 million (in 1995), all speaking the same language, Portuguese. It is the only country in Latin America in which Spanish is not the official language. Brazil is a federal republic consisting of 27 states; it has an annual demographic growth of 1.9%. Over 85% of the population are Roman Catholic. Protestant sects, however, are growing rapidly. Many people, particularly in the northeast, practice Afro-Brazilian religions that combine tribal beliefs with those of Catholicism. The Afro-Brazilian religions (*candomblé* and *umbanda*) are intimately related to "alternative treatments" for cancer and other diseases, and their treatment methods are largely diffused throughout the country.

A BIT OF GEOGRAPHY

Brazil is on the Atlantic side of South America. It is a privileged country in terms of climate and soil. A humid tropical and subtropical climate is the rule, except for a semiarid area in the northeast. There are no earthquakes, hurricanes, volcanoes, or deserts, but there is wide variation in vegetation. The north, situated below the equator, is hot, tropical; it contains the Amazon jungle that covers about one-third of the Brazilian land. The southeast and the south are richer regions with a more temperate climate. This hot/temperate climate, without major extremes, permits the poor, homeless people to sleep on the streets, under bridges, in the slums (*favelas*). The hot climate allows the Brazilian to spend a great deal of time outdoors, often just chatting with friends or watching people. As a rule, Brazilians are gregarious, friendly, warm, happy people.

A BIT OF HISTORY

Brazil was discovered (in 1500) and colonized by the Portuguese. The French, Dutch, and Spanish attempted to establish colonies but were expelled. The arrival of the Portuguese and Jesuits was a disaster for the Indians, who were not a real nation but rather sparse groupings. The Jesuits attempted to convert them to the Catholic religion, while the colonizers decided to use the indigenous population as manual workers. Incapable of submitting to the constraints of slavery, they died or fled to more distant and inaccessible areas. The Indians were almost completely decimated both numerically and culturally during the ensuing years.

An important historical/cultural aspect of Brazil is the introduction of black African slaves after the middle of the 16th century. The rest of South America, of Spanish colonization, never adopted a similar policy. Slavery in Brazil brought enormous cultural influence to the country, particularly in the northeast areas. The African influence profoundly affected the musical, religious, and folkloric characteristics of the country, and a unique culture emerged. An important difference between the slavery in Brazil and that in some other countries was that miscegenation was more naturally accepted in Brazil than in most other slave-owning countries, so that in many areas people of mixed ancestry (*mestiço*) outnumber those of pure racial stock.

Brazil proclaimed its independence from Portugal in 1822; it was one of the few (if not the only one) countries in Latin America to become independent without any bloodshed.

SOME CULTURAL ASPECTS OF BRAZIL

For a better understanding of how the diagnosis of cancer is revealed (or not) to the patient in Brazil, we believe it is important to discuss some of the important cultural habits. This is, of course, a generalized and particular opinion of the authors, who live in the southeast region of the country (Rio de Janeiro and São Paulo) and does not necessarily imply that the whole country operates as described.

In general, Brazilians do not like to obey rules and have a tendency to commit minor infractions that perhaps would not be tolerated in some other societies. They do not feel uncomfortable in telling "benign" lies if they believe these are justifiable for any reason at the particular moment.

Thus, not infrequently, family members demand from the physician a falsified histopathological and/or radiological report with the intent of hiding from the patient the diagnosis of cancer, and thereby "protecting" the patient from what the family believes to be an emotionally devastating truth.

In general, the family in Brazil is very united and has enormous power in decision making. In the situation of serious disease, such as cancer, the children "protect" the parents, the spouse "protects" the spouse, etc., from the diagnosis and prognosis of the disease. The practical repercussion of this attitude is that the family members of patients with cancer usually come to see the doctor *before* the patient and frequently ask the physician not to tell the truth about the diagnosis or even discuss the disease/prognosis with the patient. Arguments such as "he will kill himself if you tell him the real diagnosis" or "I have known my mother much longer than you, and I know her heart will not resist such bad news" are frequently used by the family to convince or intimidate physicians not to tell the truth to the patients. This feeling of "protection" is so strong that, if the physician does not agree with the family request to hide the information from the patient, not infrequently the family will change to another physician who is willing to do so.[1]

THE SOCIOECONOMIC SITUATION IN BRAZIL

Socioeconomic indicators reveal large pockets of poverty throughout the country, particularly in the northeast region. There is a large social gap between the small, privileged upper class and the masses at the bottom of the earning scale. In addition, at least one-third of the Brazilian population is illiterate. These poor people depend exclusively upon the public system for both health and education. Most of the hospitals in Brazil are public institutions, only about one-fifth being private. In terms of services available, the greater proportion of the country's doctors and hospitals are concentrated in the urban areas. Frequently, people from the north or northeast of the country go to the southern region for medical care, which may not be available to them at their home region. The Public Health System for oncology in Brazil offers reasonable resources for therapy but lacks a plan for cancer prevention. In certain areas of the country, however, it is not always easy to get a timely appointment to see a doctor or a social worker at a public institution.

In São Paulo state, the largest and richest of the country, the two most frequently diagnosed cancers in the male are stomach, and head and neck tumors; and the two most frequently seen in the female are cervix and breast tumors. Head-neck cancer in São Paulo can be considered a real tragedy given its high incidence. Moreover, advanced disease stages are seen in 75% of the patients at time of diagnosis. A large number of these patients end up not having a surgical procedure performed because of lack of available beds in the specialized public hospitals.

In Brazil, poor patients traditionally do not complain of the poor services they may get at a particular institution, unlike patients in the upper class, and rarely do they demand a change of physician. Lawsuits for medical malpractice are practically nonexistent.

ATYPICAL SITUATIONS OR REALITY?

The following examples are real situations witnessed by one of us (S.L.F.) in a public hospital in Brazil that may provide some insight into the magnitude of the problem of communication in the physician-patient relationship.

Example 1: Recently four patients with carcinoma of the larynx were referred to our department for postoperative radiotherapy following radical laryngectomy. At the time of their first consultation in our department, they all demanded an answer for the same question: "When is my voice coming back?"

This question reflects the total lack of communication between surgeon and patient before the operation and indicates how passive patients can be, undergoing a major surgical procedure without even being aware of its possible consequences. This passivity, seen more frequently among people with low earnings, emerges from the fear patients have of missing the opportunity of having the treatment performed because the doctor may get upset with one of the questions regarding the surgical treatment and/or outcome and, consequently, cancel the procedure all together. Informed consents are not routinely used in Brazil.

Example 2: In one of the largest emergency rooms in São Paulo, a woman was in the gynecology room, in the lithotomy position, ready to be examined, when the doctor finally asked her what her problem was. Very timidly she said, "Doctor, I just came to visit my husband who had a heart attack and is next door." She had mistakenly been placed in the gynecology room by a nurse who confused her with another woman, who had come to the emergency room with vaginal bleeding. Her fear of offending the institution or the health professional was so intense that she was unable to tell the nurse the real reason for her presence in the hospital.

Example 3: A 35-year-old male, upper middle class, was operated on for what was initially thought to be a gastric ulcer. The final histopathological diagnosis, however, turned out to be an adenocarcinoma of the stomach. The surgeon told the truth only to the patient's father who, to "protect" his son, did not tell him of the real diagnosis. Eventually the patient was referred to a medical oncologist, who revealed to him the final pathological findings. Thus, father and son learned about the diagnosis from different sources but were unaware of each other's knowledge of the ease. The patient's wife, who was not informed at all of her husbands real problem, found out through her children's pediatrician about the diagnosis. For nearly two years after the operation, the patient, his wife, and his father kept the diagnosis secret from one another without realizing that it was known to all of them.

LEGAL ASPECTS OF TRUTH-TELLING

In Brazil, the states have little autonomy; most of the laws are federal. This is also true for most of the laws and regulations governing the medical profession; indeed, the Medical Code of Ethics is the same for the whole country. This code, updated in 1988, is clear and objective with regard to the subject of communication between the physician and the patient.

The Patient's Right to Be Informed about and to Decide on a Treatment

Article 56: Except in an emergency, a physician must, before undertaking an investigation, treatment or research, obtain consent from the patient or his representative.

Article 59: A physician must ensure that the patient or his representative receives suitable explanations on the nature, purpose and possible consequences of the investigation, treatment or research which the physician prepares to undertake. Except for a valid reason, the physician shall not conceal a fatal or grave prognosis from a patient who requests that it be revealed to him.

Professional Secrecy

Article 102: A physician must not disclose the information obtained in the practice of his profession.

Article 107: A physician must take reasonable means with respect to his employees and the personnel about him so that professional secrecy is maintained.

Integrity

Article 110: A physician must refrain from issuing a medical certificate if he has not examined or performed any medical act on a patient.

Article 116: A physician must refrain from issuing to any person and for any reason whatsoever a false certificate of ill health or documents containing false information.

A physician who violates any of the above articles can be penalized with a temporary or even a permanent suspension of his right to engage in professional activities. However, rarely has there been any punishment of a professional who breaks the code of professional secrecy by telling the family and not the patient about the diagnosis/prognosis or who lies to a patient regarding a diagnosis.

TELLING THE TRUTH

Our experience with medical students in their last year of medical school shows us that the majority of them agree with the Medical Code of Ethics rules on patients' rights and firmly believe that the truth should always be told to the patient. However, when asked whether they observe these rules in clinical practice, the answer is an emphatic *no.* Why is the truth so frequently not told to the patient in Brazil? We believe there are at least two major reasons: (1) physicians are not really prepared for this kind of open relationship; and (2) patients are not used to demanding information from the physician and, as a rule, accept most of the decisions made on their behalf without questioning them. It is as if a tacit agreement existed between the patient and the doctor: the patient "feels" that his disease is serious but denies himself the right to know what is going on and does not ask any questions; on the other hand, the physician pretends that everything is all right, because he himself is also not prepared to deal with "bad news" and goes on with all the necessary investigations and treatments without sharing with the patient the reasons for, and consequences of, these procedures. This bizarre relationship receives full approval from the patient's family.[2,3]

In Brazil, there are three distinct situations for the relationship between the physician and the cancer patient: (1) when the diagnosis is made by the internist or general surgeon—the patient usually has not been given the diagnosis of cancer before his first visit to the doctor; (2) when the patient is referred to a medical oncologist or radiation oncologist—now the diagnosis of cancer has already been made, but the patient is frequently unaware of it; (3) when the patient is terminally ill.

The first situation—the most frequent—occurs, for example, with the pediatrician who diagnoses leukemia in a child or a gynecologist who diagnoses breast or endometrial cancer in a patient being seen regularly for a benign gynecological disease. For these physicians, cancer is only a small portion of their routine practice, and the majority of them are not prepared to deal openly with the patient. Frequently they either hide the truth from the patient, or, when they tell the patient about the diagnosis, they do so in an inappropriate and emotionally disturbing way. Here is a report from a patient on the day she went to her gynecologist's office to receive the biopsy result of a breast nodule: ". . . .the doctor was there in front of me, very nervous, trying to delay and disguise the result of the biopsy, opening and closing drawers as if he were looking for another, more comforting report. He just could not tell me I had breast cancer."

The second situation is experienced by oncologists. Most of the time, it is impossible to know how much and what kind of information the patient has received from his/her referring physician. On a number of occasions, the patient has been told that he/she has "a bit of a tumor" (the word *cancer* is avoided whenever possible) and will receive some treatment to get rid of it. The problem with such statements is that a large proportion of these patients have rather advanced disease and are beyond any possibility of cure when they are first seen by the oncologist. In our experience, only a few patients have been clearly and unequivocally informed about the diagnosis and prognosis of their cancer when they see us for possible therapy. However, the family is usually aware of the situation, having been fully informed of the disease by the referring physician. In fact, as a rule, the nononcologist referring physician expects the oncologist to deal with all aspects of the disease and believes the giving of information about the diagnosis and prognosis to the patient is a matter for the oncologist to take care of. In practice it is much more common to see the nononcologist physician than the oncologist strike a deal (a "contract") with the patient's family to avoid telling the truth to the patient.[4]

THE PROBLEM OF THE ILLITERATE

An extremely important problem in Brazil is that of communicating with totally illiterate patients of the lowest socioeconomic level. We believe this problem must exist in other countries, but it is rarely mentioned in the literature. Little is known about the illiterate, very simple person who faces major economic hardship and whose major preoccupation is to survive until the next day. Often these people live with their entire large family in a single room, amid emotional and physical violence, with little chance of comfort or privacy; incestuous relationships are not rare. The reality of these people is totally different from what is described in the textbooks. The difficulty in communicating with them is real; it is often very difficult to make them understand the rationale and consequences of a given treatment. We have experienced this problem of communication on several occasions.

One example of this situation concerns patients with carcinoma of the cervix, the most frequent cancer for women in Brazil. As part of their therapy, they have to undergo brachytherapy (uterine implant) after completion of external beam treatments. During the brachytherapy the patient remains hospitalized for approximately three days. The majority of these patients are very poor, illiterate, and intellectually unsophisticated. A few days before they are due to come into the hospital for the brachytherapy they are seen in consultation, the procedure is explained, and an information sheet is given to the patient. Immediately after the consultation with the radiation oncologist, they are seen by a social worker, who tries to get a feeling from the patient on how much she knows about the procedure to be performed as well as her social needs during her hospitalization. Despite the fact that they have the information sheet in their hands, when the social worker asks them if they have seen the doctor already or if they have received any information about the procedure, a large number just say *no,* as if the consultation never took place.

This group of patients poses a real challenge in communication. Many of them cannot stop working even during the most aggressive therapies. Some cannot even afford the economic cost of coming to the hospital daily for radiotherapy. When one tries to explain the possible side effects of a treatment to them, their reaction is minimal, and their curiosity is nil.

The disease and possible side effects of treatment are just another difficulty of life they have to face. So, how much information should be given to them, and what is the most effective way to make them understand the issues related to the disease, the treatment, and the outcome? We do not have the answers to these questions. A proper, well-designed investigation of this population is long overdue.

HOW TO TELL THE TRUTH: THE REAL ISSUE

The way the truth is told to patients varies from country to country. Several reasons may account for these variations, including cultural and religious issues, legal implications, socioeconomic differences, etc. The truth must be told not just because the law or a code of ethics demands it, but because it is a patient's right to know all about *his/her* disease. However, the fundamental issue in a patient-physician relationship is not just to tell the truth, but how to tell it. Common sense teaches one not to be insensitive and cold when telling the truth. But then how should one do it? Some physicians are naturally effective in this regard, but others are not and cause tremendous emotional disturbance in some patients.

We firmly believe that patients should know the truth, although there are times when some information may be withheld from a patient. How useful is it to tell a patient with glioblastoma multiforme, for example, that he has only a few months to live? We prefer to withhold this information unless the patient demands to know his chances of surviving the disease. Interestingly, in Brazil when we ask a patient if he/she has any questions, very seldom does the patient ask any question related to outcome. Even among people in the upper social class, it is more of an exception than the rule to ask such a question. To always tell the truth in Brazil can be very complicated. Family intervention demanding that the doctor not tell the diagnosis to the patient is so strong and frequent that to break this cultural tradition is not an easy task and, not infrequently, brings tremendous pressure and uncomfortable feelings upon the physician.[5,6]

In spite of different languages, religious beliefs, socioeconomic levels, and cultural traditions, human beings are alike and share similar emotional reactions. The essence of a patient-physician relationship is comprehension, patience, and emotional support. Unfortunately there is a great distance between the work of psychologists/psychiatrists and that of oncologists. The former write texts dealing with the emotional aspects of the patient, but with a large theoretical component and very few practical points. The latter rarely deal with emotional issues and are largely concerned with the results of treatment. Today's objective science leaves few opportunities for subjective—e.g., emotional—evaluations. There is a large group of underprivileged patients in Brazil and in other areas of the globe who do not appear to be receiving the adequate emotional support. The needs of this population must urgently be addressed.

REFERENCES

1. FARIA, S. L. 1984. Com respeito, ao paciente com cancer. Rev. Assoc. Med. Bras. **30:** 121–124.
2. FARIA, S. L. & S. S. CAMARGO. 1985. Apoio emocional a pacientes com Doença de Hodgkin: Notas sobre uma experiência. Rev. Bras. Cancer **31:** 157–160.
3. ALVES, J. G., L. SOUHAMI, J. MARSILLAC & J. MELLO. 1986. O médico, o paciente e o câncer. Ars Curandi **18:** 26–34.
4. FARIA, S. L., M. V. LEDERMAN & W. NADALIN. 1978. Emotional reactions towards radiation therapy. *In* Proceedings, Xll International Cancer Congress, Buenos Aires, Argentina, October 5–11, 1978. Vol. 2, Abstr. 18: 130.
5. FARIA, S. L. 1989. Alterações psicológicas como possivel fator prognóstico na sobrevida do câncer da mama: um papel para avaliação subjetiva do oncologista? *In* Proceedings Vl Congresso Brasileiro de Oncologia Clinica, Porto Alegre, Brazil, October 7–10, 1989: 22.
6. BARRETO, D. O. F., M. A. X. FAZOLIN & S. L. FARIA. 1994. Aspectos emocionais e éticos ligados a paciente com câncer da mama. *In* Cancer da Mama: Diagnóstico e Tratamento. S. L. Faria, L. H. S. Leme & J. A. Oliveira, Eds.: 239–250. Editora Medsi. São Paulo.
7. DE CARVALHO. M. M. M. J. 1988. Introdução a Psicooncologia. Editora Psy. São Paulo.

Ethical Dimensions and Communication Issues in Nursing Patients with Advanced Metastatic Cancer

ANN LYNCH AND CAROL BURNETT

Royal Victoria Hospital
687, Avenue des Pins Ouest
Montréal, Québec H3A 1A1, Canada

Clinical research has paved the road to many advances in technology for the treatment of cancer. These technologies may give rise to questions about the value of these treatments in simply extending life, often at considerable cost to the individual's quality of life (QOL). One such technology is bone marrow transplantation (BMT). Since the first reported successful cases in 1968 and 1969,[1] this treatment modality is now being offered to thousands of patients with advanced malignant disease. This article will explore both communication and ethical issues that are emerging with the use of autologous bone marrow transplantation (ABMT) in the treatment of advanced cancers of breast and ovary. ABMT has increasingly been considered for these types of cancers because of the poor response in obtaining long-term survival based on standard therapy.[2] Recent advances in the availability of colony-stimulating factors to assist with marrow recovery after chemotherapy have resulted in lower treatment-related mortality rates for this patient population. A BMT program has been in existence at the Royal Victoria Hospital, a 500-bed McGill University teaching hospital, since 1982. In an effort to identify key ethical issues facing nurses caring for this patient population, focus group interviews were conducted with nurses on our 20-bed inpatient Hematology/Oncology Unit and our ambulatory care setting known as Oncology Day Care (ODC). Approximately 20–30 patients are transplanted each year. The nursing care involved in the actual process of transplantation requires a three- to four-week hospitalization as well as numerous outpatient visits to the ODC for blood count and symptom control monitoring. Patients who have entered the ABMT program have previously been hospitalized on frequent occasions for conventional chemotherapy, followed in many instances by periods of febrile neutropenia. The demands that have been placed on the patients and their family are high prior to, during, and following the transplant. It was within this context that focus group discussions of ethical concerns from the nursing staff occurred. The issues of informed consent, quality of life, allocation of resources, and concept of hope were highlighted and will be explored in more detail as follows.

INFORMED CONSENT

Aggressive treatment protocols that include ABMT often involve serious potential complications such as infection, hemorrhage, pain, and peripheral neuropathies. Consequently, the patient and family need to have accurate information about these potentially life-threatening side effects.[3] Simply, informed consent implies that the patient's permission to proceed with treatment is based on a full explanation by the physician of the available options and the risks and benefits of those options. This process should involve shared decision making between the patient and his/her physician, with the physician as information provider and the patient as decision maker.[4] The process of informed consent has been explored from the perspective of both physicians and nurses caring for the BMT patients.[5] Results revealed that nurses were more concerned that patients know about the secondary effects and complications arising from transplantation, while physicians emphasized the options of treatment and possible outcomes with and without the transplant. This study also concluded that the physicians' perception of informed consent most closely matches the patients' in that most patients chose the option of transplantation based on outcome—namely, life or death. The differences in nurses' and physicians' perceptions of informed consent are, in fact, based on their different roles.[6] Nurses are involved with management of complications during transplant, while physicians are concerned with prescribing, monitoring, and evaluating the outcome of the treatment. The study further indicates that the potentially life-threatening side effects may not alter the patient's decision to choose BMT. In the patient's mind, it is often a choice between life or death. Consequently, nurses should not feel obligated to ensure that patients possess information about every possible side effect to enable them to decide upon this course of treatment. Royal Victoria Hospital nurses who participated in the focus group discussion concurred with the results concerning issues of informed consent as outlined in the study just mentioned.[6] Their comments reflected their concerns about the process of consent in this manner:

> It made me feel better to know that the patient was informed and comfortable with the decisions that she had made.

> Patients are informed about the risks of the procedure, but I think they are not always aware of what the side effects will be. The patients always say that although they have suffered, they don't regret their decision

because to accept palliation is to accept death, and many patients are not ready to do that.

Many patients say, "I'll take a chance," and we have to support them in their decision even though we feel bad when the outcome is not positive.

It is not our responsibility to provide the patients with information about the effectiveness of the treatment protocol, but we need to support them through the complications arising from it.

QUALITY OF LIFE

Studies of QOL for individuals undergoing BMT have been undertaken to understand and evaluate the outcomes of this therapy. Thirteen QOL studies of BMT survivors beyond the first year were reviewed.[7,8] These studies included patients undergoing either allogeneic or autologous BMT. These reports were analyzed on a QOL/BMT model that describes the survivorship experience in four domains: physical well-being, psychological well-being, social well-being, and spiritual well-being.[9] Most studies indicate that concerns about physical well-being and control symptoms were predominant within the first year of the transplant. However, long-term effects of BMT involving systems such as the gastrointestinal and respiratory tracts and the reproductive system continued to preoccupy as many as 25% of patients in some studies.[10,11] The issue of psychological well-being for BMT survivors has been reported as not as significant as physical well-being. Most patients report that they were happy to have survived the transplant and have another chance at life. Very few indicate regret for the decision to undergo BMT.[12,13] A study of long-term BMT survivors suggests that recovery is a dynamic, individualized process that often makes it difficult to compare QOL experience across this group of survivors.[14,15] This study also suggests the inclusion of data from the family as to their perceptions of QOL since the transplant in order to analyze if families also have "recovered" from this process.

Our discussion group commented on the quality of life of patients in several ways:

We get so close to our patients, it is sometimes upsetting to continue with ongoing treatment.

Sometimes Taxol™ is offered when the patient's quality of life seems very poor. It is hard to understand.

It is hard to face patients when there is a recurrence [after BMT]. We feel bad when things don't work out.

What would we do if we were in the same situation?

These comments demonstrate many of the dilemmas nurses face when providing care for BMT patients. The nurses' empathy for the patients' situation often makes it difficult, if not impossible, to separate their feelings about the provision of care to manage complications, and the effects that these complications are having on the patient's quality of life.

Nurses from the inpatient unit expressed more concern about this issue, as they actually see the patient through the most intense periods of treatment. As one nurse from the clinic said:

> In our area, there are time constraints; we see the patient for only five to six hours, and then they go home. Although we get attached [to them], it is not as intense an experience as hospitalization.

As a result of the dilemmas nurses encounter in their daily practice, they have developed a number of strategies to minimize the cognitive dissonance between care provider and one who extends suffering. These strategies will be explored at the conclusion of this chapter.

THE CONCEPT OF HOPE

Hope has been described as a multidimensional dynamic attribute that includes the concept of confidence in the outcome, possibility of a future, and belief in a Higher Being.[16] Hope has been identified as a key mechanism by which one can cope with the stress of being faced with a life-threatening illness such as cancer. The need for hope has been identified as one of five phychosocial needs of cancer patients.[17] Generally, one considers the need for cure or, at least, prolongation of life as an important patient goal. However, nurses often encounter difficulty in inspiring hope for this type of outcome in patients with advanced disease who are participating in experimental protocols. The concept of hope or what is hoped for may then change to hope for survival to attend an important family event, (e.g., wedding or graduation) or even hope for a peaceful death when all available treatment options have been exhausted.

Nurses involved in caring for BMT patients at our hospital expressed their views on the concept of hope for patients in several ways:

> When patients desire aggressive treatment and embark upon a protocol for metastatic disease, there is hope where none existed before—however, there is always uncertainty about the eventual outcome.

> Patients are very brave, and we have to play a role in offering hope.

> There is happiness and hope as opposed to what people outside [the hospital] think about cancer. Here, we see hope, and it makes us feel satisfied to see patients smiling again and doing well.

These comments demonstrate a more positive perspective on the nurse's role with BMT patients. Overall, nurses employed some very creative strategies to deal with the difficulties of patients enduring suffering to arrive at the outcome of either disease-free survival or ongoing disease and eventual death.

STRATEGIES TO MANAGE DILEMMAS IN CARE

Instill realistic hope. Nurses often maintained that this was difficult when the patients' cancer was progressing during the protocol; however, there was a sense of duty to carry on for the patient's sake.

> Patients tell us that they have to keep trying, and they trust us to support them and carry them through to whatever the outcome. When the patient becomes palliative, they usually stay on the active treatment floor. Although it's difficult, it is also rewarding for us to provide whatever comfort we can.

Realize that the ultimate outcome is "out of our hands." Nurses described their spirituality with this strategy in that even despite excellent technical care, certain patients do not have long-term survival. By accepting that "a higher authority" ultimately determines a patient's outcome, nurses are able to place their fate, and that of the patient, in a higher being. This strategy then permits the nurse to provide the care required to ensure that the patient's and family's goals are met.

> There is less ambivalence about the care when the patients become palliative. We are free to provide comfort care and ensure as much dignity with death as possible.

Be able to adapt care from active treatment protocol to palliation when required. Nurses commented on this:

> Care must be individualized.

> The close rapport with patients makes their death more difficult, but our role can be successful by making the patient as comfortable as possible.

> We must be advocates for the patient and keep in focus what the changing needs of the patients are. We can't feel guilty about shifting gears to

palliation and comfort care.

Support patients' decisions.

Patients trust us and need our support to carry them through to the outcome, whatever it may be. We have to make sure that we are advocates for patients in whatever decisions they make.

Alleviate patients' anxieties.

The anxiety of patients is often difficult to deal with when there are no guaranties about the outcome of the protocol.

It is helpful to encourage sharing of experiences among patients to decrease their anxiety.

Care must be individualized to respect the patient's level of anxiety related to their treatment.

COMMUNICATION ISSUES

The patient's involvement in the BMT protocol requires a certain commitment to active participation in their care. This participation is strongly encouraged by nurses in both the inpatient and ambulatory care settings. The nurse assesses the patient's goal, abilities, and strengths and endeavors to decrease anxiety through the provision of information tailored to meet that patient's needs. The individualization of psychosocial approach and symptom management ensures that standard interventions are adapted to meet each patient's situation in a more specific fashion.

The key to increased patient involvement, as we see it, is a nursing team skilled in assessment, negotiation, and support. The dynamic role of the nurse includes direct care to the patient, providing education regarding symptom management and discharge planning, and facilitating the transition to home. The patient is encouraged to question and participate in her own care. The nurse then adapts her communication style to meet the needs of the more experienced, knowledgeable patient.

It is clear that there are many challenges facing health professionals who care for this patient population. Close collaboration with the physicians on our team ensures that patients and nurses receive clear communication about the goals of the treatment plan. It is our hope in sharing these insights to challenge other health care teams to provide patient- and family-centered care that is compassionate to the needs of those who depend so greatly on us.

REFERENCES

1. THOMAS, E. D., R. STORB, R. A. CLIFT *et al.* 1975. Bone-marrow transplantation. N. Engl. J. Med **292:** 832–843, 895–902.
2. CROUCH, M. A. & J. A. ROSS. 1994. Current concepts in autologous bone marrow transplantation. Semin. Oncol. Nurs. **10**(1): 12–17.
3. DOWNS, S. 1994. Ethical issues in bone marrow transplantation. Semin. Oncol. Nurs. **10**(1): 58–63.
4. SILVA, M. C. & P. L. ZECCOLO. 1986. Informed consent: The right to know and the right to choose. Nurs. Manage. **17:** 18–19.
5. CARNEY, B. 1987. Bone marrow transplantation: Nurses' and physicians' perceptions of informed consent. Cancer Nurs. **5:** 252–259.
6. WHEDAN, M. & B. R. FERRELL. 1994. Wuality of life in adult bone marrow transplant patients: Beyond the first year. Semin. Oncol. Nurs. **10**(1): 42–47.
7. FERRELL, B. R., M. GRANT, G. M. SCHMIDT *et al.* 1992. The meaning of quality of life for bone marrow transplant survivors. Part I. The impact of bone marrow transplantation on quality of life. Cancer Nurs. **15:** 153–160.
8. FERRELL, B. R., M. GRANT, G. M. SCHMIDT *et al.* 1992. The meaning of quality of life for bone marrow transplant survivors. Part II. Improving quality of life for BMT survivors. Cancer Nurs. **15:** 247–253.
9. WOLCOTT, D. L., D. K. WELLISCH, F. I. FAWSY *et al.* 1986. Adaptation of adult bone marrow transplant recipient long-term survivors. Transplantation **41:** 478–483.
10. HENGEVELD, M. W., R. B. HOUTMAN & F. E. ZWAAN. 1988. Psychological aspects of bone marrow transplantation: A retrospective study of 17 long-term survivors. Bone Marrow Transplant **3:** 69–75.
11. SCHMIDT, G. M., J. C. NILAND, S. J. FORMAN *et al.* 1993. Extended follow-up in 212 long-term allogeneic bone marrow transplant survivors: Addressing issues of quality of life. Transplantation **55:** 551–557.
12. ANDRYKOWSKI, M. A., P. J. HENSLEE & M. G. FARRALL. 1989. Physical and psychosocial functioning of adult survivors of allogeneic bone marrow transplantation. Bone Marrow Transplant **4:** 74–81.
13. ANDRYKOWSKI, M. A., P. J. HENSLEE & R. L. BARNETT. 1989. Longitudinal assessment of physical and psychosocial functioning of adult survivors of allogeneic bone marrow transplantation. Bone Marrow Transplant **4:** 505–509.
14. HABERMAN, M. 1992. Quality of life issues for bone marrow transplantation survivors. In Proceedings of BMT Symposia at the the Seventh International Conference on Cancer Nursing: 22–24. Scutari. Middlesex, England.
15. HABERMAN, M. N. BUSH & R. YOUNG. 1993. Quality of life in adult survivors of allogeneic bone marrow transplantation. A qualitative analysis of narrative data. Oncol. Nurs. Forum **20:** 1545–1553.
16. NOWOTNY, M. L. 1989. Assessment of hope in patients with cancer: Development of an instrument. Oncol. Nurs. Forum **16**(1): 57–61.
17. YOUNG-BROCKOPP, D. 1982. Cancer patients' perceptions of five psychosocial needs. Oncol. Nurs. Forum **9**(4): 31–35.

Effective Communication with Cancer Patients

The Use of Analogies—A Suggested Approach

CHARLES L. M. OLWENY

St. Boniface Unit
Manitoba Cancer Treatment and Research Foundation
409 Taché Avenue
Winnipeg, Manitoba R2H 2A6, Canada

INTRODUCTION

The "doctor knows best" philosophy, which reigned supreme until very recently, resulted from improved technology in the understanding of the pathophysiology of disease. More recently patients have become better educated and more knowledgeable about health and disease. Consequently, "the doctor knows best" slogan is no longer acceptable to some patients. Doctors are increasingly challenged by their patients to explain the symptoms, treatment, and consequences of disease. Patients are demanding that they participate in the decision-making process. In a recent study of 150 women with recently diagnosed breast cancer in the United Kingdom,[1] 20% wanted an active role in deciding their treatment, 28% preferred to share decision making with their physician, and the remaining 52% wished their doctor to decide. Similar figures were observed in a group of Canadian women with breast cancer.[2] Women who are less than 50 years of age or women with high school education were more likely to prefer active or collaborative roles in treatment decision making.[2]

FUNCTIONS OF MEDICAL COMMUNICATION

Medical communication serves three main functions:

(1) it allows for the interchange of information between the doctor and the patient;
(2) it enables an engagement of feelings, which enhances the thera-

peutic benefit of the doctor-patient relationship by fostering trust and confidence in the doctor's capabilities;

(3) it encourages and fosters compliance.

Most problems between the doctor and the patient and between the doctor and family members are often the result of poor or failed communication. Unfortunately, communication skills are not given due prominence in the curricula of many medical schools.

Communication is a two-way process. It ought to be stressed, however, that the doctor and the patient are not equals in the setting of a consultation. Some "distance" between the two must be created and maintained. When giving information the doctor must endeavor to use appropriate language, make statements as simple as possible, and avoid medical jargon. Patients may be overwhelmed and may not absorb all that is said. It may help if the patient is accompanied by spouse, relative. or friend. However, the doctor has to avoid asking embarrassing questions in the presence of a third party. Some patients prefer to record the conversation and play it back in a more relaxed home atmosphere.[3] Doctors should realize that patients are not at ease and relaxed if they perceive their doctor to be in a hurry. The doctor should give himself or herself enough time, especially for the first visit. The doctor should appreciate that consultation time belongs to the patient and must learn to listen attentively to the patient who is narrating his/her story and indirectly telling the doctor the diagnosis. The patient should be made aware of the fact that there are other patients waiting. It may help if patients are encouraged to write down beforehand the questions they want to ask.

Just as each doctor communicates in his or her own way, each patient is different, and every situation is different and warrants a unique approach. It is imperative, therefore, that the physician determine early in the conversation what approach the patient is comfortable with. A well-informed patient such as a physician or nurse may prefer the direct use of medical terminology, while most lay persons would appreciate the use of plain language. The mistake often made is to assume that the "educated" person is familiar with medical terminology. It should be remembered that it took years of training for the physician to acquire and build this medical vocabulary.

There is no right or wrong way to communicate. All physicians have to develop an approach that suits them and is acceptable to their patients. I prefer to use common analogies, as patients are able to relate to them. Whatever approach one chooses, it is prudent to be honest and straightforward. I have used this approach in three cultural settings (in East and Central Africa, Australia, and Canada), and patients seem to like it and appear to get the points I wish to convey. The rest of this chapter will give examples I commonly use, especially in the outpatient setting.

THE NEED FOR DIAGNOSIS, STAGING, AND TREATMENT PLANNING

Cancer as an Enemy

Most persons in this day and age have been in a war situation or will recall the recent Gulf War crisis (thanks to CNN, which brought these realities to the living room). Patients often talk of cancer as an enemy—one they are going to fight and beat. I, too, often equate cancer with an enemy in trying to explain the need for diagnosis, staging, and why a certain course of action is to be preferred to another.

To successfully fight an enemy there are a few prerequisites. First, who is the enemy? A familiar enemy is preferable to one that is unknown. It is advisable to collect as much information as possible about the enemy. For instance, what are the enemy's first, middle, and last names? Does the enemy respond to a nickname? Which pub does the enemy frequent, and what soccer, football, or hockey club does the enemy support? These apparently mundane issues illustrate the details required. Similarly, it is not enough to make a diagnosis of cancer. There are over 200 different types of cancers, and to treat it properly we require as much detail as possible. Information on the organ of primary involvement is important. Is it primarily a cancer of lymph nodes (lymphoma), connective tissue and muscles (sarcoma), or blood (leukemia); or is it cancer of the body lining and skin covering (carcinoma). Is the cancer growing rapidly or slowly? Do we know the natural history of the malignancy in question? Has the doctor treated this malignancy before?

Once we believe we know the enemy, the next step is to assess the enemy's strength. This is important for two reasons. First, if we determine that the enemy is overwhelmingly strong, it might be advisable not to engage in open confrontation. In the case of the Gulf War perhaps that is what the Iraq leader should have done. He should have noted that the coalition forces (U.S.A., U.K., Canada, France, Italy) were set in battle array, and he should have signed a peace pact to avoid bloodshed. A second reason for assessing enemy strength is that such practice helps in the choice of weapons to use. If the enemy happens to be a mosquito, a piece of paper is adequate. If the enemy is a dog or a dingo, waving paper will not make it go away. In that situation a stick or stones might be used. If the enemy happens to be a polar bear or lion, then a rifle would be the appropriate weapon of choice.

Sizing up the enemy is what is referred to in medical jargon as staging disease. If we determine that the disease is far too advanced, it may be best not to treat it but to concentrate on palliative care. The tumor stage will also enable us to decide whether surgery, radiotherapy, chemotherapy, or a combination is the most appropriate therapeutic approach.

Having determined that the enemy is beatable, it is proper to enter into dialogue with allies to plan a strategy of attack. In this discussion, the reason for the fight will be explained, what is at stake, and how goals will be achieved. Similarly, before embarking on a course of treatment the goal of management must be determined. There are three important goals in cancer management—namely, to cure, to prolong survival, and to provide comfort and relieve symptoms (palliation). The chosen goal should be shared with all members of the health-care team (other physicians, nurses, social workers) and with the patient and family.[4] In the dialogue with the family, the role of each person should be stressed, with the key person being the patient. The physician's role is to advise, while the family, relatives, and friends are to provide support.

Having outlined the treatment strategy, allow the patient first to ask questions and encourage him or her to do so before you turn to the spouse or companion. The questions patients commonly ask have to do with length of survival, treatment side effects, and why radiotherapy or chemotherapy is necessary given the fact that the surgeon apparently removed all the tumor? Why is it necessary to continue treatment beyond remission?

HOW LONG DO I HAVE TO LIVE, DOCTOR?

This is a question that I get asked every day, and it is the one question I tend to avoid answering. In the past I ventured to suggest how long a patient might live, but I was often proved wrong. There are people to whom I suggested they would live for about three months who came back three years later and retorted, "Ah-ha, Doc, you said it would be three months—here I am three years!" On the other hand there are people I gave six months, and six weeks later they were dead. "I don't know," appears an honest answer. *The one with that information is listening but not talking.* My role as a physician is to alert patients when things are not going well and encourage them to put their house in order.

DOCTOR, WHAT SIDE EFFECTS SHOULD I EXPECT WITH CHEMOTHERAPY?

Bone Marrow as a Factory

It is fair to say that cancer drugs affect rapidly dividing cells of the body. They affect cancer cells because these cells are dividing rapidly, and that is why they form tumor or swelling. Unfortunately these drugs have "never been to school" and therefore cannot tell the difference between the bad rapidly dividing cancer cells and the good rapidly dividing normal body cells. Where in the body do we find normal rapidly dividing cells? First, the fingernails, which, because they grow rapidly, must be trimmed every week or so. Chemotherapy will make nails become brittle and may make them stop growing; you may actually observe lines across the fingernails representing periods of arrested growth. Second, hair also grows rapidly; hence the frequent visits to a hairdresser or barber. With chemotherapy the hair may thin out, or all the hair may fall out. However, it grows back once treatment is stopped in most instances. Other areas of the body with normal rapidly dividing cells include the lining inside the mouth, throat, gullet, stomach, and bowel. Chemotherapy may thus lead to sores in the mouth and throat, and may cause difficulty or pain in swallowing. The stomach may churn, and the patient may become nauseated and throw up or may get diarrhea.

Perhaps the most important area in the body with normally rapidly dividing cells is the bone marrow. *Bone marrow is the factory where blood is made.* Out of that factory comes three important products. There are the red cells, which make the blood red. The red blood cells carry oxygen around the body. Without enough red cells there will not be enough oxygen, and the patient may feel weak, tired, and lethargic. Then there are the white cells, which are not seen because the red cells color them red. The white cells help fight against infections; without enough white cells the patient might fall victim to simple infections. The third product of bone marrow are the platelets. We cannot see these because of their size—they are very tiny. They play an important role in helping blood to clot. Without enough platelets the patient may bruise easily and, if cut, may continue to ooze blood for a long time. Because chemotherapy drugs may affect the marrow it is necessary to check the patient's blood count regularly to make sure the doses are correct; and treatment may be delayed or drug doses modified from time to time to allow the bone marrow to recover. In addition each of the drugs has its own specific side effects: some may affect the kidney, others the heart, and yet others the lungs. Side effects are best discussed once a decision has been made as to what drugs will be used.

WHY IS IT NECESSARY TO HAVE CHEMOTHERAPY AND RADIOTHERAPY WHEN I BELIEVE THE SURGEON TOOK AWAY ALL THE TUMOR?

Breast Cancer Is Like a Tree in the Garden

I like to equate breast cancer with a tree in the garden. You do not know how old this particular tree is because it was already there when you took possession of the property. Similarly, we have no idea how long this tumor has been in the breast because we did not plant it there. You may get tired of the tree because it drops leaves in your yard; during the fall you have to sweep the yard two or three times a week, and no sooner have you swept than the wind blows down more leaves. You finally get tired of the tree and decide to cut it down. Cutting down the tree is the surgery you have just had. You know that when people cut down a tree, they do not cut it to the ground level but almost invariably leave a stump. After a while, when the weather improves and there is sunshine and rain, the stump will sprout. This is what we call local recurrence. There are two ways of preventing this. You can dig up the roots of the tree, but this will leave you with a large ugly hole or pit in your garden. In the past surgeons used to "dig up the roots" of breast cancer to prevent local recurrence. They would remove the breast, the muscles on the chest wall, and the lymph nodes; and they would open the chest and remove more lymph glands. The result was always a huge, ugly scar. The other way to deal with the stump is to set it on fire. Setting it on fire is analogous to radiotherapy. Both surgery and radiotherapy are to treat local disease (to remove local disease and prevent local recurrence).

You will also remember that we did not know how old the tree was. This tree has been producing fruits yearly and scattering seeds in the garden. Some of these seeds may fall on the driveway, will be crushed, and will not grow. Some may land on the concrete, and these, too, will not grow. However, a few will land in the soft fertile areas of the garden, and sooner or later these will begin to grow. Where are the fertile areas in the garden of the human body? In the case of breast cancer, the fertile areas include the opposite breast, the bones, lungs, liver, skin, and brain. It is for this reason that from time to time we repeat a mammogram (special X-ray of the breast) and a chest X-ray. If we are concerned, we may request a bone scan or an abdominal ultrasound to look at the liver. We now have ways to determine whether a tree is old enough to produce and scatter seeds. In the case of breast cancer there are certain features that suggest to us that the cancer has been there long enough to produce and scatter cancer seeds elsewhere. These features include the size of the breast cancer, the number of involved lymph glands in the armpit, the appearance of some of the cells under the microscope, and whether or not the removed tumor had hormone receptors. When we have a large primary tumor with involved nodes in the armpit and when the tumor does not have hormone receptors, then the patient is at high risk of the disease coming back at a distance away from primary site. In that situation we can give some additional drug treatment to prevent those seeds from germinating. In some instances we succeed, and we are able to prolong survival and improve the quality of life. Our choice of drug(s) is dependent on several factors, perhaps the most important being the age of the patient. For patients who are still menstruating and are under 50 years of age we tend to recommend chemotherapy, while for older, post-menopausal patients we recommend hormone treatment.

DOCTOR, WHAT ARE THESE RECEPTORS YOU MENTIONED?

Doors and Windows Are to Allow in Guests and Fresh Air but May Let in Undesirable Elements as Well

You probably know that breast cancer cells "feed" on female hormones just as prostate cancer cells "feed" on male hormones. To best describe that I liken breast cancer to a house. When you build a house, you install doors and windows. They may be opened to let in fresh air and allow visitors to enter. They may be closed to keep out the cold, heat, mosquitoes, and other undesirable elements, especially burglars. In the case of breast cancer, the female hormones gain access through the doors and windows. We can now count these doors and windows, and it is these that we call receptors. The more doors and windows, the better. Similarly, the more receptors on the tumor, the better. We now have drugs that block off these receptors and prevent the female hormones from gaining access to feed the breast cancer cells. One such drug commonly used is the hormone Tamoxifen. Tamoxifen blocks the doors and windows (receptors), and when the female hormone comes it bounces off the receptors. The net result is that we starve the tumor of some nutrients necessary for its growth, and it shrivels up.

YOU SAY I AM IN COMPLETE REMISSION—WHY IS IT NECESSARY TO CONTINUE TREATMENT?

When You Drive Away an Enemy, Endeavor to Strike Deep into Enemy Territory

To answer this question, I equate cancer with an enemy on the run. When the enemy is being driven out, you do not stop at the border. If you do so, the enemy will take advantage and return as soon as you turn your back. It is always advisable to penetrate deep into enemy territory and give the enemy little or no chance of coming back. Similarly, although we may have conquered the cancer and it appears to be in remission, we need to consolidate our position by giving more courses of treatment and in so doing prevent the cancer from coming back (relapse).

I AM HAVING DIFFICULTY DECIDING WHETHER I SHOULD TRY OUT A FORM OF TREATMENT— WHAT DO YOU ADVISE, DOCTOR?

The Gambling Approach Makes the Decision Easy

There are occasions when patients are ambivalent and cannot make up their mind whether to try a form of treatment or not. I find that the gambling approach helps in the decision process. Most patients have gambled at some point, and they are amazed to realize they are in good company when I tell them that I, too, gamble from time to time. Sometimes I buy a lottery ticket. If I do not buy one, then I have lost. If I do buy one, even if I have only one chance in a million of winning, I am comforted to realize that one day that chance may be mine. Similarly, if you do not try out this treatment, then you have lost. If you try, even if you have only a 5–10% chance, it might do you good. You never can tell: you may be among the 5–10% whom this treatment will benefit. Almost invariably patients will want to try out the treatment suggested.

IS THERE ROOM FOR A SECOND OPINION?

There is general agreement that the welfare of the patient is best served by the provision of more than one opinion. This is particularly so in the setting of a multidisciplinary clinic that provides for "one-stop shopping." A second opinion is reassuring to both the patient and the physician. To the patient it reveals the doctor still has an open mind. To the physician it reassures him/her that the choice by the patient was made after thorough soul searching and that the patient is truly well informed. A second opinion becomes necessary in instances when there is uncertainty about the biology of the disease and/or its treatment. It becomes mandatory if the physician senses that in spite of clear-cut recommendations doubt and uncertainty remain on the part of the patient. These may arise from lack of understanding or pressure from family or relatives to pursue a course different from that suggested by the physician. In any case patients are entitled to a second opinion and to have a choice. If the search for a second opinion leads to a change of physician, so be it. However, the process ought to be done in the open, with all parties aware of what is going on.

REFERENCES

1. FALLOWFIELD, L. J., A. HALL, P. MAGUIRE, A. BAUM & R. P. A'HERN. 1994. Psychological effects of being offered choice of surgery for breast cancer. Br.

Med. J. **309:** 448.
2. DEGNER, L.F. 1995. Personal communication.
3. DUNN, S. M., P. N. BUTOW, M. H. N. TATTERSALL, Q. J. JONES, J. S. SHELDON, J. J. TAYLOR & M. D. SUMICH. 1993. General information tapes inhibit recall of the cancer consultation. J. Clin. Oncol. **11:** 2279–2285.
4. OLWENY, C. L. M. 1991. Goals and rationale of cancer treatment. Med. J. Aust. **155:** 187–192.

Communication of the Cancer Diagnosis to Mexican Patients

Attitudes of Physicians and Patients

LAURA TORRECILLAS[a]

Oncology Service
Centro Médico de Especialidades 20 de Noviembre
ISSSTE
Mexico City, Mexico

In the health care setting the problems and challenges related to communication have special importance when we transmit a message that disrupts such basic human needs of survival as safety and comfort. To communicate to a patient the diagnosis of cancer is far from a purely medical, ethical, and legal matter; it concerns our human essence. The knowledge of a final verdict, when we inform the patient of the diagnosis of cancer, brings the most chaotic situation into his daily life: the possible nearness of death.

The idea of perishing produces fear and anxiety. Any human repudiates horrible death, this degrading and painful situation of which cancer monopolizes all the symbols.[1] Coping with this new situation involves not only the most important actor in the play, the patient, but also the family and the appropriate medical team.

The first person implicated in this sensitive issue is the physician. The act of delivering good news is easy, but to be the bringer of bad news symbolizes such different meanings as to feel like an executioner, to admit our professional ignorance, and to face a variety of new claims by the patients and his family.

Patients expect more than the technical resources that modern medicine can give. They want to explore their own situation, emotional comfort, a comprehensive explanation, and, most of all, support. In the patient-physician relationship complaints usually involve communication problems with the doctor. Patients ask for that which physicians used to offer in times when technical resources were less: dialogue, support, and kindness.

Medical training in how to tell the patient the diagnosis of cancer is completely lacking in the professional education of health care givers in

[a]Address for correspondence: Dr. Laura Torrecillas, Parras 8 Depto. 5, colonia Hipódromo Condesa, México D.F. 06100, México.

our country. It is ironic that such limited education is provided in Mexico in familiarizing professionals with what is likely to become a daily responsibility of clinical practice in oncology.

CULTURAL, GEOGRAPHICAL, AND SOCIAL BACKGROUND IN MEXICO

As physicians, history and culture have a great influence on our attitudes, especially when we care for patients who are approaching death. Consequently, the people working in hospitals are representatives of our national, ethnic, and religious backgrounds.

Our forebears practiced the ceremony of human and animal sacrifice to consecrate or invoke their gods and genius. Through the sacrifice of flesh and blood, the blessing of a holy power was obtained. Therefore, the act of dying does not arouse fear for those who find in death a sublime fecundity and the continuation of mankind. According to the Popol-Vuh (the Mayan book of the creation of humankind) the universe was born from the god's sacrifice. Thus, the need of human sacrifices did not admit of any discussion or skepticism. Sacrifice was the continuation of life, the way to maintain this world and the universal order.[2]

Spanish culture imposed on us the Christian religion, with death as a common dilemma. The terminology of suffering has existed for centuries; in the language of the Church death has been expressed through religious images such as crucifixes, and portraits of saints and martyrs. The confession ritual by a Father, the person who grants the transformation of sin into penitence through prayer, and the Holy Communion to cleanse the soul are the emancipating mechanisms of the evil human part in our country. To believe in God helps the Mexican people cope with the unknown and unfavorable circumstances of common life. "Heaven is great. God was with me this night. If it would not be that way, who knows what could happen. Because it was already night when I resurrected . . . ."[3]

Our religion is Christian in essence, but with some autochthonous shades. The character of the cross-breeding is the result of a native culture struck by a violent conquest by the Spaniards. The reminiscence of our autochthonous way of thinking is misinterpreted and colored by new ideas and customs in vogue. For example, our traditional *Dia de Muertos*—Day of the Dead—on November 2nd is a national festivity that commemorates and evokes our dead ancestors with an open invitation for the return of a departed family member or other person. Even if it appears as a pagan ceremony, it is in essence a Christian bereavement ritual to cope with death and to reduce the fear and the anxiety of our own end. Mexican people are as afraid to die as any other people in the world.

With this background, any attempt to communicate to a Mexican patient a fatal outcome should respect these religious conceptions and also social status. These issues should always be considered by the attending physician as a powerful tool to help people cope with life's end and most of all should not be regarded as a communication barrier.

DISCLOSURE OF CANCER DIAGNOSIS

Novack described in 1979 that 97% of the physicians in the United Sates of America were in favor of informing patients of the diagnosis of cancer.[4] This was a surprise after a study performed 18 years earlier, in which almost 90% of the surveyed physicians preferred not to reveal the diagnosis of cancer to their patients. The pressure imposed on health care givers by the current legal obligations, especially in developed countries, could be the real motive behind this medical viewpoint. Although this change has occurred in the United States, it is ironic that now patients from that country, who supposedly are better informed, prefer not to know their diagnosis.[5]

Today more patients feel abandoned by their doctors, because modern technology has been substituted for open communication between patient and doctor. The purpose of the patient's right to have complete information on his disease is not served by heartless truth-telling. We, as doctors, must not have any doubt about telling the truth to the patient with cancer.

The main issue of this problem is how to disclose the diagnosis of cancer. It seems that there are many ways to reveal the bad news, but that there is no single formula for a problem that depends entirely on professional experience, communications skills, cultural background, and personal interest in a human being. However, we can recognize some basic guidelines that can be considered universal communications tools to incorporate in our own practice:[5,6]

1. Look for a comfortable, quiet place, where you will not be interrupted or rushed.
2. Be aware of your nonverbal language.
3. Give the patient the opportunity to ask questions first, then the family. This reduces anxiety and promotes the development of confidence.
4. First investigate what the patient already knows and determine *what* and *how much* he wants to know.
5. Ask for the family presence during the first interview, in agreement with the patient.
6. Do not try to give all the information at the first visit, only what is most important.
7. Never use the words *cancer, death, incurable, there is no further treat-*

ment. These words often block the patient's comprehension of the information given.

8. Never define the life expectance in time.
9. In an uncurable case, never inform the patient of the imminence of death during the first visit.
10. Always be *realistic*, but never eliminate *hope*.
11. *Never lie*. The honesty of our message should never be hidden to improve its acceptance.
12. Respect the patient's and family's religion and spiritual beliefs.
13. Avoid paternalism and excessive emotional reactions.
14. Inform the patient and family that the medical team will be available for further conversation.
15. At the end, you can ask the patient: How do you feel? Why? Do you have any other questions? Is there anything else that concerns you?
16. Our first and main responsibility is to the patient, secondarily to the family.

There are three possible situations: the truth, a lie, and silence. Nevertheless, the truth cannot always be admitted, lies do not always deceive, and silence can sometimes be more eloquent and veracious than truth.[1]

The best way to proceed is to consider each patient individually. Before deciding how to handle this situation, the doctor has to fulfill the two main conditions in the management of patients with cancer: first, be certain of the diagnosis and prognosis; and second, determine exactly what the patient expects. For any well-trained oncologist the first part does not represent a challenge because studying a patient, interpreting the histological diagnosis, determining the extent of disease and the optimal treatment are the common daily activities for which we were trained. In contrast, the capacity to perceive the patient's expectations and solve his problems with adequate truth and kindness requires a human touch.

The question most frequently asked the doctor by the patient is about the stage of the disease and life expectancy. If there is a high probability of cure after treatment as in a lymphoma or germ cell tumor case, this lessens some moral weight on the doctor when revealing the diagnosis of cancer. Contrary to this situation is that with a disease with a high potentiality of causing imminent death, because to the patient this fact could be more emotionally destructive than the disease. All patients need some time to cope with their situation, and a terminally ill patient probably will not have this opportunity. For those cases, it could be more helpful to avoid elements that might deprive the patient of hope.

In the care of the terminally ill patient, it is common practice to lie about the outcome. But how much can we lie? We intentionally avoid not only the hard words, but also the topic during the patient's interview.

This practice is usually accepted by doctors because in Mexico we are not so strongly obligated by law to tell the patient his diagnosis in clear terms. The final and noble intention of the physician is to protect the patient, but it is difficult to sustain a lie until the patient's end.

Mexico does not have palliative care training; therefore, the majority of terminal cancer patients die at home without proper medical attention. Consequently, the patient-physician relationship ends when we can no longer offer the patient further cancer treatment. Confined at home, the patient copes with his death without any opportunity to protest. Thus, doctors and nurses do not live with the consequences of a presumably well-intentioned lie.

In Mexico the age and gender of the patient with cancer have special circumstances. Many women in Latin America, including Mexico—particularly the aged and those from a low social and cultural level—deny their participation as a directly involved receptor of the cancer diagnosis. Furthermore, they assign their decisions to the main family member such as husband, first son, or daughter. Frequently the attending physician participates in the patient's exclusion; during an interview he may give detailed information with words not normally used when the patient is the recipient.

Martin *et al.* reported that in Spain aged people and housewives often do not like to know their diagnosis and outcome.[7] An old patient perceives and faces her end as a natural outcome of her life. Therefore, our information about cancer not only makes this expectation real, it also brings a loss of hope for the near future. On the other hand, young people who receive unexpected news of fatal disease consider it an affront to future plans; their main reactions are anger, fear of the unknown, and a rush to experience all they can.[8,9,10]

In Latin America family support in adverse circumstances is a vital part of our social structure. Mexican society is based on matriarchy; women are usually responsible for the comfort and well-being of an afflicted family member.[11] The presence of relatives of the patient, especially the mother, wife, or daughter, is essential at the first medical interview. They will take care of the most basic matters during the evolution of the patient's disease, such as meals, cleanliness, on-time taking of drugs, and the most essential psychological and affective support. For Mexican doctors it is important to assess the family structure carefully, to allow the patient and family to retain their own coping strategies.

Cultural, social, and economic development in Mexico has marked differences among people living in the north, central and southern parts of our country. Mexicans can live in a megalopolis with more than 20 million people; or in distant, isolated places without elemental sanitary services, as do more than 50 Indian ethnic groups.[12] In these latter regions with limited access to special medical care, traditional and domestic medicine is the main health care system available and is sometimes preferred by these inhabitants.[11]

In these social groups, the mother assumes the role of the disease interpreter and primary therapist through household remedies, popular treatments, magic, and religious procedures. They use modern medical treatments as a last resort. This traditional medicine is so deep-rooted in Mexicans' psyche that it is currently practiced even by people who live in modern cities with a better educational level. Therefore the perception of cancer must be different for these people. The word "cancer" in traditional medicine embraces a wide group of dermatological, usually chronic, and nonspecific diseases. For instance, the herb "cancerina" *(Oenothera rosea)* is used primarily for active wound healing.[11] This conception might lead to confusion about cancer in a patient, because the word by itself may not be compatible for the patient with the illness that we precisely define. Hence, we need to adapt our language to words comprehensible to both patient and family.

Almost 50% of the Mexican population have health care service covered by Institutional Medicine, but with huge differences in the medical assistance rendered. Those patients who come to referral centers or third-level hospitals receive appropriate surgical, antineoplastic agent, and radiotherapy treatments according to the current status of oncology. The possibility of offering suitable treatment facilitates truthfully telling the diagnosis of cancer to the patient. Yet, contrary to the former statement, hundreds of Mexicans live not only the tragedy of having cancer but also that of poverty. Consequently, there is nothing more dramatic and frustrating for a physician than giving a curable cancer diagnosis to a patient without economic resources. Any physician in our country who does not recognize this cultural and social environment will not be able to disclose appropriately a cancer diagnosis.

THE OPINION OF MEDICAL PROFESSIONALS ON GIVING THE DIAGNOSIS OF CANCER AND ON TRADITIONAL MEDICINE

A recently reported study explored Mexican medical students' attitudes towards informing patients of the diagnosis of cancer.[8] The main results revealed that 80% of the students considered that the patient must be informed of his cancer diagnosis; but our oncology practice confirms that as active physicians these future doctors are sometimes reluctant to fulfill this task. Furthermore, 80% of these undergraduate physicians corroborated that the family should be informed because their participation is essential in the care of these patients.

I also explored the attitudes of 48 members of our medical staff, including surgeons, medical and radiotherapy oncologists, residents, and nurses. Ninety-six percent of the nurses do not use the word "cancer," compared with 35% of the doctors. Sixty percent of the medical staff and 79% of the nurses have not received any professional training related to communication of the diagnosis. This also was observed in 72% of the surveyed students.[8] However, all active specialists, nurses, and 75% of the medical students affirmed that they would like to have more training to improve their skills with this situation.

The issue of whether traditional medicine should be accepted during oncological treatment was also explored. Almost half of the routinely attended patients in our service ask if they can use traditional remedies like cat nails, snail capsules, shark cartilage, Tlacote water, and Chaina and Circulan capsules. Thirty-five percent of the physicians and 16% of the nurses do not approve of this alternative medicine and encourage patients to leave these treatments. However, 65% of the doctors and 74% of the nurses think that this popular medicine can help people accept the oncology treatments and that sometimes it is the only beneficial alternative in advanced disease. Only 10% of the nurses have a firm belief in the value of such magical substances.

A MODEL OF THE PROCESS OF COMMUNICATING THE CANCER DIAGNOSIS

The investigation and analysis of this study have led me to some conclusions about the whole process of informing cancer patients of their diagnosis. I observed that the time to inform and discuss the problem with the patient and family is fleeting in comparison with all the problems that the patient has to endure after being struck by the news. The patient's main problem begins after leaving the office or hospital. The goal of the whole process, as seen in this analysis, can be considered only the tip of the iceberg (FIG.1).

The communication basic process involves: (1) the speaker: the physician; (2) the recipient: the patient and his family; and (3) the message: cancer diagnosis information. The truthful telling of the cancer diagnosis is commonly done during a brief interview. The consequences of this is a complex cascade of situations, changes, and reactions of a magnitude beyond what would result in a longer, more reflective dialogue.

As doctors who care for cancer patients, we provide information that will be the catalyst of the patient's personal situations. We must be highly intelligent to achieve empathy in such a short time. In the proposed model (FIG. 1) the patient's concealed problems are physical, emotional, economic, and social. The physical troubles are disability, the symptoms related to the disease, toxicity, and unpleasant appearance. The emotional problems include fear, anxiety, depression, frustration, and the deterioration of self-respect. Economic difficulties are related mainly to a reduction of family income, excessive expenses, and loss of the family patrimony.

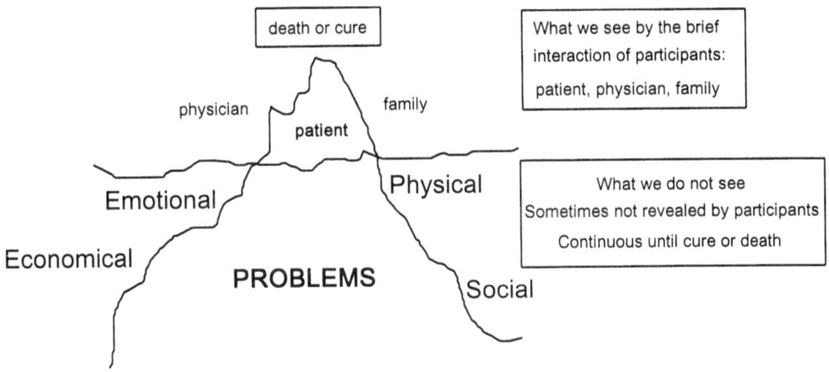

FIGURE 1. Model of the cancer diagnosis communication process.

Finally, family disintegration and rejection of the patient constitute the social problems. The patient and his family need from the physician knowledge of symptom control; help in avoiding patient carelessness; conciliation in family relations; coordination of psychological support; and responsibility for the treatment and side effects.

The development of communication skills should start from personal conviction and effort.[13] Our scientific acts must be always performed with profound sensibility and humanity. We will be better physicians as we are better persons. Our patients are our best teachers, and sometimes what we learn from them is more than the help we can give them. It is our responsibility to take advantage of our professional experience to improve the overall medical support they deserve.

REFERENCES

1. THOMAS, L. V. 1993. El hombre ante la muerte. *In* Antropologia de la muerte: 346–406. Fondo de Cultura Económica Edit. México.
2. FUENTES, C. 1992. El Espejo Enterrado: 101–106. Fondo de Cultura Económica Edit. México.
3. RULFO, J. 1994. Pedro Páramo. Fondo de Cultura Económica Edit. México.
4. LAINE, C. & F. DAVIDOFF. 1996. Patient-centered medicine a professional evolution. JAMA **275**(2): 152–156.
5. GÓMEZ-SANCHO, M. 1994. Las malas noticias. *In* Cuidados paliativos e intervencion psicosocial en enfermos terminales. M. Gomez-Sancho, Ed.: 279–287. ICEPSS. Las Palmas de Gran Canaria España.
6. J. SANZ-ORTIZ, X. GÓMEZ BATISTE, M. GÓMEZ SANCHO & J. NÚÑEZ-OLARTE, Eds. 1993. Información y comunicación. *In* Cuidados Paliativos.

Recomendaciones de la SECPAL: 35–36. Ministerio de Sanidad y Consumo Ed. Madrid.
7. MARTIN-SAN VICENTE, I., R. ALTISEN, M. ARANAZ-MOTTA, M. V. GUILLÉN-ANTÓN, U. ALVIRA & J. FERNÁNDEZ. 1994. La enfermedad terminal y la muerte: ¿Qué opinan los usuarios de un centro de salud? Med. Palliative **1**(1): 22–27.
8. DEL RÍO-ALVAREZ, A., I. PETRA, A. MOHAR-BETANCOURT, R.PEREZ-TAMAYO & A. KRAUSS-WEISMAN. 1995. Las actitudes de estudiantes de medicina ante la muerte. Psiquiatría **11**(1): 6–11.
9. CENTENO CORTES, C. 1995. Questioning diagnosis disclosure in terminal cancer patients. *In* Abstracts of the 4th International Congress of the European Association for Palliative Care, Barcelona VI. 07: 35.
10. MESENGUER, C., A. PARDI, A. D. GASCON, M. SALVADOR, A.TRIAS (PADES) & E. ESTRADE. 1995. El adolescente ante las malas noticias. *In* Abstracts of the 4th International Congress of the European Association for Palliative Care, Barcelona X.04: 83.
11. ZOLLA, C, S. DEL BOSQUE,V. MELLADO, A. TASCON & C. MAQUEO. 1992. Medicina tradicional y enfermedad. *In* La Antropologia Medica en Mexico, Tomo 2. R. Cameos, Ed.: 71–104. Universidad Autonoma Metropolitana Ed. México.
12. AGUIRRE-BELTRAN, G. 1994. El Mexicano y su biotiopologia. *In* Obra Antropologica. XIII Antropologia Medica. G. Aguirre-Beltran, Ed.: 129–168. Fondo de Cultura Económica. México.
13. FOLEY, G. V. 1995. Editorial: Everybody's talking, not communicating. Cancer Pract **2**(3): 71.

The Child with Cancer

Influence of Culture on Truth-telling and Patient Care

MARIA DIE TRILL[a,b,c] AND RIMMA KOVALCIK[a]

[a]*Dana-Farber Cancer Institute*
44 Binney Street
Boston, Massachusetts 02115

[b]*Harvard Medical School*
25 Shattuck Street
Boston, Massachusetts 02115

Culture involves sets of transmitted values, beliefs, attitudes, and habits that determine both the experiences of individuals from infancy onward and the interpretations these individuals give to their experiences. Awareness of the effect of cultural differences on behavior acquires special importance in medicine, given that cultural factors shape our experience of illness and our reactions to it. In addition, complex cross-cultural issues may not be manifested overtly by patients or their families, but can result in the misinterpretation of medical information, noncompliance with treatment, or the seeking of other physicians or treatments. Despite a growing interest in the study of cross-cultural differences in the medical field, few reports have been published on the role of culture in pediatric health care settings, where the juxtaposition of differing medical beliefs and practices can be particularly powerful. Decisions about appropriate medical intervention for one's offspring can throw into sharp relief disparities among alternative and often competing health-care models.[1] In addition to one's own medical orientation, the formulation of a treatment plan for one's child brings into play child-rearing attitudes and practices and the nature of the parent-child relationship. Because of the dependent nature of childhood, health-care providers may be less likely to accept parental decisions, particularly refusal of treatment, than would be the case with adult patients when these decisions differ from their own beliefs.[2] Compared to adult health care, communication in the pediatric setting may be further complicated by the direct involvement of three

[c]Address for correspondence: Maria Die Trill, Ph.D., Hospital Universitario Gregorio Marañón, Dept. Oncologia, Dr. Esquerdo, 46, Madrid 28007, Spain. Telephone: 1-586-6736. Fax: 1-586-8018.

rather than two parties in the patient's management: parents, ill child, and physician, all having the child's well-being as their central concern. Dealing with the potential loss of an offspring to a life-threatening disease is a catastrophic experience across cultures, disrupting the natural order of life events in which parents usually die before their children. However, when culturally defined practices come into play, the experience can be all the more devastating to the patient and his family.

This article describes cross-cultural issues that are relevant in the medical and psychological care of the child with cancer. It refers to sociocultural differences in child-rearing practices and family roles that influence the management or the pediatric cancer patient, including medical decision making and treatment planning. It describes cross-cultural differences in communicating with ill children during different stages of the disease and provides guidelines to optimize communication and patient care in pediatric health care settings.

CHILD-REARING PRACTICES: EFFECTS ON TREATMENT PLANNING

Treatment of children and adolescents with cancer requires a developmental approach embedded in the larger cultural context. The length of time that a child is cuddled, the degree of security and protection to which each child is entitled, and the extent to which adolescence is viewed as a transition period from childhood are all heavily influenced by culture and the stage of development of that culture.[3] In medieval European society children were considered petlike animals or incomplete adults for as long as they remained dependent. Increased childhood deaths led to a lack of attachments to youngsters. Only in the 18th century were children considered different psychologically and physically from adults, separate persons who constructed their own knowledge based on their active discovery of the world, and who had an important role in the family.[4]

Some developmental maturational milestones are universal and biologically determined. They most likely are the consequence of changes in the central nervous system. In addition, every community has culturally defined child-rearing beliefs and practices that determine a child's development and that are passed down through generations. For example, while the dominant value in certain cultural groups is that mothers should have primary responsibility for child rearing, children in other groups are raised more frequently by members of the extended family, nannies, or other parental substitutes.

Child-rearing practices play an important role in personality formation. Japanese child rearing is said to prolong symbiotic mothering, fostering a blurring of the boundaries between mother and child and ultimately between the self and the environment.[5–7] Japanese children do not renounce their attachment to their mothers even after they mature.[8] A major developmental task in Japan is for the child to develop a group-oriented personality, characterized by interdependency, interconnectedness, group harmony, and mutual consideration.[9] On the other hand, the importance of individuation and self-sufficiency has been described in Western cultures, where separation from the mother at early stages, from the family in adolescence, and from teachers and mentors in adulthood are stressed, accentuating the self-other differentiation and increasing firm ego boundaries.[7–10]

Differences in the behavior of children in different cultures have been observed as early as three to four months of age.[11] American infants have been shown to exhibit greater amounts of gross bodily activity, play, and happy vocalizations when compared to Japanese infants, who appeared more passive. Differences in the infants' behaviors were related to differences in caretaking styles: American moaners encouraged their babies to be active and vocally responsive, while Japanese mothers had a tendency to soothe and quiet their babies. The responses of the infants are strikingly in line with the general expectations for behavior in the two cultures. While in America the individual should be physically and verbally assertive, in Japan he should be physically and verbally restrained.

Cultural factors also play an important role during adolescence when identity formation takes place, because a major function of any culture is the transmission of a group identity. Where adolescence is traditionally viewed as a turbulent, rebellious developmental stage during which problems can be expected in some cultures, there appears to be no disturbance in personality and role functioning in other cultures where youth are not expected to revolt against authority and social independence is not encouraged.[12,13]

Differences in culturally determined child-rearing practices have significant consequences in the pediatric cancer setting. For example, the degree of involvement that children and adolescents have over the management of their disease varies greatly from one cultural group to another. In some cultures where much focus of caretaking is placed on achieving autonomy and independence, children and adolescents with cancer are encouraged to become active participants in their medical care. The pediatric bill of rights developed by the Association for the Care of Children's Health in the U.S.[14] refers to the possibility of the child's describing how he wants to take part in his treatment, and to make treatment-related choices whenever possible. Children's and adolescents' participation in medical decision making has been increasing significantly over the past years in countries such as the United States due in part to the advanced understanding of cognitive development, which has led to the belief that children comprehend much of what they go through. However, their participation in the medical decision-making process and treatment planning raises various ethical questions such as whether or not an adolescent has the right to request medical care without parental consent or to refuse potentially lifesaving treatment for cancer. In general, under the age of puberty it is still clear that parental consent needs to be obtained in the United States except in cases of medical emergency or emancipated minors (minors that are married, are in military service, or have left the family home and are self-supporting). However, minor treatment statutes and mature minor rules exist in many states and provide an age ranging from 14 to 17 years at which a minor may consent to medical treatment without parental consent. The mature minor doctrine has not been tested to support an adolescent's right to refuse treatment deemed medically necessary. Courts rarely intervene when parents support a youth's refusal of medical care.[15]

Case 1. C.L. was a 16-year-old patient who, after receiving 5 months of treatment for Hodgkin's disease, fled his home because he could not endure the cancer therapy and had faith that God would heal him without medical treatment. Despite his physician's willingness to modify the initial treatment plan, and an 80–90% cure after therapy, the teenager decided, with his parents' support, to receive alternative rather than conventional forms of treatment for his disease. The patient's parents believed that he was old enough to decide on his own. The court refused to become involved.

This stands in sharp contrast to children whose cultural backgrounds predispose them to comply with the recommendations agreed upon by their physicians and parents without questioning them. Despite reports emphasizing improved adaptation to cancer in children who are more active participants in their treatment and are consequently thought to have more control over it, clinical evidence shows that this does not necessarily apply to members of cultural groups who are expected to be more submissive and follow the recommendations of their elders. This is usually the case with pediatric cancer patients from Latin cultures, whose lesser involvement with their medical care does not necessarily lead to maladjustment to cancer, or in those of Asian backgrounds for whom living in harmony with their environment rather than attempting to control it leads to a greater degree of resignation and a more passive approach to illness.[16]

Differences in child-rearing practices may become problematic in the case of immigrants, where the child may become acculturated before the parents through school attendance. In these cases, parents will hold on to their traditional ways of child upbringing, which may differ significantly from those of their child and of the new culture, creating increased tension between patient and parents and exacerbating the distress already created by a newly diagnosed cancer.

> *Case 2.* M.L., a teenager from the Caribbean diagnosed with medulloblastoma, was referred for psychological services because of severe depressive symptoms due in great part to extreme isolation from peers. M.L. spent her days alone while her mother worked. Even though her parents were estranged, her father had a significant influence over her, refusing to allow her to socialize or engage in behaviors that were considered to be age appropriate in the new culture such as painting her nails or talking on the telephone. M.L. attributed this to child-rearing practices that took place in her country of origin, which she described as "extremely restrictive" and which exacerbated the feelings of isolation and of being "different" already created by her disease.

Child-rearing practices that may be manifested in the medical setting should not be translated into parent or child psychopathology. In some societies where child-rearing practices are more severe, authoritarian controlling and punitive forms of discipline may be viewed as a means to instill responsibility for one's actions and respect for others,[17] whereas they may be considered "abusive" among members of other cultures.

THE ROLE OF FAMILY MEMBERS IN PEDIATRIC CANCER CARE

Cultural norms include unwritten definitions of how families react to a disease and how they respond to the pediatric patient's needs. Working with culturally diverse families requires knowing how a culture defines a family. The American definition refers to the the intact nuclear family.[18] For Mediterranean cultures a family is the extended network of aunts, uncles, cousins, and grandparents, all of whom are highly involved in the patient's care.[19] Traditionally, some African societies have valued a large family and have a strong desire to have male children so that the family line, and indeed the clan, can be sustained.[20] Illness in these families will have a different meaning depending on which member it affects.

Attitudes towards family members vary with each culture. In some African cultures the observation of certain family traditions reflects a great respect for the in-laws.[20] In families of Latin background children are especially valued, and in Native American and Asian cultures respect towards elders is emphasized.[21]

The importance of understanding the hierarchy of family roles in different cultures stems from the fact that culture addresses how different members' advice is valued and which members are involved in the medical decision-making process. In most cultural groups leadership roles are assumed by the family elders. Communication and treatment planning in the context of cancer will be more effective when key members of the extended family (e.g., a grandparent) are identified and allowed to become involved in the pediatric patient's clinical management.

Case 3. D.A. was a 16-year-old southern European male who traveled with his family to the United States for the treatment of a rare tumor of the liver. D.A.'s grandfather had assumed the leading role within the family in asking questions relevant to the patient's medical care and in making decisions regarding his treatment. This created increased anger and tension between family and health-care staff, who strongly believed the parents, rather than the patient's grandfather, should be directly involved with D.A.'s medical condition. Psychological intervention was focused on helping the medical staff understand the culturally defined roles and functions of each family member.

Culture also affects the value that families place on gender. This is illustrated in studies of Lebanese families in which mothers of chronically ill boys have been found to perceive greater impact and distress of the illness on the family than mothers of chronically ill girls.[22,23]

One of the functions of the family is to help the ill child clarify conflicting values about health and health-care practices in such a way that he can choose to adopt behaviors that support wellness.[24] For example, a tendency to stop their child's cancer treatment once the patient responds initially to it has been reported in Chinese families.[25] In addition to understanding the implications of this behavior for the child's health, these families must also comprehend that early termination of treatment will most likely predispose the child with cancer to underestimate the importance of his future medical care, and will possibly interfere with his understanding of death as a likely consequence of treatment withdrawal.

Another important family role is to provide support for the pediatric patient. Cultural norms define the notion of support. Where dependency may foster closeness among family members and encourage emotional support to the patient in some cultures, it may interfere with the patient's sense of control during the course of the disease in other cultural groups.[19] Cultures with a strong family identification and a rich network of family interactions tend to foster a less strong sense of personal responsibility. Rights and responsibilities as well as medical decision making are shared, diffusing the psychological burden of assuming total care of the ill child.

Immigration imposes an additional burden on the parents of a chronically ill child. Living in a foreign country and being unable to communicate accurately or to understand the new medical system add to the psychological distress imposed on families by the diagnosis of cancer in a child. For example, adjusting to the team approach characteristic of the

American health-care system may be confusing to families who are used to medical systems that operate through patient-physician dyads.

Case 4. S.E. was a 13-year-old female from eastern Europe with metastatic osteogenic sarcoma of her right hip. Due to the patient's rapidly deteriorating condition, meetings with her parents and various members of the health-care team, including primary physician, medical residents, nurses, psychologist, social worker, and physical therapist, were regularly scheduled. S.E.'s father exhibited gradually increasing resistance to participating in such meetings. He revealed his discomfort in sharing intimate patient and family-related information with health-care staff with whom he had not established a trusting relationship, especially at a time when the patient's prognosis was poor and important medical decisions had to be reviewed on an ongoing basis. Meetings had to be adjusted to the family's psychological needs and included only S.E.'s parents and primary physician.

Conflict may also arise as a consequence of role reversal in immigrant families, as occurs in cases in which children with cancer are placed in a position of authority by health-care professionals when asked to translate medical information for their parents.

COMMUNICATING WITH THE PEDIATRIC CANCER PATIENT

Several decades ago when the prognosis of childhood cancers was very poor the main goal of the health-care team was to provide maximum comfort measures to the child and to prepare his family for the process of grieving. Recent advances in pediatric oncology have led to increased survival rates, prolonged periods of uncertainty, and in some cases the development of long-term disease and treatment-related sequelae, all of which elicit important questions and fears in a child's mind. This has led to significant modifications in truth-telling practices to ill children in some cultures.

Those who argue that children always should be told the *truth* about having cancer must recognize that the truth is susceptible to many interpretations.[26] The child's understanding about the information he receives regarding his disease and how it affects him at different stages of the illness are critical issues that require knowledge of the family's cultural background.

Communicating diagnostic and prognostic information to a cancer patient and his family may be considered one of the most emotionally charged aspects of the relationship between the physician, the patient, and his parents. It involves the resolution of a moral dilemma: how to transmit a devastating truth to both the child and his family. Due to the ethic of full disclosure between physician and patient, the current basic philosophy of oncology clinics in the United States has become to tell the truth, even if not asked.

It is difficult to keep a child with cancer from learning about his illness. His interactions with other patients in the hospital, his increased exposure to the media, where cancer is frequently discussed, and the responses of those around him to his disease will increase his awareness of the seriousness of his condition. Reluctance to disclose cancer-related information to the ill child is not uncommon in many cultures. For some it is a reflection of our own anxieties about cancer and death, and is thought to stem from our own need to protect ourselves rather than the patient from information that provokes high levels of anxiety. For others it is an extension of the belief that sharing bad news should not become a common practice in the community.[27] Among members of other cultures, withholding medical information from the ill child reflects the belief that children are not psychologically equipped to cope with such devastating news. In other cultural groups, families of pediatric cancer patients seek several second opinions, not necessarily from professionals, with the hope that one of these consultants will announce that the diagnosis was a mistake.[25]

Several variables that influence communication patterns between physician, parents, and ill child have been identified. Parents' intelligence, their level of education, the number of questions they ask, uncertainty about the prognosis, the physician's sympathy towards the family, and his anxiety about his own death have been found to be positively correlated with the administration of realistic information that parents receive.[28,29] Parents who show a greater expression of affect have been found to elicit more positive emotional comments from physicians.[30] Boys have been reported to receive more information from their physicians regarding their illness than girls.[31]

Talking to a child about his cancer is not an easy task for anyone involved in his care. An initial rule is to respect the parents' desire on what information they would like the child to have and how they want it to be transmitted.

Case 5. T.H. was a 22-year-old male of Latino descent diagnosed 4 years earlier with an osteogenic sarcoma of his left leg. It was his parents' desire since the confirmation of his diagnosis that the word "cancer" not be used in his conversations with the health-care staff. The patient's family threatened to take legal action against their physician when they were informed that, for legal purposes, due to T.H.'s age he had to be informed of the fourth recurrence of his disease. After several meetings between the family and members of the medical team, it was agreed that T.H. would be informed of his condition using terms such as "tumor progression" that his family felt more comfortable with. It was his mother's belief that had the word "cancer" been used, the patient would have "lost his hope of recovery" and "stopped fighting his disease" because of the negative connotation that the word "cancer" had in their country of origin.

Health-care professionals in the United States believe that it is important that parents provide the ill child with some explanation of why he needs to be hospitalized and receive aggressive treatments for an extended period of time. Not doing so is thought to trigger fantasies and misconceptions in the child such as the belief that he has contracted cancer because of some prior misbehavior or "bad thoughts." Parents decide who is to transmit this information to the child. It is recommended that they do this in the presence of members of the health-care team so that all of the child's questions may be answered appropriately. It is not uncommon, for example, for children to ask whether or not they are going to die when they first learn about their disease, and parents may find this too overwhelming to answer. Parents and health-care staff are advised to use a gentle, honest, and simple approach at all times. The information is usually provided upon confirmation of the diagnosis and is adjusted to the child's developmental level and cultural background. It is explained to the child that he has a serious illness that will require repeated hospitalizations and the administration of treatments that may make him lose his hair and feel initially worse. He is reassured that his hair will grow back and that the health-care team has extensive experience in treating other children with his disease, some of whom he may meet in the clinic. The child is informed that if treatment becomes painful at times, certain measures such as training in hypnosis or relaxation techniques or the administration of pain medication can be adopted to alleviate his discomfort. He is told that he may feel frightened or sad occasionally, and that it is important to let an adult know when this happens. It is also explained to the child that the treatments will temporarily interrupt school attendance and possibly participation in certain activities such as sports. Parents are encouraged to allow the child the expression of negative feelings such as anger, frustration, sadness, and fear, which are appropriate and common in response to learning about the diagnosis. In some cultural groups, the message conveyed to the child, especially boys, is that they must "be brave and behave like men," implying that if the child complains about the physical discomfort induced by the disease or its treatment, he is a coward or not manly enough. This may lead to underreporting of symptoms by the patient, who may then not be treated adequately.

If communicating with the child about his diagnosis is difficult, discussing death and dying issues is even more of an emotional burden to the family. There is no prescription as to how to communicate best with the terminally ill child about death. When choosing to do so, the use of simple, clear language tailored to the child's level of comprehension is imperative. It is best to avoid euphemisms or terms that may create confusion in the child such as "passing away" or "sleeping." Incorporating the family's religious beliefs in the discussion is usually helpful. For some families it is important to discuss life after death in order to decrease the child's fears of being alone after dying. The expression of the ill child's thoughts and questions about death and dying is strongly encouraged where discussion of death-related issues with the terminally ill child is culturally acceptable. This is usually done by questioning the child directly or by seeking professional advice.

Case 6. H.L. was a six-year-old girl with an optic glioma whose hospital friend had died of leukemia. This triggered in her a series of questions and thoughts about death and dying. One of H.L.'s beliefs was that she had to die in order to help her recently deceased friend who was "very busy" in heaven "helping the Virgin Mary cook and clean the dishes for Jesus."

Case 7. M.N. was a terminally ill nine-year-old patient with a glioblastoma who revealed to his psychologist his belief that he would meet his deceased grandfather in heaven, where they would both be able to play soccer and baseball. He had been unable to practice these activities because of the rapid progression of his disease, which forced him to remain in a wheelchair.

In certain cultural groups, discussion of death and dying issues with terminally ill children is avoided entirely. This may be due to parents' fears that such discussions will further upset and depress the child or decrease his ability to cope with a life-threatening disease, or to religious beliefs that lead them to hope for a miracle that will cure their child. In order to facilitate the family's coping in such an overwhelming situation, clinical interventions should be based on the parent's wishes for communicating with their ill child at all times.

ENHANCING COMMUNICATION AND IMPROVING PATIENT CARE

Cross-cultural conflicts between family and health-care staff may arise in the pediatric setting when there are differing beliefs about the etiology of the child's malady; the frequency of medical procedures is seen as unnecessary by the parents; or there are differing beliefs about the required treatment (antibiotics versus medicinal herbs) or about the need for medical follow-up.[1]

Language barriers may constitute additional sources of conflict. They may interfere with the establishment of an alliance between patient and physician, impose additional burdens on the patient's efforts to organize the distressing experience that a cancer diagnosis imposes, and increase patients' fears of not understanding and explaining medical information accurately. Language barriers may also complicate an accurate assessment of the child's physical and mental status.[19]

Case 8. T.W. was a four-year-old Latino girl with a supratentorial glioma for whom a psychological assessment was requested for unresponsive behavior thought to be 'due to a language barrier" by the medical staff. Upon examination in the patient's language, she was found to exhibit symptoms that included lack of speech and eye contact, limited communication skills, impaired play, and abnormal social interactions. She was diagnosed with an autistic disorder, for which she received the appropriate treatment.

The assessment of culturally different patients should focus on enhancing communication and rapport with the child and his parents, and ideally should take place in the patient's language or in the presence of a translator. It should include an understanding of why the child was brought to a health-care setting; what the child's behaviors and symptoms are that most concern the parents; what the parents believe has caused the illness and why they think it appeared when it did; how the parents believe the illness affects the child; what measures have they taken to control it, if any; how they believe the disease should be handled in the health-care setting; and what their expectations of medical care are.[1] Information should also be sought on parental fears about the disease and their perceptions of the parental role on providing health-care for the child. Dietary practices and religious beliefs and rituals including the identification of significant religious persons should be included in the initial family assessment. It is necessary to investigate the family's use of nonconventional treatments, which tends to be underreported due to parental fears of physician disapproval and to the threat that the use of such therapies creates in some members of the medical team.

In order to optimize patient care, support systems need to be tailored to the needs of each family. Involvement of professionals who are familiar with the values and lifestyles of families will facilitate the development of intervention strategies that are consistent with family characteristics.

The participation of traditional healers in the child's care should also be considered. Their role, social standing, and influence on local health practices has been gaining recognition by world health bodies.[32] The popularity of such healers among members of certain cultures stems from their speaking to patients in terms that they understand, giving them time, listening to them, and prescribing medicaments that are culturally acceptable to them.[33] Optimal patient care will be enhanced by the simultaneous use of traditional and conventional therapies. Physicians who encourage patients to actively observe traditional rites do not necessarily believe that the rite has a direct physical benefit on the patient, but rather that the maintenance of family and traditional beliefs undoubtedly speeds recovery.[34]

Coaching the younger generations to respect older generations' values and beliefs is important in immigrant families, where the diagnosis of cancer may add to intergenerational conflicts already imposed by immigration.

Cultural stereotypes must be avoided at all times. It is not uncommon when the family's behavior does not conform to the health professionals' cultural norms or medical recommendations that this be interpreted as a result of cultural differences. However, rarely is a family's adjustment to the disease and compliance with treatment attributed to the effects of culture.

Parental blaming should be avoided when parents' behavior towards the ill child is not well understood. Several studies have adopted an accusatory stance as they assess parental roles in child survival; parents, and in particular mothers, are blamed for a perceived failure to provide *adequate* care or to make *proper* health choices. However, parents in general have been found to be concerned and proactive health seekers for their children; their caretaking decisions sometimes force them to weigh concerns for an individual child against demands of the family as a whole.[35] In China, for example, children with cancer have been reported to undergo their first hospital admission during the terminal phase of the disease. This may be due to parents' unawareness of the seriousness of their child's condition or to the lack of sufficient finances,[27] rather than to lack of adherence to medical care.

SUMMARY

The definition, understanding, and shaping of childhood and adolescence vary widely. The cultural life of a community determines how children are valued and what measures will be taken to insure their health. It will also determine the family's responses to an ill child. It is for these reasons that health-care professionals should be sensitive to culturally defined health beliefs and practices that may explain behaviors such as nonadherence to prescribed therapies, the degree and quality of parents' involvement in patient care, and the family's relationship with health-care staff. Assessments of health beliefs and practices, family composition, religious rites, and beliefs about illness causation should be routinely made on each family. These assessments provide important information that will facilitate the design of treatment plans that are congruent with a family's cultural heritage.

Knowledge of cultural factors should not exclude an individualized approach to families. Each family should be evaluated in ways that allow us to identify their individual as well as culturally defined characteristics. This will eliminate the cultural stereotyping that may occur in the context of behaviors that are not well understood in a particular health-care setting.

Research studies in which health behaviors are correlated with culturally defined values and practices need to be carried out. The International Psycho-Oncology Society, through its National Representation Committee, is currently investigating oncology practices around the world. Nearly 30 countries are participating in this attempt to identify cultural variations in truth-telling, palliative care, pain control, and use of alternative medicine in oncology. The importance of this study lies not only in the results that it will yield, but also in the joint effort that it has required to share professional experiences and to enhance efficient communication among oncologists internationally. This study may also be used as a model to investigate oncology practices in pediatric health-care settings.

REFERENCES

1. KORBIN, J. E. & M. JOHNSTON. 1982. Steps toward resolving cultural conflict in a pediatric hospital. Clin. Pediatr. **21:** 259–263.
2. WHELAN, D. 1978. Blood transfusions—When the patient says no. Med. J. Aust. Aug. 26, 1978: 183–186.
3. WALDRON, J. & J. F. MCDERMOTT. 1979. Transcultural considerations. *In* Basic Handbook of Child Psychiatry. J. D. Noshpitz, Ed.: 434–444. Basic Books. New York, NY.
4. SHAHART, S. 1990. Childhood in the Middle Ages. Routledge. London.
5. DOI, T. 1985. The Anatomy of Dependency. Kodashna International, Ltd. Tokyo.
6. ROLAND, A. 1988. In Search of Self in India and Japan. Princeton University Press. Princeton, NJ.
7. SEIKO KOBAYASHI, J. 1989. Depathologizing dependency: Two perspectives. Psychiatr. Ann. **19**(12, Dec.): 653–658.
8. LEBRA, T. S. 1976. Japanese Patterns of Behavior. University of Hawaii Press. Honolulu, HI.
9. NAKAKUKI, M. 1984. Two major characteristics of Japanese culture. Presented at the 73rd Annual Meeting of the American Psychoanalytic Association. San Diego, CA.
10. SURREY, J. 1984. The self in relation: A theory of women's development. Work in Progress, Wellsley College **13:** 1–15.
11. CAUDILL, W. A. & C. SCHOOLER. 1973. Child behavior and child-rearing in Japan and the US: An interim report. J. Nerv. Ment. Dis. **157**(5): 325–338.
12. MEAD, M. 1953. A Coming of Age in Samoa: A Psychological Study of Primitive Youth for Western Civilization. Modern Library. New York, NY.
13. TSENG, W. S. & D. H. WU. 1985. Chinese Culture and Mental Health. Academic Press. New York, NY.
14. ASSOCIATION FOR THE CARE OF CHILDREN'S HEALTH. 1991. A Pediatric Bill of Rights. Association for the Care of Children's Health. Bethesda, MD.
15. HOLDER, A. R. 1988. Disclosure and consent problems in pediatrics. Law

Med. Health Care **16**(34): 219–228.

16. ADAMS, D. 1969. The monkey and the fish. Cultural pitfalls of an educational advisor. *In* The Cross-Cultural Approach to Health Behavior. L. Riddick, Ed.: 436–444. Fairleigh Dickinson University Press. Madison, NJ.
17. DEYOUNG, Y. & E. F. ZIGLER. 1994. Machismo in two cultures: Relation to punitive child-rearing practices. Am. J. Orthopsychiatry **64**(3): 386–395.
18. MCGOLDRICK, M. 1982. Ethnicity and the life cycle. *In* Ethnicity and Family Therapy. M. McGoldrick, J. Pearce & J. Giordano, Eds.: 69–90. Guilford Press. New York, NY.
19. DIE TRILL, M. & J. HOLLAND. 1992. Cross-cultural differences in the care of patients with cancer: A review. Gen. Hosp. Psychiatry. **15:** 21–30.
20. NAMBOZE, J. M. 1983. Health and culture in an African society. Soc. Sci. Med. **17**(24): 2041–2041.
21. OLNESS, K. 1992. Cultural issues in primary pediatric care. *In* Primary Pediatric Care. R. A. Hoekelman, S. B. Friedman, N. M. Nelson & H. M. Siedel, Eds.: 138–145. Mosby Year Book. St. Louis, MO.
22. KURDAHI ZAHR, L., M. KHOURY & N. B. SAOUD. 1994. Chronic illness in Lebanese preschoolers: Impact of illness and child temperament on the family. Am. J. Orthopsychiatry **64**(3): 396–403.
23. PATAI, R. 1983. The Arab Mind. Scribners. New York, NY.
24. STEELE, S. 1983. The scope of the problem. *In* Health Promotion of the Child with Long-Term Illness. 3rd edit. S. M. Steele, Ed.: 3–21. Appleton-Century Crofts. Norwalk, CT.
25. TAN, C. 1992. Treating life-threatening illness in children. *In* Chinese Americans in Loss and Separation. Social, Medical and Psychiatric Perspectives. C. L. Chen, W. C. Lowe, D. Ryan, A. H. Kutscher, R. Halporn & H. H. Wang, Eds.: 25–29. Foundation of Thanatology. New York, NY.
26. BEARISON, D. J. 1991. They Never Want to Tell You. Harvard University Press. Cambridge, MA.
27. MARTINSON, I. 1994. The reaction of Chinese parents to a terminally ill child with cancer. Cancer Nurs. **17**(1): 72–76.
28. FREEMAN, B., V. F. NEGRETE, M. DAVIS *et al.* 1971. Gaps in doctor patient communication: Doctor-patient interaction analysis. Pediatr. Res. **5:** 298–311.
29. AMIR, M. 1992. Considerations guiding physicians when informing cancer patients. Soc. Sci. Med. **24:** 741–748.
30. STREET, R. L. 1992. Communication styles and adaptation in physician-parent consultation. Soc. Sci. Med. **34:** 1155–1163.
31. PANTELL, R., T. J. STEWART *et al.* 1982. Physician communication with children and parents. Pediatrics **70:** 396–401.
32. WORLD HEALTH ORGANIZATION. 1978. International Conference on Primary Health, Alma Ata, USSR. A Joint Report by the Director of the WHO and the Executive Director of the United Nations Children's Fund.: 33. World Health Organization. Geneva.
33. PARRY, E. H. O. 1983. Making medical education relevant to health care systems. Soc. Sci. Med. **17**(24): 2037–2039.
34. MORLEY, D. 1973. Beliefs and attitudes to child-rearing and disease. *In* Pediatric Priorities in the Developing World. D. Morley, Ed. Butterworth. London.
35. FINERMAN, R. 1995. Parental incompetence and selective neglect: Blaming the victim in child survival. Soc. Sci. Med. **40**(1): 5–13.

Health Care in the United States

A Perspective from the Front Line

GLADYS GONZALEZ

Memorial Sloan-Kettering Cancer Center
1275 York Avenue
New York, New York 10021

Health care should be a basic right, not a privilege.

INTRODUCTION

In the realm of health care, the concept of communication includes honoring confidentiality, truth-telling, informed consent, and standard ethical procedures. I have worked primarily as a liaison between the physician and the patient, and between the institution and the patient. From my experience of having worked within the confines of rigid rules and regulations, I have always felt troubled by the lack of compassion and sensitivity toward the patient. Ironically, despite the aim of each institution in which I have served and each physician with whom I have worked, the human element has been compromised by the strict rules and regulations that were in effect. As a first-generation American, I am sensitive to the concerns of the non-English speaking patient, particularly to the lack of understanding among health-care personnel of patients' diverse cultural rituals and beliefs. Communication is fragile from the outset because of the dynamics of being a patient. It is important for all concerned—physicians, institutions, clinicians, technicians, and staff workers—to realize the importance of good, effective communication in the delivery of health care. In this chapter I will focus on health care in the United States, past and present, and on my experience in this field, particularly as it relates to the issue of communication.

A CULTURAL PERSPECTIVE

In the United States, the variety and mixture of cultures, nationalities, and religious beliefs can make it difficult to treat patients. Cultural and religious beliefs play an important role in how people perceive their state of health or illness. The patient's socioeconomic status and educational level may not necessarily be factors in how satisfied he/she is with his/her medical care. During the past decade, much emphasis has been placed on cost containment, providing optimal care, and improving access to health care for all United States citizens and residents. But although it is a central concern of the medical community to reach out to the community at large, the medical community fails to adequately meet the needs of the culturally diverse population. Within our multicultural, diverse communities, the probability of compromise of health care is much greater when patients and physicians do not share the same language, ethnicity, value system, and class. Sensitivity to patients' diversity strongly influences the delivery of care. Failure to recognize the importance of the rituals and customs of a patient's ethnic group can lead to misdiagnosis and poor adherence to treatment regimens and follow-up care. In addition, lack of knowledge of a patient's belief system and how that patient perceives his or her illness or health may be interpreted by the physician or health-care practitioner as an annoyance and may create a barrier to effective communication. An American-trained physician may, for example, give the impression that Western medicine is superior when treating an Asian patient who has a high regard for his own traditional medicine. It is becoming more important in health care to view the patient holistically, considering ethnicity along with other factors.[1–6]

I was reared in one of the largest cities in the United States. Within a ten-block radius lived members of at least four very different ethnic groups. Each group had very different belief systems and worldviews. No doubt each group had a different view of health, illness, and medicine. This was evident in the milieu of the local clinic or emergency room. It took me years to fully understand the anecdote I will now relate.

> A friend's four-year-old sister had been sick for a few days. The child had become pale and weak from vomiting. In a short while the child could no longer walk. Her mother fed her warm homemade soups and swaddled her in blankets. The mother practiced folkloric medicine, feeding the child warm liquids, and prayed for her to get better. I could not comprehend why the child's mother did not take her to see a doctor. Finally, she did take the child to the local emergency room. The child was immediately admitted for acute appendicitis. Luckily, the child's appendix was surgically removed before it could rupture, and she became well.

The mother's reason for not seeking professional medical attention sooner was her lack of confidence in the American health-care system. This was a result of harsh treatment she had received as an immigrant. In addition, she strongly believed that her folkloric remedies would cure her child and would also spare her the embarrassment of not speaking good English.

In some physician practices, support staff workers take an active role in patient care. Receptionists, secretaries, or line staff may have to ask a variety of private, personal questions during an office visit or telephone call. This screening process serves as a means of efficiency and to aid the physician. If the physician knows at the outset the reason for a patient's visit or telephone call, he can better assist or comfort the patient. This screening also has financial and administrative advantages. A physician can see more patients when his support staff has thoroughly screened calls and patients. With information provided by the patient, the support staff can direct the call or patient to a technician or nurse. It is unusual for a patient to speak to a physician before going through such a screening process.

Some patients find this acceptable. However, the screening practice may be seen in some cultures as an invasion of privacy, an outright violation of confidentiality. Some patients may be reluctant to seek medical care under such conditions.[3–5]

We Americans live in a consumer-driven society.[5] As part of the self-help movement, we are encouraged to take on some of the responsibility for our care.[4] Patients have a bill of rights, there are patient advocates in hospitals, we go for second opinions, do research, check doctor's credentials, and question procedures and charges. But in some cultures, the physician is viewed as a strict, authoritative figure. To question him is to show disrespect.[1]

It is typical to find a variety of ethnic groups working together in the health-care field with the goal of providing optimal care. However, how can this goal be attained if there is a lack of understanding or appreciation of ethnicity? Cultural differences often create misunderstandings, misinterpretation, and conflict in health care and sometimes result in inferior care.[1–3,5,7–9] In order to bridge the gap between the health-care system and the population it serves, there is a need to address the issue of communication.

HISTORICAL OVERVIEW OF HEALTH CARE AND HOSPITALS IN THE UNITED STATES

Hospitals are shaped by the needs of the society, its attitudes, beliefs, values, and economy. In early America hospitals were primarily religious and charitable institutions, established to provide care for the sick, rather than medical care as such. The earliest hospitals were actually almshouses or poorhouses that housed the indigent and incurable.[8–12]

The traditional physician was of the affluent class, because only the wealthy could afford the high cost of medical school.[8,12] The family doctor would treat a person from infancy through adulthood. In effect part of the extended family, he knew the entire family history.[5,8] The relationship between physician and patient was largely based upon the priestly, paternalistic model. In this traditional model, the patient did not actively take part in his/her health care. The family as a whole was considered first and took an active role in making decisions. Often the dominant person in the family would be responsible for the patient's care.[4–6]

The period around the turn of the century was one of rapid growth in the health-care field, specifically in inpatient care (hospitalization). The advancement of industrialization led to advancements in medical technology and biomedical science. Medical care that was once practiced by a physician making house calls with his black leather bag was now being moved into a hospital setting, where special equipment was available. The medical specialist was becoming essential. Nursing as an occupation changed, too, becoming more supportive of the work of physicians. Voluntary hospitals and hospitals specializing in specific diseases became more common during this period, which also saw the development of religious and ethnic hospitals.[8,9,11]

World War II began another period of evolutionary change in the health-care system in the United States. The health-care field was becoming very lucrative. That, along with advances in technology and government support, persuaded more individuals to become physicians. The rapid growth in the number of physicians required the support of other disciplines in the health-care field—e.g., technicians, clinicians, and nurses.[8,9,11]

As a result of giving large numbers of people physical examinations prior to induction into military service, the government became increasingly aware of the population's poor health. Government health programs were created to provide benefits for the poor. The Medicaid and Medicare programs were initiated in the 1960s. Medicaid is mandated by the federal government to provide care for the poor and is administered by the federal, state, and city governments. Medicare is a federal program to provide care for the elderly and the catastrophically ill; it is administered by state and local governments. There has been a long-term effort on the part of the government to control disease, ensure health, and apply uniform standards.[2,8–11]

For the most part, health care in the United States is a free enterprise, provided by nonprofit organizations. Health care became a vast enterprise, particularly in the area of hospitalization. Hospital insurance developed rapidly to cover the high cost of hospitalization; a patient's entire life savings could be consumed by expensive hospital care.[13] The rapid growth of hospital insurance was a major factor contributing to the increased use of hospitalization.[2,9]

THE HEALTH-CARE SYSTEM IN THE UNITED STATES TODAY

We now have two distinct agents in the health-care field: administrators and health-care managers on the one hand, and the clinical entity on the other. The administrators focus on finance, operations, facilities management, and risk management (quality assurance and utilization review). The clinical entity consists of physicians, nurses, technicians, and other health-related occupations.[9]

The health-care system in our society is divided into four interrelated components: ambulatory care, inpatient care, long-term care, and mental health services.[9] Of these four components, in-patient care is the most costly and the most in need of change. There are five types of hospital systems in the United States: (1) *Teaching hospitals* are research oriented, highly technical, and complex; they are funded by federal grant. They provide care for the indigent. These are large institutions, located in urban areas. (2) *Multisystem:* one umbrella institution has two or more hospitals serving under a lease or legal incorporation, under the direction of a board. (3) *Public hospitals* are owned by agencies of the federal, state, or local governments. Typically these hospitals provide specialized care for American Indians, government personnel, and veterans. State hospitals are typically designed to provide long-term care for the mentally or chronically ill. (4) *Private hospitals* vary in size; most are much smaller than the types mentioned above. They focus on specialized care and tend to have a revenue margin. (5) *Rural hospitals* are smaller, nonurban institutions that focus on the needs of their surrounding community. They have less access to federal funds.[8,11]

As a result of the escalating cost of hospitalization, the DRG (diagnostic related groups) system was implemented by the government in 1983. Originally, hospitals and physicians were paid or reimbursed on a per diem basis. This permitted overcharging and too much latitude. The DRG system provides for payment by the case in order to control costs and budgeting. The DRG system, which is heavily regulated, defines appropriate care for each type of case. The DRG system was later amended to better suit the needs of society. Hospital reimbursement went from a retrospective cost-based system to a prospective payment system based primarily on DRGs of specific illnesses.[2,8,9,11–14]

Despite the worthy intentions of the DRG system, it has led to many problems. It imposes time limits on hospitals and physicians for carrying out specific routines. As a result, it can lead to premature discharge from the hospital and readmission.[2,3,8,9,12,13]

Currently there are two distinct ways for a person obtain health-care services: fee-for-service and managed care. Under fee-for-service a patient is referred, or refers himself, to a physician; care is delivered; a bill is generated; the patient pays and awaits reimbursement from his insurance carrier, or the provider of health care is paid directly by the insurance carrier. Fee-for-service allows the patient freedom to choose his physician, all services are available, and costs are covered. However, it can lend itself to fragmentation of patient care—for instance, where there is a lot of diagnostic testing, with results going to several different physicians for analysis. Fee-for-service does not encourage or facilitate continuity of care or cost containment.[2–4,8,9,12,13]

Managed care is any system that manages health care delivery and controls costs. Managed care programs, characteristically known as health maintenance organizations (HMOs) cover most medical expenses provided that the patient uses physicians and hospitals within the organization's network. The patient's financial obligation is usually a nominal fee, known as a copayment. Most managed care models work as a comprehensive medical plan that provides or arranges all care for plan members. They do not provide benefits for care outside of the contracted provider network except in cases of emergency. Managed care involves controlling the utilization of hospital and physician services via preadmission screening. The basis of a managed care system is the development of a doctor-patient relationship. The primary care physician, the "gate keeper," makes referrals to other physicians or services for the patient, the patient is given care, and a bill is circulated and paid. The primary care physician acts as case manager. Managed care emphasizes preventive services and the early detection and treatment of medical problems. States across the nation have been looking at managed care as a vehicle to reduce costs for publicly insured patients.[4,13]

Despite the efforts to implement a comprehensive plan providing primary care at reduced cost and with improved access, managed care has not rectified all past problems, has worsened some, and has created new problems as well. Managed care programs often restrict freedom of choice. Not all services may be available. The cost of services is covered only if they have been coordinated by the primary care physician. Costs are still inflated. Managed care programs attempt to route patients into their own assigned hospitals or clinics for treatment. However, many patients are not aware of exactly how the program operates and how it can best suit their needs, and some revert to the fee-for-service system. In effect, managed care programs have sent many patients back into city hospital emergency rooms, where they receive acute care and often leave a large unpaid bill.[2,4,8–10,12,13]

Managed care physicians are prepaid a lump sum for the number of patients they see. The physician's income does not come directly from the patient but from the managed care program. There is little incentive for managed care physicians to educate and treat their patients, because the physicians will get paid the same amount anyway. The developers of managed care programs did not anticipate the human element. It is difficult to modify human behavior. Most people go to the doctor when they are sick. Most patients want quick relief, disregard information, and continue to seek medical services as they had previously—for many, in a hospital emergency room.[2–5,8,9,12,13]

Currently, the philosophy of health care in America is changing. Patients are inreasingly being treated in an ambulatory-care setting rather than in an inpatient-care setting (hospital). As a nation we are focusing more on preventive medicine. Health care in our society is viewed as a commodity—an unwanted commodity. Managed care and health maintenance organizations (predominantly business and finance oriented) are becoming the model for combating the high cost of health care. They are also viewed as a solution to the problem of restricted access to health care for United States citizens and residents. Managed care raises many ethical issues in the health-care delivery system. Modifications of the system are continually being proposed, discussed, and enacted. One such modification is the point of service (POS) plan. This is like an HMO in that most medical services are covered in full (there is a copayment) as long as the patient uses the organization's network of physicians and hospitals. Unlike an HMO, the patient can also obtain care from nonnetwork providers and still receive some benefits.[2,9,10,13]

The ever-changing health care delivery system is affecting the way physicians are treating patients and the relationship between doctor and patient. Doctors are losing their autonomy, as insurance carriers are becoming the driving force in heatlh care. Cost-saving strategies not only restrict patients but contribute to the increasing fragmentation of medical care.[2,12,13]

GAPS IN COMMUNICATION

Repeated Giving of Medical Information

The trend toward managed health care, whether in the form of an HMO or of an insurance carrier managing or monitoring the health care of a patient, means, among other things, that the patient has to divulge his medical condition and history to several people before seeing the physician. This is problematic, because (1) most patients do not have information about their medical history readily available, and they become frustrated by the need to repeat it; (2) one's medical history becomes less and less confidential as the information is processed; (3) the clerical or line staff, though trained and expert in their jobs, are often inexperienced in dealing with the psychosocial impact of health-care delivery; and (4) most patients feel very uncomfortable having to divulge their medical problems and history to nonmedical personnel.

Despite the increased use of HMOs, many patients do not have a primary care physician or general internist. A patient may seek medical advice or treatment from several different doctors simultaneously. When a patient gives his medical history to several physicians, he may be inconsistent in giving vital historical and anecdotal information, because the patient may forget or may think that certain information is irrelevant. Patients are not given much time to communicate their history. In addition, a patient's ability to articulate his condition may be influenced by the condition itself. When physicians rely heavily on modern technology to make their assessments, verbal communication between patient and doctor may become minimal. The physician's desire to make effective use of his time may also minimize communication with the patient, who may quickly be referred to other colleagues for highly technical care. Often a patient is left unclear as to who will give follow-up care, and medical records may not necessarily be sent to the physician who manages the patient's care. It becomes difficult to establish a relationship with your physician when your care is so fragmented.[2–5,8,12]

Confidentiality of Medical Information

Not many years ago, a doctor's office used to consist of the doctor and a nurse, with the nurse undertaking all the clerical responsibilities; or the doctor and his secretary, with the secretary often acting as his medical assistant. The overall setup of the doctor's office was personal. There was one-on-one contact between patient, physician, and staff. The secretary or nurse would be responsible for filing insurance claims to the guarantor. There would be a set fee for services regardless of the complexity of the visit. A diagnosis or explanation would be placed on insurance claim forms even if the patient had come in for a routine visit. Filing forms allowed for the physician to be paid or the patient reimbursed.

Today's doctor's office is usually a group practice of three or more physicians, where typically there is a receptionist, secretary, billing manager, office manager, laboratory technician or clinician, medical assistant, and registered nurse. When making an appointment, you speak with the receptionist, who schedules your appointment and informs you of the fee and whether or not their group participates in your insurance plan. When you go for your visit, you meet and speak to several staff members on your way in and out of the office, reiterating the reason why you are there. There is no feeling of continuity of care when you must make an appointment with one person, negotiate a bill with another, discuss insurance matters with an office manager, and get instructions from a nurse or clinician.

In addition, throughout the patient's visit his/her personal, private life is revealed in the presence of the staff and other patients in the waiting area. This lack of privacy is often aggravated by the architecture of the office: the staff's work area is built into the waiting area.[3,4] Often other patients can overhear the conversations of the technicians and other workers pertaining to another patient's life. The office setting does not promote satisfactory communication or confidentiality.

Through the years, the health-care field has become more and more complex. Insurance carriers or HMOs have become the authorities in managing the care of the patient, as the direct result of their reimbursement policies. When a patient signs his name on a claim form for payment to the physician or reimbursement, he is authorizing the release of information about his medical condition and history.[8,12] That information can then be reviewed and disclosed to a hospital or health-care service plan so that it may process his claim.[13] The authorization could also permit disclosure to the patient's employer for the purpose of utilization review or financial audit. Even though much emphasis is placed on confidentiality, the insurance filing system, like the overall office structure, does not allow for privacy.

Increased Direct Involvement of Clerical and Line Staff with Patients

Clerical and line staff are becoming increasingly involved in patient care. Staff members who assist physicians or health-care practitioners are often not equipped to handle the emotional demands of the situation. Rather than being formally taught how to handle stressful situations, they learn through day-to-day experience. This may have serious repercussions for both patient and workers. When patients are ill or in pain, it is quite normal for them to behave irrationally. They may become impatient, nervous, annoyed, demanding, even hysterical. They may become uncooperative, aggressive, or hostile toward the physician or staff. It is the duty and responsibility of the clerical staff not only to maintain and manage the office, but also to defuse any difficult situations that may develop, always treating the patient with dignity and respect. When confronted with an aggressive or hostile patient or family member, the health-care worker may feel that in some way he/she provoked the patient and blame him/herself for not having been better able to prevent an embarrassing scene.[2–5]

A staff worker who is not experienced in handling difficult situations may worsen a situation by inadvertently disclosing confidential information. I vividly recall a situation in which I was involved some years ago that was very troublesome to me. I was working for the chief of service in an internal medicine department. He was an older doctor, an expert in his area who was able quickly to diagnose his patients. He maintained a heavy patient schedule and generally spent little time with his patients.

> A well-groomed, well-spoken twenty-year-old man came in for a consultation because of a dry cough. He had swollen lymph nodes in his neck. As he was leaving the office after his visit with the doctor, I was given his chart and was asked to schedule an appointment for a CT scan. This test was routinely used to rule out lymphoma. The young man became annoyed because he did not want to make the appointment. I tried to convince him that it was necessary, that the doctor needed the test

in order to make an accurate diagnosis. The patient adamantly told me that he had not wanted to come in to see the doctor in the first place; that he came only because his mother had urged him to. He felt the test was unnecessary because he felt fine. He told me that I should contact his mother and forward the bill to her. The young man spoke condescendingly to me, as he refused to make the appointment. He placed me in awkward position.

Once again, I tried to explain that it was important to schedule the CT scan appointment. Assuming that the doctor had given him a thorough exam and had already explained the need for the test, I told him that the test was necessary because if there was a tumor surrounding the mediastina, the CT scan would be the only way it could be detected. I did not intend to alarm the patient but to help him understand the importance of the test. Needless to say, he then scheduled the appointment without further hesitation.

Later that afternoon, just before the office closed, I received a telephone call from his mother. She was extremely upset and anxious and asked me in a concerned voice, "Does he really have a tumor? Does he have cancer?"

I was terribly upset because I realized I had caused the mother unnecessary grief. My responsibility was to schedule the CT appointment. Had this young man left without making the appointment, I knew there would be no follow-up. I knew I needed to convey the importance of the CT scan. I was disappointed in myself for not having known a better way of dealing with the situation. I then realized how important effective communication skills are for front line workers.

The next day, I told a senior co-worker of the incident. She was an older women and had been working with the doctor for more than ten years. I thought that she would have understood my position, but instead she reprimanded me for mentioning the "T word." I had innocently made a mistake.

Although I blamed myself, I felt strongly that had I been trained to deal with such a situation, I would have been better able to handle it. I also felt that the doctor should have spent more time with his patient and explained to him the importance of having the CT scan. I know from experience that a patient may behave differently with a doctor than with staff members: he may be subdued with the former, but aggressive with the latter.

CONCLUSION

Communication can start at a simple level—being courteous.[4] This should be incorporated into the daily routine at every level of the medical hierarchy. In my opinion, training and development programs on communication should address such topics as compassion, understanding, and respect for each patient's individuality—his culture, class, sexual orientation, education level, and religious beliefs. Training programs should also include training in crisis intervention, stress management, and ethics.[5] These programs should be geared not only to health clinicians, but also to front-line staff, such as receptionists, secretaries, and clerical personnel. Continuing education addressing communication can effectively lower the cost of medical care by contributing to determining and providing for patients' needs more quickly and accurately. All participants in health care should learn to view the patient as a unique individual, a contributing member of their community.

ACKNOWLEDGMENTS

I would like to thank my outstanding instructor Dr. Lin Lombardi for her time and guidance. I would also like to thank many friends for their contributions and assistance, particularly Nancy Weinstock and Richard Stiefel. Mostly, I am indebted to Dr. Antonella Surbone for giving me the privilege of joining the eminent contributors to this volume and also for her help and encouragement. Finally, I ask my son's forgiveness for the time I stole from him in order to write this.

REFERENCES

1. GALANTI, G. 1991. Caring for Patients from Different Cultures. Case Studies from American Hospitals. University of Philadelphia Press. Philadelphia, PA.
2. PETE, L. 1994. Urban primary care. Classroom discussion. New York Univerisity. New York, NY.
3. TAHIR, L. 1994. Health psychology. Classroom discussion. New York University. New York, NY.
4. TAYLOR, S. 1991. Health Psychology. 2d edit. McGraw-Hill. New York, NY.
5. WEINSTOCK, N. 1996. Personal communication.
6. GARRET, T. M., H. W. BAILLIE & R. M. GARRETT. 1993. Health Care Ethics. Principles and Problems. 2d edit. Prentice Hall. Englewood Cliffs, NJ.
7. FREIDSON, E. 1991. Medical Work in America. Essays on Health Care. Yale University Press. New Haven, CT.
8. LOMBARDI, L. 1993. Health care: The government's role. Classroom discussion. New York University. New York, NY.
9. LOMBARDI, L. 1993. Health-care managment. Classroom discussion. New York University. New York, NY.
10. GREEN, L. 1990. Community Health. 6th edit. Time Mirror/Mosby College Publishing. St. Louis, MO.
11. KOVNER, A. R. *et al.* 1990. Health Care Delivery in the United States. 4th edit. Spring Publishing Co. New York, NY.
12. FRASER, L. 1995. Health-care technology and delivery systems. Classroom

discussion. New York University. New York, NY.
13. LOMBARDI, L. 1995. Financial management in health services. Classroom discussion. New York University. New York, NY.
14. BECK, D. 1989. Basic Hospital Financial Management. Aspen Publishers. Rockville.

The Psychological Repercussions of New York State's Do-Not-Resuscitate Law

An American Experience with Mandated "Truth-telling"

MARGUERITE S. LEDERBERG

Memorial Sloan-Kettering Cancer Center
1275 York Avenue
New York, New York 10021

HISTORICAL BACKGROUND

The thrust toward "truth-telling" is older and more socially accepted in the United States than in other parts of the world. It has been molded in part by international events such as the Nazi doctors' abuses and the Nuremberg trials, in part by sociopolitical factors embedded in the nation's history.

Technological Backlash

Recent decades have seen a growing suspicion of technology prominent in the most developed countries. Disappointments have been particularly concrete in personal health. The medical profession's own enthusiasm has encouraged high expectations, with enough justification that the public can be described as "doing better and feeling worse"[1] as its hunger for near-magical results remains unquenchable.

One unfortunate consequence of this mind-set was that cardiopulmonary resuscitation (CPR) became automatic in hospital deaths. This included the expected ones, for which CPR had never been intended, and for which it was more traumatic than useful.

Cardiopulmonary resuscitation had its beginnings with two important medical developments in the 1950s. The first was the development of resuscitation techniques that brought back to life previously healthy individuals who had suffered from a cardiac arrhythmia or a drowning accident. The second was the development of "iron lungs," which provided long periods of respiratory support to victims of bulbar polio, who usually recovered completely after their infection had run its course. The results of both these interventions seemed nothing short of miraculous at the time, and it was not long before the techniques were applied more and more often to sicker and sicker patients, until it seemed questionable not to attempt to resuscitate any patient, no matter how grave the prognosis. Medical sophistication improved sufficiently that temporary success was the rule rather than the exception. Technology had indeed captured both staff and patients.

Development of Bioethics

The burgeoning development of bioethics in the United States has followed in part from the loss of public trust in the medical profession; but bioethicists have positioned themselves as outsiders, defending patient autonomy against entrenched medical paternalism.[2] Truth-telling is a nonnegotiable issue in this framework, philosophically buttressed by a more-or-less Kantian justification of the overarching primacy of individual autonomy.

American Legal System

Aspects of the American legal system contribute to making bioethics important in American public life. They include the ease of undertaking a lawsuit, the universal access to a jury trial, and the importance of case law in setting precedents and molding social policy. This has enabled a few determined clients and lawyers to translate private beliefs into public policy. Through the media, it has also enabled the country to carry on a spirited public discussion that continues to promote substantive social change.

In that forum, truth-telling is already an accepted dogma, and the new frontiers revolve around euthanasia and physician-assisted suicide, to mention only the most controversial issue in which patient autonomy is a key element.

Use of Expert Opinion Reports

In this heated climate, government leaders have sought methods of consensus building. The president of the United States and several state governors have made use of expert advisory groups to help them shape policy.

The President's Commission for the Study of Ethical Problems in Medicine and Biomedical and Behavioral Research published several influential reports between 1981 and 1983.[3] One of them formalized mandatory informed consent for all human research subjects and led to the development of Institutional Review Boards (IRB's), which are now an indispensable fixture in all research institutions. (These are called ethics committees in other countries, but in the United States ethics committees deal mainly with individual cases rather than routine oversight of research protocols.)

History of the Informed Consent Doctrine

The development of the requirement for informed consent in clinical practice has been a slow process.[4] The earliest principle invoked was that of assault and battery in the case of nonconsensual touching. However, this was less powerful than one would have expected because it was not accompanied by a well-developed right to full information. After the late 1950s, cases were decided on the basis of the principle of negligence. This addressed issues of fraud and misrepresentation. But it still demanded only that physicians behave in a manner accordant with their peers. Since doctors were not in the habit of talking much to their patients, this resulted in a continuation of what some have called "a conspiracy of silence", although "unexamined consensus" is probably a more accurate term. Subsequently, the principle of self-determination was invoked (Canterbury vs. Spence, 1972)[4] and has been widely quoted since then.

However, the real enfranchisement of all patients came through world attention focused on the rights of experimental patients, in settings such as the Nuremberg trials, the Helsinki Declaration,[5] and the Presidential Commission reports.[3]

Two key points were affirmed by the Presidential Commission. The first is the absolute right of a competent patient to refuse any treatment, even a life-saving one. The second is the moral equivalence of not starting a treatment and stopping it, as long as the conditions for not starting it are met in both situations.[6]

Role of the New York State Gubernatorial Commission

In 1985, Governor Mario Cuomo created the New York State Task Force on Life and the Law, to advise him and state lawmakers on bioethical controversies.

The first Commission Report established a legal definition of brain death, which was adopted by the legislature.[7] This set the stage for further deliberations on terminal care issues and for further Task Force reports. These have played an important role in shaping medical care in the state.

THE EXPERIENCE OF A TERTIARY CARE HOSPITAL

What follows is a description of a tertiary hospital's experience in adapting to the many changes required of it as it struggled into the latest era of terminal care. It is a particular story, but its basic elements were replayed throughout the State of New York.

It is important to realize that the New York State experience is not that of the United States as a whole. As of this writing, only the State of Missouri labors under the kinds of constraints that will be described below. Other states have much more flexible statutes. However, the story bears telling, as an interesting example of the complex interplay between politics, law, medicine, and the media—an interrelatedness that is becoming inevitable in many situations and many countries.

Use of the MGH Classification

In 1976, the Massachusetts General Hospital (MGH), in a groundbreaking effort to stem the inappropriate use of CPR and to give official support to physicians trying to avoid it, published a classification of different levels of acceptable terminal care,[8] which can be summarized as follows.

A. Maximum therapeutic effort:

Example: C.A. is a 22 year-old mother of a young child, and is receiving chemotherapy for acute lymphocytic leukemia. She is in a good prognosis group, but with the expected bone marrow depression, she has developed acute sepsis. She will receive aggressive treatment. If she has a cardiac arrest, she will be resuscitated and transferred to the intensive care unit.

B. Maximum effort with daily re-evaluation:

C.A. responded to her first course of therapy, but has relapsed and received a bone marrow transplant. Her prognosis is further dimmed by the development of a fungal infection, which is not responding well to treatment, and is causing respiratory insufficiency. In the presence of anemia and severe infection, she is at high risk for hypoxia. It has been explained to her and her husband that the future hinges on a bone marrow response, and on the effectiveness of antifungal treatment. Until it is clear that these have failed, she will still receive aggressive treatment and have an attempt at resuscitation (CPR).

C. Selective limitation of certain therapeutic measures:

C.A. is in relapse, and dyspneic at rest. However, she is still alert and lucid and eager for a little more time with her family, especially her child, to whom she is trying to say good-bye, and a sister who is flying home from abroad. No further active treatment for the leukemia is contemplated, but she will receive antibiotics and blood products as long as she is lucid and at least until her sister arrives. While the benefit of resuscitation is questionable, it would probably be attempted, at least for now.

D. Comfort care only:

C.A. is becoming delirious. Her family have gathered and are keeping someone at her beside at all times. It has been agreed in discussion with the staff that she will receive only comfort measures, such as pain medications and neuroleptics for her delirium. She is now clearly a "DNR" patient—that is, a patient who has a "do-not-resuscitate" order.

These guidelines were adopted by many institutions, including Memorial Sloan-Kettering Cancer Center. Decisions were reached by physicians without always consulting patients and families formally, since it was a routine exercise of their clinical judgment. But it should not be assumed, as outsiders sometimes have, that these decisions were being hidden from patients or families. When categories were changed on short notice, as in the middle of the night or during an unexpected crisis, it was usually in the direction of more, rather than less, treatment. The decisions were reached in an open setting, and were executed by numerous colleagues in nursing and medicine. The system worked because it revolved around common shared assumptions about futile interventions.

Role of a Journalistic Exposé

In March 1984, a reporter and photographer from a metropolitan daily newspaper made their way into one of the house staff offices where patient assignments and resuscitation status were routinely displayed. An "exposé" appeared the next day, claiming "A Secret Grade System for Cancer Patients at a Top Hospital," and stating that "a chalk mark on this blackboard could mean the difference between life and death".[9] It was wrong and mischievous on just about every count. In particular, to state that CPR meant "the" difference between life and death was to perpetuate the public's magical beliefs about CPR, the very falsehood that the classification system was trying to address. Its only accurate point was to identify a lack of one-on-one medical accountability, which was then standard medical management, but which was to become unacceptable over the next several years.

Institutional Responses

Immediate

The article generated feelings of hurt and betrayal in the staff. There was a swift administrative response: the classification was withdrawn, and new guidelines were issued, specifying a presumption for CPR unless there was a documented, formal "do-not-resuscitate" (DNR) discussion with the patient and family.

The number of resuscitations increased, and the special care unit (SCU) was initially crowded with dying patients on life supports. Their doctors were not used to requesting permission for DNR orders when they thought it would not be well tolerated. This generated increased stress between the SCU and the wards. Stress is contagious; hence there were also increased tensions within the SCU staff, between the consult fellow and other staff, between doctors and nurses, between attendings and trainees, and between SCU and ward attendings. The common denominator in all of these conflicts was a perception by one group that the other group was not intervening actively enough to prevent "inappropriate" resuscitations.

The amount of physical traumatization involved in "futile" resuscitations is unknown outside the medical profession, and there has been little empathy for the brutalizing effect it has on staff and for their sense of being forced to behave unethically. Ironically, a verbal segment of the public accuses doctors of wanting to "torture" patients.

The responsibility for explicit DNR discussions was ultimately the attending physician's, at a time when such discussions were not part of their training. The learning process was slow and painful for some, although others adapted easily. The difficulty of the task was underestimated by many non-attendings, and the pressure from house staff and nurses mounted steadily over the need for DNR orders in individual cases.

Long-term

The institution mounted longer-term responses. In 1984, a DNR Committee was created to help the institution adjust. In January 1985 a task force recommended the creation of an Ethics Committee and outlined its mandate. In June 1985, the Ethics Committee began to meet and took over the functions of the DNR Committee among other duties.

It developed detailed guidelines concerning all terminal care. It carried out an extensive educational program that included ward meetings, teaching tapes, grand rounds presentations, nursing meetings, and house staff conferences. Lastly, it studied the implementation of the guidelines and the impact of the educational programs.

Passage of the New York State DNR Law

On April 1, 1988, a new factor brought the rest of the state into the same situation as the index hospital: the New York State regulation concerning DNR orders went into effect.[10] It established a legal presumption for CPR unless explicitly refused in a formally witnessed discussion. Thus, it perpetuated the magical expectations of CPR, and formalized the mistrust of the attending physician, who was specifically excluded from being named by the patient as a decision maker. Lastly, it introduced, for the first time, a patient or family's legal right to demand a futile treatment. Its positive impact was to take DNR orders out of the closet, to promote a more open attitude toward the reality of dying patients, and to prod doctors into having more meaningful communications with their patients.

The history of this regulation is an interesting cautionary tale about the vicissitudes of the political process. The law was based on the second report of the New York State Governor's Commission on Life and the Law,[11] which was a response to frequent complaints by patients and families that doctors insisted on resuscitation, and was meant to give legal support to patients' right of refusal. However, by the time the report became law, strong religious interests had intervened to insure that CPR was always offered, and remained the default position.

It was, and still is, extraordinary for consent to an intrusive, potentially harmful and ineffective medical procedure to be assumed unless it is specifically rejected. With both parties using patient autonomy as their practical guiding principle, one group wanted to protect patients from resuscitation, while the other insisted that patients be resuscitated. The latter group prevailed, turning the State of New York into a natural experiment.

Psychological Repercussions of the Law

Many SCU's throughout the state were now inundated with intubated patients. Staff reactions were again complex. One could not attend a state medical meeting without hearing anger at loss of autonomy, bitterness at wasting one's skills, guilt at inflicting pain, shame at practicing inappropriately, and a general undermining of professional self-esteem.

A few members of the legal profession claimed that doctors were overreacting and had more leeway than they were exercising. But given the tone of journalistic debate and after a careful reading of the law, many doctors, and more importantly many risk managers, suggested very cautious interpretations.

A subtle but significant new dynamic was introduced in the doctor-patient relationship. Many families and patients developed an increased sense of entitlement: for example, if CPR, why not dialysis? Physicians felt that families had been given power without responsibility, while they retained responsibility without power.

Attendings holding mandated discussions without training or natural aptitude ran into repeated difficulties. At a state-of-the-art treatment center, early and mid-stage discussions would be experienced as talk of "defeat without waging a good fight." Patients often felt confused, betrayed, threatened, or angry. Late-stage discussions took two forms. In the first, the patient felt put upon in an acute crisis and became angry. In the second, the family was approached after the patient became incompetent, felt put upon, and became angry. In either case, when the discussion took place so late, the treatment team was angry. The alternative was to avoid discussion altogether: resuscitation occurred, and only the staff was angry.

This semifacetious description should not blind one to the real anguish experienced by patients and families making resuscitation decisions. Even when a seasoned physician outlines the options very realistically, the decision carries a symbolic meaning that goes far beyond its practical implications. Many family members carry away with them the feeling that death occurred because they gave permission for it to occur.

ETHICS COMMITTEE INTERVENTIONS

Numerous interventions continued to be carried out by the Ethics Committee. They could be broken down into:

1. In-house education to create a common understanding and cut down intrastaff scapegoating: this included continuation of interventions described earlier and creation of special forms and information booklets that were distributed on all floors.
2. Support for the attendings in the front line: this included instruction, information, moral support, and especially on-the-spot help with conflict resolution. It is interesting to note that most ethics consult requests during this period came in as emergencies.
3. Special education programs for house staff and fellows, pending the development of more numerous senior role models. The ones already present cooperated in giving lectures and making demonstration tapes. In recent years, developing good communication skills has become a part of the formal curriculum in many training centers, and the object of several research projects. We currently have an ongoing seminar in which fellows discuss terminal issues.
4. Ongoing unit-based support programs: Ethics committee members gave many teaching sessions at attending rounds, multidisci-

plinary rounds, "pizza rounds," and in any other available setting.

5. Creation of an institutional mechanism for resolution of disputes: The Ethics Committee itself was selected by the administration to perform this function. Since then, such an arrangement has been legally mandated in all hospitals throughout the nation.
6. Ongoing monitoring: The committee used feedback from staff at all levels to maintain an informal monitoring process. It tracked the number of deaths, resuscitations, and problem situations.[12] Compliance with the law was found to be excellent. Within one year discussions were held in more than 85% of possible cases, supported by appropriate documentation, and with very few ambiguous situations. However, many discussions were held with families after the patient had become incompetent. This has been observed repeatedly in other centers and other states. Its resistance to change throughout the country is one of the reasons why so much current theory and research addresses the problems of surrogate decision making.
7. Community education to change the social climate: Interested staff members were active in conferences and media events to raise the level of public understanding of the law's strengths and weaknesses.
8. Activism to improve the current regulations: Medical professionals also worked directly with Commission members and staff, as well as state legislators.

Passage of the New York State Health Proxy Law

The latter activities, multiplied in many centers, bore fruit when, in 1990, some of the difficulties inherent in the DNR law were improved with the passage of the New York State Health Proxy Law,[13] following publication of a state commission report.[14] It permitted patients to select an individual who would have the legal power to make health decisions for them when they were unable to do so for themselves. It did not override the DNR law, and excluded the withdrawal of food and nutrition, but nevertheless gave patients an emotionally less demanding way of leaving advance directives. It also gave more authority to the proxy, thus easing the ambiguity that often burdened family members who had become unofficial proxies under the earlier system.

Role of the Patient Representative Department

The use of advance directives has been promoted by the Ethics Committee and carried out effectively by the Patient Representative Department, whose members have become skilled at conflict mediation and are trusted by both the medical staff and patients and their families.

Patient representatives function as ombudsmen, directly available to receive any patient or family complaint, and to guide it through the hospital system. Many of their cases have an ethical dimension. In recognition of this, the Ethics Committee recently voted to have ethics consults directed to the Chair of the Patient Representative Department, an active Committee member, who now screens them for further disposition to the Committee.

CURRENT UPDATE

A review of the number of ethics consults received by the Committee graphed against the significant social and legislative developments that have impinged on them, gives one reason to be encouraged.[15] They show a steep rise in the number of consults during the early years, then a steady drop that tracks the development of educational programs, the change in social climate, and the passage of the Health Proxy Law. The medical staff understand the options better, are more comfortable with the requirements and work more effectively with patients and families to enable them to use advance directives. Painful as it was to adjust, the basic requirements of the DNR law are now taken for granted.

The number of educated consumers is also rising, although not as fast as one might expect. This is due in part to continuing magical beliefs that are directly or indirectly promoted by the media and to some extent by the unreality of some abstract ethical discourse. But most of all, it is embedded deep in the human psyche's response to death.

Potential Conflict between Patient Freedom and Judgments about Medical Futility

The Ethics Committee continues to receive a steady trickle of problem cases, which are very difficult because conflicts between staff and patient/family surrogates are often at the core of the problem. They usually consist of a patient and/or family member demanding that resuscitation be offered indefinitely. Given the skill of intensive care personnel, this can, in certain cases, result in prolonged existence, and in a use of medical resources that the staff experience as wasteful at best, unethical and repugnant at worst.

Under the current law, New York physicians are limited in their ability to respond. In the rest of the country, they have more freedom, but are still constrained by the claims of patient autonomy. This is reflected in the medical literature by the lively dialogue about:

1. the issue of medical futility: many complex issues are subsumed under this heading, but one of them can be described as addressing the physician's claim to professional autonomy.
2. the issue of the responsibilities of patients and surrogates: discussions on this topic explore (and frequently reject) possible limitations on consumers' claims to autonomy.

Nevertheless, there is a thrust, in bioethics, toward examining the overvaluing of autonomy more critically, especially in terminal care situations.[16]

Physicians' claim to expert judgment in terminal care situations has been strongly defended[17,18] and just as strongly attacked.[19] Regardless of the beliefs espoused, several studies have demonstrated that physicians regularly consider many factors in their decision making. Some of these seem to relate to personal beliefs,[20,21] others to unacknowledged evaluations of medical futility.[22]

Physicians' accuracy in guessing their patients' preferences has not been good;[23] but family surrogates have hardly been any better.[24–26] Hence, the whole concept of substituted judgment, (which is, historically, the primary legal principle under which surrogates are empowered), has come under attack.[27,28] More to the point, even patients themselves may have difficulty formulating advance directives in a way that can be trusted to correspond to their choices in a time of crisis.[29,30] Furthermore, three years after passage of the Federal Patient Self-Determination Act, only 15–20% of patients avail themselves of the option, unless very labor intensive programs are in place to increase their number.[31–33] Attempts are underway to improve methods of obtaining patient preferences,[34–36] but for now, families and physicians still play an important role in making decisions for patients who have not prepared advance directives at all.

CONCLUSION

The current system works best for patients who have given some forethought to their mortality and have laid out clear advance directives, and for doctors who are skilled at delicate communication.

Increasing emphasis on patient-doctor communication must remain an important goal in medical education. It is not unreasonable to hope that, as good role models become more common, medical students will be effectively socialized, just as they used to be in the paternalistic era.

Similarly, efforts at improving patient participation must continue. But there will always remain a subgroup of patients and families for whom enfranchisement comes at the price of having hard decisions thrust on them that they cannot digest, and that they feel to be unbearably stressful. They will still experience it as a betrayal of trust, will be hurt, angry, frightened or guilt ridden, and may react with a desperate denial of the inevitable.

Negotiating a new balance to ease the lot of this subgroup remains an important task for the future. Patients and families must not lose the enfranchisement that has been so hard earned. Yet it is counterproductive to disenfranchise doctors in situations where medical realities are such a powerful determinant. The inequality inherent in the New York State example has been its main drawback. Ideally, one should provide effective support and help for patients and families in coming to terms with finality, without asking them to make quasi-medical, pseudo-decisions. This exercise is as psychologically unsound as it is ethically appealing.

Meanwhile, living through this period of adaptation has demonstrated, yet again, that change is difficult, that policy decisions are never simple in their genesis or their implementation, that a mechanism such as an ethics committee can be an effective agent of transformation, and that institutions can adapt to changing times.

REFERENCES

1. KNOWLES, JOHN H., Ed. 1977. Doing Better and Feeling Worse: Health in the United States. Norton. New York, NY.
2. ROTHMAN, D. J. 1991. Strangers at the Bedside: A History of How Law and Bioethics Transformed Medical Decision-Making. Basic Books. New York, NY.
3. THE PRESIDENT'S COMMISSION FOR THE STUDY OF ETHICAL PROBLEMS IN MEDICINE AND BIOMEDICAL AND BIOBEHAVIORAL RESEARCH. 1983. Summing Up. U.S. Government Printing Office. Washington, DC.
4. KATZ, J. 1984. The Silent World of Doctor and Patient. Collier-Macmillan. London.
5. World Medical Association Declaration of Helsinki. 1984. Recommendations Guiding Medical Doctors in Biomedical Research Involving Human Subjects. Adopted by the Eighteenth. World Medical Assembly, Helsinki, Finland.
6. THE PRESIDENT'S COMMISSION FOR THE STUDY OF ETHICAL PROBLEMS IN MEDICINE AND BIOMEDICAL AND BIOBEHAVIORAL RESEARCH. 1983. Deciding to Forgo Life-Sustaining Treatment. U.S. Government Printing Office. Washington, DC.
7. The New York State Task Force on Life and the Law. 1986. The Determination of Death. The New York State Task Force on Life and the Law. New York, NY.
8. THE CLINICAL CARE COMMITTEE OF THE MASSACHUSETTS GENERAL HOSPITAL. 1976. Optimum care for hopelessly ill patients: A report of the Clinical Care Committee of the Massachusetts General Hospital. N. Engl. J. Med. **295:** 362-364.
9. New York Post, March 23, 1984. p.1
10. New York Public Health Law. Sections 2960 to 2979 (McKinney 1994 & Suppl. 1995).
11. THE NEW YORK STATE TASK FORCE ON LIFE AND THE LAW. 1986. Do Not

Resuscitate Orders. The New York State Task Force on Life and the Law. New York, NY.
12. MISBIN, R.I., D. O'HARE, M. S. LEDERBERG & J. C. HOLLAND. 1993. Compliance with New York State's do-not-resuscitate law at Memorial Sloan-Kettering Cancer Center: A review of patient deaths. N.Y. State J. Med. **93:** 165–168.
13. THE NEW YORK STATE TASK FORCE ON LIFE AND THE LAW. 1987. Life-Sustaining Treatment: Making Decisions and Appointing a Health Care Agent The New York State Task Force on Life and the Law. New York, NY.
14. New York Public Health Law. Sections 2980 to 2994 (McKinney 1994 & Suppl. 1995).
15. HOLLAND, J. C. Chairperson's Annual Report. Memorial Hospital Ethics Committee. New York, NY.
16. CALLAHAN, D. 1993. The Troubled Dream of Life: Living with Mortality. Simon & Schuster. New York, NY.
17. FINSTER, S, N. THEAKER, R. RAPER & M. FISHER. 1994. Surrogates' decisions in resuscitation are of limited value. Br. Med. J. **309:** 953.
18. CURTIS, J. R., D. R. PARK, M. R. KRONE *et al.* 1995. Use of the medical futility rationale in do- not-attempt-resuscitation orders. JAMA **273:** 124–128.
19. NELSON, J. L. 1994. Families and futility. J. Am. Geriatr. Soc. **42:** 879–882.
20. COOK, D. J., G. H. GUYATT, R. JAESCHKE, J. REEVE *et al.* 1995. Determinants in Canadian health care workers of the decision to withdraw life support from the critically ill. JAMA **273:** 703-708.
21. ASCH, D. A., HANSEN-FLASCHEN & P. N. LANKEN. 1995. Decisions to limit or continue life-sustaining treatment by critical care physicians in the United states: Conflicts between physicians' practices and patients' wishes. Am. J. Respir. Crit. Care Med. **151:** 288–292.
22. HANSON, L. C., M. DANIS, E. MUTAN & N. L. KEENAN. 1994. Impact of patient incompetence on decisions to use or withhold life-sustatining treatment. Am. J. Med. **97:** 235–241.
23. MORRIS, B. A., S. E. VAN NIMAN, T. PERLIN, K. S. LUCIC *et al.* 1995. Health care professionals' accuracy in predicting patients' preferred code status. J. Fam. Pract. **40:** 41–44.
24. EMANUEL, E. J. & L. L. EMANUEL. 1992. Proxy decision-making for incompetent patients: An empirical and ethical analysis. JAMA **267:** 2067–2071.
25. SECKLER, A. B., D. E. MEIER, M. MULVIHILL *et al.* 1991. Substituted judgment: How accurate are proxy predictions? Ann. Intern. Med. **115:** 92–98.
26. HARE, J., C. PRATT & C. NELSON. 1992. Agreement between patients and their self-selected surrogates on difficult medical decisions. Arch. Intern. Med. **152:** 1049–1054.
27. SUHL, J., P. SIMONS, T. REEDY & T. GARRICK. 1994. Myth of substituted judgment: Surrogate decision-making regarding life support is unreliable. Arch. Intern. Med. **154:** 90–96.
28. LAYDE, P. M., C. A. BEAM, S. K. BROSTE, A. F. CONNORS *et al.* 1995. Surrogates' predictions of seriously ill patients' resuscitation preferences. Arch. Fam. Med. **4:** 518–524.
29. COHEN, L. M., M. GERMAIN, A. WOODS, D. GILMAN & J. D. MCCUE. 1993. Patient attitudes and psychological considerations in dialysis discontinuation. Psychosomatics **34:** 395–401.
31. SEHGAL, A, A. GALBRAITH, M. CHESNEY, P. SCHOENFELD *et al.* How strictly do dialysis patients want their advance directives followed? JAMA **267:** 59–63.
32. Federal Patient Self-Determination Act, Pub. L. 101–508, Sections 420-6,

4751(OBRA), 42 U.S.C. 1395 cc(a) et seq (1990).
33. EMANUEL, L. L., M. DANIS, R. A. PEARLMAN & P. A. SINGER. 1995. Advance care planning as a process: Structuring the decisions in practice. J. Am. Geriatr. Soc. **43:** 440–446.
34. EMANUEL, L. L., M. J. BARRY, E. J. EMANUEL & J. D. STOECKLE. 1994. Advance directives: Can patients' stated choices be used to infer unstated choices? Med. Care **32:** 95–105.
35. LYNN, J. 1995. Procedures for making decisions for incompetent adults. JAMA **267:** 2082–2084.
36. SCHEIDERMAN, L. J. & A. G. KALMANSON. 1995. Who decides who decides? Arch. Intern. Med. **155:** 793–796.

Walking a Difficult Path Is Easier with a Friend

Thoughts from a Practicing Oncologist

MARGARET A. TEMPERO

UNMC/Eppley Cancer Center
University of Nebraska Medical Center
600 South 42nd Street
Box 986805
Omaha, Nebraska 68198-6805

INTRODUCTION

As an academic oncologist, I have spent my career providing and analyzing data. I use and teach the data to support management decisions for cancer patients. But I have been asked to provide a perspective on communicating with cancer patients. For this, I have no data. I have only my personal viewpoint on what works and what does not.

What follows reflects my own style of communication, which has developed from a deep conviction about the importance of the doctor-patient relationship in cancer care.

BEARING BAD NEWS

Long ago, I accepted the fact that referring doctors would often leave the unpleasant job of defining prognosis and limitations of treatment to the consulting oncologist. Frequently, as a young consultant, I would arrive in the patient's room announcing that I had been called in to consult with them about their diagnosis of cancer only to learn that the patient either had not been told or had not understood the information given. My shocking revelation often took them by surprise and impeded progress in working together toward a management plan. I now have a softer approach. I begin by asking what the patient understands about their illness, asking them (not the family) to retell the story of their diagnostic workup. Once they have used the word "cancer," I am home free. If this does not happen, I gently ask the patient whether the attending physician thinks that they have cancer. Almost uniformly, the answer is yes, and I can build on that.

I personally do not care for hospital-based consultation. Being hospitalized and dependent upon others makes patients vulnerable. Many patients find themselves on busy hospital floors in semiprivate rooms without adequate privacy. Patients who have recently undergone surgery may be medicated and incapable of completely comprehending the discussion. The timing of our consultation visit often does not coincide with the visit of family members on whom the patient depends for support. Sadly, these problems cannot always easily be solved. My working rule is simply to remember this and be sensitive to it. I always arrange for a follow-up visit in a more quiet environment such as an outpatient clinic with the patient's family present. At that point, I assume that anything I said in the hospital was not retained, and we retell the story together. The patient has now had some time to contemplate the diagnosis and consider the questions that need to be asked; the outpatient interchange is much more productive.

During the consultation process, I try not to rush. Many times, the same question will be asked repeatedly but in a different context; the consultant must be patient and consistent in his or her responses. If possible, we let the patient end the interview by telling us that we have answered all their questions.

WHOSE FAULT IS IT?

Guilt can be a problem for many cancer patients. Did they do something to deserve this terrible illness? Did they ignore early signs and symptoms and cheat themselves out of a chance for cure? We know that most cancers are biological accidents and that one cannot always assign a cause and effect related to lifestyle or our environment. Patients need to be reassured that having cancer is not their fault. Furthermore, many cancers do not have early signs and symptoms; even for those that do, a two- or three-month delay in seeking a medical evaluation usually does not make the difference between a curable and an incurable lesion. While the majority of patients will not vocalize this, they do worry about it and appreciate the reassurance that they did the best that they could. A medical team can sometimes inadvertently add to patients' guilt. We often short-circuit our communication and relay that "he or she failed treatment." Nothing could be farther from the truth. Our therapies often fail the patient, but our patients certainly never fail the therapy. Our patients succeed when they take advantage of useful options. It is not their fault if the management failed to control their disease.

EMPOWERING THE PATIENT

The majority of patients are excellent consumers. They can understand the goals of treatment. They can weigh the risks and benefits. They can choose wisely. Considering this, I often think of myself as a skilled servant whose job is to teach the patient the information they need to know and then to guide them through the management plan. Part of empowerment is continued access to information. It is important not to place barriers before the patient. You and your staff must be available for continued counsel.

Setting the goal of treatment is critical. The risks that one might accept decline as one moves through the goals of cure, prolongation of life, palliation, and the acquisition of new knowledge. Patients need to understand the goal in order to decide how much they are willing to risk. Sometimes the goals of treatment are not clear, and patients must choose between the option of no therapy (avoiding risk) and therapy (for uncertain gain). I am often asked what I would do if I were in their shoes or what I would recommend for my loved one. My answer is simple: I do not know. The truth is that none us of can predict how we would react in a difficult, life-threatening situation. How often have we heard a young person proclaim that losing an arm or a leg or being disfigured would be so hideous that they would prefer to die. Yet we know the power of the human spirit, and, in fact, very few patients take, or request assistance in taking, their own lives.

The clinical setting in which care is delivered can have an important impact on a patient's sense of control. Involving the patients and their families in the process can have a strengthening affect. For many reasons, our institution has focused on strategies that minimize hospitalization time and rely on the patients (or appropriate family members) to take increasing responsibility in their care.[1,2] It has been our group's impression that patients are not only willing but actually eager to play an active role. Of course, this demands that we in turn provide a support system, which includes a day hospital opened for extended hours seven days a week and a knowledgeable home care team. Examples of patient independence include the self-administration of chemotherapy, antibiotics, and growth factors. In some cases, patients learn to self-draw blood samples from central venous access devices, which further minimizes trips to the hospital or clinic.

Patients who cannot look forward to potentially curative therapy particularly need to be in charge of their own care. The decisions are not easy; the choices are often not appealing. They need to learn as much as they can. Our job is to teach. Often, the only good decision is the one the patient is comfortable with.

ALL OR NONE

Teaching patients the statistics about their illness is a very delicate business. I have lost count of the times that I have chided students or residents about telling a patient they had "six months to live." I ask how they know. The typical response is that they read in the textbook that the median survival for this selected cancer was six months. So I then point out that the statistic means 50% of the patients died at six months, but 50% of the patients lived longer. Are they seeing a glass as half-empty or half-full? And what do statistics about a group of patients really predict for a single individual? For that patient, it is all or none. There is no mean, median, average, or even range. The student then counters that patients need to know how long they are going to live so they can make plans and get their affairs in order. I agree that they do need to know the range of possibilities. A frank, level discussion about the possibility of cure (or not) and the usual natural history of the disease is education enough. Mature adults (and the majority of our patients are) make provision in case of a catastrophe. Once done, we need to walk in hope.

FRAMING THE TRUTH

There is no doubt that cancer consultation is an art. Patients can hear the same message from different consultants; yet one consultant can leave them devastated, and another can leave them hopeful.

I have already mentioned the importance of empowering your patient with information. The consultant can ease the process by appearing less authoritative. Having a relaxed manner and sitting during the consultation process is important. If possible, a quiet consultation room with ample seating for family members provides a level playing field. It is less intimidating for patients than an examination room and permits them to be more composed and controlled.

The truth must always be told, but the consultant can frame the truth in the best possible light. While it is true that a colon cancer patient with periaortic node metastases will not be cured and is destined to die of their disease, the mere presence of the distant node metastases is not immediately life threatening. Even patients with liver metastases, a potentially life-threatening problem, can often be reassured that the normal synthetic function of the liver is still present. While these nuances may seem trivial to those of us who are healthy, this knowledge can be of great comfort to those of us who are not.

I feel certain that the care giver's attitude can profoundly effect the patient.

> Bill was a successful professional diagnosed with metastatic cholangiocarcinoma at the age of 42. He accepted his diagnosis with resignation. He had great faith and chose to avoid treatment. He enjoyed being upbeat

> and cheerful and elected to live his last few months with that spirit. When he was hospitalized, a parade of students, residents, and attending physicians scolded me for not telling Bill "the truth." They could not comprehend that he could understand his fate and still have a cheerful attitude. Bill, on the other hand, confided to me that this was the most miserable group of doctors he had worked with. They were all depressed and could find nothing to talk about but how poorly they expected him to do.

Patients who wish to be happy and hopeful should certainly be permitted to do so. We are charged with delivering good medical care but not with the responsibility of taking away someone's hope. This integral part of the human spirit should always be protected. I once asked a senior colleague how to respond to a patient with a terminal illness who said they hoped they would get better. Without hesitation, she replied, "I tell them I hope they get better too."

Patients often do not hear enough good news. We try to show interest in them and in their lives. We welcome them as a friendly visitor when they arrive at our clinic. When possible, we commend them on their achievements: handling the toxicity of treatment, maintaining their weight, staying active, and so on. If they achieve a remission, even a partial one, we rejoice with them.

GIVING UP VS. MOVING ON

For many terminal patients, choices eventually have to be made about the wisdom of pursuing therapies with extremely small chances of benefit. In fact, many patients pressure physicians to treat even with techniques or drugs that have no proved value or have been proved to be useless. In the past, under fee-for-service arrangements and with very little oversight, this practice pattern was common. The constraints on practitioners and patients to spend less money and to operate under managed care plans will necessarily streamline our treatment guidelines in the future.

However, cancer patients must be taught that stopping therapy is not the same as giving up. In these circumstances, the cancer specialist must be very sensitive to maintaining a close link with the patient and to avoid the appearance of abandonment. One can view avoiding useless therapy as avoiding unnecessary risk and protecting one's self from harm. For highly motivated patients, this is an excellent opportunity to participate in experimental treatment and provide a gift of information for others. Above all, stopping therapy does not mean that we too, as providers, have lost hope that the patient will get better.

AFTER THE STORM

I have not mentioned much about the family and friends of the patient. They are the unsung heroes as they stand quietly by providing emotional support or assist actively in the consultation process by recording and interpreting information. They are part of the team and need to be recognized as such by professionals in the health care team. They need to be reassured that their difficult task is worthwhile, and they need to commended for standing by during trying times. Over the years, it has been our practice to continue to reach out to them after the patient's death through periodic contact and notes of condolences.

GIFTS

The practice of oncology has been an unique opportunity for me. Early in my career there was no doubt about my professional goal. These patients needed me, and, somehow, I needed them. I have learned and continue to learn from each one. Each is like a flower. I am not sure how long they will be with us but I have powerful appreciation for the beauty they bring. I am profoundly grateful for the education they have given me.

REFERENCES

1. TEMPERO, M., A. BERG, M. BLOCK, M. HUTCHINS, R. LANGDON, D. MORAVEC, C. TWEEDY & J. ANDERSON. 1994. A phase II trial of protracted therapy with 5-Fluorouracil and daily oral leucovorin in metastatic colorectal cancer. J. Infusional Chemother. **4:** 112–115.
2. BENNET, C., J. L. ARMITAGE, G. O. ARMITAGE, J. M. VOSE, P. J. BIERMAN, J. O. ARMITAGE & J. R. ANDERSON. 1995. Costs of care and outcomes for high-dose therapy and autologous transplantation for lymphoid malignancies: Results from the University of Nebraska 1987 through 1991. J. Clin. Oncol. **13:** 969–973.

Communication with the Cancer Patient in China

SIDE LI[a] AND JIA-LING CHOU[b,c]

[a]*Shanghai Cancer Institute*
Shanghai, China

[b]*Memorial Sloan-Kettering Cancer Center*
1275 York Avenue
New York, New York 10021

The population in China reached 12 billion in February 1995. With the improvement of living conditions and health care over the last several decades, the life expectancy reached 75.97 years of age in 1993. Endemic spread of certain infectious diseases is no loner the major threat to life as it used to be. On the other hand, the proportion of cancer deaths is on the rise. For example, new cases of cancer patients in Shanghai are about 15,000 per year,[1] and in the whole country new cases approximate 3.2 million annually. Lung cancer is the most common malignancy, and its annual incidence was 57 per 100,000 persons.[1]

Such a large number of cancer patients have an immense impact not only on the health-care system but also on patients' families, their friends, and the whole society. Management of these patients requires expertise and relies on good communication with the patients. Chinese medical ethics are certainly different from Western ethics. To understand the differences it helps to examine some unique features of the Chinese cultural background and traditions.

Before Western medicine was introduced into China, Chinese medicine had been in practice for more than 2,000 years. Chinese traditional medical ethics were thought to have an equivalent to the Hippocratic Oath outlined in a treatise entitled *On the Absolute Sincerity of Great Physicians* by a physician named Sun Simiao (A.D. 581–682) of the Tang Dynasty in the section "The Important Prescriptions Worth a Thousand Pieces of Gold."[2] Another important treatise, "Five Admonitions and Ten Maxims for Physicians," was written by Chen Shigong (A.D. 1555–1636) of the Ming Dynasty.

The principles in these treatises can be summarized as follows. A human life is sacred. Physicians must make every effort to rescue and extend life without conditions. Physicians should not in any circum-

[c]Corresponding author.

stance seek wealth or aim to profit from their career because of their expertise. All patients should be treated on equal grounds, and physicians should respect and be conscientious in serving their patients.

Chinese medical ethics are quite different if they are viewed from the standard and conduct of modern biomedical research. The Chinese medical texts that deal with ethics are concerned principally with the good behavior of a practicing physician.[3] An essential component of ethics that is developed in the Chinese medical texts is that of "humaneness." The formulation of humaneness reflects a general idea of ethics as based on the proper behavior of good individuals rather than on a system of rules. The ethical perspective is clearly virtue oriented, as a result of the long history of the influence of different culture schools and religions.

In addition, there is no comparative biomedical research conducted in this country. Consequently the context, even the meaning, of such terms as informed consent, use of placebos, and alternative forms of therapy are very different from those used in Western ethics.

During the past two decades, several issues of medical ethics have attracted much attention in China. That stage of development can be marked by a conference on the philosophy of medicine held in Canton in 1979.[4] Issues that raised great interest were death, euthanasia, and the delivery of medical care without discrimination.

While much publicity is focused on these issues, communication between medical staff and patients has not received adequate attention. This is nevertheless an important subject in medical ethics. In the treatment of cancer patients, almost every step of case management from the time of initial diagnosis requires skillful communication between healthcare personnel and patients.

The majority of cancer patients in China are cared for at community hospitals, as there are only a few major cancer hospitals in large cities. Subspecialities such as medical or surgical oncology do not exist, and patients who have solid tumors are seen by surgeons initially if the tumors appear to be resectable. For example, patients who have lung cancer are seen by thoracic surgeons, those who have gastrointestinal cancer by general surgeons, etc. If adjuvant chemotherapy is indicated, patients will then remain in surgical wards for further treatment. Those who require radiation therapy will be referred to radiation departments. Patients who have hematologic malignancies, on the other hand, are treated by hematologists.

INFORMATION ABOUT CANCER DIAGNOSIS

How do doctors tell patients the diagnosis of malignancy? This is a very delicate issue, and it is usually dealt with individually. For those who have potentially curable diseases or a high probability of being cured, doctors find no difficulty in discussing diagnosis, management, and prognosis directly with patients. Patients who have a good educational background appear to be able to accept the diagnosis and treatment in more or less an expected way, although many doctors prefer to break the news gradually. For those patients who have only one choice, such as inpatient chemotherapy, it is inevitable that they will learn the diagnosis sooner or later. In such cases physicians choose to break the news to them either directly or through their family members. For those who have highly malignant tumors or disease already at an advanced stage, the usual practice is for doctors not to tell patients about their cancer diagnosis, but to tell their spouse or other close family members first.

Traditionally, people in this country believe that psychological factors play an important role in fighting diseases. If one is not aware of a terminal disease, he may remain hopeful and optimistic. If, on the other hand, one knows that his life may last no more than a few months, he may collapse immediately upon learning the diagnosis. He may not eat normally or he may refuse further treatment even if treatment may turn out to prolong life. In most cases, patients' families also do not want doctors to reveal the news to the patient without first discussing it with the family. The root cause of this practice is that, traditionally, family structures remain the center of life. The elderly and the mentally or psychologically handicapped are cared for by family members rather than in institutions. Psychological shock, as when a cancer diagnosis is disclosed, is usually absorbed, shared, and dealt with by the whole family. Some family members would rather bear the bad news among themselves than share it with the patient. Traditionally patients in this country do not exercise their right to self-determination. Some patients may even prefer not to be informed about a bad diagnosis and allow their family members to make decisions. Such wishes are respected in medical practice.

Doctors may also choose to tell a cancer diagnosis to the patient's employer first; as a result of the welfare system developed over the last 45 years or so. There is no private insurance system. Employees who are hired or retire from government-owned enterprises—whether they be factories, shops, offices, or schools—are covered by the public health insurance for almost all the medical expenses. Large sums for medical expenses and subsidies for the sick and deceased have to be approved by the enterprise in cases where patients are unable to pay.

From the historic point of view, China has very stable social and family structures that were developed over a long period. Certain practices of daily life are deeply rooted in everyone's mind; it may take a long time for people to accept new ideas in modern ethics.

PATIENTS ON PROTOCOL TREATMENT

In order to assess the results of a new treatment, such as a novel combination of chemotherapeutic agents, random assignment trials need to be conducted. Patients who are eligible for, and agree to enter, such trials are randomly assigned to one arm. As mentioned above, the concept of informed concept is different in this country from that in Western countries. It is accepted practice for doctors to accept "verbal consent" from patients or their families. Once treatment is started, the patients are usually told about side effects, but they may not be told in which arm they are enrolled, as some doctors fear that psychological factors may interfere with the interpretation of results.

CONFLICTS BETWEEN INDIVIDUAL AND PUBLIC INTERESTS

Chinese medical ethics dictate that physicians make every effort to save a patient's life. However, the role of physicians in making treatment decisions is challenged when individual patients' interests conflict with others'. The current insurance system cannot cover all the best therapeutic options available. This means that even if one kind of chemotherapy is known to be effective and prolong life but is expensive, patients may be given another, less effective treatment at a lower cost. It is understandable that when patients are insured by a small enterprise that has only limited funds, spending too much on a few patients may jeopardize other employees' medical coverage. It is an extremely difficult and delicate task to balance such interests and maintain a fair system. Such decisions are not made by physicians but by patients' employers. It certainly requires good communication between patients and their employers.

DEATH AND RESUSCITATION

For cancer patients dying at hospitals there are usually no complicated legal issues involved. There are usually no legal guardians who dictate what is done. Doctors and nurses do not have to go to patients or families for their decisions about resuscitation. In general legal intervention is involved in medical cases only on rare occasions.

It is understood by both dying cancer patients and their families that prolonging life by resuscitation is most unlikely to be beneficial to patients. It is generally accepted that nature should be allowed to take its course, especially when a patient is dying of a terminal disease. Many Chinese value the quality of life. While many people pay attention to keeping a healthy lifestyle, even practicing *t'ai-chi* at six o'clock every morning, they may not like the idea of being confined to a bed in the intractable pain of a terminal disease. To them what is important is not life itself but living in an ideal way. Prolonging the life of a dying patient is no more than extending suffering.

It is, however, more difficult for young patients and their families. It is also hard for parents if the patient is their only child and they are no longer able to bear children (the majority of young families now have only a single child). However, the issue regarding resuscitation might not be raised in the case of young cancer patients as it might with young people dying of diseases such as an infection. The families of young cancer patients would accept the idea that no resuscitation should be performed provided that all necessary measures had been effectively taken.

Opposed to this is a traditional view that life should be valued and preserved at all cost and that physicians should do their best to save lives.[5,6] It also must be pointed out that not every hospital has an intensive care unit; even when one is available, it has only a few beds, which usually would not accommodate cancer patients at the terminal stage.

Cancer patients at an advanced stage may not be admitted to hospitals, especially in view of the shortage of beds relative to the vast population. In Shanghai 13 hospices were recently opened to accommodate terminal cancer patients. Basic supportive care is administered, usually without specific cancer therapy.

The issue of whether to carry on long-term supportive care such as tube feeding or parenteral hydration at the terminal stage is often raised in clinical practice. If medical expenses can be fully covered, the patients and their families are usually in favor of continuation of treatment. If, on the other hand, the expenses have to be paid by the patients, they and their families usually request withdrawal of supportive care.[5] Such withdrawal can be done without a court order. The decision is usually made after a consensus is reached between doctors, the patient, the family, and the employer.

In the traditional family there is a close link between each member of the family. For example, even if a person is married, his or her parents are still considered family members. If a patient's life can be saved, most family members and even close relatives do what they can to give financial support, even if that sometimes means selling property and personal belongings. However, if that kind of financial support can be translated only into maintaining life without meaningful quality, the patient or family may forgo such life-support measures so that the family does not suffer financially. If a patient chooses this course, he or she is performing an act of compassion that is highly regarded. It should also be pointed out that in Chinese philosophy the right to choose death has existed for a long time.[7] According to Taoism and Confucianism, life is the result of interaction between *Yin,* which comes from mother and the earth, and *Yang,* which comes from father and the heavens. Death is no more than a return of *Yin* to the earth and *Yang* to the heavens. This is simply a natural event.

Recently there has been discussion about euthanasia, one of the issues raised in the 1979 conference mentioned above.[4] A poll was conducted in China in 1985, when the idea was still new to many people, regarding opinions about euthanasia for cancer patients dying in intractable pain. Thirty-nine percent were in favor of it.[8] However, in practice it appears to be difficult to implement active euthanasia, because of the centuries-long influence of various schools and religions. Those who follow Buddhism believe that to save or extend a life is to do good and that this will be rewarded in their next life; to kill or shorten a life is evil, and this will be punished in their next life. This is partly based on the Buddhist precept that prohibits killing. According to the Confucian principles of filial piety, children should keep their parents alive as long as possible.

Physicians observing Chinese medical ethics on the sanctity of life are reluctant to forgo treatment and assist in death. Most lawyers in China are opposed to euthanasia. However, health-care workers and the public have become increasingly aware of the importance of quality of life, and there is evidence that the number of people in China who approve of passive euthanasia is increasing.[6]

With the increasing awareness of the quality of life, the issue of patients' autonomy and self-determination will probably soon be on the agenda for change. With the gradual changes in industrial and financial structures and cultural exchange with the outside world, one may expect a gradual change in people's views of modern ethics. It has been noted that increasing attention is focused on medical ethics in the education of medical students.[9]

Obviously, there has been much less exchange of information with the West in the field of medical ethics than in the application of modern medicine's new diagnostic and therapeutic techniques. There has not been adequate exposure of health-care workers to the theory and practice of Western medical ethics. The issue of what roles patients' rights and autonomy play in the care of the sick remains debatable. This issue has been a pivotal one in determining the attitude toward the care of patients and certainly influences many aspects of communication with cancer patients.

REFERENCES

1. JIN, F., S. S. DEVESA, W. ZHENG, W. J. BLOT, J. F. FRAUMENI, JR. & Y. T. GAO. 1993. Cancer incidence trends in urban Shanghai, 1972–1989. Int. J. Cancer. **53:** 764–770.
2. SUN, S. The Important Prescriptions Worth a Thousand Pieces of Gold. Printed in the period of Wanli's reign, Ming Dynasty **1:** 9–11.
3. WU, Z. H. 1994. Conflicts between Chinese traditional ethics and bioethics. Camb. Q. Healthcare Ethics **3:** 367–371.
4. QIU, R. Z. 1982. Philosophy of medicine in the 1970's. *In* Studies in Philosophy of Science: 281–331. Knowledge Press. Beijing.
5. QIU, R. Z. 1991. Morality in flux: Medical ethics dilemmas in the People's Republic of China. Kennedy Inst. Ethics J. **1:** 1627.
6. PU, S.D. 1988. Euthanasia in China: A report. J. Med. Philos. **16:** 131–138.
7. XU, T. M. 1990. China: Moral puzzles. Hastings Cent. Rep. **20:** 24–25.
8. QIU, R. Z. 1985. The concept of death and euthanasia. Med. Philos. **1:** 77–79.
9. LU, Y. H., X. Y. MENG & X. LIU. 1994. Professional behavior of medical school graduates: An analysis. Med. Educ. **28:** 296–300.

From Paper to Practice: Quality of Life in a Developing Country

The Challenges That Face Us

GILLY BURN

World Health OrganizationCollaborating Centre for
Palliative Cancer Care
Sir Michael Sobell House
Churchill Hospital
Oxford OX3 7LJ, United Kingdom

Our growth and its essential support depends above all upon our capacity and readiness to listen to our patients and their families. It was from them that the vision first came, and as we continue to pay them our full attention, we will discover how to go on.[1]

My experiences and observations of some of the daily challenges that face those who live and work in a country where not only is the health budget a minute percentage of the gross national product, but cancer and palliative care are low priorities within that budget, are many and varied. They are based on interactions with Indian colleagues but above all on the comments and shared experiences of Indian patients and families.

My first visit to India in a professional capacity was as a temporary advisor to the Cancer and Palliative Care Unit of the World Health Organization (WHO) in 1989. Subsequently I have been working in India for increasing lengths of time, always in collaboration with the WHO, but not funded by them.[2] The more I am there, the more I realize how little I know and the more humble and, indeed, overawed I feel. In a recent letter to the *Journal of Palliative Care*, Dr. Charles Olweny relates a famous saying that: "If you visit a country for a week, you become an expert and can write a book. If you stay for a year you might write a paper, and if you stay longer you do not know enough to write anything."[3] I can echo those statements. What I communicate with you is what I have seen, heard, and experienced and my unsophisticated thoughts.

India is a country of such color and contrast! It has luxurious five-star hotels with every amenity, to match or better those in the West; and outside a family are spending their lives in the gutter, surviving on the waste of the Western-style monstrosity in whose shadow they live. The problems are great, and there are no easy solutions.

In India it is estimated that there are 1 million new cancer patients each year, with 750 thousand to 800 thousand incurable at diagnosis.[4] The incidence of cancer is between 1.5 million and 1.7 million people in a pop ulation of around 900 million. The most common cancer is preventable and tobacco related, affecting the head, neck, and lungs (approximately 50% of all cancer patients). In women, cancers of the cervix and breast are the most common. For a variety of reasons, nearly 80% of the patients are incurable at diagnosis. Reasons for late presentation include ignorance of the disease process and warning signs, fear of the diagnosis, and poverty, which renders the patient unable ever to afford to seek medical treatment. Very often local or ayurvedic treatments have been tried; there is frequently an innate fear of hospitals. The tertiary referral center may be several hundred kilometers from the village where the patient lives. Most of the patients presenting at a late stage have a predictable spectrum of symptoms.[5] In India there is no social security system, so no work means no money. If it comes down to feeding one's family or seeking medical help, the family will come first. The distances from the hospital may be long, and there may not be any means of mechanized transport, so bullocks and carts or bicycle rickshaws may be the only means of transport for several kilometers.[6] The Indian family is a strongly knit unit; if one member is ill, the whole family may come to the hospital to support the ill person. The public transport system consists mainly of overcrowded buses, the passengers packed inside like sardines and hanging onto the sides and roof. Once they are on the bus, arrival safe and alive is not a certainty. There are several fatal accidents every day: the hurry of the West has reached India's roads, but the road system does not have the capacity to meet the need. There are no motorways, and most major trunk roads are one lane in each direction. The monsoons and the heat often render the road's surface dangerous, and this danger is compounded, particularly at night, by other forms of transport, which are not illuminated.

In India there are now 11 regional cancer centers, which treat only about 10% of cancer patients. There are over 100 district hospitals, which offer different levels of oncology service.[7] Not all the hospitals have functioning radiotherapy or brachytherapy equipment. If a machine breaks down, it may be months or even years before it is repaired or replaced. One hospital I visited had not had functioning radiotherapy equipment for over nine months. Of its 96 beds, approximately 12 were occupied by people who were too ill to return to their village but who nevertheless were not able to receive any treatment. In that particular hospital there was no oral morphine available and no palliative care services. There are other centers offering palliative care, some of which, although well intentioned, are wholly inadequate.[8]

Contrasted to this, in one of the regional cancer centers I visited, there were patients nearing death and existing by means of artificial support.

> One man, in his 70s, with multiple abdominal metastases, was being artificially ventilated and receiving highly sophisticated, expensive treatment, including chemotherapy. The physician was unable to give a clear

> outline of the treatment goals. Although the patient was paralyzed and being ventilated, he did not have constant nursing attention. Because the patient was in an intensive care unit, his family members were not allowed in; so while he died alone without nursing care in a spiritually hostile environment, his family suffered quietly outside in the grounds of the hospital.

Patient and family were separated at the time in life when people most need to be together. What was it like for that man to die alone? What memories are the family left with? How do they cope with their grief? What about the patient? Did he have any *real* choice? What about his unfinished business? Were there family issues that needed to be talked about and resolved? It is difficult to communicate when one is paralyzed and being ventilated. Can we even begin to imagine what it must be like for people who can hear everything going on around them but are incapable of communicating what *they* want? And what about the cost —not only the emotional cost, but the financial cost of this highly inappropriate care?

I have seen many families sell their houses, land, cow, everything in order to strive for an unattainable cure. The family of this particular patient was paying over 300 dollars a day for him to spend his last hours on a machine. The love of the family drives them to what they feel is best for the patient. Very often there is a feeling in developing countries that everything coming out of the affluent West must be the best, and there is a tendency to copy what may be inappropriate even in a setting with greater material resources. The West is often a bad model for poorer countries. Our death-denying attitudes and belief that we are omnipotent, our lack of spiritual direction have often meant that money is seen as power, and money has become our God. With money we believe all things are possible, but money cannot stop someone dying whose time has come. How do patients end up where the legacy they leave behind is one of bankruptcy for generations to come?

From my experience it seems that most patients in India are not told the truth about their advanced disease. There appear to be two extremes. They may be told that they are curable when quite clearly that is not a possibility, barring a miracle. Very often I am told that in order to maintain hope it is necessary to lie to the patient. Lying has rightly been dubbed "intellectual shortsightedness" by Dr. Robert Twycross. I am convinced, again by what I have experienced, that it is not *what* is said, but *how* it is said that is more important. The same words can sound so different as a result of the different intonation, body language, and context in which they are spoken.

The other extreme is telling the patient, "Go away, there's nothing more to be done." Often the fear of being abandoned, pain, and desperation to have *something* done lead a patient to seek second and third opinions, often hundreds of miles from his home. However, it is usually not a cure that the patient is seeking, but relief from his suffering, from his terrible pain, or from the smell of his fungating lesion. *Any* treatment seems better than no treatment, and at least while he consents to treatment, albeit inappropriate, there is still a chance to interact with the doctor for a few minutes. Very often it is just the contact with the doctor that the patient and family are paying for. They do not want to trudge that last, lonely, painful journey alone and abandoned. For the majority, palliative care is simply not available.

I have seen many compassionate, competent doctors in India spend quality time on quality communication with their patients. It is a joy to behold. Very often these are the doctors who are brave enough to tell the truth in a gentle, sensitive manner. These are the ones, also, who know that something more *can* be done in terms of palliative care and comfort measures. These are the doctors who try and see their patients in the greater social context, who weigh the benefits and disadvantages of aggressive therapy.[9,10] They struggle with ethical issues like truth-telling and informed consent, aware that they are very likely to lose a patient to a colleague in so doing. And there are doctors who are striving to increase their repertoire of palliative care skills, are avid readers of the latest books and journals, and really are trying to *listen* to what the *patient* wants.

I am reminded of a patient I saw in a clinic in Orissa.

> A man in his early forties with a large solid tumor on his neck, he had already had a tracheostomy for obstruction, his neck was solid with tumor, and he was unable to turn his head. Above his tracheostomy was a large, gaping, fungating tumor about two inches across. During examination it emerged that he had received several courses of aggressive chemotherapy, to which his tumor was not responding. In order to receive the treatment the patient was staying over 150 kilometers from his home. His wife was with him, but he was separated from his two teenage daughters. Treatment, which cost in the region of 600 dollars a month. was paid for in part by more wealthy members of his family. The patient was then attending the pain clinic, suffering from pain, dysphagia, and insomnia.
>
> After the physical consultation the relatives asked if they could speak to the doctor. The doctor, visiting at the time from a hospice in the United Kingdom, agreed only with the patient's permission. (Quite clearly this was an unexpected response from a doctor—it is the norm to inform the relatives and not the patient.) The relatives asked how long the patient had to live. The doctor reflected the question back and asked what they had been told; "Five to seven years," was the response. The doctor informed the relatives that this was not the case, and that he probably had only a matter of months.
>
> The doctor then inquired about the cost of the treatment. The relatives responded that it did not matter—they were prepared to pay anything. However, the doctor's next question was to ask if the patient had children,

and daughters in particular. Realization suddenly dawned across the brother's face. "Yes," he said, "if the treatment is doing no good, we could use the money toward the dowries of the daughters." (Although officially illegal in India, the dowry system still exists, whereby the family of the bride has to present money, jewelry, saris, and other expensive items to the groom and his family.) The relatives thanked the team for being honest and said they would now go away to discuss with the patient *what he wanted.*

The positive outcome was that he decided not to have more treatment and to return home to his family for the rest of his life. One of the tragedies, however, was that oral morphine tablets are not available in that area of India, so he probably died without receiving adequate pain control.

One of the outrages in trying to deliver effective pain relief and palliative care in India is that, despite the fact that India is one of the major growers of opium in the world, India's cancer patients cannot get cheap morphine. This is so despite the considerable efforts by Dr.Stjernsward of the WHO.[11] The narcotics control laws are so stringent that it is extremely difficult to use morphine legally.[2,9] I am reminded of a wonderful oncologist working in a cancer hospital in Kerala who was determined to get good pain relief for his patients and struggled for nine months to get a supply of 1000 morphine tablets costing only five dollars. After the supply ran out, it took another five years to get the next consignment.

Every state in India has different laws, and special permits must be obtained to transport morphine from manufacturer to hospital and to store, supply, and prescribe it. Some states decree that you can prescribe or hold only a certain amount, or so many doses of morphine, and those may be inadequate for the patient's needs.[12] Some hospitals will allow only in-patients to have morphine, and others may prescribe only a one- or two-week supply to be sent home with the patient. If the patient lives in a rural area, hundreds of kilometers from a hospital, the logistics of getting morphine are daunting. It may mean a return journey of two days on a bumpy road. If the patient has pain and bone metastases, one has only to imagine the horrors of such a journey.

As I have already mentioned, high-tech treatments appear to be much more appealing to medical staff. This is due in part to the difficulties of obtaining oral morphine and the long distances that make follow-up difficult; but a great deal more education is needed regarding the use of oral morphine. Its use is accompanied by enormous fears on the part of the patient, the family, and the doctor: fear of addiction, of theft of the drug, and of prosecution. Respiratory depression and the misconception that morphine is synonymous with death and should only be used *in extremis* are common. These fears are entrenched, and my own belief is that theoretical teaching alone is insufficient to dispel them. Workshops, which may have a 15-minute to half-hour session on the use of morphine, are expected to result in widespread use. One director of a regional cancer center said to me that he was disappointed that more doctors in the state were not using morphine. He had gone to great lengths to arrange for 300 doctors to have training sessions in palliative care. Upon enquiry about what the training comprised, it turned out that it was a two-hour session on all aspects of palliative care, including the use of morphine. A valiant effort, but how far will it have changed practice?

In another center, which has had access to oral morphine since the end of 1992, the cancer hospital has utilized less than half of the tablets that were allocated. When I first visited the hospital, in April 1993, while being shown around,

> I saw a patient who was clearly moribund, eyes rolling, being wheeled out of the hospital on a two-wheeled wheelchair, his distressed family around. To my subsequent regret I asked the doctor accompanying me what was wrong with the patient. At that, he ordered that the patient be taken back to his bed. The poor man was respiratorily distressed. He would have been better off sitting up, as he was dyspneic, but there were no pillows. It turned out that he had lung cancer with multiple secondaries, and he was clearly dying. He had been anuric for over 24 hours. In order to relieve his respiratory distress, I suggested a small dose (2.5–5 mg) of morphine, which could be repeated as necessary, but the suggestion was greeted with absolute horror. Instead, the patient was given 80 mg iv frusemide, and an intravenous infusion was set up together with antibiotics and respiratory stimulants. The patient died in distress a few hours later, with his wishes to return home unfulfilled.

Sadly, in that hospital morphine is still not used to its fullest potential.

Another major problem is the lack of communication between carer and patient, and among the members of the multidisciplinary team. The status of the nurse in India is low. Only a few nurses who go into the profession actually *want* to nurse. I started to survey the nurses in a B.Sc. and M.Sc. nursing course, asking them (in groups of 50–100) how many chose to take up nursing. Only 4% on average responded positively; most really wanted to become doctors, but when they did not get into medical school, they automatically went for a degree in nursing. Nurses with degrees almost without exception go into teaching. The diploma nurses who receive three years' training tend to be bedside nurses, so that normally the nurse who is actually delivering direct care tends to be of a lower status. The nurses who end up teaching the diploma nurses may only just have finished their degree, so they have had much less patient contact and clinical involvement. Verbal communication between nurse and patient is rare. Part of the reason for this is the great shortage of nurses—often only one trained nurse per 40–60 patients. It is difficult to have meaningful communication in these circumstances because of the constraints of time and status, and patient advocacy on the part of the nurse is a rarity. Meaningful communication between doctor and nurse is also not commonplace. Nurses are expected only to obey the doctor's orders and not to challenge the status quo.

It is interesting to note the hierarchical system and how it tends to hinder effective communication. This still exists to a certain extent in the West, but more and more, people are being encouraged to challenge and question, and this is seen more as a positive attribute than a threat. Sadly, the hierarchical system can stifle enthusiasm and a genuine quest for learning. Promotion is often by dint of age rather than aptitude for the job, and so the healthy element of competition is lost. Things are slowly changing, however, and one of the exciting outcomes of teaching in India is that there are now many more multidisciplinary workshops. Palliative care and communication skills are taught by a nurse/doctor team in both the clinical and theoretical settings. The healthy interaction between the facilitators serves as a role model.[13] After identifying the needs of health care professionals in India, the United Kingdom–based organization Cancer Relief India has taken up the education of doctors and nurses in the areas of palliative care and communication skills.[14]

One of the fascinating observations in the clinical setting is to watch the way in which patient and doctor communicate. This can be superbly carried out, with the doctor communicating respect for the patient by the fact that he greets him, sits down (and offers the patient a seat), and asks his permission to be examined, or if visitors like myself can be present. When one sees this respect for a patient (whatever his caste or creed) by a doctor or nurse, the communication channels flow. To observe the doctor's skill in ascertaining the patient's real concerns and to watch active listening and the fact that the doctor or nurse may use appropriate touch to communicate a message are very encouraging.

One doctor in North Kerala, after completing a special 10-week course in palliative care[13] in the United Kingdom that I organize, was asked what he was going to change in his practice subsequent to the course. He replied, "I'm going to write 'Listen' above the door opposite where I sit, and I'm going to sit by the patients who are bedridden" (as opposed to standing over the patient or at the end of the bed.) He is now doing just that. He is not offering cure, but he is communicating that he cares; and from my observation, whatever the caste or status of the patient, the communication that conveys that a person is valued opens up infinite therapeutic channels. In the first year of its being, the new pain and palliative care clinic at his hospital has had nearly 400 referrals. This is a phenomenal achievement for a new service in a system that does not normally function comfortably in collaborative work. I believe this has to do with the effective communication skills of the doctor concerned, which encourage trust from both his colleagues and patients. There are also several volunteers working in the same clinic. This is, in fact, very unusual in

India—volunteer work is not undertaken on anything like the same scale that it is in the United Kingdom.

. At the other end of the spectrum, I have seen patients treated with total indifference. Fingers are poked at tumors and in orifices in a callous and painful manner without ever acknowledging the patient beforehand. There is huge interest in the tumor and its biological behavior, but often little regard for the human beneath and the effect of the cancer on his life. The patient's story is not listened to, his real and human anxieties ignored or not addressed. So often in the fear of destroying hope the truth is not communicated in words. But the actions of the doctor reveals to the patient all he needs to know. It is interesting to note how the same health care professional communicates with patients of different status or social backgrounds.

As a final illustration,

> I am reminded of a man in his early 50s (Mr. A) with carcinoma of the junction between the esophagus and stomach. He had been operated on in a major cancer center and was told that he was now cured and that there was no need to return for further treatment. The relatives, in contrast, had been told that his cancer was inoperable and that "nothing more could be done." Mr. A had a wife, two sons—one in America, one married and living in Mr. A's small apartment with his pregnant wife—and a daughter of 24. At the time I met Mr. A, I was due to present a paper at a conference and was staying at a hotel in Bombay.
>
> The patient's wife and daughter came to see me at the hotel, clutching a large bundle of the patient's notes in which his terminal cancer was diagnosed. They asked if I would come and see Mr. A. He was not eating, they knew he would die in the not-too-distant future, and they were adamant that he should not be told that he had cancer. I listened and said that I would see him but that if he wanted to know about his condition I would not lie to him, nor would I blurt out "You have cancer." I would listen to the patient and go at his pace.

The difficulty for me was that I knew I would never see the patient again and that it is difficult to build trust in a short interview.

On the way to the house, I thought how difficult it must be for the wife and daughter to keep up the pretense, and I inquired how they were coping with the strain of it all. This simple enquiry evoked a flood of tears and an acknowledgment that it was, indeed, difficult to keep up the pretense. In fact, relationships between all the family members had become strained, particularly with the pregnant daughter-in-law, who had not long been married to their son.

I arrived at the house to find a good-looking but weak man sitting in a chair. I met the other family members and asked if I could spend some time alone with Mr. A. This evoked obvious discomfort in the wife and daughter, but Mr. A seemed quite happy to have the privacy. At frequent intervals during the interview plates of food were brought in, which neither I nor Mr. A could manage to eat (giving food to guests is a very great Indian tradition, as is eating meals together—food is prepared with love). I carried out a routine physical assessment on Mr. A, inquiring about pain and other symptoms. His main problem was weight loss (around 15 kg in 2 months) leading to weakness, lethargy, and anorexia. He found the anorexia particularly distressing because his family appeared to want to force-feed him. His wife prepared all his favorite foods, spending hours in the kitchen. When the food was presented, he just could not eat it, and he felt a mixture of remorse, fear, and guilt—remorse and guilt because of all the effort his wife was making and the fact that the food was being wasted, and fear at the horrifying significance of not being able to eat. This was compounded by the fact that his wife seemed to present him larger and larger portions "to build him up." The more food he saw, the less he could face it. His wife, too, had feelings of guilt at not being able to prepare the "right" food and anger that her efforts at care were being rejected.

Simple explanation and information to both parties at discharge could, perhaps, have alleviated much of the unnecessary heartache.

> Mr. A then expressed concern at "the funny atmosphere" in the house. "Nobody talks in the same way any more; it seems everyone is trying to be jolly." This echoed with what his wife and daughter had said about the strain of keeping up the pretense.
>
> I then asked what I believe to be a key question in assessment: "How are you sleeping?"

Sleep is often a good indicator of the physical, emotional, and spiritual status of a person. This is not always the case, but very often if people do not sleep it is due to physical or emotional symptoms of the disease.

> Mr. A.'s response to my question was, "I don't sleep very well at all." "What keeps you awake?" "Worry," he replied. "What are you worried about?" "I'm worried I won't see my daughter married before I die." This was his biggest worry. Asked if he was afraid of dying, he replied, "No, but I have to get things done first."

It seemed to me this was an odd conversation from a man who apparently did not know his diagnosis and probable prognosis. Remembering the family's anxiety about my blurting out the truth, I did not feel comfortable about delving into his diagnosis. He knew his time was limited, and he indicated this in his comments about finding a husband for his daughter. In retrospect I did what I felt best at that time and in those circumstances. I did not want to destroy hope, and I did not want to lie; he needed an achievable goal.

One of the advantages of working in India is that on the whole the nation has a strong religious and spiritual foundation. People are not embarrassed, as we are often in the West, when talking about God.

> In response to Mr. A's anxiety about his daugher, I felt I had to reveal the human side of our professional role. I said that we never know when our God will take us and that we need to be prepared for that day whenever it is. So many lives are full of regrets for things not done or said.[1,15] Since I had begun traveling so much, the precious gift of life had become more evident together with the fragility of it. Whenever I leave my mother, I tell her I love her and attempt not to have any "unfinished business" in case one or the other of us should die before we meet again. In the same sort of analogy I suggested that if there was "business" Mr. A wanted to sort out, there was no time like the present; perhaps now was the time to look for a suitable husband for his daughter.
>
> The other thing he really wanted to do was get out of the house and go to the beach. His family had cocooned him inside in their efforts to protect him and do "what was best."

Somehow there was an unspoken truth between us, yet I never revealed the diagnosis or prognosis. Perhaps it was what I did not say that let him know. But I believe he knew all along that his life was limited. He and his family were playing games trying to protect one another.

> Before I left, the daughter came in, and I was able to tell her how much her father loved her and how he wanted to find a husband for her. To his wife I communicated the need for small meals of what Mr. A could manage to eat and "gave permission" for him to go to the beach and to live life as he wanted. This was obviously quite a difficult concept for her to grasp. I then left to go and speak at the conference, enriched by the encounter. The next day, I telephoned Mr. A's daughter. Her father had slept well and had been to the beach and had enjoyed himself.

There is a wonderful sequel to the story.

> Five months later I received a letter from my friends who had introduced me to Mr. A. Mr. A's son in America married my friend's daughter. The son came home for his wedding, which Mr. A was able to attend. During the last months of his life he found a charming husband for his beloved daughter, and he danced at her wedding four days before he died.

Cicely Saunders advocates to those involved in the care of dying people "openness, scientific rigor together with personal concern and freedom for the spirit."[1] They are key elements in building palliative care. The challenges of establishing quality palliative care demand all the above, with the overriding need to attend to the individual patient and his family. We need to use all our senses, to be human, to take off our protective professional armor, and to enter into our patient's world. As Saunders has indicated, our patients and their families are our greatest teachers.

From my work with patients in both the United Kingdom and India it seems to me that the basic human needs are the same. Granted, there are cultural differences, but behind every label of caste, creed, or color the basic human condition remains the same. Our dreams, hopes, and fears are very similar. I believe the key to good quality of life is good communication—what we say, how we say it, but more importantly how we hear, how we listen, and how we interpret what we hear.

I leave you with a thought for us all from Ralph Waldo Emerson: "To laugh often and love much, to win the respect of intelligent persons and the affection of children. To earn the approbation of honest critics and to endure the betrayal of false friends. To appreciate beauty, to find the best in others, to give oneself; to leave the world a bit better, whether by a healthy child, a garden patch or redeemed social condition To have played and laughed with love and exultation. To know even one life has breathed easier because you have lived, this is to have succeeded."[16]

REFERENCES

1. SAUNDERS, C. 1993. Some challenges that face us (closing address of the 2nd Congress of the European Association for Palliative Care). Palliative Med. **7**(Suppl. 1): 77–83.
2. BURN, G. L. 1990. A personal initiative to improve palliative care in India. Palliative Med. **4:** 257–259.
3. OLWENY, C. L. M. 1994. Ethics of palliative care medicine: Palliative care for the richer nations only. J. Palliative Care **10**(Autumn): 17–22.
4. STJERNSWARD, J. 1993. Palliative medicine—A global perspective. *In* Oxford Textbook of Palliative Medicine. D. Doyle, G. W. C. Hanks & N. MacDonald, Eds. Oxford University Press. Oxford.
5. SEBASTIAN, P. *et al.* 1993. Evaluation of symptomatology in planning palliative care. Palliative Med. **7:** 27–34.
6. JEFFREY, D. 1995. For whom the bell tolls—Palliative care in the third world. J. R. Soc. Med. **88:** 307–310.
7. MUMFORD, J. W. & S. P. MUMFORD. 1988. The care of cancer patients in a rural South Indian hospital. Palliative Med. **2:** 157–161.
8. FOX, R. 1994. Mother Theresa's care for the dying. Lancet **344:** 17,9.94.
9. 1994. Proceedings of the First International Conference of the Indian Association of Palliative Care, Varanasi. 27–29.1.94.
10. JEFFREY, D. 1994. Palliative care in India: An educational challenge. Proc. R. Coll. Physicians Edinb. **24:** 462–465.
11. 1994. Cancer Pain Relief: A Guide to Opioid Availability in Palliative Cancer

Care: Pain Relief and Other Symptoms. Cancer and Palliative Care Unit, WHO. Geneva.
12. JORANSON, D. 1993. Availability of opioids for cancer pain: Recent trends, assessment of system barriers, new World Health Organisation guidelines, and the risk of diversion. J. Pain Symptom Manage. **8:** 353–360.
13. BURN, G. L. 1994. Palliative care in India. Cancer Care (WHO Geneva)**1:** 1.
14. WEBB, P. 1993. Cancer relief in India. Eur. J. Cancer Care **2**(2): 53–54.
15. BURN. G. L. 1993. Spiritual care. Practice Nursing 16.3-5.4.93, p17f.
16. EMERSON, R. W. 1906. Works of Ralph Waldo Emerson. Nimmo, Hay & Mitchell. Edinburgh.

Communication with the Cancer Patient in Iran

Information and Truth

ARDESHIR GHAVAMZADEH[a,b] AND BABAK BAHAR[b]

[a]Department of Oncology and Hematology, and
[b]Bone Marrow Transplantation Center
Shariati Hospital
School of Medicine
Tehran University
Karger Avenue
Tehran 14114, Iran

Confrontation with death or its possibility is a horrible shock for most people, especially if this occurs as a result of a cancer diagnosis and if the patient is young and active or is for any other reason not psychologically ready for this confrontation. In Iran most cancer patients are referred by internists, general practitioners, or surgeons. Some of these patients feel anxiety or fear when they are informed that they are being referred to a cancer specialist, so sometimes the physician in charge does not inform the patient or patient's family that they are being referred to an oncologist; therefore, the cancer diagnosis or its possibility is left completely unsaid.

Our patients come from a very wide spectrum of educational level, economic support, cultural background, and religious belief. Rural patients from these points of view are more homogeneous. Despite these differences, the common point of all Persian patients is the form and meaning of "family." Iranian families are nuclear and, in some areas, extended. Familial relations and sentiments are very important and strong. The successes and difficulties of any family member affects all other members, and sometimes the expression of feelings is very strong. So cancer strikes not only the patient but the family as well. Today the course of cancer is often prolonged and draining and is punctuated by crises, with alternating periods of hope and despair, often ending with loss. The emotional cost, as well as the cost in time, money, lost resources, and family disruption, is great.

The family and its meaning is very important, indeed, pivotal, for oncologists dealing with cancer patients in Iran. We will consider this in conjunction with other aspects of caring for Iranian cancer patients.

DEATH AND ITS MEANING IN OUR CULTURE

Apart from state of emotional well-being and individual experiences with death, which can differ among our adult patients, the cultural milieu and social background are common for our patients; and this so-called sociocultural background regarding death and dying is more homogeneous in our country than in countries like India. The constellation of forces bearing on familiarity with death and associated with religious beliefs are said to be the most important sociocultural influences on attitudes toward death.

Iranians are familiar with death. Many old people live with their families, and many of them die at home. All or most family members are involved in burial rites. Religious beliefs in our country strongly and explicitly deal with the fact of death. Despite these background influences, when a patient is informed directly or indirectly that he or she has cancer, his or her psychological balance is severely disturbed. Even when one member of a family, such as a husband or wife, is informed about the cancer of another family member, he or she sometimes cannot tolerate this and is so severely struck that the patient realizes that a bad thing has happened even though he or she has not been informed. These reactions, which can endanger the medical situation and the treatment process, are not completely dependent upon the educational level or economic class of our patients. Sometimes, when the diagnosis is found out by more than one or two members of a family, all the family members, especially the adults, become socially paralyzed or their social functioning becomes weakened for a short or not-so-short period. In contrast with these patients, some patients with strong religious beliefs encounter their diagnosis with restraint; but these patients are in the minority, and in time their emotional control breaks down. Iranians react very emotionally individually and as a group when they are faced with cancer diagnosis and prognosis.

THE TRUTH

For a long time the tradition among physicians of Iran has been to reduce information to cancer patients and patients with poor prognosis and to respond to their questions in a very general way. Although nowadays some patients press doctors to get more and more-detailed information about the meaning of their diagnosis, the cause of their disease, and its prognosis, experienced oncologists withstand this and do not provide information about cancer and poor prognosis except when they are legally required to.

A common practice is to tell selected members of the family—selected according to who seems able to know the diagnosis and prognosis and yet remain stable and cooperate with the doctor in providing information to the patient's relatives who are legally important for decision making and economic support. A patient's son-in-law, daughter-in-law, or grandson may provide such liaison. Finding such a person is sometimes difficult; Questionnaires filled out by the doctor's secretary, a ward nursing staff, or admission personnel are in part designed to help find such a person, which is sometimes difficult.

If the patient is a child, for legal reasons we disclose the diagnosis to his or her parents as soon as possible. And if such therapeutic options as bone marrow transplantation are chosen, doctors are forced give the diagnosis to the legally responsible person (but preferably not to the patient).

We generally disclose the diagnosis to only one member of family because when the number of persons informed increases, a potentially confusing system of double accountability between what the therapeutic team thinks and what the family thinks may arise. It is sometimes said that this condition forms part of the adaptive mechanism of the patient, who plays his part by not revealing what he has understood on his own. However, this equilibrium is disturbed when difficult treatment decisions present themselves. Moreover, sometimes intrafamily conflicts occur, and these may have a very bad effect on the patient-doctor or family-doctor relationship. So we prefer to inform only one member of the family and insist that the information not be spread. We know that not haveing access to sources of basic information sometimes depresses or aggravates patients and may even leads to a state of unreality or a syndrome of sensory deprivation; but this is not usual among Iranian patients.

When the doctor decides to disclose information and the diagnosis to a patient, he or she should consider the following:

(1) what the patient already knows of the disease;
(2) what conclusions the patient has already been able to draw (including any misunderstandings that may have been formed);
(3) the structure and nature of the patient's family;
(4) the social milieu to which the patient belongs;
(5) the patient's age, intelligence, and emotional stability.

Informed consent in Iran can be signed by a first-degree relative of the patient who is at least 18 years old and psychologically normal. When a patient is admitted to any hospital ward, including an oncology ward, a general informed consent should be signed by the patient or her or his legal sponsor. When a chemotherapy regimen is prescribed, some oncologists add another informed consent to the hospital's general-purpose informed consent. This one explains the possible side effects of chemotherapy (such as the cardiac side effect of adriamycin). This informed consent, too, can be signed by the legal sponsor of the patient, so the diagnosis need not be disclosed to the patient. Legal rules in Iran support this kind of informed consent, and the patient's family prefers that the diagnosis not be disclosed to the patient. When bone marrow transplantation is planned, first of all it is explained to the patient's family; if they agree to it, then it is suggested to patient. It is in this situation that the diagnosis and prognosis are disclosed and the benefits and side effects of bone marrow transplantation are completely explained to the patient. Only in this situation should informed consent be signed by the (adult) patient himself, because the procedure needs a cooperative, well-informed patient.

COMMENTS

Without any doubt we agree that every patient has the natural right to know about her or his disease prognosis and to have an active role in treatment and medication programs. But first of all he or she should be able to tolerate the truth with minimal psychological and somatic damage. A prerequisite of such tolerance is knowledge of new achievements of modern oncology, increased treatment methods and successes, and also side effects. We think such knowldege should be part of the cultural background and popular knowledge. It can be transferred to people's beliefs only by national governmental teaching programs, through school programs, television programs, and other large-scale mass education strategies.

This needs time; the beneficial effects of such teaching programs will appear in future generations. Such teaching can sometimes be carried out between physician, patient, and family members. In most Iranian cases in our daily practice this is still uncertain and sometimes causes delays or breaks in treatment.

REFERENCES

1. HIGGS, R. 1990. A case conference revisited: Commentary 2: An obstructed death and medical ethics. J. Med. Ethics **16**(2): 90–92.
2. BYRNE, P. 1990. A case conference revisited: Commentary l: Comments on an obstructed death. J. Med. Ethics **16**(2): 88-89.
3. HELM, A. 1995. Truth telling, placebos, and deception: Ethical and legal issues in practice. Aviat. Space Environ. Med. **56**(1): 669–672)
4. SURBONE, A. 1993. The information to the cancer patient: Psychosocial and spiritual implications. Support. Care Cancer **1**(9, Mar.): 89–91.
5. MIYAJI, N. T. 1993. The power of compassion: Truth-telling among American doctors in the care of dying patients. Soc. Sci. Med. **36**(3, Feb.): 249–264.
6. DUYNBAR, S. & S. REHM. 1992. On visibility: AIDS, deception by patients, and the responsibility of the doctor. J. Med. Ethics **18**(4, Dec.): 180–185.
7. DALLA-VORGIA, P, K. KATSONYANNI, T. N. GARANIS, G. TOULOUMI & P. DROGARI. 1992. Attitudes of a Mediterranean population to the truth telling issue. J.

Med. Ethics **18**(2, Jun.): 67–74.

8. HOSHINO, K. 1992. Bioethical issues and principles in cancer treatment. Gan-To Kagaku-Ryoho **19**(3, Mar.): 281–285.
9. HEBERT, P. C. 1994. Truth-telling in clinical practice. Can. Fam. Physician **40**(Dec.): 105–113.
10. GUYEX, P. & H. GOODARE. 1994. An Introduction to Psycho-oncology. Routledge. London.
11. KAPLAN, H., SADOCH & J. GREES. 1994. Synopsis of Psychiatry: 76–86, 767, 770. Williams and Wilkins. [city?]

The Impact of Perceived Behavior on Patient-Physician Satisfaction

LEA BAIDER,[a] BEATRIZ UZIELY,[a] AND
ATARA KAPLAN DE-NOUR[b]

[a]*Sharett Institute of Oncology*
Hadassah University Hospital
Jerusalem, P.O. Box 12000
Israel, 91120

[b]*Department of Psychiatry*
Hadassah University Hospital
Jerusalem, P.O. Box 12000
Israel, 91120

INTRODUCTION

Cancer is often perceived as painful and terminal. The disease and even the word itself have a profound impact on the way we see and respond to our social milieu and medical institutions. As Cassileth expressed it, "Cancer is much more than cellular dysfunction. It is a historical event; a conceptual bias; a social, economic and ethical dilemma."[1]

It is not surprising that psychological distress among cancer patients is often very high. Various studies have reported that 47% of the patients exhibit symptoms of distress such as adjustment disorders, anxiety, and depressive disorders.[2–4] Less, however, is known about the specific factors that make patients vulnerable to distress or about those that are potentially protective.

In the past two decades, two groups of possibly protective factors have received theoretical attention: medical communication and social and emotional support. Both have been found to play a key role in helping patients cope, leading to better adaptation and improving physical health and even survival rates. Several studies have suggested that social support or, more accurately, perceived social support modifies and ameliorates distress in cancer patients.[5–7] Other studies have focused on the importance of informing patients and involving them in decision making. Physicians and patients, therefore, are being seriously studied and their interaction is being reformulated.[8–10]

While research often notes cultural and societal values in cancer management, few studies have examined the influence of culture on the interaction and perception of physicians and patients. Each researcher approaches the relationship with his/her own beliefs, attitudes, knowledge, and opinions about the rules governing the exchange.[11–14]

The germinal work of Glaser and Strauss[15,16] suggested that a physician's ideology concerning disclosure could be of paramount importance in determining the form and content of communication. Discussion of what to communicate to patients, therefore, requires consideration of the socially and culturally conditioned values and beliefs held by physicians—who share societal restraint about open disclosure of "unpleasant news"—and by patients. Previous attempts to examine physician communication practices and the rationale behind them have concentrated on a unidirectional account of what they reported or did not report. Few systematic attempts have been made to examine physician ideologies and values on communication and on their patient-physician mutual perception.

For the cancer patient, the relationship with the physician has particular significance. The illness may threaten a patient's sense of connection to others and to his/her own world. It has been our clinical impression that the physician is the most important social support to the patient struggling with fear and anxiety related to the illness and coping with severe side effects from treatments. The ability of a physician to establish an empathetic relationship with the patient could be a major factor in controlling and reducing the symptoms of psychological distress. Pain, loss of function, and lost sense of control can disrupt ordinary means of building an egalitarian relationship with the physician, thus intensifying the isolation and the power gap in the physician-patient relationship.

A few studies have examined the satisfaction of different patient populations with their physicians.[17–19] In these studies, a list of physician behaviors is provided, and patients are asked to rate their degree of satisfaction or dissatisfaction with these behaviors. Our approach differs. In order to examine the patient-physician relationship, we studied not only patient perceptions but also physician perceptions. We avoided direct questions about satisfaction. Instead, we asked patients and physicians to describe physician behavior along a number of items—first on the perceived or the actual physician and then on the expected or the ideal physician.

The following hypotheses were formulated:

a. There will be a significant difference between the perception of patients and physicians of the ideal physician.
b. There will be an even greater difference in the perception of the actual physician.
c. Within the physicians' group, the discrepancy between the actual and ideal physician will be small; that is, physicians are satisfied with their behavior and feel it approximates their ideal.
d. Within the patients' group, the discrepancy between the actual and ideal physician will be large; that is, patients are not satisfied with

their physicians.

e. Dissatisfaction with the physician will contribute significantly to the patient's psychological distress.

SUBJECTS AND METHODS

Both patients and physicians participated in the study. Two hundred and five patients were selected randomly during a six-month period from among Israeli patients attending the Out-Patient Department of Oncology, Hadassah University Hospital, Jerusalem. Seventy-three percent were women, and 72% of the total sample were married. Their mean age was 54.3 (SD 12.9), and on average they had 13.3 (SD 4.3) years of schooling.

Patients on their first visit to the Out-Patient Department were excluded. Those patients selected had been ill for different lengths of time, with a mean of 7.7 months (SD 30.7).

On the whole, the patients were in good physical condition, with a mean Karnofsky score of 95.6 (SD 8.8).[20] The most frequent diagnoses, in descending order, were: breast cancer, 83 (40%); colon cancer, 25 (12%); melanoma, 17 (8%); cancer of the rectum, 11 (5%).

All 27 physicians working in the Department of Oncology, 14 of whom were women, participated in the study. Their ages ranged from 30 to 53, with a mean of 40.5 (SD 7.91).

The assessment was done by a questionnaire developed for a similar study.[12] The eight behaviors consisted of four on information and four on the empathetic aspects of the relationship. The two sets of questions were combined and included the following:

1. Explanation of the disease
2. Explanation of the planned treatment
3. Patient's participation in the planned treatment
4. Explanation to family members
5. Ability to talk freely to a physician
6. Ability to approach the physician with problems
7. Encouragement by the physician
8. Ability to rely on the physician

The patients were first asked to describe their oncologist along these eight behaviors. A four-point scale was used, from "my physician does/is not . . . at all" to "very much so." This description provided the patient's perception of the oncologist, referred to as the "actual" physician. Using the same eight behavior questions, the patients were then asked to describe how they would like their physician to be—the "ideal" physician.

The questionnaire seems fairly valid, with internal reliability

(Cronbach's alpha value) of 0.775 for the ideal and 0.845 for the actual physician. We suggest that the discrepancy between the two descriptions represents patient satisfaction with the physician—the bigger the discrepancy, the greater the dissatisfaction.

The physicians answered the same questionnaires, which were phrased "I do . . ." for the actual and "It is important that the physician . . ." for the ideal.

The questionnaires were administered anonymously to the patients by a psychologist working in the Out-Patient Department, and to the physicians by an oncologist. There were no refusals. Patients were administered the Brief Symptom Inventory (BSI)[21] to assess psychological distress. Statistical analysis included comparing the actual and the ideal within each group by paired *t* test and across groups by *t* test. Stepwise Multiple Regression was carried out with BSI as the dependent variable.

RESULTS

We began by comparing patient and physician perceptions of the ideal physician (TABLE 1). The differences were much smaller than expected, with no differences found in the "emotional" behaviors. On the cognitive items, three significant differences were found; the patients perceived the ideal physician as one who would explain the disease more to them and less to their families, and would include them more in the treatment planning.

While only few differences were found between the patient and physician ideal perceptions, many differences were found on the perceived actual physician. The patients described their physicians as less explanatory than the physicians described themselves and also less encouraging and less approachable.

We then compared the actual and the ideal within each group (TABLE 2). As expected, only a few discrepancies were found in the physician's group: they explain the disease somewhat less than necessary, they encourage the patients somewhat less than they should, and they expect more trust from the patients. In other words, the physicians were quite satisfied and described their actual behavior as close to their ideal behavior. The patients, however, had a very different opinion—that their physicians fell short of the ideal on all items.

The last question concerned the effects of patient dissatisfaction with their oncologist on their psychological distress. The total score on the BSI-GSI was 57.4 (SD 10.2), which suggests moderate psychological distress and was reported in cancer patients who are in good medical condition and not in active chemotherapy.

Multiple Regression was done with GSI as the dependent variable, introducing into the equation the background variables (sex, age, marital

TABLE 1. Comparison of Physicians' and Patients' Perceptions of the Ideal and the Actual Physician

Item	Ideal			Actual		
	Physician	Patient	*t* Value	Physician	Patient	*t* Value
Explains disease	2.56	2.84	-2.47[a]	2.22	2.17	NS[b]
Explains treatment	2.89	2.88	NS	2.78	2.16	6.24
Includes in planning	1.78	2.71	-3.88[d]	2.07	1.75	2.32[a]
Explains to family	2.81	2.41	3.79[d]	2.85	1.77	10.5[c]
Can talk freely	2.85	2.88	NS	2.74	2.04	5.74[c]
Can be approached with problems	2.81	2.85	NS	2.74	2.08	6.06[c]
Encourages	2.86	2.66	NS	2.59	1.76	6.43[c]
Can be trusted and relied on	2.85	2.92	NS	2.27	2.11	NS
X for 8 items	2.68	2.77	NS	2.54	1.99	8.10[c]

[a]Significance .05.
[b]NS = not significant.
[c]Significance .000.
[d]Significance .001.

status, education), the medical variables (Karnofsky score and length of sickness), and I-A discrepancy.

To our surprise, none of the variables significantly influenced the psychological distress, and the multiple *R* was only .145 with an *R* square of .020. We thought this negative result could be due to mixing highly distressed with nondistressed patients. In other words, one could suggest differences in the variables that influence the two groups. The patients were, therefore, divided into two groups; one (137 patients) with a GSI cutoff point of up to 62, suggesting psychological distress, and the other (68 patients) with a GSI of 63 and above, suggesting psychopathology.

On Multiple Regression, the results were again negative. Even in the high-distress group with a multiple *R* of .306 and an *R* square of 0.094, the F value was far below statistical significance. We also ran the same Multiple Regression, introducing the patient's perception of the actual physician instead of the discrepancy, with the same negative results.

DISCUSSION

Traditional views of the relationship between physician and patient cast it as hierarchical: the physician was decision maker, and the role of the patient was to comply. In the past several decades, however, there has

TABLE 2. Patients' and Physicians' Actual-Ideal Discrepancies

Item	Patients			Physicians		
	A-I	*t* Value	*p*	A-I	*t* Value	*p*
Explains disease	0.68	11.47	.000	0.33	2.55	0.17
Explains treatment	0.73	12.43	.000	0.11		NS
Includes in planning	0.95	13.62	.000	-0.30		NS
Explains to family	0.66	8.00	.000	-0.04		NS
Can talk freely	0.85	12.78	.000	0.11		NS
Can be approached with problems	0.77	11.25	.000	0.07		NS
Encourages	0.90	12.13	.000	0.26	2.27	.032
Can be trusted and relied on	0.85	14.47	.000	0.58	4.19	.000

been a change in the nature of the patient-physician relationship. This change has led to what Suchman and Matthews[22] describe as the "connectional dimension" between patient and physician. Suchman and Matthews[22] suggested that a feeling of connectedness with the physician, of being thoroughly understood, reduces the feeling of patient isolation and incompetence. Independent of whatever biotechnical treatment is offered, this open, transpersonal connectedness is the basic ingredient for mutual cooperation and a therapeutic patient-physician relationship.

In a summary of 41 studies[23] containing objectively measured physician behavior and patient outcome, it has been shown that patient satisfaction is related to the quantity of information provided by physicians, their greater technical and interpersonal competence, increased partnership-building, more positive and less negative exchange, and more overall communication.

Although there has been a trend toward greater patient participation in illness management in recent years, it has not been well defined, nor is much known about how it may affect patient-physician interaction. A review of patient-physician communication studies suggests that compared with poorly informed patients, well-informed patients who actively participate in treatment planning are more likely to adhere to treatment regimens, cope with their illness, and achieve better recovery. Information about the disease and its treatment reduces a patient's uncertainty and increases a sense of control over events.[24–26]

In any human interaction, two critical components should be addressed: power and control. The attitudes, perceptions, and values inherent in the patient-physician relationship are some of the crucial dimensions of medical care, contributing not only to patient satisfaction but also to the ultimate outcome of patient compliance. Active participation in decision making and assumption of responsibility for treatment have been suggested as possible contributors to the control of disease and recovery.[27,28]

However, it is well known that when physicians do convey information to patients, it is often neither understood nor retained. Cassileth *et al.*,[29] in an early study of 200 patients, found that only 60% could correctly recall what their treatment entailed; 41% could not list a single major treatment risk; and only 27% could remember other treatment alternatives. It has been suggested that lack of patient comprehension may be associated with the severity of the illness. Desire for information and input into medical decisions are negatively associated with age and sex; older male patients are less likely to want active participation.[30] On the other hand, female patients, better educated patients and those of higher socioeconomic status are seen to absorb more information than other patients.

Several researchers have described the importance of medical information as a form of support. They examined helpful and unhelpful behaviors toward cancer patients from potential support providers. Sharing medical information was the most frequently cited helpful behavior from physicians, with the least helpful being the giving of insufficient medical information. Of 98 patients randomly selected by Truckett *et al.*,[31] three-quarters had questions that they did not put to their physician. They felt there was insufficient time and, thus, were reluctant to ask.

More recently, a study by Manfredi *et al.*[32] explored patient information-seeking behavior. Telephone interviews were conducted with 257 cancer patients and their relatives who called the National Cancer Institute Information Service for information. Results indicated that these patients were generally satisfied with their communication with their treating physician, were well informed, and wanted to participate in their treatment planning. These patients, who themselves contacted the Cancer Institute, were also better educated, better informed, younger, and less sick.

In our study, we found that the ideal of both physicians and patients was very high. On a scale of 0 to 3, the ideal behavior scored more than 2.5. However, contrary to our hypothesis, differences between the ideals of patients and physicians were small: there were no differences on any of the "empathy" items (trust in the physicians, ability to talk to them freely, to approach them with problems, and to receive encouragement from them).

Some differences were found on the "information" items, with patients expecting the ideal physician to explain the disease more to them and less to their families. Further, patient expectations of inclusion in treatment planning were higher than those of physicians. It should be stressed, however, that these expectations of ideal behavior are strongly determined by culture. In a study of cancer patients recently arrived from the former U.S.S.R. and treated in the same out-patient oncology department, expectations were significantly lower even though the majority had been diagnosed with cancer after immigration.[12]

Our second hypothesis concerning the behavior of the actual physician was borne out by the study. There were significant differences between the way in which patients and physicians described physician behavior on most items. No differences were found on only two items: how far patients trust their physicians (which is, in fact, patient rather than physician behavior) and the degree to which physicians explain the disease.

On all other items, very significant differences were found: patients perceived the physicians including them less in treatment planning and explaining the disease more to their families than to the patients themselves. Further, patients reported that they can talk to or approach the physicians less and are encouraged by physicians far less than perceived by the physicians themselves.

This finding raises the question as to whose perception is correct. Is the error with patients or physicians? Do patients wrongly perceive the behavior of physicians, or do physicians use denial and see themselves far nearer to their ideal? Other studies, too, have found discrepancies between the way physicians and patients describe each other's behavior.

In a British hospital, Williams[33] found that more than 305 of patients surveyed said they had not been informed about anesthesia or operating room procedures and had not been given advice about fitness, diet, and other treatments.

Similarly, in the United States, Cleary *et al.*[34,35] found in a telephone survey of 6,455 discharged patients that 44.9% said they had not been advised about daily routine, 38.7% said they had not had a relationship of trust with hospital staff, and 31.8% were not told whom to ask for additional medical help if needed.

Mosconi *et al.*[36] compared the perception of patients and oncologists about the information imparted. Only some 60% of patients, whom physicians claimed had been told about their cancer, agreed this was so. It could, of course, be said that this finding relates to a common mechanism of denial in the patients. However, less than 50% who were told they were free of cancer agreed they had been so informed. Almost the same number claimed they had received more information. It, thus, seems there is a wide gap between the behavior of physicians as described by themselves and as described by patients. The obvious question as to whose perception is correct cannot be answered on the basis of the present study.

The data strongly support our third hypothesis, that in the physician's group the discrepancy between ideal and actual is small. In other words, physicians perceive they live up to their ideal and, it can be assumed, are generally satisfied with their behavior. Nevertheless, they see room for improvement in being more explicit about the disease, more encouraging, and wanting their patients to trust them more.

The fourth hypothesis, that patients believe their physicians fall far short of their ideal, was, regrettably, also confirmed. Patients asserted that their physicians explain far less and are less empathetic than they would like them to be. They also wish they could trust their physicians more.

Most other studies do not support our finding of a high discrepancy, which we interpret as "high dissatisfaction." With all due caution, we suggest that the high satisfaction found by other studies could often be due to imprecise methodology. In a recent study, Ford *et al.*[37] found that most oncologists are blind to their patients' psychological distress. Only one out of five oncologist assessments of psychological distress correlated with patient reports of such distress. In that particular study, physicians tended to underrate patient distress and record satisfaction with their own performance. It should be noted that this '"blindness" to emotional conditions and needs is not limited to patients diagnosed with cancer.

Joos *et al.*[38] studied 243 patients with chronic diseases and found that patient satisfaction was more strongly related to whether the physician met their need for information and effective support, rather than whether the physician accommodated their need for examinations, tests, medications, and other treatment.

Kindelan *et al.*[39] asked patients, prior to their visit to a physician, to rank their order of preference for information about etiology and prevention, diagnosis, prognosis, treatment, and social effects of the illness. The resulting report indicated that satisfaction from a visit has four components: distress relief, rapport, communication, and compliance. The physicians also completed a questionnaire about their satisfaction with the consultation, indicating the type of information the patients desired. In this study, both patients and physicians were satisfied with the visit, though with little correlation between the two groups. Highly significant was the difference between the information the patients said they wanted and the perception of the physicians as to what type of information the patients wanted. The most interesting finding in that study is that the hypothesis was not supported. Higher satisfaction was not found in the group of patients whose physicians perceived correctly what type of information they wanted.

This brings us to a central problem that needs to be highlighted. We found a very high discrepancy in the patient's description of the ideal and actual physician, suggesting that the patients are basically dissatisfied with their physicians. In contrast, most studies reported high satisfaction. We suggested that perhaps these studies had used inadequate methods to assess satisfaction. As corroborating evidence, we cited Ford's study suggesting that patients cannot be satisfied when their physicians fail to per ceive their psychological distress. Also, in Kindelan's findings, despite physician failure to perceive patient information needs, the patient's high satisfaction with the doctor was not affected.

It should be pointed out that the measurement of patient-physician satisfaction poses a number of methodological and conceptual problems. Carr-Hill[40] observed that when an overall satisfaction score is "c," high levels of dissatisfaction regarding information given to the patient could be masked by high levels of satisfaction with multiple aspects of care. Cleary *et al.*[35] paradoxically found that patients who expressed a preference for more involvement in their care were more dissatisfied and gave more negative evaluations of their physician's care than did patients without this preference.

The fifth and most important hypothesis, dealing with patient dissatisfaction with the patient-physician relationship, has been that a discrepancy between the ideal and actual physician will correlate significantly with patient anxiety. The assumption relates to the concept of directionality, such as satisfaction versus dissatisfaction affecting levels of psychological distress in the patient. However, the hypothesis was not supported: the discrepancy between actual and ideal did not contribute significantly to psychological distress. These disappointing results, which should not have been a surprise, were repeated when we analyzed the data separately for patients with high distress and for those with low distress.

Some recent studies presented similar results. Dermatis *et al.*[41] studied patients before bone marrow transplants and found no relationship at all between psychological distress (measured by the same instrument as in our study, BSI) and the perceived quality of patient-physician communication.

On the other hand, Roberts *et al.*[42] measured psychological distress (by the SCL90) and satisfaction with physicians by the Cancer Diagnostic Interview Scale. Patient satisfaction was, on the whole, high, and did have significant protective effect on psychological distress.

We began our study hoping to show the importance of the patient-physician relationship and to prove that physicians' unawareness of this contributes to patients' psychological distress. Based on our findings, it is clear that there is a significant problem in the patient-physician relationship. Paradoxically, however, the negative effect of this relationship does not contribute to a patient's psychological distress.

It seems that the concept of satisfaction with medical care is an ambiguous one. Also, the impact of satisfaction on patients' psychological adjustment is not well documented. Better understanding of this complex concept related with medical care can be achieved only when sufficient consideration is given to the emotional, psychological, social, and cultural factors of the patient's and family's milieu.

REFERENCES

1. Cassileth, B. R. 1979. The Cancer Patient: Social and Medical Aspects of Care. Lea and Febiger. Philadelphia, PA.
2. Derogatis, L. R., G. Morrow, J. Fetting, D. Penman, S. Piatesky, A. M. Schmale, M. Hendricks & C. Carnicke. 1983. The prevalence and severity of psychiatric disorders among cancer populations. JAMA **249:** 751–757.
3. Razavi, D. & F. Siefel. 1994. Common psychiatric disorders in cancer patients. Supportive Care in Cancer **2:** 223–232.
4. McDaniel, J. S., D. L. Musselman, M. R. Porter, D. A. Reed & C. D. Nemeroff. 1995. Depression in patients with cancer. Biology, diagnosis and treatment. Arch. Gen. Psychiatry **52:** 89–99.
5. Waxler-Morrison, N., T. G. Hislop, B. Mears & L. Kan. 1991. Effects of social relationships on survival for women with breast cancer—A prospective study. Soc. Sci. Med. **33:** 177–188.
6. Ward, S., H. Leventhal, D. Easterling, C. Luchterhand & R. Love. 1991. Social support, self-esteem and communication in patients recurring chemotherapy. J. Psychosoc. Oncol. **9:** 95–116.
7. Gustafson, D., M. Wise, F. McTavish, O. J. Taylor, W. Wolberg, J. Stewart, R. V. Smalley & K. Bosworth. 1993. Development and pilot evaluation of a computer-based support system for women with breast cancer. J. Psychosoc. Oncol. **11:** 69–93.
8. Blanchard, D. C., M. Labraque, J. Ruckdeschel & E. Blanchard. 1990. Physician behaviors, patient perceptions, and patient characteristics as predictors of satisfaction of hospitalized adult cancer patients. Cancer **65:** 186–192.
9. Shores, A. D., H. R. Rubin, M. E. Haisfield, D. B. McGuire, J. R. Zabora & S. Krumm. 1993. Health care providers' and cancer patients' preferences regarding disclosure of information about advance directives. J. Psychosoc. Oncol. **11:** 39–53.
10. Bloch, R. 1994. Disclosing cancer diagnosis to a patient. J. Nat. Cancer Inst. **86:** 868–870.
11. Baider, L. 1985. The oncologist and his patient: An inquiry into their relationship. J. Psychol.—Judaism **9:** 46–57.
12. Baider, L., P. Ever-Hadani & A. Kaplan DeNour. 1995. The impact of culture on perceptions of patient-physician satisfaction. Isr. J. Med. Sci. **31:** 179–185.
13. Surbone, A. 1993. The information to the cancer patients: Psychosocial and spiritual implications. Supportive Care Cancer **1:** 89–91.
14. Pfeffer, R. M. 1993. Ethics and the oncologist. Med. Law **12:** 235–240.
15. Glaser, B. G. & A. L. Strauss. 1965. Awareness of Dying. Aldine Publishing Co. Chicago, IL.
16. Glaser, B. G. & A. L. Strauss. 1968. Time for Dying. Aldine Publishing Co. Chicago, IL.
17. Brody, D., S. M. Miller, C. E. Lerman, D. Smith, C. G. Lazaro & M. J. Blum. 1989. The relationship between patients' satisfaction with their physicians and perceptions about interventions they desired and received. Med. Care **227:** 1027–1035.
18. Steptoe, A., I. Sutcliffe, B. Allen & C. Coombes. 1991. Satisfaction with communication, medical knowledge and coping style in patients with metastatic cancer. Soc. Sci. Med. **32:** 627–632.
19. Burton, M. V. & R. W. Parker. 1994. Satisfaction of breast cancer patients

with their medical and psychological care. J. Psychosoc. Oncol. **12:** 41–63.

20. KARNOFSKY, D. A. & J. H. BURCHENAL. 1949. The clinical evaluation of chemotherapeutic agents in cancer. *In* Evaluation of Chemotherapeutic Agents. C.M. Macleod, Ed.: 199–205. Columbia University Press. New York, NY.
21. DEROGATIS, L. R. & P. M. SPENCER. 1982. The Brief Symptom Inventory (BSI). Administration, Scoring and Procedures Manual. Clinical Psychometric Research. Baltimore, MD.
22. SUCHMAN, A. L. & D. A. MATTHEWS. 1988. What makes the patient-doctor relationship therapeutic? Exploring the connexional dimension of medical care. Ann. Intern. Med. **108:** 125–130.
23. HALL, J. A., D. L. ROTER & N. R. KATZ. 1988. Meta-analysis of correlates of provider behavior in medical encounters. Med. Care **26:** 657–675.
24. GOFFMAN, T. E. & L. DACHOWSKI. 1992. The strategic management of serious news. Mil. Med. **157:** 424–426.
25. FALLOWFIELD, L. J. 1993. Giving sad and bad news. Lancet **341:** 476–478.
26. FALLOWFIELD, L. J., S. FORD & S. LEWIS. 1994. Information preferences of patients with cancer. Lancet **344:** 1576.
27. SCHAIN, W. S. 1990. Physician-patient communication about breast cancer. Surg. Clin. North Am. **70:** 917–935.
28. PELLEGRINO, E. D. 1993. The metamorphosis of medical ethics. JAMA **269:** 1158–1162.
29. CASSILETH, B. R., R. V. ZUPKIS, K. SUTTON-SMITH & V. MARCH. 1980. Information and participation preferences among cancer patients. Ann. of Intern. Med. **92:** 832–836.
30. ROTER, D., M. LIPKIN & A. KORSGAARD. 1991. Sex differences in patients' and physicians' communication during primary care. Med. Care **93:** 354–357.
31. TRUCKETT, D. & A. WILLIAMS. 1984. Approaches to the measurement of explanation and information giving in medical consultations. Soc. Sci. Med. **18:** 571–580.
32. MANFREDI, C., R. CZAJA, M. BUIS & D. DEREK. 1993. Patient use of treatment related information received from the Cancer Information Service. Cancer **71:** 1326–1337.
33. WILLIAMS, O. A. 1993. Patient knowledge of operative care. J. R. Soc. Med. **86:** 328–331.
34. CLEARY, P. D., S. EDGEMAN-LEVITAN, M. ROBERTS, T. W. MOLONEY, W. MCMULLEN, J. D. WALKER & T. L. DELBANCO. 1991. Patients evaluate their hospital care: A national survey. Health Affairs **10:** 254–267.
35. CLEARY, P. D., S. EDGMAN-LEVITAN, W. MCMULLEN & T. L. DELBANCO. 1992. The relationship between reported problems and patient summary evaluations of hospital care. Qual. Rev. Bull. **18:** 53–59.
36. MOSCONI, P.,B. E. MEYEROWITZ,M. C. LIBERATI & A. LIBERATI. 1991. Disclosure of breast cancer diagnosis: Patient-physician reports. Ann. Oncol. **2:** 273–280.
37. FORD, S., L. J. FALLOWFIELD & S. LEWIS. 1994. Can oncologists detect distress in their out-patients and how satisfied are they with their performance during bad news consultations? Br. J. Cancer **70:** 767–770.
38. JOOS, S. K., D. H. HICKMAN & L. M. BORDERS. 1993. Patient desires and satisfaction in general medicine clinics. Public Health Rep. **108:** 751–759.
39. KINDELAN, K. & G. KENT. 1987. Concordance between patient's information preferences and general practitioners' perceptions. Psychol. Health **1:**

399–409.
40. CARR-HILL, R. A. 1992. The measurement of patient satisfaction. J. Public Health Med. **14:** 236–249.
41. DERMATIS, H. & L. LESKO. 1991. Psychosocial correlates of physician-patient communication at time of informed consent for bone-marrow transplantation. Cancer Invest. **9:** 621–628.
42. ROBERTS, C., C. E. COX, D. S. REINTGEN, W. BAILE & M. GIBERTINI. 1994. Influence of physician communication on newly diagnosed breast cancer patients' psychologic adjustment and decision-making. Cancer **74:** 336–341.

Telling the Truth to Cancer Patients and Patients with HIV-1 Infection in Japan

HIROAKI MITSUYA

Experimental Retrovirology Section
Medicine Branch
Division of Clinical Sciences
National Cancer Institute
National Institutes of Health
Bethesda, Maryland 20892

TELLING THE TRUTH TO PATIENTS WITH CANCER IN JAPAN

In May 1995, the Ministry of Health and Welfare of Japan (MHW) reported the results of its study of family satisfaction with truth-telling to cancer patients. The report revealed that 56% of the families of patients who were informed of the diagnosis and died of cancer felt that it was satisfactory to have let those patients know that they had cancer; however, 44% of the families were not certain whether it was worthwhile or thought that the patients were better off unaware of the diagnosis. By contrast, 67% of the families of patients who were not informed of the cancer diagnosis felt satisfied that the diagnosis was not disclosed to those patients. In Japan, the MHW task force on care for terminally ill patients recommended in 1989 that informing cancer patients of their diagnosis and life expectancy was essential.[1] However, the view that patients should be given full information about their diseases has not yet been well accepted in Japan. In the previous MHW report, presented in 1992 on the same subject, a similar percentage (59%) of the families of cancer patients viewed that it was rewarding to have let the patients know their diagnosis. Apparently, there was no significant change in the percentage of families who found that disclosure was satisfactory in the 1995 report as compared to the report in 1992, although the number of patients who desire to know the truth is gradually increasing.[2] It is worth noting, however, that there is a double standard in truth-telling in Japan: in a newspaper survey in 1981–1985, 53–56% of respondents expressed their desire to be informed of their own cancer diagnosis, while only 10–12% of respondents preferred to inform the patient of the diagnosis if one of their family members has cancer.[3] A recent international survey has shown that the notification rate of identified cancer to patients is as low as 29.5% in Japan, compared to 87.3% and 51.9% in the United States and Italy, respectively.[4] Historically, changes toward truth-telling took place quite rapidly in the United States. Studies in the United Sates up to the mid-1960s show that the diagnosis of cancer had not been disclosed to most patients, while a study done in 1977 revealed that 97% of physicians had disclosed cancer diagnosis to patients.[5] Several factors appear to account for the difference between Japan and the United States.

First, there is in Japan a persistent belief that the disclosure of cancer diagnosis only brings about a loss of hope and unwanted emotional distress to patients. There exists a concern that after knowing the diagnosis of metastatic and untreatable cancer, patients may isolate themselves, become desperate, and even commit suicide. The authoritarian and paternalistic elements in the Japanese health care system apparently reinforce the belief that the disclosure of cancer diagnosis produces only "bad results." In Japanese culture, even if one does not explicitly ask a favor, others are often expected to infer his/her intention and act accordingly.[6] Thus, the preferred ethical principle is nonmaleficence compounded with paternalism, which prohibits disclosure of "harmful" truth to terminally ill patients.[7] Such reluctance of health care providers to disclose "bad news" to patients is noted in other cultural areas such as eastern and southern Europe and Africa.[2,4] Goodgame reported that an AIDS diagnosis is often not disclosed to patients in Uganda because of the health care providers' fear of adverse psychological reactions of patients.[8] It is worth noting that paternalism in Japan can be well illustrated even on ordinary checkups in hospitals. Physicians tend not to fully explain the reason for planned examinations and the subsequent results to patients. Patients' attempts to obtain a second opinion from other doctors are often considered an insult to the primary doctor. The drugs prescribed by doctors are often provided to patients with their labels removed.

Second, the decision-making process in Japan tends to be group oriented.[7] In the setting of terminal health care, physicians most often consult with principal family members, but not with patients. In this respect, obedience to the wishes of spouses, family members, or family elders is appreciated in Japan, and free choices offered by health care providers may contradict such cultural "norms."[9] This may explain, at least in part, why as much as 67% of the families of patients felt satisfied that the diagnosis was not disclosed to patients. In this respect, Gostin has recently noted that autonomous decision making established in Anglo-American cultures may counter family-centered values and the social meanings of competency in certain ethnic cultures.[10] In the United States, ethical issues in medicine have evolved around the principle of patient autonomy. This principle asserts the rights of patients to be informed of their diagnosis, prognosis, and the risks and benefits of therapies, and to be allowed to make informed decisions about treatments and withholding resuscitation. In the United States, autonomy has become a moral absolute. In this respect, Pellegrino lists several reasons, including improved education of the public, a strong tradition of privacy rights and personal liberty, a distrust of authority and the possibilities of medical technology, and the loosening of family and community identification in the United States.[11] Pellegrino then proposes that the fundamental issue in the controversy over truth-telling is not a culturally bound phenomenon, but a universal phenomenon of conflict between traditional values and the contemporary Anglo-American concept of autonomy.[11] Analysis only of cultural differences may fail this critical issue. It is worth noting that the right to autonomy or self-determination may be inconsistent with the belief systems of other cultures and ethnic environments. For example, Blackhall et al. have recently reported that Korean-American and Mexican-American individuals were more likely to hold a family-centered model of medical decision making rather than the patient-autonomy model favored by most African-American and European-American individuals.[12] One has to use caution that Korean can be substantially different from Japanese ethnicity; however, culturally Japan is closer to Korea than to the United States. Miyaji argues that many physicians in Japan have an act-utilitarian or contextualist attitude in regard to patient autonomy.[13] Indeed, in a recent study, as many as 36% of physicians contend that introduction of informed consent should be determined in a "case-by-case" manner; and 23% of them as yet believe that it is difficult to introduce informed consent to Japan, while only 36% of them believe that it is required.[14]

Third, physicians tend to argue against truth-telling and reason that no assistance or advice is readily available from trained counselors, social workers, psychotherapists, or such to respond to the psychological crisis of patients who are informed of cancer diagnosis. Physicians also argue that patients generally feel rather uncomfortable with referral for counseling, since it often means such patients suffer mental weaknesses or illnesses, one of the societal stigmas in Japan. It should be noted, however, that establishing a psychiatric liaison program first may be essential even under these circumstances. Indeed, it is reported that psychiatric consultation substantially increased in a medical unit where a psychiatric liaison program was established and a number of patients were informed of their cancers.[15] Larger studies are required, however, to clarify this issue in Japan.

It should also be pointed out that only a nominal fee is allowed to health care providers by the National Health Insurance schedule in Japan. One report in 1988 describes that the medical service fee for physician consultations and technical services is approximately one-tenth of that in the United States.[16] This low medical service fee schedule tends to reinforce health care providers' tendency not to spend time for lengthy consultations and explanations. The judicial precedents in Japan, at least in part, contribute to the sluggish move to truth-telling in Japan, which grants health care providers substantial power in handling medical documents. Indeed, the Japanese Supreme Court has recently ruled that physicians are not obliged to inform cancer patients of the nature of their condition, upholding earlier rulings by district and high courts.[17] Other factors include an emphasis on cure and treatment per se, less emphasis on the patient-physician relationship in medical education in Japan, and the limited number of physicians who have an interest in palliative care.[18] The cultural tendency in Japan and other Asian countries to avoid open confrontation with death may also contribute to the preservation of the status quo and the sluggish changes.

TELLING THE TRUTH TO HIV-INFECTED PATIENTS IN JAPAN

There has recently been a report in Japan that as many as 66 (28%) of 168 institutions and hospitals that are associated with the Japanese Government–sponsored acquired immunodeficiency syndrome (AIDS) treatment group have not informed their patients of their human immunodeficiency virus type 1 (HIV-1) positivity.[19] This study also revealed that at least 33 individuals have been identified as having transmitted HIV-1 unknowingly to their partners, although it is not clear as to when these secondary infections occurred. Twenty-one (68%) of the 33 secondary HIV-1–infected cases were associated with hemophiliac patients.

In Japan, the number of HIV-1–infected individuals and patients with AIDS is as yet relatively smaller than in other industrialized countries such as the United States and European countries. As of November 1995, the number of reported AIDS cases was 1,063 nationwide and that of reported HIV-1–infected cases was 3,471, according to the official report from MHW, although the latter number is thought to be substantially underrepresented. The unique feature of HIV-1 infection in Japan is that as high as 50–60% of HIV-1–infected individuals and patients with AIDS are hemophiliacs.[20,21] In March 1983, following the initial report that AIDS is caused by HIV-1,[22] the use of heat-treated concentrated clotting factors was approved. and the administration of unheated factors was banned in the United States to halt the spread of HIV-1 infection through blood products. In Japan, the clotting factor product called "Creo" or "AHF" made of blood from a few blood donors was the therapy for hemophiliac patients in the 1970s; however, the profitability with "Creo" and "AHF" was modest, and they were not mass-produced. In 1976, unheated concentrated clotting factors made from a pool of human blood from a few hundred thousand donors in the United States were introduced and brought about a significant profit to pharmaceutical firms in Japan. From 1983 to 1985, when the danger of transmitting the virus through concentrated blood products was at its height, the use of heat-treated blood products was still banned; and efforts to market unheated concentrated clotting factors, which had been suspected to contain contaminating HIV-1, were continued, resulting in a sudden, sharp increase in the importation of HIV-1–contaminated clotting factors from the United States.[23] During this period, approximately 2000 of 5000 hemophiliacs were infected with HIV-1 in Japan. In July 1985, heat-treated blood products were finally approved for domestic use in Japan, two years and four months after their approval in the United States. Two lawsuits against both MHW and five pharmaceutical companies—three Japanese (Green Cross, Nippon Zoki Pharmaceutical, and Chemosero Therapeutic Research Institute) and two foreign (Baxter and Bayer Institute)—had been filed in Tokyo and Osaka District Courts, alleging that they allowed contaminated blood products into Japan despite their knowing that such products were dangerous and were banned in the United States and Europe. The two groups involved in the lawsuits consisted of a total of 161 plaintiffs, who are the victims or their family members. On October 6, 1995, both the Tokyo and Osaka District Courts recommended that the Japanese Government and the drug firms accept responsibility and pay each plaintiff Y45 million ($450,000), a sum far less than the Y115 million ($1.15 million) originally sought.[24] No party would have to admit fault. No criminal prosecutions have been sought in Japan. Other victims and family members who have not been involved in the litigation will also have to be relieved and somehow compensated.

Due to the unique demography of HIV-1 infection in Japan, there may be certain aspects common to truth-telling to cancer patients and to patients with HIV-1 infection. It is worth noting that some physicians who provided long-term care and administered the HIV-1–contaminated blood products to their hemophiliac patients without knowing the danger of transmission of HIV-1 have a sense of complex guilt and have been quite hesitant to or have failed to disclose the fact to their patients. When HIV-1–infected patients are juvenile victimized hemophiliacs, the parents often request that physicians not tell the diagnosis or the status of HIV-1 infection to their children. In the worst cases, physicians have not even performed an HIV-1 antibody test for hemophiliac patients because of their fear of the results. In some cases, patients express that they do not want to know the diagnosis. In other cases, physicians judge by themselves that not giving information will be beneficial to the patients, sometimes refusing to inform even young adult patients of HIV-1 status.[25] In cases of heterosexual and homosexual transmission, physicians may inform patients of HIV-1 positivity more often; however, the report by Matsuda and Yamada observes that even nonhemophiliacs are not informed of HIV-1 infection in some cases.[19] Taking all these cases into consideration, the general attitude of physicians who do not disclose HIV-1 status to infected patients appears to represent more evidence of the persistent authoritarian and paternalistic elements in the current Japanese medical establishment. In the context of truth-telling to cancer patients, the contradiction between the physicians' moral duty to protect patients and their respect for the patients' autonomy may be resolved to a certain extent by their interpretation of principles of truth, rights, duties, and hope.[7] In the case of HIV-1 infection, however, such paternalistic elements in truth-telling can produce quite devastating consequences: patients may not have the advantage of antiviral therapy that can retard the progress of HIV-1–related illnesses and prolong their survival;[26,27] patients may refuse the administration of therapy against AIDS and HIV-1 infection, which is often accompanied by side effects; and patients may unintentionally transmit HIV-1 to their partners. Thus, one can conclude that paternalism combined with contextualism in the care of HIV-1–infected individuals represents only digressive "information control" over the patients.

OBSTACLES TO TELLING THE TRUTH TO HIV-1–INFECTED PATIENTS

Health care providers note various obstacles to truth-telling of HIV-1 positivity to their patients. These include the lack of a counseling system to support patients after disclosure, improper environments for doctors to inform their patients, and the possible breach of confidentiality of the patients' status. Interestingly, all of these obstacles have been used as circumstantial reasons why Japanese physicians are reluctant to inform patients of a cancer diagnosis. Indeed, the report by Matsuda and Yamada[19] observes that Japanese physicians are hesitant to inform patients of HIV-1 positivity for quite similar reasons as for not disclosing a cancer diagnosis to patients.

LACK OF A COUNSELING SYSTEM FOR HIV-1–INFECTED PATIENTS

Counseling is a basic component of care for HIV-1–infected individuals, to assist them to face the diagnosis, to fight the disease, and to reduce the chances of transmission of HIV-1 to others.[28] Counseling is critical when patients are informed of their HIV-1 positivity, when they progress from asymptomatic status to AIDS-related complex, and when they develop frank AIDS.[29] In some areas in Japan, anonymous and walk-in counseling systems are available prior to receiving HIV-1–antibody testing. However, in most cases, physicians who care for patients with HIV-1 infection and inform them of their HIV-1 positivity or their disease status are not professionally trained to provide appropriate counseling. It has been pointed out that when doctors do not have a "counseling mind", truth-telling becomes only "a short notice" to patients.[25,30] It should be noted that providing mere information or fact is only a way of delegating the entire burden of medical decisions to the "informed" patient, thus limiting medical responsibilities on the side of the physician.[31] Physicians should never feel relieved of medical and legal responsibilities by informing patients of the simple truth.[32] Patients and physicians should be reciprocally collaborating partners to attain their mutual goal, the treatment of illness.[33]

PRIVACY AND HIV-1 INFECTION

In general, patients' privacy is protected poorly in Japan as compared to the United States, primarily due to the nature of hospital facilities. In Japan, almost all outpatient clinics, whether university, private, or public, do not have a private room where patient and family can talk to and consult with health care providers. Unlike most examination rooms in the United States, which are divided by full floor-to-ceiling walls, patients in Japan almost always have to talk to health care providers in a cubicle partitioned only by curtains or wooden or plastic screens. Patients and families can easily overhear conversations of other patients with physicians and nurses. This situation also exists for other types of health care giving, including gynecological outpatient services. While an attempt to preserve a private room for interviewing and medical examinations of potentially HIV-1–infected individuals has been made in some hospitals, it is often argued that it is difficult to allocate private rooms for only a few HIV-1–infected patients. When patients are informed of their HIV-1 positivity, disease progress, or development of frank AIDS, they suffer from the shock, despair, and fear of death. Some patients cry for hours, and become absent minded and confused. Obviously, counseling is needed for patients prior to and after such disclosure. The lack of private rooms in most hospitals and institutions has been a critical obstacle to the assurance of adequate privacy for patients with HIV-1 infection. It should be stressed that the lack of private rooms has also posed problems in caring for outpatients with cancer and other illnesses as well.

It should also be pointed out that the privacy of HIV-1–infected individuals is sometimes, if not often, poorly maintained outside the clinics. The diagnosis of AIDS or asymptomatic HIV-1 infection is sometimes leaked to others by nonprofessional workers at hospitals and even by professional staff. Privacy tends to be more facilely breached by nonmedical workers in medical insurance departments of employers. It is obvious that health care providers should not discuss the private matters of patients in public places where others may overhear. Likewise, health care providers should not attempt to satisfy their curiosity about patients who are not in their care. Furthermore, when hospitals or institutions apply for reimbursement through medical insurance, meticulously documented medical records such as diagnoses and medications used are transmitted to nonprofessional workers and clerks. Hospital billing offices obtain both financial and medical records and curious individuals could make accurate deductions about the patients' diagnosis. The introduction of third-party payers poses more serious problems. Fearing possible disclosure of their diagnosis in the work place and the potential consequences, a number of patients with HIV-1 infection choose to purchase costly antiretroviral drugs out of their own funds and do not seek reimbursement from health insurance. When such medical records are held by employers or life insurance companies, patients may fall victim to immediate discrimination because of HIV-1 infection. Routine and systematic training of health care providers and those working in the health insurance field is needed in order to reinforce the principle of confidentiality in the clinical setting.

REFUSAL TO TREAT HIV-1–INFECTED PATIENTS

The report by Matsuda and Yamada also observes that surgeons in 45 of 208 (22%) hospitals refused to treat HIV-1–infected patients whose antibody status was known, and internists in 6 hospitals (3%) refused to see those patients.[19] Such hospitals or doctors contend that the major reason for refusal of patients with HIV-1 infection is that such hospitals may not cover liability in cases of inadvertent HIV-1 infection to health care workers. Of 237 hospitals in which HIV-1–infected individuals were treated, 112 hospitals have reported incidents of needle stick or exposure to HIV-1–tainted body fluids, although none of those exposures resulted in HIV-1 infection. Considering that no unique or special equipment or facilities are required for treating patients infected with HIV-1 in most circumstances, a number of physicians and medical staff appear to view AIDS and its related diseases as an unusual and special illness.

Another tacit anxiety of such hospitals and physicians is that treating patients with HIV-1 infection may result in loss of other patients who are wrongfully afraid of contracting AIDS by visiting such hospitals through encounters with HIV-1–infected patients or sharing medical equipment. Obviously, such fear and anxiety of lay people are derived from ungrounded misconception and a lack of medical knowledge. To assure that patients with HIV-1 infection readily receive medical care, MHW has recently launched a plan that each prefecture establish "base (mainstay)" hospitals in its major cities, although the establishment of such hospitals seems to be tardy and has raised some controversy, including whether it is necessary to establish such hospitals.

CONCLUSIONS

In Japan, the number of HIV-1–infected patients is still relatively smaller than that in other industrialized countries. This may contribute in part to the as yet relatively poor ambience for the care of HIV-1–infected individuals in that country. With respect to truth-telling, it seems obvious that the attitude of physicians who are reluctant to disclose the diagnosis is based on reasons that are common to the settings of both cancer and AIDS. The issue of truth-telling to patients with HIV-1 infection has, however, posed a number of fundamental challenges to contemporary medical ethics in Japan. Whether or not to inform patients of HIV-1 positivity and the status of HIV-1–related illnesses challenges health care providers more acutely and directly than in many cancer cases in that delaying and avoiding telling the truth to HIV-1–infected patients may produce quite devastating and irreversible consequences. Simple paternalism or contexualism is by no means justified in the setting of truth-telling to HIV-1–infected patients. As in the case of cancer, truth-telling to HIV-1–infected patients is not an easy task, however. One has to seriously consider the situation in which patients contracted AIDS in Japan, although the magnitude of the tragedy of AIDS is the same for all individuals worldwide. In addition to truth-telling to HIV-1–infected individuals, the patient-physician relationship has to be rigorously examined; the counseling system has to be tightly coordinated; the patients' privacy has to be strictly assured; and the education of health care providers, lay people, and other patients on the biology and medical aspects of HIV-1 is absolutely required. Earnest efforts should also be made to fight against any possible discrimination to HIV-1–infected patients. Health care providers must remember that merely providing simple information is only a way of delegating the entire burden of medical decisions to the "informed" patient; that they should never feel relieved of their medical and legal responsibilities by informing patients of the simple truth.[31,32] Indeed, truth-telling to HIV-1–infected patients is a real touchstone for medical ethics in Japan.

ACKNOWLEDGMENTS

The author is grateful to Drs. Antonella Surbone and Rihito Kimura for encouragement and kind advice; Drs. Naoko Miyaji, Junki Takamatsu, and Takuma Shirasaka for helpful discussions; and Mr. Mark Kavlick for critical reading of the manuscript.

REFERENCES

1. JAPANESE MINISTRY OF HEALTH AND WELFARE AND THE JAPAN MEDICAL ASSOCIATION. 1989. The report for terminal care. Chuo Hoki Shuppan. Tokyo.
2. AKABAYASHI, A., M. D. FETTERS & GEN OHI. 1995. Truth-telling of the cancer diagnosis in contemporary Japan: A discussion and analysis. *In:*

Proceedings of the Second International Congress of Psycho-Oncology: 93–100. Kobe, Japan, October 19–22., 1995.
3. MORIOKA, Y. 1991. Informed consent and truth telling to cancer patients. Gastroenterol. Jpn. **26:** 789–792.
4. KOINUMA, N. 1995. An international perspective on full disclosure. *In:* Proceedings of the Second International Congress of Psycho-Oncology: 84. Kobe, Japan, October 19–22, 1995.
5 NOVACK, D. H., R. PLUMER, R. L. SMITH, H. OCHITILL, G. R. MORROW & J. M. BENNETT. 1979. Changes in physicians' attitudes toward telling the cancer patient. JAMA **241:** 897–900.
6. DOI, L. T. 1963. Some thoughts on helplessness and the desire to be loved. Psychiatry **26:** 266–272.
7. MIYAJI, N. T. 1993. The power of compassion: Truth-telling among American doctors in the care of dying patients. Soc. Sci. Med. **36:** 249–264.
8. GOODGAME, R. W. 1990. AIDS in Uganda: Clinical and social features. N. Engl. J. Med. **323:** 383–389.
9. LEVINE, R. J. 1991. Informed consent: Some challenges to the universal validity of the western model. J. Law Med. Ethics **19:** 207–213.
10. GOSTIN, L. O. 1995. Informed consent, cultural sensitivity, and respect for persons. JAMA **274:** 844–845.
11. PELLEGRINO, E. D. 1992. Is truth telling to the patient a cultural artifact? JAMA **268:** 1734–1735.
12. BLACKHALL, L. J., S. T. MURPHY, G. FRANK, V. MICHAEL & S AZEN. 1995. Ethnicity and attitudes toward patient autonomy. JAMA **274:** 820–825.
13. MIYAJI, N. 1994. Ethical discourse of Japanese and American physicians on truth-telling in the care of dying patients (in Japanese). J. Japan Assoc. Bioethics **4:** 94–99.
14. SCOPE/INFORMED CONSENT. 1995. From the front of 317 physicians. Scope **400:** 12–25.
15. UCHITOMI, Y., J. SUGIHARA, M. FUKUE, Y. KURAMOTO, T. AKECHI, N. OOMORI & S. YAMAWAKI. 1994. Psychiatric liaison issues in cancer care in Japan. J. Pain Symptom Management **9:** 319–324.
16. IGLEHART, J. K. 1988. Japan's medical care system (Part 2). N. Engl. J. Med. **319:** 1166–1172.
17. NEWS. 1995. Japanese court rules against informing the patients. Ann. Oncol. **6:** 511.
18. KASHIWAGI, T. 1991. Palliative care in Japan. Palliative Med. **5:** 165–170.
19. MATSUDA, J. & K. YAMADA. 1995. Present situation of health care setting for patients living with human immunodeficiency virus type-1 in medical institutions of Japan. Jpn. J. Clin. Hematol. **36:** 451–456.
20. YAMAMOTO, N. 1994. Present status of AIDS and AIDS research. *In:* Guides to AIDS/HIV Infection. S. Kimura, & N. Yamamoto, Eds.: 10–18. Nankodo. Tokyo.
21. NEWS. 1995. Update on HIV infection in Japan (in Japanese). Nihon-Iji-Shimpo **3737:** 95.
22. BARRE-SINOUSSI, F., J. C. CHERMANN, F. REY, T. NUGEYRE, S. CHARMARET, J. GRUEST, C. DAUGUET, C. AXLER-BLIN, F. VEZINET-BRUN, C. ROUZIOUX, W. ROZENBAUM & L. MONTAGNIER. 1983. Isolation of a T-cell lymphotropic virus from a patient at risk for the acquired immunodeficiency syndrome (AIDS). Science **220:** 868–871.
23. EXECUTIVE COMMITTEE OF THE COALITION FOR HEMOPHILIAC ORGANIZATION IN

JAPAN FOR AIDS. 1994. Global suffering in hemophiliac communities and HIV contaminated blood products. Brochure in a Satellite Symposium to the Tenth International Conference on AIDS. Yokohama, Japan, August 7–12, 1994.

24. GUEST, R. 1995. Settlement for tainted blood. Br. Med. J. **311:** 1044–1045.
25. ISHIGAMI, W., K. YASHIKI, S. SHINSHYO & J. KOYANO. 1993. Care for people with HIV and the infringement of human rights (in Japanese). Nippon Rinsho (Jpn. Clin. Med.) **51**(Suppl.): 565–569.
26. MITSUYA, H., R. YARCHOAN & S. BRODER. 1990. Molecular targets for AIDS therapy. Science **249:** 1533–1544.
27. MITSUYA, H. & R. YARCHOAN. 1994. Development of antiretroviral therapy for AIDS and related disorders. *In:* Textbook of AIDS Medicine. S. Broder, T. Merigan & D. Bolognesi, Eds.: 721–742. Williams & Wilkins. Baltimore, MD.
28. WENGER, N. S., L. S. LINN, M. EPSTEIN & M. F. SHAPIRO. 1991. Reduction of high-risk sexual behavior among heterosexuals undergoing HIV-antibody testing: A randomized clinical trial. Am. J. Public Health **81:** 1580–1585.
29. KOBAYASHI, M. & K. UEDA. 1993. The counseling for persons with HIV infection (in Japanese). Nippon Rinsho (Jpn. Clin. Med.) **51**(Suppl.): 578–583.
30. NEGISHI, M. 1993. Explanations, guidance, and advises how to fight against HIV infections for PWAs (in Japanese). Nippon Rinsho (Jpn. Clin. Med.) **51**(Suppl.): 575–577.
31. SURBONE, A. 1992. Truth telling to the patient. JAMA 268: 1661–1662.
32. SURBONE, A. 1990. Truth in medicine: Telling the truth to the patient—The essential step. *In:* Proceedings of American-Italian Foundation for Cancer Research, 1990: 37–39. [Au: Place of publication?]
33. KIMURA, R. 1987. The patients-physicians relationships. *In:* Bioethics: Thoughts of Life: 93–104. Nihon-Hyoronsha. Tokyo.

Truth-telling Practice in Cancer Care in Japan

YOSUKE UCHITOMI[a,b] AND SHIGETO YAMAWAKI[c]

[a]*Psycho-Oncology Division*
National Cancer Center Research Institute, East
6-5-1, Kashiwanoha
Kashiwa, 277, Japan

[c]*Department of Psychiatry and Neurosciences*
Hiroshima University School of Medicine
Kasumi 1-2-3, Minami-ku
Hiroshima 734, Japan

INTRODUCTION

Japanese physicians are taught to consider the Hippocratic obligation as requiring them to do that which is expected to have the best consequences for the patient, and they usually consider themselves the final authority regarding medical treatment for their cancer patients. However, the decision whether to disclose the cancer diagnosis is left to family members, who usually do not tell the truth.

In the 1980s, the policy with regard to telling the truth was influenced by the introduction of hospice care in Japan and was accelerated mainly by a majority of the nurses and a limited number of physicians caring for terminally ill cancer patients[1] because of issues related to providing aggressive treatment for terminally ill patients who had not been informed of the cancer diagnosis. This situation had resulted in impaired communication between patient and family, lack of symptom management for cancer patients with pain and emotional distress, and so on. In 1989, a Japanese Ministry of Health and Welfare task force advocated that physicians inform the terminally ill patient not only of the cancer diagnosis but also of their limited life expectancy, and further recommended that telling the truth be considered a necessity.[2] The trend toward full disclosure of the diagnosis has progressed extremely slowly in Japan.

To clarify issues regarding truth-telling practice in cancer care in Japan, this paper briefly introduces two national surveys of physicians

[a]Corresponding author.

and bereaved family caregivers, regarding truth-telling practice in cancer care in Japan[3,4] and reports on the guidelines for telling the truth to terminally ill patients proposed by the Japanese Ministry of Health and Welfare.[2]

TWO NATIONAL SURVEYS OF PHYSICIANS AND BEREAVED FAMILY CAREGIVERS REGARDING TRUTH-TELLING PRACTICE IN CANCER CARE IN JAPAN

Bereaved Family Caregiver Survey

To clarify cancer care issues in Japan, the Japanese Ministry of Health and Welfare surveyed family members who had cared for cancer patients who subsequently died to determine their opinion regarding informed consent and quality of life.[3]

All of the cancer patients between the ages of 40 and 64 years in 11 prefectures of Japan who had died of cancer between March and April 1992 were identified by the Vital Statistics Division, Statistics and Information Department, Japanese Ministry of Health and Welfare. In October 1992, investigators visited the bereaved families under the leadership of directors from the respective local health centers and requested the family member who had cared for the cancer patient to respond to a questionnaire that included questions related to truth-telling practice. The response rate was 68.3% (1918/2810). The age and gender distributions of the 1918 cancer patients and the bereaved family caregivers are shown in TABLES 1 and 2. The relationship to the cancer patient of the family caregivers responding is shown in TABLE 3.

Of 1918 bereaved family caregivers who had cared for the cancer patient, 18.2% reported that the patient was informed of the cancer diagnosis, while 81.3% reported that the patient was not (TABLE 4). Of care-

TABLE 1. Age and Gender of Cancer Patients

			Gender	
Age (yr)	Number	Percent	Male	Female
40–49	327	17.1	162	165
50–59	822	42.8	522	300
60–64	769	40.1	549	220
Total	1918	100	–	–

TABLE 2. Age and Gender of Bereaved Family Caregivers

			Gender	
Age (yr)	Number	Percent	Male	Female
<39	269	14.0	95	173
40–49	339	17.7	97	242
50–59	759	39.6	169	590
>60	536	27.9	227	308
Not indicated	15	0.8	–	–
Total	1918	100	–	–

givers caring for patients who had been informed of the cancer diagnosis, approximately two-thirds reported that the patient was given the cancer diagnosis by the physician, one-fourth by the family, and the others by the physician and the family. Among 81.3% of patients who were not informed of the cancer diagnosis, 42.5% of caregivers reported that the patient might have suspected cancer; 25.1% reported that the patient was not aware; 12.6% reported no idea as to whether or not the patient was aware. According to the subclassification of the 11 prefectures, 22.6% of the 664 cancer patients who used to live in large urban centers with populations over one million were given the diagnosis; 17.8% of 818 patients in small urban cities; and 12.2% of 436 patients in rural districts. There was a slightly higher trend toward disclosure of the cancer diagnosis in urban centers compared to that in rural areas.

Family caregivers were also asked whom the physician informed of the patient's condition and about the therapeutic program apart from the cancer diagnosis. All family caregivers reported that the physician informed them of the condition and therapeutic program, although only

TABLE 3. Relationship to Cancer Patient of Responding Family Caregiver

Relationship	Number	Percent
Spouse	1527	79.6
Child	232	12.1
Parent	43	2.2
Sibling	41	2.1
Other extended family member	57	3.0
Unrelated person	14	0.7
Not indicated	4	0.2
Total	1918	100

TABLE 4. Informing Patients of a Cancer Diagnosis and Patients' Awareness of Having Cancer[a]

	Number	Percent
Patient informed of cancer diagnosis	349	18.2
By physician	237	12.4
By family	96	5.0
By physician and family	16	0.8
Patient not informed of cancer diagnosis	1560	81.3
Suspected cancer	815	42.5
Was not aware	481	25.1
No idea	241	12.6
Other	23	1.2
Not indicated	9	0.5
Total	1918	100

[a]The 1918 respondents were the bereaved family members who had cared for the cancer patients. Data modified and used by permission from Reference 3.

22.5% of the cancer patients were informed (TABLE 5). Of the family caregivers, 72.5% reported that they were informed by the physicians and could understand the information regarding the condition and therapeutic program; 13.8% were informed but failed to understand; and 5.8% could not understand due to insufficient physician's explanation (TABLE 6).

In Japan, all family members are informed by physicians of the cancer patient's diagnosis, condition, and therapeutic program, before the cancer patient is told the truth. Then, all family members except the patient discuss whether the cancer diagnosis should be disclosed, and the entire family makes a final decision about the truth-telling policy. This decision

TABLE 5. Persons Informed by the Physician of the Cancer Patient's Condition and Therapy Program[a]

	Number	Percent
Patient	431	22.5
Family member	1882	98.1
Other	226	11.2
No idea	4	0.2
Not indicated	4	0.2

[a]The 1918 respondents were the bereaved family members who had cared for the cancer patients. Data modified and used by permission from Reference 3.

TABLE 6. Family Caregivers' Understanding of the Information from the Physican Regarding the Cancer Patient's Condition and Therapy Program[a]

	Number	Percent
Informed	1852	96.6
Given full information and could understand well	1391	72.5
Given full explanation but could not understand	264	13.8
Could not understand due to insufficient explanation	111	5.8
Other	46	2.4
Not indicated	40	2.1
Not informed	60	3.1
Not indicated	6	0.3
Total 1918	100	

[a]The 1918 respondents were the bereaved family members who had cared for the cancer patients. Data modified and used by permission from Reference 3.

is usually respected by the physicians. Japanese physicians usually rely on the substitute consent of the family, while the family usually rely on the physician's decisions regarding medical treatment. Overall, approximately one-fifth of the patients were informed. Approximately half of the patients who were not informed of the diagnosis, however, suspected they had cancer. Usually, they never say the word "cancer" to family members or their physician. It is feared that disclosure of the truth would break communication and the relationship among the patients, families, and health-care providers and that the patients would ignore the families' and physicians' decisions to conceal the cancer diagnosis.

This most common practice in Japan may be related to Japanese cultural characteristics that guide how people relate to one another. The group will is respected rather than the individual, since the sense of belonging to the family is strong. Cancer patients who were not informed but suspected that they had cancer might agree with the families' and physicians' policy of not telling the truth, which families and physicians consider a protection of the patient from disappointment and confusion.

Physician Survey

To clarify the psychiatric issues involved in developing a relationship between cancer patient and physician in Japan, we surveyed physicians' and psychiatrists' attitudes and practices regarding cancer care for terminally ill patients.[4]

TABLE 7. Japanese Physicians' Practice with Regard to Informing a Terminally Ill Patient of the Diagnosis of Cancer[a]

	Number	Percent
Never tell the diagnosis of cancer	182	55.5
Seldom tell	57	17.5
Sometimes tell	44	13.3
Tell approximately half of the patients	12	3.5
Tell over half of the patients	34	10.2
Total	329	100

[a]Data show the responses of 329 physicians at 31 teaching hospitals, including national and local cancer center hospitals in Japan, at which it is the policy to inform cancer patients of their diagnosis. Terminally ill patients were defined as those whose prognoses were presumed to be less than six months. Data used by permission from Reference 4.

In August 1989, questionnaires were sent to each department of all cancer center hospitals and the departments of psychiatry at all teaching hospitals certified by the Japanese Ministry of Health and Welfare; 225 chief physicians at 31 teaching hospitals, including 21 national and local cancer center hospitals and 10 affiliated hospitals, and chief psychiatrists at 197 general teaching hospitals were included. Responses were obtained from 329 physicians from 130 departments and 156 psychiatrists from 87 departments. Since we had requested the chief of each department to make the appropriate number of copies for their staff, the precise response rate cannot be calculated. Questions surveyed the physician's opinion, attitude, and practice during the prior year (1988) concerning care for terminally ill cancer patients whose prognoses were less than six months. The average ages of the 329 physicians and 156 psychiatrists who participated were 40.7 and 41.0 years, respectively. The male-to-female ratios of the physicians and the psychiatrists were 321:8 and 143:13, respectively.

Physicians were asked whether they informed terminally ill patients of the cancer diagnosis. In response, 55.5% indicated they never gave their patients the cancer diagnosis; 17.5% seldom; 13.3% sometimes (TABLE 7). The majority of physicians usually concealed the diagnosis from the terminally ill cancer patient, although their families, of course, were fully informed of the diagnosis and prognosis.

Most physicians (69%) reported that they frequently or sometimes felt troubled by the patient's psychiatric problems during the management of terminally ill patients. One of the reasons that they felt troubled might have been related to the fact that they could not use the word *cancer* to communicate with terminally ill patients. Other words commonly substituted for cancer in Japan are those that imply an inflammation, unclean tissues, or precancerous change that will become malignant if left untreated. Therefore, most physicians conceal the truth while treating cancer and caring for terminally ill patients.

Both physicians and psychiatrists reported that the psychiatrists' participation in caring for terminally ill patients was essential or occasionally necessary. However, actual psychiatric consultation referrals were below what would be expected for psychiatrist's participation in cancer care. In the United States the majority of cancer patients referred for psychiatric consultation tend to have advanced disease and a poorer prognosis.[5,6] Only 6% of the physicians reported giving frequent referrals for psychiatric consultation; 29% sometimes gave referrals. Furthermore, over half of the physicians reported that the word "psychiatrist" was usually avoided in referring patients. Words commonly substituted for psychiatrist were counselor, insomnia specialist, or psychosomatic physician. Thus, there are great problems that interfere with appropriate psychiatric consultation referral for terminally ill cancer patients in Japan.

Some physicians pity patients referred for psychiatric consultation. In Japan, there is still great stigma and fear of both mental illness and terminal cancer. Most Japanese people feel that doing one's best is a matter of maintaining good relations with members of one's group. Tsuji,[7] a Japanese senior psychiatrist, indicated that Japanese people think that being a cancer patient will cause them to become isolated and to be treated as an outsider. It was further suggested that being referred for psychiatric consultation will also cause the patient to be ostracized and treated as an alien.

Usually, cancer patients who are not informed but suspect that they have cancer repress their emotions, sometimes denying their illness, and try to behave like a healthy person or an honor student in the oncology unit to avoid being treated as an outsider. Only patients expressing disturbed emotions or behaving abnormally toward nurses and physicians are referred for psychiatric consultation. Kashiwagi[8] reported from personal experience that the majority of psychiatric diagnoses in cancer patients involved adjustment disorders with anxious mood since most of the patients had repressed the fear of asking their physicians for their diagnoses. He found that "irritation," one of the prominent features of anxiety, was observed in patients who were not given a cancer diagnosis.

However, 3.5% and 10.2% of the 329 physicians responding reported that they gave half and over half of the terminally ill patients the cancer diagnosis, respectively (TABLE 7). In recent years, oncologists at the National Cancer Center Hospital in Tokyo have fully disclosed the cancer diagnosis to terminally ill patients. Although informed consent has been introduced in the trial of preclinical drugs, written consent for treatment including anticancer agents has just begun to be invariably practiced by all oncologists at National Cancer Center Hospitals in Tokyo in April 1995. It is suggested that these trends are influenced by the basic ethical principles of respect for persons, which was introduced from the United States. The trend toward full disclosure of the diagnosis has progressed extremely slowly in Japan, since almost none of the university hospitals have an oncology department or an educational program regarding clinical oncology and palliative medicine.

REPORT ON GUIDELINES FOR TELLING THE TRUTH TO TERMINALLY ILL PATIENTS AS PROPOSED BY THE JAPANESE MINISTRY OF HEALTH AND WELFARE

In 1989, after two years of discussion, the Japanese Ministry of Health and Welfare task force on care for terminally ill patients advocated informing patients of their limited life expectancy as well as the cancer diagnosis.[1] The task force recommended that telling the truth to such patients be considered a necessity. Health-care providers in Japan do not usually tell patients their cancer diagnosis, since they think that the disclosure of terminal cancer would result in a loss of hope and emotional distress for the patient. The guidelines for informing terminally ill patients of their limited life expectancy are as follows: (a) the possibility of a stable psychological state after the disclosure of the truth—e.g., patients' willingness to know the diagnosis, their inability to deal with family affairs and manage work, avoiding quarrels over inheritance, patient's ability to cope and adapt to emotional distress, good compliance with treatment; (b) patients can make decisions related to their care; (c) the prior existence of a good relationship among health-care providers, the patient, and family; (d) arrangement of a good support system to manage the physical and psychological aspects of the terminally ill patient after being told the truth. Other than these guidelines, there has been no legislation regarding the practice of truth-telling in Japan.

On April 25, 1995, the Japanese Supreme Court issued its first decision regarding whether the patient should be told the cancer diagnosis.[8,9] The case involved Kazuko Makino, a 50-year-old nurse. She visited a hospital in January 1983, and died of gallbladder cancer in December 1983 after having been told by her physician in March that she had gallstones. Her physician suspected cancer and recommended hospitalization for surgery. She promised to return to the hospital after a trip planned for the end of March, but she did not return to the hospital immediately, and by June the cancer had spread to her liver. Although recognizing that telling a patient of the cancer diagnosis during the initial consultation process would have an impact on the patients and their treatment, the Supreme Court judged that physicians are not irrational in concealing from patients that cancer is suspected. The Supreme Court also explained that physicians should be careful not to diminish the severity of illness when giving a substitute diagnosis. In this case, the Supreme Court found that the physicians were not negligent. This decision has met with heavy criticism from the oncology community. Although in 1983, the vast majority of patients in Japan were not told their cancer diagnosis and it was common practice for physicians to conceal cancer from them, this case has had a great impact on Japanese physicians.

CONCLUSION

In Japan, a diagnosis of cancer is still considered the equivalent of a death sentence. Although the truth-telling practice in cancer care in Japan is recommended by the Japanese Ministry of Health and Welfare,[2] it has been accepted extremely slowly by physicians caring for terminally ill cancer patients. Kashiwagi,[10] who was a member of the task force, reported that the truth-telling practice in cancer care has been hampered by several factors, including the strong emphasis on cure, the limited number of physicians who are interested in palliative care, the lack of educational programs regarding palliative medicine, the lack of profit in hospice care, and the death taboo.

Other factors may be related to Japanese cultural characteristics that guide how people relate to one another. The surveys discussed here[3,4] revealed that the family's decision is respected more than the individual's. Disclosure of the cancer diagnosis makes most Japanese people feel that being a terminally ill cancer patient will cause them to be isolated and treated as an outsider. The predominant ethical principles in Japan are based not only on respecting the patient's decisions but also on protecting the patient's fears of harming their relationship with their family.

However, some reports,[1,3,4,11] including two national surveys, revealed a small but clear trend toward the disclosure of cancer diagnoses in Japan. Japanese patients and their physicians are expected to begin to cooperate in fighting cancer as they do in Western countries.

REFERENCES

1. Suzuki, S., J. M. Kirschling & I. Inoue. 1993. Hospice care in Japan. Am. J. Hosp. Palliative Care **10:** 35–40.
2. Japanese Ministry of Health and Welfare and the Japan Medical Association. 1989. The Report for Terminal Care. Chuo Hoki Shuppan. Tokyo. (In Japanese.)
3. Japanese Ministry of Health and Welfare. 1993. FY 1992 report on the socioeconomic survey of vital statistics; malignant neoplasms. Statistics and Information Department, Minister's Secretariat, Japanese Ministry of Health and Welfare. Tokyo. (In Japanese.)
4. Yamawaki, S., Y. Uchitomi, H. Fukuda, S. Wakamiya & S. Okajima. 1990. A study of psychiatric consultations for terminally ill cancer patients. *In* Annual Report of the Cancer Research (1-30) of Japanese Ministry of Health

and Welfare FY 1989. K. Hiraga, Ed.: 117–124. Japanese Ministry of Health and Welfare. Tokyo. (In Japanese.)
5. MASSIE, M. J. & J. C. HOLLAND. 1987. Consultation and liaison issues in cancer patients. Psychiatr. Med. **5:** 343–359.
6. MCCARTNEY, C. F., P. CAHIL, D. B. LARSON *et al.* 1989. Effect of a psychiatric liaison program on consultation rates and on detection of minor psychiatric disorders in cancer patients. Am. J. Psychiatry **146:** 898–901.
7. TSUJI, S. 1990. Psychological aspects of dying patients. *In* Shi no Rinsho, Vol. 1. Japanese Society of Death and Dying, Eds.: 114–127. Ningen to Rekishi Sha. Tokyo. (In Japanese.)
8. ASAHI NEWSPAPER. 1995. The Japanese Supreme Court issued its first decision regarding whether the patient should be told the cancer diagnosis. ASAHI Newspaper. April 26, 1995. (In Japanese.)
9. DILLNER, L. 1995. Japanese Court rules against informing the patients. Ann. Oncol. **6:** 514–515.
10. KASHIWAGI, T. 1991. Palliative care in Japan. Palliative Med. **5:** 165–170.
11. HOLLAND, J. C., N. GEARY, A. MARCHINI *et al.* 1987. An international survey of physician attitude and practice in regard to revealing the diagnosis of cancer. Cancer Invest. **5:** 151–154.

APPENDIX

In May 1995, the fiscal year 1994 report on the socioeconomic survey of vital statistics conducted by the Statistics and Information Department, Minister's Secretariat, Japanese Ministry of Health and Welfare, revealed that 20.2% of the bereaved family caregivers reported that the patient was informed of the cancer diagnosis, while 79.8 % were not.

Communication with Cancer Patients

Experiences in Pakistan

IMTIAZ A. MALIK[a] AND ASMA FOZIA QURESHI[b,c]

[a]*Department of Medical Oncology*
National Cancer Institute
Clifton
Karachi, Pakistan

[b]*Department of Community Health Sciences*
The Aga Khan University
Karachi, Pakistan

INTRODUCTION

Pakistan is a southern Asian country situated to the northeast of the Indian subcontinent. With a population of 128 million, it is the seventh most populous country in the world. Administratively, there are four provinces—Punjab, Sindh, North West Frontier Province (NWFP,) and Balochistan—as well as the federally controlled Tribal and Northern Areas and the State of Azad Jammu and Kashmir.[1] The population of Pakistan has increased from 32.5 million in 1947 to 128 million in 1993, with 66% of the people living in rural areas. The population is unevenly distributed among the provinces. Punjab is the most densely populated province, with about 26% of the total land area and more than half (56%) of the total population. Balochistan, on the other hand, is the largest province in area (44% of the total land area), with only 5% of the population. Sindh comprises 18% of the land area and 32% of the total population. Karachi is the largest city in the country; its population is estimated to be over 10 million.

[c]Address for correspondence: Dr. Asma Fozia Qureshi, Professor, Department of Community Health Sciences, The Aga Khan University, Stadium Road, P.O. Box 3500, Karachi 74800, Pakistan. Telephone: (92) 21 493-0051. Fax: (92) 21 493-4294. e-mail: chsaku@biruni.erum.com.pk (AF Qureshi).

PEOPLE, CULTURE, RELIGION, AND LANGUAGE

Though the population of Pakistan is predominantly Muslim (96.7%), important religious minorities include Christians, Hindus, Ahmadis, Zoroastrians, Sikhs, and Buddhists. There are eight main languages listed in the census, with several dialects.[2] The lingua franca and medium of education in many schools is Urdu, but English continues to be used for education particularly in the professional colleges. Both are official languages; however, Urdu is recognized as the national language.

Pakistan historically attracted migrants from many nations in the northwest and the northeast. These included Dravidians, Aryans, Greeks, Turks, Persians, Afghans, Arabs, and Moguls. The dominant racial type in Pakistan is Indo-Aryan. There is a rich social and cultural diversity among its people. There are wide variations in customs, traditions, code of conduct, manners, dress, food habits, and cooking methods. This is not surprising, as geographic and climatic conditions vary from one of the highest mountain ranges in the world to deserts and extensive coastal areas.

Overall literacy is low, but there are wide variations from highly literate urban clusters (90% or more) to the appalling, low rates among rural women (4%).[1] Economically, Pakistan ranks 132nd on the UNDP Human Development Index.[3] A third of the population lives below the poverty line. There is a great need for human and social development, especially in the areas of health, education, housing, the environment, and in rural-urban and female-male inequalities.

HEALTH SERVICES AND PATTERNS OF HELP SEEKING

The allocation to the national health budget is 0.70% of the GNP, and only 55% of the population has access to health services.[4] The public sector provides approximately 20% of the health services; the great majority of people use the private sector, where health-care providers include chemists, formally trained allopathic doctors, paramedical health workers, and traditional practitioners of various systems of medicine—homeopaths, *Hakims* (*Unani* or Greek traditional healers), and holy men.

Health-seeking behavior is determined largely by perceptions of illness, cost, quality of care, and access to health facilities. In traditional societies such as Pakistan, people often seek help for illness from diverse sources. Illness management is initially in the home and is controlled by family members. The more serious an illness, the more likely is the use of multiple sources of health care and frantic switching from provider to provider. Generally, cultural patterns govern a respectful attitude towards knowledgeable persons and seniors. Questioning is often considered a threat to authority and is discouraged. While physicians are frequently seen as omnipotent, hospitals are often associated with death and dying.

INCIDENCE OF CANCER AND AVAILABILITY OF ONCOLOGICAL SERVICES

At present there is no population-based tumor registry in Pakistan. Although recently some work was started in Karachi, most of the previously available data are based upon institutional records. According to World Health Organization estimates, it is expected that Pakistan would have 150 thousand new cancer cases per year.[5] However, the total number of patients registered at recognized cancer-care facilities is estimated to be between 25 to 30 thousand. This suggests that a large number of cancer patients never reach the cancer-care facilities. There are approximately 20 facilities dedicated to the care of cancer patients. Most of the physicians providing cancer care are radiotherapists. There are only six trained medical oncologists for adults and two pediatric hematologist/oncologists in the whole country. There are significant variations in types of cancers observed in Pakistan as compared to Western countries. In men squamous cell carcinoma of the head and neck and lymphomas are relatively more common. In women cervical cancer is less common as compared to other developing countries; however, gallbladder and ovarian carcinomas are relatively more common. Although in certain cases these variations may be attributable to health habits (e.g., tobacco chewing), for most cases the underlying causes remain unknown.[6,7]

SPECIAL ISSUES RELATED TO CANCER

Perceptions and Awareness of Cancer and Problems with Physician-Patient Communication

There is a general lack of awareness about cancer. It is still considered as taboo and invariably fatal. Lack of awareness among patients is illustrated by a recent study that was conducted on patients with breast cancer. In this study, 117 consecutive patients presenting in 1994 with histologically confirmed breast cancer were interviewed by the same physician. The breast lump had been accidently discovered by 94% of the patients. None of the women carried out regular self-examination of their breasts. Five percent of the lumps were discovered by the physicians, and only 1% were found by screening mammography. The average size of the lump at the time of diagnosis was 3.65 ± 2.26 cm with a range of 1 to 10 cm. There was a long delay (average 37.1 months) between initial awareness of the lump and its recognition as a health hazard. Patients preferred to consider the lump as a minor problem caused by trauma, clotting of milk, or infection. There was a further average delay of 9.6 months between visit to the doctor and confirmation of the final diagnosis. The common reasons for this delay were patient refusal of the diagnostic procedure (51.2%), use of unconventional methods of therapy (37.6%), and inappropriate therapy by general practitioners (11.2%).

Additionally, cancer is perceived as a fatal disease, and the diagnosis is often hidden from the patient by the family members. The vast majority of patients are unaware of their diagnosis at the time of presentation to the oncologist. In almost all cases, the family requests that the patient not be informed of the diagnosis. They feel that it will be psychologically detrimental to the patient and will worsen the quality of life. They also fear that awareness of the diagnosis is likely to cause or hasten death.

Physicians have generally adopted the attitude of not discussing the disease or its treatment with the patient. They give several reasons to justify this approach. These include the presence of extensive family support, strong family ties, fear of introducing misconceptions, a general sense of helplessness and despair while dealing with cancer, and ill effects of therapy. This situation differs markedly from that in Western countries, where patients are always told of the diagnosis and the disease and its treatment are discussed in detail. The authors have generally taken a more individualized approach. If the patient is literate, desires to know the diagnosis and its treatment, and would gain from this knowledge, we provide full information to the patient. It is our observation that this improves compliance with therapy. On the other hand, if discussion of the disease and its therapy is likely to result in lack of compliance, abandonment of therapy, or utilization of unconventional treatments, only minimal and necessary information is provided. In these cases, instead of using the word "cancer," relatively vague terms such as "tumor," "growth," "lump," or "germs" are often used in patient communication. If the overall objective of therapy is the physical and psychological well-being of the patient, sometimes this approach helps to achieve treatment objectives.

Use of Unconventional Methods of Care

Unconventional, alternative, or unorthodox therapies are difficult to define. However, from a sociological standpoint, unconventional therapy refers to medical practices that are not in conformity with the standards of the medical community.[8,9] In a traditional society like Pakistan, several types of therapies are in common use. These include homeopathy, which adheres to a system of medical care introduced in Germany by Dr.

Hannemann in the late 1700s. In this method, tiny quantities of substances are administered on the principle that "like is cured by like."[10] Other methods in common use include *Hikmat,* in which practitioners called *Hakims* use therapy based on the humoral theory of Hippocrates. It is also referred to as *Unani* (Greek) medicine. In Pakistan, *Hakims* rely mainly on herbs for treatment. A third system of therapy, practiced by holy men or *Pirs,* provides spiritual therapy either personally or through a designee; patients visit their tombs for the purpose of therapy. People also believe that cancer can be caused by spirits (*Jinns*) who cast their shadow or *saya* on the patient. They strongly believe that in this situation management should be spiritual rather than biomedical. They often visit *Pirs* for this purpose, who either provide an amulet (*taviz*) or read holy verses and blow the words towards the patient, a procedure called *dam.*

We carried out a study of the prevalence of unconventional methods of treatment in cancer patients (TABLE 1). One hundred fifty-eight cancer patients visiting the oncology clinic were interviewed by the same physician. The mean age of the patients was 45.8 ± 16.7 years. There were 66

TABLE 1. Use of Unconventional Methods of Treatment by Cancer Patients

Clinical Characteristics	Number (n = 158)
Age in years ± SD	45.8 ± 16.7
Sex	
Male	66
Female	92
Marital status	
Single	27
Married	124
Widow/divorcee	7
Educational status	
Illiterate	35
Primary/high school	67
College	56
Number of persons in household ± SD	7.7 ± 5.3
Awareness about cancer	
Yes	121
No	37
Type of unconventional methods used (%)[a]	
Homeopathy	60.5
Hikmat (herbs)	31
Spiritual (pirs, tombs)	40
Relaxation/prayers	10.5
Physical abuse (torture)	5

[a]Several patients used more than one type of unconventional method.

males and 92 females. Most of the females were housewives. The average number of people in the household was 7.7. Overall 48% of the patients had used some kind of unconventional method of therapy before visiting the physician—most of them homeopathy or *Hikmat.* In this study, we also established that almost 70% of the patients were aware of their diagnosis. The use of unconventional methods of therapy did not correlate with the socioeconomic or educational status of the patients. This is unlike the situation in Western countries, where unconventional methods are more frequently utilized by better-educated patients belonging to the higher socioeconomic groups.[8,9] In general, frequency of use of unconventional therapy in our patients correlated with family size. This probably reflects the variability of opinions and suggestions expressed by different family members in large households. The average length of time spent receiving these unconventional therapies in our study was 6.6 months. This may be one of the major factors responsible for late presentation and poor outcome of cancer patients in developing countries.

Perceptions about Chemotherapy

In Pakistan, influenced by the Greek and the Ayurvedic systems, people commonly consider most Western allopathic medicines "hot" (*garam*) and consider most traditional herbs "cold" (*thanda*). Cancer chemotherapy is considered *garam.* Patients believe that cytotoxic drugs will have severe side-effects and may, indeed, be intolerable. We recently carried out a study of 100 cancer patients regarding their perceptions about chemotherapy before and during treatment (TABLE 2). The mean age of the patients was 43 years; the majority were females. Thirty-four percent of the patients were college graduates, and the majority belonged to the middle class. Most patients (84%) were aware of the diagnosis of cancer. Others thought they were receiving treatment for nonmalignant conditions such as infection, gallstones, fracture, etc. Only 4% of the patients receiving chemotherapy were concomitantly using unconventional methods of therapy. Thirty-eight percent of the patients had some idea about chemotherapy before the treatment was started. In terms of frequency, the most dreaded side effects were alopecia, vomiting, nausea, anxiety, and economic burden. When these patients were interviewed while on therapy or immediately afterwards, there was only a slight change in their perception of side effects (TABLE 3). Most interestingly, 94% of the patients said that if needed they would take therapy again, and almost all felt that when indicated they would recommend chemotherapy to others. This suggests that at least in cancer patients on chemotherapy, there is increasing awareness about the importance and benefit of chemotherapy.

TABLE 2. Cancer Patients Participating in Study of Perceptions of Chemotherapy

Clinical Characteristics	Number (n = 100)
Age in years (range)	43 (10–84)
Sex	
Male	22
Female	78
Educational status	
Illiterate	16
Primary school	12
High school	24
College graduate	34
Professional school	14
Socioeconomic group	
High	18
Middle	64
Low	18
Marital status	
Single	72
Married	26
Widow/divorcee	2
Average number of persons in household (range)	7 (1–14)
Level of support at home	
Good	64
Fair	20
Poor	16
Type of underlying cancer	
Breast	38
Lymphoma	16
Ovarian	8
Lung	4
Miscellaneous	34
Stage of cancer	
I	4
II	24
III	52
IV	20
Awareness about cancer	
Yes	84
No	14

Ethical Issues in Cancer Therapy and Research

In Pakistan, there is no mechanism to monitor and maintain the quality of clinical care. State regulatory authorities are ineffective, and no

TABLE 3. Perceptions and Experiences Regarding Side Effects of Chemotherapy in Cancer Patients: The Most Dreadful Side Effects in Order of Frequency

Number	Before Chemotherapy	During and After Chemotherapy
1	Alopecia	Vomiting
2	Vomiting	Nausea
3	Nausea	Alopecia
4	Anxiety	Weakness
5	Economic burden	Anxiety
6	Chills/fever	Mood changes
7	Pain	Mouth soreness
8	Problems with social interaction	Anorexia
9	Anorexia	Economic burden
10	Weight loss	Chills/fever

other pressure groups exist to question the type of care provided. Litigation is almost nonexistent. Similarly, ethical issues in clinical care and research are practically never addressed. Most health-care institutions do not have Human Subjects Protection Committees and informed consent for clinical care and research is rare.

There are several physician- and patient-related factors that significantly affect delivery of care to cancer patients. Physician-related factors include the small number of trained specialists, lack of adequate physician training facilities, absence of integrated cancer care facilities, and a general attitude of despair and hopelessness. Even well-trained physicians do not interact with patients very well. This is due partly to the high patient load. However, physicians often have a preconception that patients will misinterpret the information they provide and that it is better to withhold it. All these factors result in lack of communication between patients and physicians, and the truth is often hidden from patients.

It is also important to emphasize that patient-related problems are often cultural and related predominantly to large, overprotective families. Unlike the situation in the West, where patients are by themselves, families in Pakistan feel that a large number of other people are available who can cushion the patient from psychological distress; they take it as a responsibility on themselves to "protect" the patient as much as possible. This often involves hiding the truth. In case of serious illness, decisions about therapy are frequently made collectively by the family. Patients also tend not to confront the problem head-on. They hide their health problem for as long as possible until it becomes visibly apparent. The reasons for these attitudes are many, including lack of understanding, fear of surgery and chemotherapy, lack of trust in the medical system, and a strong desire on part of the patient not to add another burden to the family. Although, in general, there are gender differences in access to medical care, in case of women—particularly in relation to breast and gynecologic problems—the availability of a very limited number of appropriately trained female doctors can further compound the problem.

In conclusion, it is quite apparent that there is increasing awareness about cancer and its treatment. Although a large number of patients still remain unaware of their underlying diagnosis, this usually does not interfere with their care. Similarly, awareness about side effects of chemotherapy has improved significantly. Continuing efforts at public education and physician training will improve the situation even further. Patients are increasingly inquisitive about their disease and its treatment. However, a lot remains to be done to meet Western standards.

ACKNOWLEDGMENTS

The authors are grateful to Mr. Sulaiman Gilani for his help in preparation of this manuscript.

REFERENCES

1. National Institute of Population Studies. 1992. Pakistan Demographic and Health Survey 1990/1991. National Institute of Population Studies. Islamabad. IRD/Macro International, Inc. Columbia, MD.
2. Population Census Organization. 1984. 1981 Census Report of Pakistan. Population Census Organization, Statistics Division, Government of Pakistan. Islamabad.
3. United Nations Development Programme (UNDP). 1994. Human Development Report. Oxford University Press. New York, NY.
4. United Nations Children's Fund (UNICEF). 1995. The State of the World's Children. Oxford University Press. Oxford.
5. Parkin, D. M., Ed. 1986. Cancer Occurrence in Developing Countries. International Agency for Research on Cancer. Lyon.
6. Jafarey, N. A. & S. H. M. Zaidi. 1987. Cancer in Pakistan. J. Pak. Med. Assoc. **37:** 70–72.
7. Ahmed, M., A. H. Khan & A. Mansoor. 1991. The pattern of malignant tumours in Northern Pakistan. J. Pak. Med. Assoc. **41:** 270–273.
8. Eisenberg, D. M., R. C. Kessler, C. Foster, F. E. Norlock, D. R. Calkins & T. L. Delbanco. 1993. Unconventional medicine in the United States. N. Eng. J. Med. **328**(4): 246–283.
9. Lerner, I. J. & B. J. Kennedy. 1992. The prevalence of questionable methods of cancer treatment in the United States. Ca. Cancer J. Clin. **43**(3): 181–191.
10. Mull, J. D. & D. S. Mull. 1988. Mothers' concepts of childhood diarrhea in rural Pakistan: What ORT Program planners should know. Soc. Sci. Med. **27**(1): 53–67

Communicating with Cancer Patients in Saudi Arabia

DEREK YOUNGE,[a,b] PAUL MOREAU,[b] ADNAN EZZAT,[c] AND ALAN GRAY[c]

[b]*Department of Orthopedics*
[c]*Department of Oncology*
King Faisal Specialist Hospital and Research Centre
Riyadh 11211, Saudi Arabia

INTRODUCTION

Saudi Arabia has a population of approximately 17 million people, 13 million Saudi Nationals and 4 million expatriates. The average family has 7 children, and one half of the population is under the age of 16. The population has the highest growth rate of any country in the world, with the Saudi population increasing at 3.5% per year. The country's oil-based economy has transformed it from a mainly nomadic to a predominantly urban society with a sophisticated infrastructure, all within the period of 20–30 years.

Consistent with the rapid improvements in nutrition, sanitation, housing, and effective vaccination programs, the population is undergoing an epidemiologic transition in which the morbidity and mortality patterns are changing from those associated with infectious diseases and nutritional deficiencies to the "age of degenerative and man-made diseases" such as cancer, and heart and cerebrovascular disease. It can be reasonably predicted that this transition, combined with the prolongation of life expectancy, will lead to an absolute increase in the number of cancer cases occurring in the Kingdom, with an increasing proportion occurring in older people. In Kuwait and Bahrain, where population-based statistics on cancer are available, cancer is already the third commonest cause of death.[1] A population-based cancer registry was begun in 1994, but the true incidence of cancer in Saudi Arabia is not yet known.

[a]Address for correspondence: Derek Younge, M.D., Department of Orthopedic Surgery (MBC 77), King Faisal Specialist Hospital and Research Centre, P.O. Box 3354, Riyadh 11211, Saudi Arabia.

HOW THE PUBLIC PERCEIVES CANCER

The word for tumor in Arabic is *waram*, which has the same meaning as tumor formerly did in English—i.e. "swelling". This is then qualified as to whether it is benign or malignant. Most patients seem to assume that a tumor is benign. In some areas of the country there is a local custom of using the terms "male" or "female" to describe whether the tumor is malignant or not. The word for cancer in Arabic is *saratan*, which also means crab, giving the impression of a monster with many arms that can devour. It is not surprising, therefore, to find that the public has a similar fear of the diagnosis of cancer as in the West, where it is the most feared of all illnesses.

Bedikian and Saleh[2] interviewed 100 Saudi patients with cancer and reported that 93% had an adverse reaction to the diagnosis, with a median duration of symptoms for 3–5 months. None received professional assistance for these problems, and the authors recommended that psychosocial support be available to patients as part of their entire management. Bedikian,[3] in a further study, interviewed 250 healthy Saudis on their attitudes and knowledge of cancer, revealing a considerable degree of fear and anxiety about this disease. Similarly, Ibrahim *et al.*[4] interviewed 600 adults on their knowledge and attitudes towards cancer and confirmed the high level of fear and misperceptions about the disease. Both groups of authors called for more comprehensive health education and awareness of cancer as a treatable disease.

RELATIONSHIP BETWEEN THE DOCTOR AND THE PATIENT

The relationship between the doctor and the patient in Saudi Arabia is different from that in Western countries. In the West, health care systems are based on the individual, and patients are treated as autonomous agents capable of receiving information on which they make decisions about their own future.

It is no longer considered ethical in Western countries to withhold vital information from the patient, and informed consent is a subject of wide public debate. Patients are seen as health care consumers with rights to information, interaction with health professionals, and participation in decision making regarding their health. Informed consent is considered an essential right for each individual, and only by attempting to understand the nature of their illness, its implication for their future, and the advantages and disadvantages of treatment options can patients fully participate in their treatment and thereby regain some control over their destiny when faced with a potentially fatal illness.

In contrast, in Saudi Arabia, the predominant principle is one of "beneficence," where the patient is viewed as one member of the larger family and the family is responsible for the patient. The consent for the patient's treatment is usually a substitute consent given by the family, whose purpose is to avoid disturbing the patient emotionally. In this way, the family feels that they are protecting the patient from harm by making efforts to secure his or her well-being and ensure that the patient is treated in an ethical manner (beneficence). If patients are told the truth, then they will need to understand the situation and act accordingly, but in Saudi Arabia it is assumed by many that an ill person will not adapt to the true situation of a serious illness, resulting in a loss of hope that may lead to an earlier death than may otherwise occur. This policy of beneficence also relies on health professionals as authority figures who can be trusted to do what is best for the patient, as seen from the point of view of the family.

This concept of denying the patient information on his/her illness is shared by other countries,[5] and a similar attitude prevailed in Western countries until only 20 years ago. The introduction of modern technology, however, and particularly the ability to effectively treat cancer have also changed the relationship between patient and doctor. Such technology has a "cost" to the patient in terms of toxicity and complications as well as major benefits. Increasingly, doctors in this country dealing with cancer or other major illnesses insist that the patient be fully informed and give their consent before starting a treatment that can have side effects. Already many cancer patients in this country are well informed about their illness and have some idea of their prognosis, and this trend is steadily increasing.

Serious problems can arise when the patient is denied knowledge of his or her disease when the treatment carries significant morbidity. The side effects or complications of chemotherapy or radiotherapy can be significant, but the patient could theoretically be led to accept these risks without necessarily being told that he has cancer.

Two of the authors are expatriate Westerners involved in the surgical treatment of sarcomas, usually by means of limb-salvage surgery. When there is a question of major surgery, lack of informed consent can be a real dilemma. The complication rate for limb-salvage surgery approaches 50%, and in almost every case a joint is lost, with either an arthrodesis or a total joint prosthesis being the result. Compared to amputation, limb-salvage surgery may seem marvelous to the operating surgeon, but the result compared to a normal limb resembles nothing less than mutilation to the patient. This "mutilation" and all its associated morbidity can be quite acceptable to a patient facing death or amputation as an alternative, but to a patient who does not know or at least suspect that he/she has a very serious cancer, this can be devastating.

We still have some situations where children and even adults are not informed of the serious nature of their tumor by their family and may be told that a planned limb-sparing operation or even an amputation is a minor procedure. Consequently, they have great difficulty accepting any morbidity as a result of this surgery, or in trusting the physician again. The family often asks that we not tell the patient that an operation will be necessary, in order that they may tell the patient gradually, and thereby "soften the blow." Unfortunately, this may mean that they will not be told at all. As a result, we are very reluctant to admit a patient to hospital unless we know they have been told about their cancer and have consented to surgery in advance. This can be extremely difficult for the family to do, even though we routinely use the services of Saudi workers to help in this task. On the other hand, the practice in the adult medical oncology clinics has shown a marked improvement of disclosure of diagnosis over the past 5–6 years. This has resulted in a decrease in the rate of "lost to follow-up" patients from the tumor registry by about 40%.[6]

The aims of a good health service should be "to provide treatment or restore patients to as near a normal quality of life as possible under the circumstances" or, more simply, "to maximize the patient's well-being."[7] The patient's perception of this is that they will: (a) be restored to normal health; (b) have their symptoms relieved; and, if neither (a) nor (b) is possible, (c) have their suffering relieved. It is the duty of health professionals to explain not only the benefits but also the limits of treatment in ways the patient can understand and accept. It may take several sessions to explain this to a patient, and it may eventually result in both the patient and the doctor silently agreeing to avoid the issues. Patients use denial when the truth is too painful to bear. It is always important to respect such resistance—it is there for a purpose.[8]

Doctors may also "collude" with the relatives to "protect" the patient from the knowledge of cancer. There may be several reasons why doctors avoid telling their patients: (a) the doctor may not know what to say or how to say it when dealing with such a problem; (b) the doctor may wish to avoid the difficulties of having to cope with a patient who is upset and disturbed as a result of this information; (c) the doctor may consider dying patients a personal "failure"; (d) the doctor may feel that patients simply will not cope; (e) it takes too much time and patience out of a busy work schedule.[8] Health professionals should be aware of these weaknesses and their own biases. Surveys in the Western world consistently show that patients want to know,[9] and there is no evidence that Saudi patients feel any differently.

PROFESSIONAL COMMUNICATION

The emphasis for cancer patients in Saudi Arabia is on "curative treatment," and it is not always recognized by physicians that the patient with advanced disease is sometimes more appropriately treated with palliative care. While there is now ample evidence that patients cope better with a serious illness if they have been informed,[10] many patients remain in ignorance of the extent and prognosis of their disease. Saudi patients continue to travel overseas at considerable cost with unrealistic expectations, often receiving treatment that may be neither necessary nor appropriate. Local physicians are expected to do follow-up care, of course, as well as they can.

It is important that physicians be taught that they must bear some responsibility for the quality of their patients' deaths also.[11] In advanced cancer, 80% of patients will suffer pain, and in 60% this will be severe and require strong analgesics of the morphine type.[12] There is a general lack of knowledge of pain relief in the Kingdom, and in many hospitals adequate outpatient narcotic analgesics, particularly morphine, are simply not available.[13] There is an unreasonable fear of morphine among patients and their families, despite the fact that studies have convincingly shown that addiction is never a problem in a terminal illness.

CULTURAL ASPECTS

Foreign health professionals are constantly impressed by the strength of the family in the Kingdom. The family unit is the structural foundation of Saudi society. One has the impression that patients here cope better with terminal illness while living at home than do patients in other parts of the world. This is because of the close family involvement and their strong Islamic faith, which allows them to accept death as an expression of God's will. It is a religious duty to provide for parents and children in need in order to make their lives as comfortable as possible. Most major decisions in the Saudi family are taken by or at least involve the senior male member of the family.

An example of the problems of looking after a chronic illness in Saudi Arabia is a study by Watts,[14] which describes how 22% of new patients to a pediatric orthopedic clinic had cutaneous cautery (*al-kawi*), which is not considered an effective form of treatment and can have complications. He found no association between cautery use and the parents' educational levels. Watts makes the point that the majority of patients receiving cautery did so after they had already been seen in modern medical facilities. He reports that this is in keeping with the old Arabic belief that cautery is reserved as a last resort, and he suggests that it reflects patients' disappointment with modern medical care. He suggests that this is due to the overly high expectation of what is possible; and perhaps if doctors spent more time explaining to patients or their relatives the nature of the disease and the appropriate expectations, the patients' never-ending search for cures for many of the chronic diseases could be decreased.

For the foreseeable future, care will be provided by foreign nurses and, for some time, partly by foreign doctors, who must be educated in the social and cultural life of the Kingdom. Their task, however, is aided by the ritual of hospitality, which is such an important part of Saudi life.

DILEMMAS AND MISCONCEPTIONS ABOUT PALLIATIVE CARE

There is an impression that palliative care of a terminal illness is confused with euthanasia.[15] The two are opposites. Palliative care is the moral and ethical alternative to euthanasia. The motive for euthanasia is life without hope. This society sets great store on hope. Good palliative care, by relieving the patient's symptoms and providing support and knowledge, restores the hope that tomorrow may be more comfortable than today.

Another misunderstanding is that using morphine medically can be a form of euthanasia by shortening life. In an Islamic society there are severe punishments for people using addictive drugs, especially alcohol or narcotics. The patient is often reluctant to use morphine, but written information on its benefits, provided to the patient and his relatives, has made this a more accepted treatment option.

Relatives often ask for extreme treatment procedures as the patient is dying. The question of "withholding treatment" in a terminal illness has become a moral dilemma for Islamic authorities.[15] Some Islamic scholars believe that everything possible should be done to keep the patient alive, while others disagree and state that the use of unnecessary and ineffective measures is not appropriate when the patient is clearly going to die. At King Faisal Specialist Hospital and Research Centre, the hospital has a protocol of "No Code" similar to the "Do Not Resuscitate" order in the West. When such patients die, the emergency resuscitation team is not called. Death is allowed to occur with dignity. However, most other hospitals in the Kingdom do not have a similar protocol for managing terminal illness. Part of the art of medicine is to decide when life sustainment is futile and when to allow death to occur without further impediment.[11] Many doctors in Saudi Arabia are still unwilling to exercise this judgment of "appropriate" care.

SUMMARY

The following factors are relevant to the communication problems that exist in this country:

1. *Cultural aspects:* The impression is that patients here cope better with terminal illness at home than do patients elsewhere. The extended family, with its strong ties, and the strong Islamic faith that encourages its members to provide for parents and children in case of need mean that

any input by health professionals is magnified by the family in the care of the patient. At first, it was uncertain if foreign health professionals would be accepted into Saudi homes (which are intensely private and protected for the family) for the purpose of caring for patients. This has proved unfounded. Hospitality is a very important part of Saudi society; nurses and doctors are welcomed and respected. Much of this success is due to the use of Saudi men as drivers and translators. These people provide 24-hour service, act as social workers assessing the needs of the family, and are the link between the patient and family, the nurse, and the doctor.

2. *"Cure" or "palliation":* The emphasis for cancer patients in Saudi Arabia is still on "curative treatment," even after any realistic hope of a cure is gone. The problem this causes is compounded by many patients being excluded from the decision-making process. Decisions made by the family may not always reflect the patient's wishes. Greater communication is needed to guide treatment decisions.

3. *Truth-telling:* Denying information of the patient's illness is probably more a historical than a cultural phenomenon. Similar attitudes prevailed until very recently in practically all other countries. In this very conservative country, people are committed to preserving Islamic culture in the face of Western technology. As medicine continues to demonstrate its effectiveness as well as its limitations, people will come to realize that the right of patients to know and understand their illness allows them to cope much better, and is compatible with the responsibility of the family to care for them.

4. *Work force:* The government employs 14,500 doctors, but only 12% are Saudi nationals. Nearly all the 33,000 nursing work force are expatriates. There is a constant turnover of expatriate staff. The commitment to continuing care with proper communication that is required for the whole of medicine is likely to be fully realized only when the majority of the workforce are Saudi nationals.

5. *Primary, secondary, and tertiary care services:* The Kingdom is well served by a system of 174 public hospitals and numerous private clinics. However, for a patient with a chronic or terminal illness, continuing care, even in the community, tends to be provided by the hospital service; whereas the polyclinics and health centers seem to provide mainly crisis management. The aim should be to develop community care for chronic illness as part of the primary health care system.

The impact of Western medicine on Saudi society has been dramatic and sudden, as evidenced by the high growth rate of the population. There is now widespread interest in matching the culture to the technology. Much of the drive to change the attitudes of both patients and health professionals comes from young Western-trained Saudi doctors, who are in the best position to merge the strengths of both cultures in this sensitive area.

REFERENCES

1. WORLD HEALTH ORGANIZATION. 1995. Cancer Control in the Eastern Mediterranean Region. EMRO Technical Publications, Series 20. WHO Regional Office. Alexandria.
2. BEDIKIAN, A. Y. & V. SALEH. 1985. An evaluation of the need for psychosocial counselling for Saudi cancer patients. King Faisal Specialist Hosp. Med. J. **5:** 91–98.
3. BEDIKIAN, A. Y. & S. E. THOMPSON. 1985. Saudi community attitudes towards cancer. Ann. Saudi Med. **5:** 161–167.
4. IBRAHIM, E. M., F. A. AL-MUHANNA & I. SAIED *et al.* 1991. Public knowledge: Misperceptions and attitudes about cancer in Saudi Arabia. Ann. Saudi Med. **11:** 518–523.
5. SUZUKI, S, J. M. KIRSCHING & I. INOUE. 1993. Hospice Care in Japan. Am. J. Hospice Palliative Care July/August 1993: 35–40.
6. DEPARTMENT OF ONCOLOGY, KING FAISAL SPECIALIST HOSPITAL AND RESEARCH CENTRE. 1993. The 1993 Annual Report of the Tumor Registry. King Faisal Specialist Hospital and Research Centre. Riyadh.
7. The American President's Commission for the Study of Ethical Problems in Medicine and Biomedical and Behavioral Research. 1983. Washington, DC.
8. BUCKMAN, R. 1988. I Don't Know What to Say—How To Help and Support Someone Who Is Dying. MacMillan. London.
9. SUTHERLAND, H. J., H. A. LLEWELLYN-THOMAS, G. A. LOCKWOOD, T. L. TRICHLER & J. E. TILL. 1989. Cancer patients: Their desire for information and participation in treatment decisions. J. R. Soc. Med. **82:** 260–263.
10. MANUEL, G. M., S. ROTH, F. J. KEEFE *et al.* 1987. Coping with cancer. J. Hum. Stress **13**(4): 149–158.
11. CALLAHAN, D. 1994. Ethics and the medical ambivalence towards death. Humane Med. **10:** 172–183.
12. GRAY, A. J., A. EZZAT & S. VOLKER. 1995. Developing palliative care services for terminally ill patients in Saudi Arabia. Ann. Saudi Med. **15**(4): 370–377.
13. DOYLE, D. 1991. The Provision of Palliative Care. An Internal Report by the Medical Director, St. Columbia's Hospice, Edinburgh, to the Administration, King Faisal Specialist Hospital and Research Centre, Riyadh.
14. WATTS, H. G. 1989. Cutaneous cautery (Al-Kawi): A study in a pediatric outpatient clinic in Central Saudi Arabia. Ann. Saudi Med. **9:** 475–478.
15. The Seventh Conference of the Islamic Fiqh Academy. Arab News. May 16, 1992.

Communication with Cancer Patients in Culturally Diverse Societies

PHYLLIS N. BUTOW,[a,b] MARTIN H. N. TATTERSALL,[c] AND DAVID GOLDSTEIN[d]

[b]*Medical Psychology Unit*
Department of Medicine
University of Sydney
Sydney, Australia

[c]*Department of Cancer Medicine*
University of Sydney
Sydney, Australia

[d]*Department of Medical Oncology*
Prince of Wales Hospital
Sydney, Australia

INTRODUCTION

The importance of doctor-patient communication in the practice of cancer medicine is now well recognized, and a large number of relevant articles are published each year. In a recent Medline search of the period January to December 1994 using the key words "neoplasms and psychology," communication was the third most common topic, representing 27% of the 610 articles retrieved. However, very few of these articles address the particularly complex issues raised by the management of cancer patients within a multicultural society. This chapter attempts to combine a general review of communication in cancer medicine, with a consideration of these multicultural issues.

COMMUNICATION: IS IT IMPORTANT?

There is a universal fear of cancer that results from its association with images of extreme debility and pain and the fear of death. These fears have been well documented in Western and several other cultures.[1-3] With

[a]Address for correspondence: Dr. Phyllis Butow, Medical Psychology Unit, Department of Medicine, University of Sydney, Sydney, NSW, 2006, Australia.

the advent of aggressive cancer therapies, often accompanied by debilitating physical and psychosocial side effects, the cost-benefit ratio of treatment to outcome has become harder to evaluate, especially in those patients where the goal of treatment is palliation and/or prolongation of life. Many physicians now seek to maintain optimum quality of life (QOL) by incurring a minimum of side effects without depriving the patient of the potential palliative and curative effects of treatment.[4] In these scenarios, both doctor and patient need to weigh up complex issues of cost and benefit. Successful treatment of patients with malignancy either to improve survival, maximize quality of life, or reduce psychological distress, requires effective communication between the doctor and the affected individual.

Cancer patients place effective doctor communication high on their list of priorities for care. In an Australian study assessing the perceptions of 232 ambulatory cancer patients, doctor-patient communication dominated the top 10 aspects of care regarded as important.[5] Over 99% of patients emphasized such aspects as the quality of information provided about their cancer and the opportunity to ask their doctor questions.

Equally, the amount and kind of information patients should be given and the ways in which it should be delivered have been the subject of considerable debate within the medical community, suggesting that this is an issue of great interest to doctors.[6–12] A recent survey of 393 British medical oncologists found that 28% suffered from clinical levels of anxiety and depression; the clinicians themselves viewed communication difficulties as contributing significantly to their stress levels.[13]

Legislation and consensus guidelines concerning medical communication have also been developed. Most countries have adopted as a guiding principle the Declaration of Helsinki, which states: "In any research on human beings, each potential subject must be adequately informed of the aims, methods, anticipated benefits and potential hazards of the study."[14] In the United States this principle has been embodied in legislation that requires doctors to obtain fully informed consent from patients taking part in trials.[15] While similar regulations do not yet exist for treatment decision making, the trend has been towards encouraging a similar level of frankness in clinical treatment discussions. The National Health and Medical Research Council of Australia, for example, recommends: "Patients should be encouraged to make their own decisions about medical treatments or procedures and that to do that effectively, they should be given adequate information about all pertinent matters, including even low probability or mild risks, in a form which promotes understanding."[16]

Achieving the elusive balance between underinforming and overloading the patient is important. The outcomes of patient dissatisfaction with communication are noncompliance with medical advice,[17] "doctor shopping,"[18] exploration of alternative medicine treatments,[19] poorer coping,[20] and general dissatisfaction.[21]

WHAT DO PATIENTS WANT?

Evidence regarding patient preferences suggests that an inflexible approach to information delivery is not ideal. While the majority of cancer patients in most Western countries (up to 85%) state that they want all information, good or bad,[22] a minority still prefers to receive minimal information only. When it comes to decision making, a larger percentage prefer to abdicate this role in favor of the doctor.[22,23] In a recently completed Australian study of 80 cancer patients seeing a medical oncologist, while 29 patients (36%) favored an equal and collaborative role in decision making, only 18 (23%) sought the dominant role. A sizable minority (41%) preferred to leave decision making in the hands of the doctor.[24]

Several studies have identified stable predictors of information and involvement preferences, such as age, gender, and education.[22,25] In the Australian study mentioned above,[24] only locus of religious control, a subscale of the Cancer Locus of Control scale,[26] was significantly related to preference. Those who believed that God can influence the development and progression of their disease wanted less information ($p < 0.0001$). This finding reflects the significant influence that religion and culture can have in determining attitudes not only to information, but to the roles of the physician, the patient-physician interaction, and the family when a member is ill.[27]

For example, Ali *et al.*[28] note that in Egypt the "patient must be dependent and nurtured, and is not to be involved in decision-making . . . . It is the family that makes decisions in Egypt because dignity, identity and security are bounded by belonging to the family." Therefore, "disclosure of the exact serious diagnosis to a patient by the physician is a socially unacceptable behaviour and an untactful act. However the family is informed of the diagnosis and the plan of care." Egyptians also believe that physicians have enough education to treat their diseases; therefore, "the patient cannot contradict or question the physician's orders because this would imply impolite behaviour, or interference in the physician's work or lack of respect from subordinate to superior." However, in some Asian cultures where there is much less emphasis on the individual, patients may respond to illness with denial, depression, dependency, and passivity. This response may be associated with noncompliance despite a belief in doctors as figures of authority to be held in awe.[29,30] These approaches are in contrast to the American culture of individualism, consumerism, and positive thinking, which generates quite different approaches to illness.

Another source of cultural difference comes with the relatively widespread practice in Asia of self-medication, which arises from a strong tradition of self-care.[31] Similarly, belief in reincarnation and in miracles means that both Asian and Arab families do not plan for death.[31] The understanding of causation is also different, with illness in some Asian cultures being seen to be due to loss of body equilibrium[32] and in Egyptian society as a divine punishment for sin, to be accepted with stoicism and some sense of shame.[28] While it is very important to avoid cultural stereotyping and recognize individual differences,[33] these cultural contexts clearly have an impact on doctor-patient communication.

Charlton[34] collated a number of studies exploring patients' views on being told their diagnosis, which revealed considerable within- and cross-cultural diversity. For example, in studies spanning from 1978 to 1990, the percentage of cancer patients definitely wanting to be told their diagnosis varied from 49% in the United Kingdom and 54% in Denmark to 93.6% in the U.S.S.R. and 90% in Germany. Such variation can make it extremely difficult in multicultural societies like Australia and America for doctors who are trying to negotiate between the dominant sociocultural attitude, the views of the patients and their families (sometimes expressed forcefully), and the medicolegal environment. Unfortunately there have been very few studies examining current experiences of communication, preferences, or interventions from the refugee patients' and doctors' perspectives. If we are to deliver health care in a culturally sensitive manner, it seems increasingly clear that there is a need for more information about cross-cultural differences in communication needs and attitudes to cancer, in both indigenous and migrant populations.

WHAT DO DOCTORS TELL?

Within this climate of concern about communication how do doctors find their way along the fine line between paternalism and insensitivity? Empirical data show that until the 1970s, the trend was firmly in the direction of not disclosing the cancer diagnosis to the patient, although even back in the 1940s opinion was divided. Seelig[35] and others[36,37] felt that the patient should not be told that their disease was cancer except in exceptional circumstances. Seelig stressed the great shock and distress this sudden knowledge might induce in the patient. These findings reflected the trend in medicine to withhold any information that might severely upset patients.[38,39] Others felt the patient should be told the whole truth.[40,41]

In the 1960s, arguing that physicians' covert attitudes can have a profound influence on patients' well-being, Oken[39] said, "When doctors lose hope their patients know it. If doctors communicate the feeling that cancer is dreadful and irremediable, how can patients fail to despair? And frightened and despairing, how can they deal with the possibility they have cancer?" He investigated current practice in a study of 219 cancer physicians in 1961. Ninety percent of physicians in this study reported that they never told the patient about their diagnosis. Specific words such as "cancer" and "malignancy" were almost never used. The majority of these doctors believed that most patients really do not want to know their diagnosis, regardless of what they say. The argument against telling centered on the anticipation of profoundly disturbing psychological effects and the need to maintain hope.

This rationale was still being cited in the 1970s. On the basis of a survey of consecutive admissions to a Scottish teaching hospital in 1976, McIntosh[42] concluded,."There will always be anxiety associated with cancer, whether it is grounded in uncertainty or in patients' knowledge of their condition." He suggested that many patients chose the anxiety resulting from uncertainty as it allowed them hope; if necessary, the patient could pick up the facts via indirect means, such as identifying the name of the treatment center. A policy of routinely informing all patients was considered distressing to most and largely unnecessary to the remainder.

A contrary view put by the then editor of the *British Medical Journal* suggested that euphemisms and prevarication often leave patients and families with an enormous barrier of deceit, and the removal of this "web of deception" is met with great relief.[43] Smith said, "the malignant reputation of cancer is enhanced by the secrecy surrounding it." By this time, at least in the United States, this view appeared to have gained precedence. Using the same questions as Oken had employed, Novack *et al.*[44] found that the number of doctors revealing the diagnosis had increased from 10% in 1961 to 97% in 1979.

While there has been change reported in doctor attitudes over time, there has also been considerable variability reported in the way bad news is broken in different countries.[45,46] In the United States and Australia, hope is given in the context of disclosure of prognosis and an outline of a treatment plan. In other places, such as Italy and Japan, the disclosure of the diagnosis of cancer is seen as incompatible with successful treatment, as it precludes hope.[47] It is not known to what extent this variation reflects attitudes among the doctors or the doctors' response to attitudes among their patients. Certainly there is considerable cross-cultural variability in patient preferences, as discussed above.

A small number of studies have examined wider issues than disclosure of the diagnosis in the bad news consultation.[48–51] These pilot studies have identified considerable variability in both how the diagnosis of cancer is communicated and in patients' preferences. For example, 11% of patients in one study[49] were told their diagnosis by their general practitioner (GP), whereas 86% of patients in another[51] preferred the GP to tell. Most (84%) patients preferred to have a relative present,[49] whereas only 38% of Peteet *et al.*'s[50] sample were accompanied by a relative when told their diagnosis.

In a recent Australian study,[52] we found that 27% of patients were told about prognosis, whereas 57% wanted to discuss this. Thirty-five percent of patients reported talking about the effects of cancer on other aspects of life, while 63% expressed a preference for discussing this topic. Most patients wanted all available information and wanted a close relative but no other health professional present at the initial diagnostic interview. The majority of dissatisfied patients wanted more information, better emotional support, and a shorter time period between seeking help and confirmation of cancer. Patient experiences and preferences from this sample are shown in TABLES 1 and 2. The variability in patient preferences shows that a list of prescriptions for how to disclose a cancer diagnosis is too simplistic an approach. Guidelines for clinicians should be derived from patient-based data rather than clinical opinion and should emphasize the variability in patients' preferences.

Seventy percent of patients in this study endorsed the idea of a sheet providing sample questions commonly asked by patients facing a cancer diagnosis. In previous studies we have found that patients appreciate and use communication aids such as a tape of the consultation and a sheet listing questions often asked about cancer.[53,54] These patient-preferred procedures would be inexpensive additions to clinical practice and merit introduction and review.

ETHICAL CONSIDERATIONS

Modern medical ethics emphasize the patient's right to be fully informed of his or her medical condition, and to participate in decisions about treatment. Truth-telling, once regarded as cruel and insensitive, is now thought by many to be morally and legally obligatory.[55,56] The rationale for this approach is to safeguard the autonomy and integrity of the individual and to ensure that the patient plays an active role in decisions about his or her care. Some doctors have suggested that in the attempt to fulfill perceived moral and/or legal obligations, the individual patient's true wishes and best interests may be overlooked.[6,57]

Ethical decisions involve weighing up a number of ethical principles.[58] The traditional principles adopted by medicine have been beneficence (behaving for the good of others) and autonomy (respecting the rights and freedom of others). The principle of beneficence underpins the practice of paternalism, wherein the doctor takes responsibility for acting in his or her patients' presumed best interests. The assumption behind paternalism is that sickness makes the patient incompetent, and therefore the responsibility for deciding what constitutes benefit or harm should rest firmly upon the doctor. Providing information that portrays a bad prognosis or revealing that the doctor and the medical profession in general do not know which treatment is best may cause psychological distress in some patients, albeit temporary; therefore, it is advisable to "first, do no harm" and withhold information. The consequence of this view may be coercion and usurpation of decision making.[59] This may be done in subtle ways, such as by ignoring what the patient says, failing to pre-

TABLE 1. Communicating the Diagnosis: Patient Recollections

Question	Answer	Percent
Who told?	Surgeon	41%
	GP	27%
	Cancer specialist	21%
	Other specialiast	8%
	Relative, secretary, other	3%
How told?	Face-to-face	74%
	Telephone	25%
	Other	1%
Where told?	Doctor's rooms	52%
	Home	22%
	Inpatient hospital ward	15%
	Outpatient hospital clinic	5%
	Treatment area	2%
	X-ray clinic	2%
	Other	2%
Privacy?	Private room	68%
	Curtained area within an open room	13%
	Open area with others in view	8%
	Other	11%
Spouse/relative present?	Yes	38%
	No	62%
Other health professional present?	Yes	15%
	No	85%
Perception of doctor's attitude?	Caring/sympathetic	76%
	Comfortable	31%
	Uneasy	14%
	Worried	14%
	Rushed	7%
	Judgmental	1%
Prepared for cancer diagnosis?	Complete surprise	36%
	Unexpected	20%
	Partly unexpected	20%
	Confirmation of suspicion	24%

TABLE 2. Comparison of Patient Experiences and Preferences in Empirical Studies

	Patient Experiences	Patient Preferences
Told by surgeon	41% (B); 74% (L)	—
Told by GP	27% (B); 11% (L); 33% (P)	86% (S)
Told face-to-face	74% (B); 77% (L); 84% (P)	77% (B); 84% (S)
Relative present	38% (B); 38% (P)	57% (B); 84% (S)
Other health professional present	15% (B)	13% (B)
Alone to hear diagnosis	49% (B); 43% (P)	38% (B); 75% (S)
Told about cancer support services	46% (B)	75% (S)
All information given	—	78% (B); 80% (L)

NOTE: B = Butow *et al.*[43] L = Lind *et al.*[40] P = Peteet *et al.*[41] S = Sardell *et al.*[42]

sent the options, or slanting information in such a way as to guarantee the result preferred by the doctor.[59]

The principle of autonomy, on the other hand, recognizes the need to respect the patient's integrity and right to self-determination. The assumption behind this model is that the patient wants information and involvement in decision making and is competent to assume this role. At the extreme, autonomy means that the patient has the right, on the basis of proper and adequate information, to reach decisions that may seem wholly irrational by the standards of medicine or to the community in general.[60,61] This may be the outcome, for example, when there is conflict between a migrant's traditional views of health care and those of the doctors treating him or her.

Neither paternalism nor complete autonomy offer an ideal basis for medical decisions. Paternalism is not ideal because the doctor cannot know all the patient's wishes, goals, and values; and a patient may well choose not to disclose circumstances, objectives, and judgments that influence his/her information needs.[62] Several recent studies have reported that doctors are *not* very good at estimating the amount and sort of information patients want,[63,64] or how well the patient has understood information they have imparted.[65] Furthermore, paternalism is open to an abuse of power if an assumption of superiority is wrongly made.[59]

Autonomy, on the other hand, fails to acknowledge the differences between wellness and sickness. The sick person is not simply a well person with a disease, but rather is qualitatively different, not only physically but also socially, emotionally, and even cognitively.[66] At a time when they may feel physically unwell and overwhelmed with anxiety, many patients appear to sanction a degree of paternalism in decision making, by opting to exercise their "autonomous choice of dependency."[67] Degner and

Sloan[68] found that perceptions of the general public are often quite different from those of actual patients: 59% of patients versus 36% of the non-patient public preferred to leave treatment decisions to the doctor.

Physical and mental weakness may also compromise the patient's ability to make an autonomous choice. This issue was recognized in a recent document produced by the Health Department of New South Wales, Australia,[69] which suggested that discussions about significant medical decisions be held early in an illness because "at this stage, a patient is more likely to have the time and energy to think through the alternatives and discuss them with family members." In some circumstances, directing the patient to make a treatment decision may be interpreted as moral abandonment.[59,70]

In a European context, perhaps the ideal is a compromise between these two extremes. Both doctor and patient bring essential knowledge and values to the clinical decision, and a mutual, active, knowledge-sharing approach is best.[58,71] By contrast, in other cultural groups the ideal approach remains to be defined. This complexity is further aggravated by the patient's degree of acculturation, which is related to years of residence.

CONCLUSIONS

Despite conflicting evidence, the majority of data support an open, negotiated exchange of information with European patients. In order to identify and accommodate those patients who prefer minimal involvement, it has been suggested that doctors should measure patients' information and involvement preferences more objectively; a variety of questionnaires have been developed for this purpose.[22,25] Another strategy to minimize patient discomfort without compromising autonomy is to inform patients of the psychological risks associated with full disclosure and involvement in medical decisions; then patients can decide on their preferred role accordingly.

The evidence suggests that communication skills that allow the doctor to determine how much patients want to know, to deliver the information in a positive, supportive way, and to confirm that patients have understood the information they sought may in the end be more important than objective counts of the amount of information presented. Properly conducted randomized trials of strategies and interventions in all areas of communication to confirm these hypotheses are urgently required. As there is no available evidence concerning the efficacy of such strategies, randomization is an ethical and necessary procedure to ensure that such research is methodologically sound. The approach to providing services within a multicultural society remains uncertain and requires intensive qualitative and intervention research.

REFERENCES

1. HOLLAND, J. C. B. 1976. Coping with cancer: A challenge to the behavioral services. *In* Cancer: The Behavioral Dimensions. J. W. Cullen *et al.*, Eds. Raven Press. New York, NY.
2. LONG, S. O. & B. D. LONG. 1982. Curable cancers and fatal ulcers: Attitudes toward cancer in Japan. Soc. Sci. Med. **16:** 2101–2108.
3. DOMINO, G. & M. P. REGMI. 1993. Attitudes towards cancer: A cross-cultural comparison of Nepalese and US students. J. Cross-cultural Psychol. **24:** 389–398.
4. COATES, A. S., V. GEBSKI, J. BISHOP *et al.* FOR THE AUSTRALIAN AND NEW ZEALAND BREAST CANCER TRIALS GROUP. 1987. Improving the quality of life during chemotherapy for advanced breast cancer. A comparison of intermittent and continuous treatment strategies. N. Engl. J. Med. **317:** 1490–1495.
5. WIGGERS, J. H., K. O. O'DONOVAN, S. REDMAN & R.W. SANSON-FISHER. 1990. Cancer patient satisfaction with care. Cancer **66:** 610–616.
6. TOBIAS, J. S. & R .L. SOUHAMI. 1993. Fully informed consent can be needlessly cruel. Br. Med. J. **307:** 1199–1201.
7. LIND, S. E., D. M. GOOD, S. SEIDEL *et al.* 1989. Telling the diagnosis of cancer. J. Clin. Oncol. **17:** 583–589.
8. GOLDBERG, R. J. 1984. Disclosure of information to adult cancer patients: Issues and update. J. Clin. Oncol. **2:** 948–955.
9. HOLLAND, J. C. 1989. Now we tell—but how well? (Editorial) J. Clin. Oncol. **7:** 557–559.
10. BREWIN, T. B. 1986. Truth, trust, paternalism. Lancet **ii:** 490–492.
11. TATTERSALL, M. H. N. & R. J. SIMES. 1992. Issues in informed consent. *In* Introducing New Treatments for Cancer: Practical, Ethical and Legal Problems. C. J. Williams, Ed.: 79–90. John Wiley & Sons. New York, NY.
12. BAUM, M. 1986. Do we need informed consent? Lancet **ii:** 911–912.
13. RAMIREZ, A. J., J. GRAHAM, M. A. RICHARDS, A. CULL, W. M. GREGORY, M. S. LEANING, D. C. SNASHALL & A. R. TIMOTHY. 1995. Burnout and psychiatric disorders among cancer clinicians. Br. J. Cancer **71:** 1263–1269.
14. WORLD MEDICAL ASSOCIATION. 1964. Declaration of Helsinki: Recommendations Guiding Medical Doctors in Biomedical Research Involving Human Subjects. World Medical Association. Helsinki.
15. UNITED STATES FOOD AND DRUG ADMINISTRATION. 1982. Code of Federal Regulations (DHEW Publication 191-21). U.S. Government Printing Office. Washington, DC.
16. NATIONAL HEALTH AND MEDICAL RESEARCH COUNCIL. 1988. NHMRC Statement on Human Experimentation and Supplementary Notes. NHMRC. Canberra.
17. HAYNES, R. B., D. W. TAYLOR & D. L. SACKETT, Eds. 1979. Compliance in Health Care. John Hopkins University Press. Baltimore, MD.
18. KASTELER, J., R. KANE, D. M. OLSEN & R. THETFORD. 1976. Issues underlying prevalence of "doctor-shopping" behaviour. J. Health. Soc. Behav. **17:** 328–339.
19. PLOYN, J. F. A., R. M. RIJCKMAN, C. J. VAN BRUNSCHOT & H. W. VAN DEN BORNE. 1985. Cancer patients' personality characteristics, physician-patient communication and adoption of the Moerman diet. Soc. Sci. Med. **20:** 831–847.
20. MOLLEMAN, E., P. J. KRABBENDAM, A. A. ANNYAS, H. S. KOOPS, D.T. SLEIJFER & A. VERMEY. 1984. The significance of the doctor-patient relationship in coping with cancer. Soc. Sci. Med. **18:** 475–480.

21. COHEN, F. & R. S. LAZARUS. 1979. Coping with the stresses of illness. *In* Health Psychology. G. C. Stone, F. Cohen & N. E. Adler, Eds.: 217–254. Jossey-Bass. San Fransisco, CA.
22. CASSILETH, B. R., R. V. ZUPKIS, K. SUTTON-SMITH & V. MARCH. 1980. Information and participation preferences among cancer patients. Ann. Intern. Med. **92:** 832–836.
23. SUTHERLAND, H. J., A. J. LLEWELLYN-THOMAS, G. A. LOCKWOOD, D. L. TRITCHLER & J. E. TILL. 1989. Cancer patients: Their desire for information and participation in treatment decisions. J. R. Soc. Med. **82:** 260–263.
24. BUTOW, P. N., M. MACLEAN, M. H. N. TATTERSALL & S. M. DUNN. The dynamics of change: Cancer patients' preferences for information, involvement and support. Unpublished manuscript.
25. HACK, T. F., D. F. DEGNER & D. G. DYCK. 1994. Relationship between preferences for decisional control and illness information among women with breast cancer: A quantitative and qualitative analysis. Soc. Sci. Med. **39:** 279–289.
26. WATSON, M., S. GREER, J. PRUYN & B. VAN DEN BORNE. 1990. The cancer Locus of Control scale. Psychol. Rep. **66:** 39–48.
27. GORDON, D. 1990. Embodying illness, embodying cancer. Cult. Med. Psychiatry **14:** 275–297.
28. ALI, N. S., H. Z. KHALIL & W. YOUSEF. 1993. A comparison of American and Egyptian cancer patients' attitudes and unmet needs. Cancer Nursing **16:** 193–203.
29. TRILL, M. D. & J. C. HOLLAND. 1993. Cross-cultural differences in the care of patients with cancer: A review. Gen. Hosp. Psychiatry **15:** 21–30.
30. NICHALKOVIT, T., J. M. HILL & J. C. HOLLAND. 1993. The effects of culture on illness behaviour and medical care: Asian and American differences. Gen. Hosp. Psychiatry **15:** 41–50.
31. MANIO, E. B.& R. R. HALL. 1987. Asian family traditions and their influence in transcultural health care delivery. Children's Health Care **15**(3): 172–177.
32. RAMIREZ, A. J., M. R. BOGDANOVIC & M. JASOVIC-GASIC. 1991. Psychosocial adjustment to cancer: Cultural considerations. Eur. J. Psychiatry **5:** 9–18.
33. MULLER, J. H. & B. DESMOND. 1992. Cross-cultural medicine a decade later: Ethical dilemmas in a cross-cultural context: A Chinese example. West. J. Med. **157:** 323–327.
34. CHARLTON, R. C. 1992. Breaking bad news. Med. J. Aust. **157:** 615–621.
35. SEELIG, M. G. 1943. Should cancer victims be told the truth? J. Mo. State Med. Assoc. **40:** 33–35.
36. SACHS, B. 1942. Be an optimist. J. Mt. Sinai Hosp. **8:** 323–325.
37. PIATT, L. M. 1946. Physician and the cancer patient. Ohio State Med. J. **42:** 371–372.
38. FITTS, W. T. & I. S. RAVDIN. 1953. What Philadelphia physicians tell patients with cancer. JAMA **153**(10): 901–904.
39. OKEN, D. 1961. What to tell cancer patients. A study of medical attitudes. JAMA **175**(13): 1120–1128.
40. LIND, C. C. 1946. Doctor, patient and the truth. Ann. Int. Med. **24:** 955–959.
41. UNDERWOOD, F. J. 1949. Early cancer is curable. Miss. Doctor **26:** 280–281.
42. MCINTOSH, J. 1976. Patients' awareness and desire for information about diagnosed but undisclosed malignant disease. Lancet **7980**(2): 300–303.
43. SMITH, A. 1976. Should a doctor tell the truth when a patient has cancer? The Times. London.

44. NOVACK, D. H, R. PLUMER, R. L. SMITH *et al.* 1979. Changes in physicians' attitudes towards telling the cancer patient. JAMA **241:** 897-900.
45. HOLLAND, J. C., A. MARCHINI & S. TROSS. 1986. An international survey of physician practices in regard to revealing the diagnosis of cancer. 14th Int. Cancer Congr. Abstr. Lect. Symp. Free Commun, Vol 3 (Abstract No. 3964). Karger. Basel.
46. UCHITOMI, Y., J. SUGIHARA, M. FUKUE, Y. KURAMOTO, T. AKECHI, N. OOMORI & S. YAMAWAKI. 1994. Psychiatric liaison issues in cancer care in Japan. J. Pain Symptom Management **9**(5): 319–324.
47. GARRO, L. C. 1990. Culture, pain and cancer. J. Palliat. Care **6**(3): 34–44.
48. ROBERTS, C. S., C. E. COX, M. D. REINTGEN, W. F. BAILE & M. GIBERTINI. 1994. Influence of doctor communication on newly diagnosed breast patients' psychologic adjustment and decision-making. Cancer Suppl. **74:** 336–341.
49. LIND, S. E., M. D. GOOD, S. SEIDEL, T. CSORDAS & B. J. GOOD. 1989. Telling the diagnosis of cancer. J. Clin. Oncol. **7**(5): 583–589.
50. PETEET, J. R., H. E. ABRAMS, D. MURRAY ROSS & N. M. STEARNS. 1991. Presenting a diagnosis of cancer: Patients' views. J. Fam. Pract. **32:** 577–581.
51. SARDELL, A. N. & S. J. TRIERWEILER. 1993. Disclosing the cancer diagnosis. Cancer **72:** 3355–3365.
52. BUTOW, P. N., J. KAZEMI, L. J. BEENEY, A. M. GRIFFIN, M. H. N. TATTERSALL & S. M. DUNN. 1996. When the diagnosis is cancer: Patient communication experiences and preferences. Cancer **77:** 2630–2637.
53. DUNN, S. M., P. N. BUTOW, M. H. N. TATTERSALL, Q. J. JONES, J. S. SHELDON, J. J. TAYLOR & M. D. SUMICH. 1993. General information tapes inhibit recall of the cancer consultation. J. Clin. Oncol. **11**(11): 2279–2285.
54. BUTOW, P. N., S. M. DUNN, M. H. N. TATTERSALL & Q. J. JONES. 1994. Patient participation in the cancer consultation: Evaluation of a question prompt sheet. Ann. Oncol. **5:** 199–204.
55. LANTOS, J. 1993. Informed consent: The whole truth for patients? Cancer Suppl. **72:** 2811–2815.
56. GOLDBERG, R. J. 1984. Disclosure of information to adult cancer patients: Issues and update. J. Clin. Oncol. **2:** 948–954.
57. 1995. Your baby is in a trial (Editorial). Lancet **345:** 805–806.
58. SIMES, R. J. Ethical issues in clinical trials. A review. Unpublished Ph.D. dissertation.
59. POLLARD, B. J. 1993. Autonomy and paternalism in medicine. Med. J. Aust. **159:** 797–802.
60. GIESEN, D. 1993. Legal accountability for the provision of medical care: A comparative view. J. R. Soc. Med. **86:** 648–652.
61. SHELP, E. E. & M. PERL. 1985. Denial in clinical medicine: A reexamination of the concept and its significance. Arch. Intern. Med. **145:** 697–699.
62. LORD SCARMAN in Sideway v. Bethlem Royal Hospital (1985). Cited in D. Giesen. 1993. Legal accountability for the provision of medical care: A comparative view. J. R. Soc. Med. **86:** 648–652.
63. BLANCHARD, C. G., M. S. LABREQUE, J. C. RUCKDESCHEL & E. B. BLANCHARD. 1988. Information and decision-making preferences of hospitalised cancer patients. Soc. Sci. Med. **27:** 1139–1145.
64. WIGGERS, J., K. O'DONOVAN, S. REDMAN & R. SANSON-FISHER. 1990. Cancer patient satisfaction with care. Cancer **66:** 610–616.
65. MACKILLOP, W. J., W. E. STEWART, A. D. GINSBERG & S. S. STEWART. 1988. Cancer patients' perceptions of their disease and its treatment, Br. J. Cancer **58:**

355–358.
66. CASSELL, E. Cited in B. J. Pollard. 1993. Autonomy and paternalism in medicine. Med. J. Aust. **159:** 797–802.
67. WILLIAMSON, C. 1992. Whose standards? Consumer and professional standards in health care. Open University Press. Buckingham, U.K.
68. DEGNER, L. F. & J. A. SLOAN. 1992. Decision making during serious illness: What role do patients really want to play? J. Clin. Epidemiol. **45:** 941–950.
69. NEW SOUTH WALES HEALTH DEPARTMENT. 1993. Dying with dignity: Interim guidelines on management. New South Wales Health Department. Sydney.
70. PELLEGRINO, E & D. C. THOMASMA. 1987. The conflict between autonomy and beneficence in medical ethics: Proposal for a resolution. J. Contemp. Health Law **3:** 23–46.
71. CONNOLY, T. J. 1981. Willing participant or exploited patient? Med. J. Aust. **1:** 172–174.

Talking with Patients Suffering from Malignant Melanoma

G. W. MILTON

Skin and Cancer Foundation Australia
277 Bourke Street
Darlinghurst, N.S.W., Australia 2010

Australia is a multicultural society. Prior to the Second World War our population was mainly from the United Kingdom, although there were small groups from other countries. In the early postwar years, the generation most likely to get melanoma now, the immigrants, came largely from the United Kingdom, Greece, Italy and Yugoslavia. At present large numbers of immigrants are from Asia.

One way of demonstrating the fact that Australia is a multicultural society is by investigating the country of origin of overseas-trained medical graduates at present resident in Australia as immigrants, who apply to practice in this country. In order to do this they have to take the Australian Medical Council examination to obtain medical registration. According to the Australian Medical Council Annual Report 1993–1994, immigrant doctors living in Australia at that time came from 61 different countries. The largest number of applicants came from India, followed in order by Egypt, Philippines, the United Kingdom, Sri Lanka, Pakistan and China (equal), and Iraq. This variety of country of origin is not unique to medicine, so the population of this country originated in many different places. Unfortunately, figures are not available to give the country of origin of all patients who develop malignant melanoma, but from my personal experience malignant melanoma in aboriginals and dark skinned races is either unknown or exceedingly rare. However, one feature of public life that has developed in the last 20 years in Australia has been widespread and effective public education on the nature of malignant melanoma and its dangers.

Any person who has a malignant melanoma is frightened, especially in Australia where public education about the dangers of the disease has resulted in a moderately well-informed public. At various stages of their illness patients fear various things. First, there is the fear of a sinister, mysterious, evil illness: "What caused this? I have always been healthy. I don't deserve it." Most people fear the treatment, even if it is successful. The prospect of an operation is frightening, especially if the patient has no symptoms, such as pain, that require to be relieved by surgery. Now that lawyers have made us divulge all possible complications of surgery, this fear is enhanced. The patient may fear the mutilation caused by surgery. It could make them unattractive or prevent them from doing their normal job or enjoying their usual recreation.

The expense of surgery and other treatment is alarming to many people. Then there is the fear of dying, of being dead, of showing cowardice, of leaving relatives and friends, of being an object of pity, a "thing" rather than a person. The fact that they have to trust a stranger either to make or help them make vitally important decisions that may profoundly affect their lives is not easy to bear. People are also fearful of the loneliness of dying from illness: "It is all very well for you, you will go on living whatever happens to me." Finally, they fear that those around them will not be honest with them and so be untrustworthy when discussing their illness.

Of course, these apprehensions are not all present in the patient at the first interview, but the physician who sees the patient and his family at the start of his illness must be aware of the fears the patient will have to surmount. The physician's manner and conduct from the first day must lay the basis for all the future relationship between the patient and his family and physician. Hence, there are some rules for the early interviews, which will presumably take place in a strange environment for the patient—i.e., in a hospital or physician's office.

1. If at all possible, the patient should not be alone, but have his partner or family member with them. The reason for this is that the patient is suffering from mixed apprehensions and will not "hear" all that is said to him, and consequently will often misunderstand or later forget relatively simple explanations. Also the patient will be unlikely to think of all the questions he may want to ask now or later; and again patients tend to forget or become confused with the answers. The partner is more likely to ask appropriate questions and later when back home to be able to reassure the patient of the physician's replies.

Another reason for having the partner present is that if the physician sees the patient separately from his family, one of two events may follow. When the patient gets home he will often give a confused or inaccurate account of his interview, and this will not reassure either him or his family. If the physician communicates separately with the family, the patient will immediately, and often correctly, guess that he is not being told the whole truth, which he will assume to be worse than the story he has been told. Both patients and family practically always accept this explanation and approve of combined interviews. Both parties should understand the reason for the combined interview from the start and know that all future important decisions will only be made after mutual discussion. If the disease later progresses and becomes very dangerous and possibly fatal, it is most important that the patient, his family, and his physician completely trust each other; this will not come about if what is said to the patient differs from what is said to his family.

The policy of telling the truth (more on truth later) to the patient and family occasionally leads to difficulty if, before the interview, a relative asks to see the physician separately and states that the patient must not be told the truth because they could not bear it. The answer to this should be that the physician's first responsibility is to the patient, and he must be allowed to communicate with the patient as he thinks best. If the physician is deliberately deceptive to the patient, the result for the patient will be worse that the truth, because the subsequent behavior of family and friends will rapidly convince the patient that the very people he needs to trust most are deceiving him. This thought in the patient's mind makes him feel more and more isolated and alone. As long as the family knows that they will be present at all important interviews, they will nearly always accept this arrangement.

If at the first interview the patient presents with a lesion that is obviously a dangerous melanoma but is apparently quite unaware of the seriousness of his situation, it is desirable that he should be warned that the lesion does not look trivial and that the diagnosis will need to be confirmed by biopsy, the results of which will take a few days. The reason for allowing a few days rather than getting the result immediately is to give the patient time to become "acclimatized" to his danger, and to make sure he has family with him when the results of the biopsy are discussed.

It is helpful to have a brochure to give the patient that sets out in simple language the facts about melanomas and skin cancer. The brochure should also have a list of the most commonly asked questions with appropriate answers. In addition it is helpful to have a glossary of technical terms to explain medical language, so that the patient and his family can understand what words like nevus, tumor, benign, malignant, secondary, and metastasis mean. When the patient comes for his next interview, he will have at least some understanding of what is going on and some question he wishes clarified. At all interviews the physician must have enough time, free of interruptions, to devote his whole attention to the patient and his family and try to answer honestly all their questions.

2. The second rule when discussing melanoma is never to tell a direct lie, because once lied to, most of us are reluctant to trust the speaker again completely. As the illness progresses the need for trust between patient and physician is vital for both parties.

To be sure there are grades of truth. It is important not to be brutal. "You will be dead by Christmas" may be the absolute truth, but only someone with a slightly sadistic mind would say this.. Another equally truthful answer to the question "How long have I got?" would be, "It is difficult to predict this in any one person because there is considerable variation in how rapidly this disease progresses"; or "Very rarely even quite advanced disease will be inactivated by the body's defences, and sometimes the disease will not progress rapidly." Such an answer may appear somewhat long-winded; but the person you are talking to is looking into the black hole of oblivion and none of us relishes this prospect. However, if the patient asks specifically by stating that he has personal affairs to settle, it is important that he know as accurately as possible how long he will be able to manage his affairs. In this case, the truth about the chances of survival must be given directly, but some ray of hope can be given by stating quite truthfully that very rarely even advanced disease may regress. Very unfavorable statistics—such as if the person has a 7-mm-thick lesion, the chances of his survival is less than 20%—need not be emphasized when talking to the patient; very favorable statistics that apply to patients with very thin lesions can be stressed.

3. Another question frequently asked by the patient is, "What symptoms should I look out for?" The most appropriate answer is not to list all possible symptoms of recurrent disease; because there are so many, it is impossible to predict in any one patient what will be the site of internal recurrence and hence what symptoms might develop. Most patients appreciate that if they are given a complete list of all possible symptoms, they are likely to develop some of them because of anxiety. However, the patient should be warned that if he develops some unexplained symptom such as cough or abdominal cramps, he should see his physician. The patient should also be warned that the commonest site for regional recurrence is either in the draining lymph nodes, the scar of the original excision, or the tissue in between. The patient should also be told that if the nodes become involved, they are usually felt by the patient himself when washing or stretching, as a painless lump that has developed apparently overnight. If he feels such a lump, it may not be related to the melanoma, but he should get it checked immediately: even if it is due to spread of the tumor, there is still a reasonable chance that it can be successfully treated.

4. When the disease becomes incurable, the apprehension of both patient and family increases, and one or more of the fears mentioned at the beginning of this chapter will come into the patient's mind. Now, more that ever, it is important that the patient's natural feelings of loneliness and isolation not be made worse by bad managment.

At this stage of his illness the patient is usually cared for by a team rather than by an individual surgeon or physician. From the patient's point of view there are advantages to having, say, an oncologist and oncologically trained nurses, or highly trained neurosurgeons and surgical staff who have access to other specially trained and experienced personnel in charge. But one disadvantage of team management for the patient and family is that they may not know whom to turn to for advice, help, support or information. The names of the various specialities are confusing: "What is an oncologist?" "What does palliative care mean?" Another disadvantage for an individual of being managed by a team is that most medical teams are, quite rightly, anxious to acquire knowledge about the conditions they treat as well as looking after the patients under their care. This leads to clinical trials, and talk of "going on a trial" can be far from reassuring to an individual patient. To be sure, most people are pleased to help in the advance of medical knowledge, but to be told "We don't yet know whether treatment X is better than treatment Y, and so we have this clinical trial to find out" does not reassure someone facing a possibly terminal illness. It tends to suggest that the patient is of more interest to the team as a statistic than as a person.

Both these disadvantages of a team can be overcome by a good team: to do so all the members of the team must understand how their patient's mind is working. To be a good team, its members must know and trust one another. All members must know what the others do or say and how they say it. For example, if the patient is told by one member of the team that he (the patient) has a secondary deposit in the lung, and another refers to this as a metastasis, and a third is reluctant to discuss the problem at all, the patient and family will become confused. From the patient's point of view the "captain" of the team may be a somewhat remote superspecialist who is not only very important, but also very busy and more interested in the trial than in him. Hence, the importance of less exalted team members having the time, willingness and ability to talk with the patient and family and help them at this very difficult period of their lives.

The team must always have at least one co-opted member who will probably never be present when the team discusses the patient but who must be made to feel a member of the team nevertheless. The co-opted member is the patient's family physician. The family physician may have known the patient and family for years, and it is to him that both patient and family are likely to turn and feel more comfortable when in distress. The central team members should be aware of this and keep the family physician fully informed, not only by letter but also by telephone contact, especially when major decisions or events have taken place. If the chief of the team feels that he cannot spare the time to give the family physician a call and explain what is happening to his patient, then a trusted team member such as a younger physician or nurse should do so. In this way the central team keeps the family physician informed about events as they happen and in addition can learn how the patient and family are coping at home. This information may be extremely useful in palliative care.

One of the reasons that many patients with advancing cancer seek help from charlatans who claim a cure for cancer by some weird process or secret drug is that in the clinic with the magic "cure" all talk is favorable and positive, any uncertainty is diluted, and there is no word of double-blind trials. No one likes to be told there is *nothing* more that can be done.

5. Another problem arises as the disease advances: "What do we tell the children?" As a vital part of the family, the children should be told the truth like the others, for at least three reasons . First, the love and support of children, even young children, can be very helpful to the sufferer and his partner, but they cannot offer much support if they can only guess at what is going on by the behavior of their parents. The commonest mis-

take made with children at times like this is to underestimate how much they can comprehend and how much help they can be. Second, if children are excluded from all discussions about their parent's illness and the patient subsequently dies, the child may very much regret in later life how they behaved towards their parent at the end of his life. Third, children are less likely to make the home environment worse by knowing the truth and being included in the family than they are if they feel they are on the outside. Even young children can and do respond remarkably well to the fact of approaching death as long as they feel they really are part of the family. Children must not be forbidden to say what they think. In one of his discussions on life and death, the late Lord Bertrand Russell said words to the effect that, as one approaches the end of one's life, it is important to be interested in events that will take place after your death. This certainly applies to a sick parent talking with his children. They are his continuity; how can he talk sensibly with them if he has to always pretend things are not what they seem.

6. Patients frequently ask, "What can I do to beat this thing, should I have some special diet?" A sensible answer seems to be, to live a healthy life and eat good food, but no one has shown any advantage can be gained by a special diet or vast vitamin supplements. In short, live the way you enjoy living, do the things you enjoy doing, and eat the things you enjoy eating.

Talking with patients takes time and requires thoughtful consideration for the people to whom you are talking; but the rewards in terms of appreciation and friendship are enormous.

Psychological Training for Health-Care Professionals in Oncology

A Way to Improve Communication Skills

NICOLE DELVAUX[a] AND DARIUS RAZAVI[b]

[a]*Unité de Psycho-Oncologie*
Institut Jules Bordet
1 rue Héger Bordet
B-1000 Brussels, Belgium

[b]*Service Médico-Psychologique*
Hôpital Universitaire Saint-Pierre
Rue Haute 322
B-1000 Brussels, Belgium

INTRODUCTION

A 47% prevalence of psychiatric disorders has been reported in cancer patients populations.[1] Among these, adjustment disorders are the most frequent. They are often related to the risk of therapeutic failure, type and length of therapy, treatment impact on quality of life, coping problems, and availability of social support. It is obvious that cancer patients who do not meet DSM-III criteria for psychiatric disorders also experience distress.

Several studies provide evidence that psychosocial interventions reduce patients' psychological distress.[2] Sanson-Fisher and Maguire[3] also argue that the way doctors communicate with their patients affects not only the adequacy of the clinical interview and the detection of psychological disturbance, but also patients' compliance and satisfaction with care. Unfortunately, a substantial proportion of the problems developed by cancer patients remain untreated.[4–6] This failure to identify many of the patients' problems seems related mostly to insufficient psychosocial knowledge and deficient communication skills among health professionals who care for these patients and their families.

Nowadays, medicine in general and oncology in particular are confronted not only with an exponential growth of scientific knowledge, but also with numerous questions regarding their clinical applications. Medical progress has created many new difficulties in the process of decision making and communicating with patients and their relatives. Some new clinical situations, such as organ transplantation, which implies approaching the donor's family, or patients' requests to hasten death, need to be resolved with high-quality communication.[7,8]

Moreover, it is often recognized that cancer care is highly stressful.[9,10] Stressors are usually cumulative in oncology: critical decisions, errors yielding important consequences, communication of bad news, numerous therapeutic failures, administration of treatments with serious side effects, contacts with mutilated/disfigured patients, emotionally loaded relationships, death of patients. A lot of these stressors imply communication with patients, relatives, and colleagues. They may lead to the development of burnout, which may influence quality of care, occupational life, and/or institutional functioning.

Interventions and strategies have been proposed to help staff deal with cancer care: staff selection, financial and organizational facilities, and also training and research opportunities. Training is probably one of the most cost-effective ways of reducing stress in cancer care and of improving satisfaction with care and enhancing quality of care.[11]

The term "psychological training program" (PTP) will be used here to describe all teaching strategies developed in order to help health care professionals deal with communication problems in oncology. The importance of PTP is often acknowledged. It is being implemented more and more frequently in general hospitals and other health care settings. However, elaboration of content, form, and techniques vary with the experience and personal options of the trainer.[12–15] There have been several studies regarding their effectiveness. This paper will discuss the potential benefit of PTP and its impact on psychosocial care.

OBJECTIVES

Health professionals are confronted with numerous clinical situations in which communication cannot be avoided: diagnostic disclosure, uncontrolled chronic pain, compliance problems during curative treatments, aggressive patients, informed consent, euthanasia request, suicidal risk, and breaking bad news (like poor prognosis or death). The main objective of PTP remains to make health care professionals sensitive to communication problems with patients and relatives. These problems are influenced by personal difficulties in coping with fear of death, fear of the unknown, fear of being unable to respond to patients' questions, and fear of reactivating patients' distress. PTP should help health professionals develop their communication skills and cope with these complex clinical problems.

Basic communications skills can also be useful in other daily professional situations such as obtaining a case history, conveying information about treatment, reassuring patients, achieving patients' satisfaction, and monitoring patients and relatives' adaptation to illness and treatment. In clinical practice, some health care professionals still find it hard to elicit psychosocial as well as physical problems, or to do it without taking too much time. They frequently express a need for communication strategies and guidelines.

In medical communication, two types of behaviors are considered important: instrumental and socioemotional behaviors.[16] They correspond to the main purposes of the medical consultation: on one hand exchanging information—including taking and giving information—which is necessary for solving clinical problems, and on the other hand creating a therapeutic relationship, which is necessary for obtaining the patient's trust. More specifically, communication with cancer patients and their families has support as a third purpose.

In clinical practice and during training sessions, information and emotional support are often used without any previous information taking and assessment of patients' needs. A major objective of PTP in oncology is thus to develop an understanding of the needs of patients and families. It should enable one to identify patients' objectives and requests, to detect emotional distress, and to evaluate patients' understanding of transmitted information. Each communication function is achieved by using evaluative, informative, and supportive strategies. For assessing patients' problems, evaluative strategies may use open questions, clarification, and checking. Training may help health care professionals improve their ability to clarify the exact nature and extent of the problems encountered by patients, and feel and recognize their emotional reactions. Information has a well-known function in clinical practice but is used most often without elaboration of what has been understood. PTP allows participants to experiment with the advantages of progressive information. It also highlights the need for basic but often neglected strategies such as introducing oneself and ending the interview. Support includes many verbal and nonverbal strategies such as setting up the interview and the relationship, and the use of silence and empathy. It has been experienced in training sessions that all these supportive strategies often facilitate the evaluative function.

If the potential effect of PTP is the enhancement of communication skills (FIG. 1), there are still many questions related to other potential effects such as: the impact of training on health care professionals—their attitudes, quality of care, coping with stress, professional growth; and the impact on patients—their satisfaction with care, detection of their needs, compliance with treatment, quality of life. The effects of training on communication skills and attitudes could be linked with a better quality of care (with higher diagnostic and therapeutic competencies) and with more effective coping with occupational stressors met in oncology; however, there is not enough empirical evidence of these relationships.[17] FIGURE 1 schematizes the expected impact of psychological training on patients and carers through an improvement of communication skills.

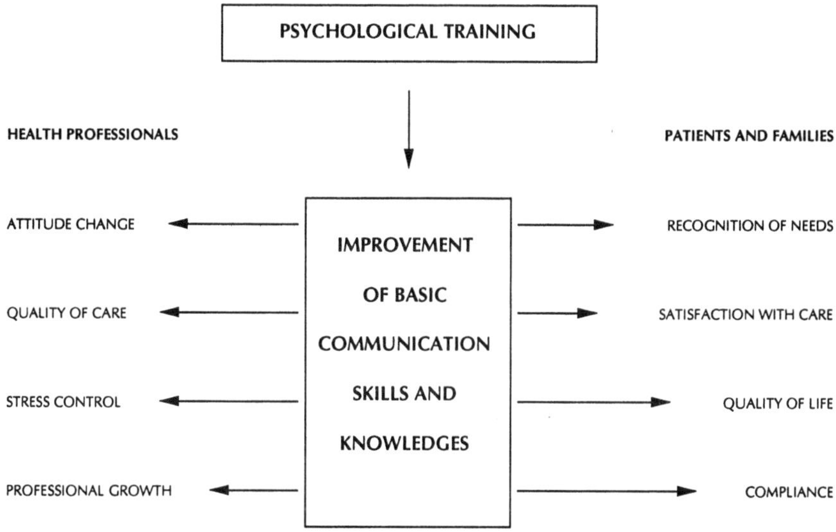

FIGURE 1. Psychological training.

TECHNIQUES

To be effective, PTP in oncology needs to be connected with clinical practice, and training techniques should be active. Available techniques are cognitive, behavioral, experiential, supportive. Cognitive techniques include theoretical information, courses, seminars, and lectures. Cognitive approaches in PTP should give health care professionals an understanding of psychosocial aspects of cancer and help them develop a method of communicating with patients. During training sessions, trainers often give theoretical input. But there is a risk of reducing active participation and transmitting too simplistic information about complex facts or concepts. Homework and journal clubs are therefore useful. Reading materials on the most important concepts in the field are now available. International scientific journals are complemented by several books: the *Handbook of Psychooncology*,[1] the *Oxford Textbook of Palliative Medicine*,[18] and, in French, the *Abrégé de Psycho-oncologie*.[19]

Experiential techniques include case history discussions, staff observations, and supervisions. During a training session, case history observation gives the opportunity to present, discuss, and analyze practical situations in their complexity. It outlines the personal strategies in communication and heightens the self-awareness of health care professionals. It clarifies which areas are important to explore in order to determine the nature and extent of the patients' problems. It also offers opportunities for exchanges with colleagues about psychosocial matters—opportunities that are often lacking in clinical practice. To be effective, this technique has to be used in small group sessions in order to stimulate discussion. Helping the participants present the clinical situations seems useful: the methodology for presentation should include information on the purpose of the interview, the history of the patient, the history of the present illness, specific physical and psychosocial problems, attitude towards illness, available support. The clinical presentation should end with a question from the participant in order to induce discussion.

Behavioral techniques include role playing exercises, patients' interviews under observation, and walking rounds. Role playing exercises have been widely used for teaching communication skills.[20] This consists of asking participants during a training session to play different roles (patient, family, nurse, physician, etc.) and to discuss the simulated interview. The identification with played roles enables participants to observe and analyze feelings, attitudes, perceptions, and behaviors induced by clinical practice. It helps to experiment with communication strategies, such as setting up the interview, getting the patient to talk, controlling an interview, using assessment questions before informing and counseling. Role playing exercises are perhaps one of the most formative techniques. But trainers have to use them very carefully, with clear instructions, in the secure context of small group sessions. When scripts are proposed, they should be as close as possible to clinical practice and usual situations. The use of audiovisual techniques such as videotaped role playing exercises and video- or audiotaped patient interviews should be encouraged.

Staff support and stress management programs include stressor identification, symptom recognition and monitoring, occupational and personal objective clarification, discussion of communication problems, and sometimes behavioral techniques (relaxation). Staff support programs benefit from a small number of participants (no more than 8 to 12). The good atmosphere of group support is also related to participants' motivation, positive inputs from the authorities, experienced leadership, and regular and convenient meeting times and places.[21]

PROGRAMS

General professional training remains essentially targeted to technical care, with limited concern for the psychological problems generated by cancer diagnosis and treatment. Few doctors and nurses involved in cancer care receive any formal training in basic interviewing, assessment, and counseling skills. Even if they had received some such training, it is usually limited to nondirective methods such as listening and reflecting. While such methods are of value in some situations, they can be counterproductive with cancer patients.[22]

In order to help some specialists (such as those involved with breast cancer care, stoma care, pain and symptom control, care of children with cancer, etc.), the training programs should also focus on the psychological dimensions of supportive care and rehabilitation. Various training programs are now being proposed. The need for specific training in palliative care is now also acknowledged.[23–29] Efforts have been made to train future professionals during their undergraduate period.[12,30–37] This is often not enough, because basic education is focused mostly on technical care and, because of time limitations, does not allow extensive focus on psychosocial matters.[38–40]

PTPs are being developed for several groups of professionals involved in cancer care (physicians, nurses, mental health professionals) working in institutions (cancer centers, general hospitals, hospices, etc.) or in-home care programs.

PTPs range from one-day courses to longer specific curricula that require mild to intensive involvement of participants. Most of them are residential workshops and take place during the weekend and are less often organized in the working environment. All these PTPs vary in form, content, and duration. They include basic and postbasic trainings.

In Great Britain, for example, three- to five-day residential workshops in small groups are proposed for physicians, nurses, social workers, and chaplains.[22] Videotaped interviews and structured role playing exercises are used. Sharing experiences and discussing them give insight into how a patient or a relative may feel, outline the positive aspects of coping with stress, help the participants identify the risk of projective attitudes, and also offer alternative communication strategies. As participants progress through the workshops, they start wondering about how they can apply their new skills within their own work and still survive emotionally.

Another PTP using cognitive, experiential, and behavioral techniques was proposed in Belgium to health care professionals working with terminal patients.[41] These modules were flexible in their schedule in order to allow attendance by busy doctors and nurses. They lasted 12 hours spread over 4, 6, 8, or 10 sessions. Their aims were to develop a better understanding of death and dying issues related to cancer and to foster more positive attitudes toward care of the dying.

For those who offer workshops or short training programs, a key challenge is to help participants apply in their clinical practice what they have learned. Attempts to organize consolidation modules have been made. Peripatetic teachers may organize regular short workshops for already trained participants working together.[19] Remote learning approachesmay be used for individual feedback of audiotaped material; new miniature two-way radios enabling health care professionals to be supervisedduring their live interviews with patients or relatives are also being developed.[22]

Longer PTPs are increasingly being recommended. Several groups are working on this topic in the United States and Europe. Full-time curricula are now available.[27,42] The European School of Oncology organizes fellowships of several weeks in supportive and palliative care. The Memorial Sloan-Kettering Cancer Center in New York and the Jules Bordet Institute in Brussels propose a two-year curriculum in psychooncology. These two years are dedicated to training in clinical practice and research. This curriculum may benefit from a third year for consolidating the skills acquired and for training teachers.

EFFECTIVENESS

Up to now, little has be done to evaluate existing training for health care professionals dealing with cancer patient.[43] Training effectiveness can be evaluated by attitudinal, behavioral, or cognitive changes. Psychological stress–related symptoms are supposed to be another variable because of their potential influence on quality of occupational life and on quality of care.

Several authors have considered changes in attitudes towards cancer or death as a result of participation in training groups. Results reported are usually positive, but evaluation is often informal.[13–15,44–46] More formal assessment of training effectiveness does not always support the perceived success of the training program.[47–49]

Several other methodological and theoretical problems are still unresolved—e.g., what are the short- and long-term emotional, cognitive, and behavioral changes induced by training? Are attitude changes linked with behavior changes? What are the optimal content and duration for effective PTP?

In a controlled study, the effectiveness of a 12-hour PTP was assessed with a semantic differential attitude questionnaire. The assessment was made just after the end of the training and one year later.[41,43,50] The results showed that post-training changes were particularly significant for subjects reporting negative attitudes before training. However, one year after training, post-training changes were no longer noticed.

In order to improve effectiveness, longer modules were tested. In one of these studies, 72 oncology nurses were randomly assigned to a 24-hour PTP or to a waiting list.[51] Attitudes assessed by a semantic differential questionnaire,[47] occupational stress assessed by the Nursing Stress Scale,[52] and communication skills assessed by standardized videotaped role playing exercises were used to compare trained and control subjects. The results show a significant training effect on attitudes, especially on those related to self-concept, and on the level of occupational stress related to inadequate preparation. Limited changes were found regarding post-training communication skills. Trained subjects were significantly more in control of the interview compared to control subjects. The results show that a 24-hour PTP is effective. Results show that post-training changes in

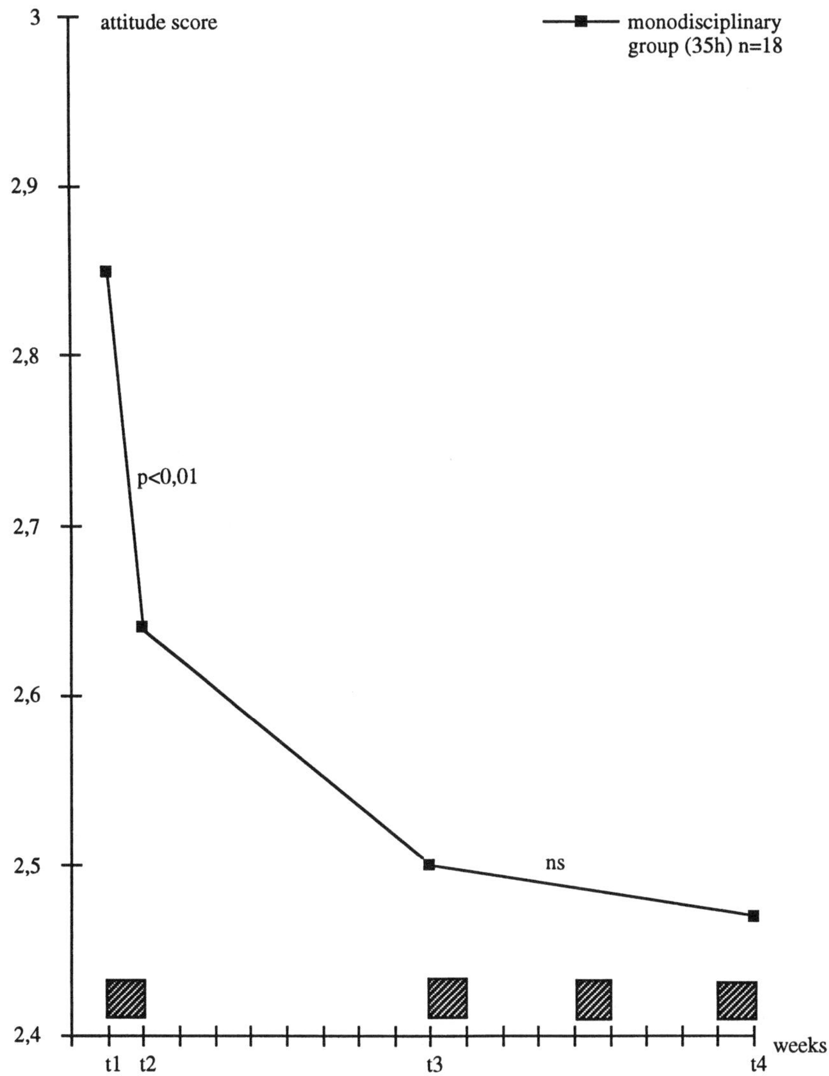

t1 : before training
t2 : after training
t3 : before first consolidation training week
t4 : after third consolidation training week

FIGURE 2. Training effectiveness and consolidation of attitudes.

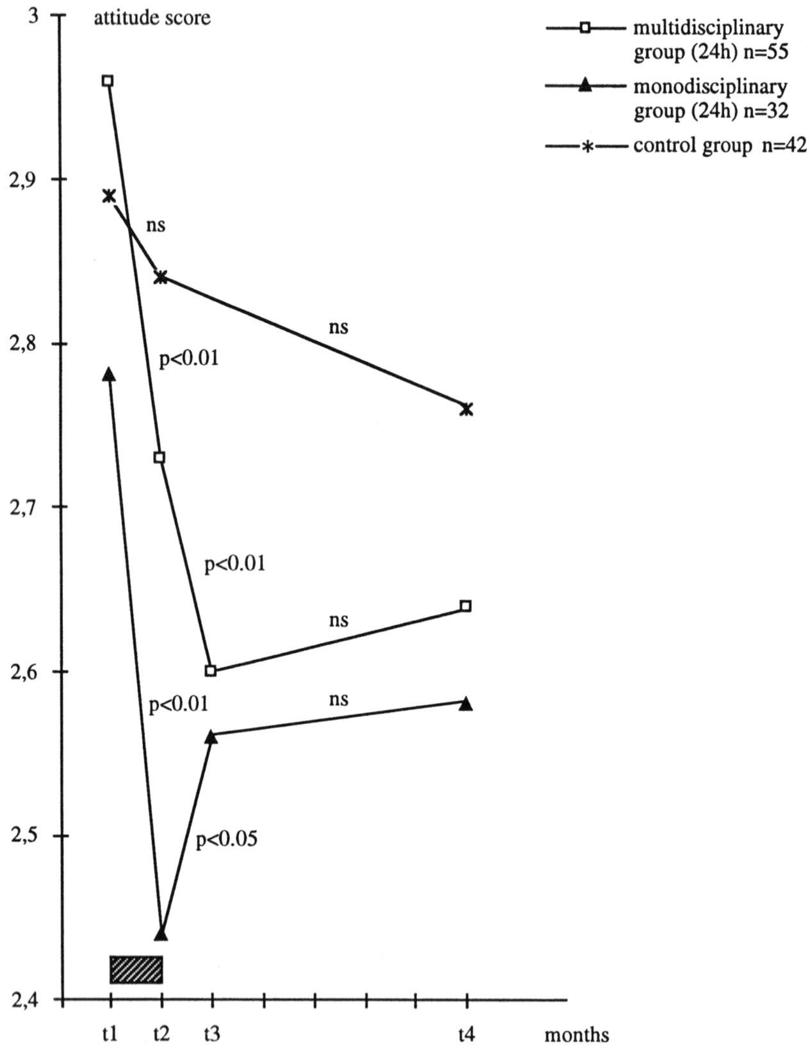

t1 : before training
t2 : after training
t3 : two months after training
t4 : twelve months after training

FIGURE 3. Training effectiveness on attitudes: comparison of multidisciplinary versus monodisciplinary groups.

attitudes were no longer noticed two months after training. The same trend was observed for post-training Nursing Stress Scale scores.[51]

The lack of consolidation observed two months after training may be explained by the loss of the "peer support group effect." It can also be hypothesized that the trained participants do not find support and/or time in their institutions to give them the opportunity to practice their skills.

Therefore, the question of whether or not PTP should be longer and/or consolidated by several follow-up sessions should be investigated. Different questions related to the optimal number of sessions and the duration and content of the training remain unanswered. In an unpublished pilot study, consolidation modules (three monthly full-time weeks of 35 hours) were assessed after an initial 35-hour training week. Consolidation modules enabled more behavioral training techniques to be used (such as case discussions and role playing exercises) and implementation of skills in everyday work to be discussed. The results show a significant consolidation effect of post-training attitude changes. FIGURE 2 illustrates immediate (just after the end of the training) post-training attitude changes and shows significant consolidation (8 and 17 weeks after training) of these attitude changes. A statistically significant decrease of a mean attitude score means a "positive" attitude change.

Other possible predictors such as the benefit of multidisciplinary versus monodisciplinary groups should also be investigated. A pilot study assessing post-training changes of multidisciplinary training groups shows that attitude changes were still noticeable not only just after training, but also two months later. FIGURE 3 illustrates 2 and 12 months post-training attitude changes in a trained group compared with a control group of health care professionals. An increase of mean attitude score two months after the end of the training is found in monodisciplinary training groups. A statistically significant increase of a mean attitude score means a "negative" attitude change. An advantage of multidisciplinary versus monodisciplinary groups may thus be also hypothesized.

CONCLUSION

To improve the psychological and social care of cancer patients, health care professionals must be trained in basic interviewing, assessment, and counseling skills. PTP should therefore give the ability to detect, clarify, and organize key verbal and nonverbal cues that patients and relatives give about their problems, to control the interview and maintain its focus, to acquire precision in assessment strategies and open directive questions (e.g., dates, names, symptom intensity), and to explore emotionally loaded areas (e.g., the wish to die, prognosis, death) in a helpful and not-too-painful way.

PTP should be available in all health care settings devoted to cancer care. Consolidation training programs should also be available to stimulate the implementation of learned skills. A special effort should also be devoted to broader competence and skills in order to respond more adequately to complex problems encountered in oncology. Ethical issues, for example, are numerous in oncology. They are often related to psychological, social, legal, and spiritual matters. Ethics education may focus specifically on problems that are not targeted by PTP. Ethics education should aim at improving clinicians'—mostly physicians'—ability to identify and discuss ethical problems with patients, relatives, and colleagues.[53] This specific training should prepare health care professionals to analyze and cope with the complexities of difficult clinical situations such as truth-telling, informed consent, active and passive euthanasia, do-not resuscitate orders, deciding curative and palliative treatments, etc.

Developing full-time curricula in psychooncology is another way to improve standards in quality of care. It should also help deal with the significant lack of experts in this area. Moreover, there are not enough well-trained professionals who can provide PTP at the present time. For this reason, training key persons in teaching methods is a priority. Finally there are also obstacles to implementing PTP, such as the skepticism of health care professionals (especially physicians) about its usefulness. Research on training effectiveness should also be developed. These studies should aim at assessing effectiveness of PTP by measuring the impact of communication skills improvement on quality of care and patients' quality of life. This will convince not only skeptical health care professionals but also hospital managers to invest time and money in this type of training.

REFERENCES

1. HOLLAND, J. C. & J. H. ROWLAND, Eds. 1989. Handbook of Psychooncology. Oxford University Press. Oxford.
2. HILL, D. R., K. KELLEHER & S. SHUMAKER. 1992. Psychosocial interventions in adult patients with coronary heart disease and cancer. Gen. Hosp. Psychiatry **14** (Suppl.): 28–42.
3. SANSON-FISHER, R. & P. MAGUIRE. 1980. Should skills in communicating with patients be taught in medical schools? Lancet **ii:** 523–526.
4. MAGUIRE, P. 1984. Communication skills and patient care. *In* Health Care and Human Behaviour. A. Steptoe & A. Matheews, Eds.: 153–173. Academic Press. London.
5. DAWN CAMP, L. 1988. A comparison of nurses' recorded assessments of pain with perceptions of pain as described by cancer patients. Cancer Nurs. **11**(4): 237–243.
6. FORD, S., L. FALLOWFIELD & S. LEWIS. 1994. Can oncologists detect distress in their out-patients and how satisfied are they with their performance during bad news consultations? Br. J. Cancer **70:** 767–770.
7. STEIN, A., T. HOPE & J. D. BAUM. 1995. Organ transplantation: Approaching

the donor's family. Br. Med. J. **310:** 1149–1150.

8. BLOCK, S. D. & J. A. BILLINGS. 1994. Patient requests to hasten death. Arch. Intern. Med. **154:** 2039–2047.
9. DELVAUX, N., D. RAZAVI & C. FARVACQUES. 1988. Cancer care, a stress for health professionals. Soc. Sci. Med. **27**(2): 159–166.
10. RAMIREZ, A. J., J. GRAHAM, M. A. RICHARDS, A. CULL, W. M. GREGORY, M. S. LEANING, D. C. SNASHALL & A. R. TIMOTHY. 1995. Burnout and psychiatric disorder among cancer clinicians. Br. J. Cancer. **71:** 1263–1269.
11. FALLOWFIELD, L. 1995. Can we improve the professional and personal fulfilment of doctors in cancer medicine? Br. J. Cancer. **71:** 1132–1133.
12. ANDERSON, J. A. 1979. Practical approach to teaching about communication with terminal cancer patients. J. Med. Educ. **54:** 823–824.
13. BERTMAN, S. L., H. GREENE & C. A. WYATT. 1982. Humanistic health care education in a hospice/palliative care setting. Death Educ. **5:** 391–408.
14. SHINN, M., M. ROSARIO, H. MORCH & D. E. CHESTNUT. 1984. Coping with job stress and burnout in human services. J. Pers. Soc. Psychol. **46:** 864–876.
15. ZIEGLER, J. L., N. KANAS, W. M. STRULL & N. A. BENNET. 1984. Stress discussion group for medical interns. J. Med. Educ. **59:** 205–207.
16. HALL, J. A., D. L. ROTER & N. R. KATZ. 1987. Task versus socioemotional behaviors in physicians. Med. Care. **25**(5): 399–412.
17. STEWART, M. & D. ROTER. 1990. Communicating with Medical Patients. Sage Publications. Newbury Park, CA.
18. DOYLE, D., G. W. HANKS & N. MCDONALD, Eds. 1993. Oxford Textbook of Palliative Medicine. Oxford University Press. Oxford.
19. RAZAVI, D. & N. DELVAUX, Eds. 1994. Psycho-oncologie. Masson. Paris.
20. MCMANUS, I. C., C.A. VINCENT, S. THOM & J. KIDD. 1993. Teaching communication skills to clinical students. Br. Med. J. **306:** 1322–1327.
21. LEDERBERG, M. 1989. Psychological problems of staff and their management. *In* Handbook of Psychooncology. J. C. Holland & J. H. Rowland, Eds: 631–646. Oxford University Press. Oxford.
22. MAGUIRE, P., D. RAZAVI & R. ZITTOUN. 1990. Training in psychosocial oncology. *In* Psychosocial Aspects of Oncology. J. C. Holland & R. Zittoun, Eds.: 137–142. Springler-Verlag. New York, NY.
23. SAINSBURY, M. J. & G. W. MILTON. 1975. The nurse in a cancer ward. Med. J. Aust. **2:** 911–913.
24. VACHON, M. L., A. L. LYALL & S. J. J. FREEMAN. 1978. Measurement and management of stress in health professionals working with advanced cancer patients. Death Educ. **1:** 365–375.
25. DICKINSON, G. E. & A. A. PEARSON. 1980. Death education and physicians' attitudes toward dying patients. Omega **11:** 167–183.
26. DOYLE, D. 1982. An education center for professionals. Death Educ. **6:** 213–226.
27. JELLINEK, M. S., M. DIE TRILL, S. PASSIK, F. I. FAWZY, M. BARD & A. WEISMAN. 1992. The need for multidisciplinary training in counseling the medically ill: Report of the training committee of the Linda Pollin Foundation. Gen. Hosp. Psychiatry **14**(Suppl.): 3–10.
28. DIMAGGIO, J. R. 1993. Educating psychiatry residents about death and dying: A national survey. Gen. Hosp. Psychiatry. **15:** 166–170.
29. WEBER, J. 1994. New directions in palliative care education. Support. Care Cancer **2:** 16–20.
30. BLOCH, S. 1975. Teaching medical students how to care for the dying. Med.

J. Aust. **2:** 902–903.
31. BLOCH, S. 1976. Instruction on death and dying for the medical student. Med. Educ. **10:** 269–273.
32. BARTON, D., M. K. CROWDER & J. M. FLEXNER. 1979. Teaching about dying and death in a multidisciplinary student group. Omega **10:** 265–270.
33. MARKS, S. C. & S. L. BERTMAN. 1980. Experiences with learning about death in the undergraduate anatomy curriculum. J. Med. Educ. **55:** 48–52.
34. BENOLIEL, J. Q., Eds. 1982. Death Education for the Health Professional. McGraw-Hill. New York, NY.
35. GOODELL, B. W., J. I. DONOHUE & J. Q. BENOLIEL. 1982. Death education in medical school: A seminar in terminal illness. Death Educ. **5:** 363–389.
36. ZELINSKY, L. F. & J. A. THORSON. 1983. Educational approaches to preparing social work student for practice related to death and dying. Death Educ. **6:** 313–322.
37. Channon, L. D. 1984. Death and the preclinical medical student: I. Experiences with death. Death Educ. **8:** 231–235.
38. LIEFF, J. D. 1982. Eight reasons why doctors fear the elderly, chronic illness and death. J. Transpers. Psychol. **14:** 47–60.
39. MCLEAN, U. 1979. Learning about death. J. Med. Ethics. **5:** 68–70.
40. POPE, S. 1992. Fundamentals for a new concept of oncology nursing in the professional nursing education program. Cancer Nurs. **15**(2): 137–147.
41. RAZAVI, D., N. DELVAUX, C. FARVACQUES & E. ROBAYE. 1988. Immediate effectiveness of brief psychological training for health professionals dealing with terminally ill cancer patients: A controlled study. Soc. Sci. Med. **27**(4): 369–375.
42. FORBES, F. J. 1994. Towards an optimal teaching programme for supportive care. Support. Care Cancer **2:** 7–15.
43. DELVAUX, N., D. RAZAVI, C. FARVACQUES & E. ROBAYE. 1988. The effectiveness of a psychological training designed for health care professionals dealing with terminal cancer patients. *In* A Safer Death. Multidisciplinary Aspects of Terminal Care: 171–184. Plenum Press. New York, NY.
44. SHANFIELD, S. B. 1981. The mourning of health care professionals: An important element in education about death and loss. Death Educ. **4:** 385–395.
45. WISE, T. N. 1987. Training oncology fellows in psychological aspects of their speciality. Cancer **39**(6): 2584–2587.
46. SCOTT, J. F. & N. MACDONALD. 1993. Education in palliative medecine. *In* Oxford Textbook in Palliative Medicine. D. Doyle , G. W. Hanks & N. Macdonald, Eds.: 761–780. Oxford University Press. Oxford.
47. SILBERFARB, P. M. & P. M. LEVINE. 1980. Psychosocial aspects of neoplastic disease. II. Group support for the oncology nurse. Gen. Hosp. Psychiatry. **33:** 192–197.
48. MILES, M. S. 1980. The effects of a course on death and grief on nurses' attitudes toward dying patients and death. Death Educ. **4:** 245–260.
49. AMARAL, P., A. M. NEHEMKIS & L. FOX. 1981. Staff support on a cancer ward: A pilot project. Death Educ. **5:** 267–274.
50. RAZAVI, D., N. DELVAUX, C. FARVACQUES & E. ROBAYE. 1991. Brief psychological training for health professionals dealing cancer patients: A one-year assessment. Gen. Hosp. Psychiatry **13:** 253–260.
51. RAZAVI, D., N. DELVAUX, S. MARCHAL, A. BREDART, C. FARVACQUES & M. PAESMANS. 1993. The effects of a 24-hour psychological training program on attitudes, communication skills and occupational stress in oncology: A ran-

domized study. Eur. J. Cancer **29A**(13): 1858–1863.
52. GRAY-TOFT, P. & J. G. ANDERSON. 1980. The nursing stress scale: Development of an instrument. J. Behav. Assess. **3:** 11–23.
53. BYRNE, P., Eds. 1990. Medicine, medical ethics and the value of life. John Wiley & Sons. Chichester, U.K.

Improving Communication with Cancer Patients

A Challenge for Physicians

DARIUS RAZAVI,[a] NICOLE DELVAUX,[a]
AND PENNY HOPWOOD[b]

[a]*Unité de Psycho-Oncologie*
Service Médico-Psychologique
Hôpital Universitaire Saint-Pierre
Rue Haute 322
B-1000 Brussels, Belgium

[b]*CRC Psychological Medicine Group*
Stanley House
Christie Hospital
Wilmslow Road
Withington
Manchester M20 9BX, United Kingdom

INTRODUCTION

In Europe and the United States the number of cancer diagnoses is steadily increasing. Early detection techniques and effective treatments have improved cure rates, but this progress is often associated with invasive diagnostic investigations and with aggressive treatments. Even though much progress has been made in achieving better tolerance of these investigations and in controlling treatment side effects, patients and their families still have a considerable burden to bear. Clinical interventions ranging from surgical reconstruction to patient education programs are often necessary to help patients preserve their psychological and physical integrity or to cope with reversible or irreversible damage. Preserving the best possible quality of life for cancer patients and their families has become a major goal in cancer care.

Good communication between professionals and their patients, together with appropriate information, education, and support, facilitate patients' adjustment. Moreover, it has been claimed that professional communication is a major source of patients' dissatisfaction. Communication is part of a complex process in the patient-physician relationship. Communication is influenced by characteristics of both the patient and the health professional, by the nature and background of their relationship, and by the communication and surroundings that bring them together.

For example, physician-patient communication may vary depending on the physician's desire to inform and the corresponding need of the patient to be informed. If the balance between these two is wrong, it is likely to lead to dissatisfaction and poor quality of life. Communication can thus be viewed from the point of view of the carer's "formal" communication, the recipient's efforts to obtain information and the way he integrates it, and the informal channels that come into play.[1] Although much literature has been devoted to this, there still are many unanswered questions and uncertainties concerning the best way to give information about diagnosis, treatment and its side effects, and prognosis.

This paper discusses and presents factors influencing communication with cancer patients and problems raised by giving and receiving information. The potential positive effects of good communication skills are highlighted, and the need for training health care professionals in general and physicians in particular is emphasized.

FACTORS RELATING TO HEALTH CARE PROFESSIONALS

Physicians' Attitudes

It has been suggested that physicians fall into three groups with regard to giving information.[2] The first is characterized by a tendency to actively seek an opportunity to inform the patient about cancer. The second is characterized by an active tendency to conceal all information. The third group is an intermediate one, combining the passive withholding of information with the provision of carefully chosen facts according to the circumstances. There has been an increasing proportion of doctors using the third strategy in recent years.

Attitudes toward giving information have changed over the last twenty years. In 1974, 78% of physicians felt that patients should be told the nature of their disease.[3] In 1979, 97% of physicians were in favor of communicating a diagnosis of cancer to patients.[4] The results of a study made in 1982 assessing North American physicians' attitudes show that more than 80% of interviewed physicians felt that the diagnosis should be communicated to patients in clear terms as quickly as possible.[5]

This change in attitudes was probably due to medical progress but was determined also by the action of media, the movements in defense of patients' rights, and the development of palliative care in Great Britain and the United States. Another important factor was the change from a predominantly paternalistic and authoritarian kind of physician-patient relationship to a relationship in which they feel equal partners.[6] Despite the changes observed, attitudes toward giving information remain very different all over the world. This cultural difference in attitudes is illustrated by a study done in Greece in which it is reported that 73% of the practitioners surveyed were not in favor of communicating the diagnosis.[7] In Belgium, attitudes towards telling the truth may be classified in the middle.[8] These figures differ significantly from those reported above concerning North American attitudes.

Physicians' attitudes may also vary according to whether they are disclosing a diagnosis or prognosis. Two studies found that about 70% of doctors surveyed were in favor of communicating a diagnosis, but that they were reluctant to communicate the imminence of death: 45% to 95% of health care professionals were not in favor of communicating a poor or fatal prognosis.[9,10]

Status and Experience

Clinical experience was also found to influence communication of the diagnosis.[10] With increasing clinical experience, physicians previously opposed to informing patients of a diagnosis become more inclined to do so.[9] The same trend was found by comparing the opinion of oncologists with that of dermatologists, who are rarely confronted with cancer patients.[11] The amount of experience seems, however, to have little influence on the communication of an unfavorable prognosis.

In a study involving different groups of health professionals,[8] an unfavorable attitude toward giving full information to the patient was evident when the prognosis was poor. Greater reluctance was also noticed with a higher level of direct responsibility for patient care. Increased responsibility due to professional status generally tended to increase the emotional involvement in care and may thus affect negatively communication with the patient. This study shows also the influence of prognosis on telling the truth to patients and families. In case of a bad prognosis, the percentage of physicians reporting never telling the truth increases when they communicate with the patient and decreases when they communicate with the family. FIGURE 1 illustrates this tendency.

Disease and sociodemographic characteristics may also play a role. In a study assessing the quality of information given in Italy to 1262 women with breast cancer,[12] the factors associated with providing complete information were: early-stage disease, patient's age, educational level similar to that of the health professional, and certain characteristics of the institutional milieu in which the health professional practiced.

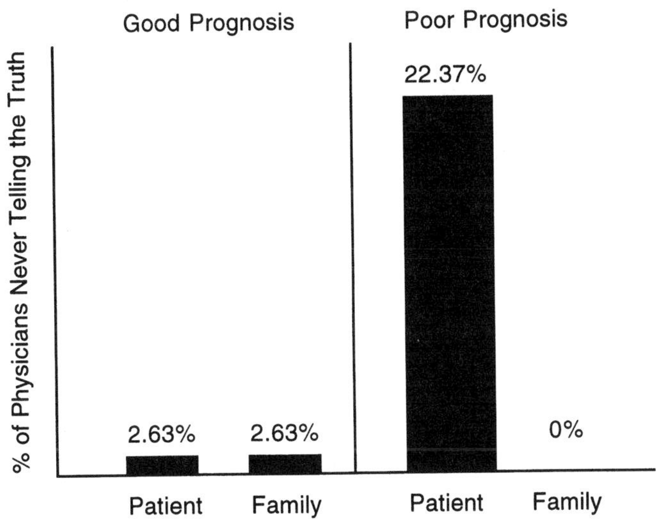

FIGURE 1. Influence of prognosis on telling the truth to patients and families in Belgium.

Emotional Factors

Reluctance to give information can also be due to the fear of precipitating extreme psychological reactions (anxious, depressive, aggressive, or suicidal) in patients. The frequency of these reactions is not high, but the impact of such experiences on health professionals may explain why some of them take refuge in avoiding breaking bad news, probably in order to protect themselves from a repetition of these traumatic reactions.

Furthermore, there is often reluctance to explore patients' concerns, in case this may trigger anxiety or distress, which is often perceived by doctors and nurses as negative and damaging. There is genuine concern to avoid making things worse for the patient, without due consideration of the need for information; and even if it is bad news, they underestimate patients' capacity to cope with such information and the benefits of expressing feelings in the process of adjustment. Physicians may overestimate the patients' worry about their prognosis. An explanation may be that they identify with the patient's expressed or implicit question "How long have I got to live?"

These existential concerns are central for patients in the weeks following the diagnosis.[13] However, although these preoccupations are important for certain patients during the diagnostic phase, during which an important effort to obtain information may often be observed, they frequently become less important later. If health professionals do not notice these changes in the patients' concerns, they are likely to remain unaware of the diversity of personal and interpersonal problems produced by cancer and its treatment.

Blocking Tactics

It has been suggested that doctors and nurses consciously distance themselves from their patients' concerns, especially their psychological distress, as a means of preserving their own emotional well-being. Valid concerns that result in using these blocking tactics should not be discussed lightly, since they highlight a clear need for improved training and support.

Practical Considerations

Practical considerations like time constraints, workload, and lack of privacy in medical settings are other factors that may influence communication. This does not mean that good working conditions may influence positively the quality and quantity of communication. However, these factors explain why health care professionals who have acquired communication skills by training may lose them in working conditions that do not support a good atmosphere for communication.

FACTORS RELATING TO PATIENTS

Educational Level

Evaluation of the intellectual level of the patients also determines the level of communication. The information needs of patients with limited intellectual ability often vary, both quantitatively and qualitatively, when compared to those expressed by other patients. These differences stress the need to develop a strategy tailor-made to each patient, to define their individual needs, and to give the information in the simplest way possible. Indeed, when a patient's intellect is limited, understanding complex medical information is difficult. This difficulty may shape the physician-patient relationship into an authority-submission axis. This type of relationship may foster distrust in the long run, which may result in poor treatment compliance.

Emotional Concerns

Emotional concerns are not frequently disclosed by cancer patients. The reluctance is probably linked to the fear of being viewed as ungrateful or as wanting to discontinue treatment. There is also a fear of stigmatization by being labeled neurotic. The reluctance may also be secondary to a sense of failure if distress is revealed, or to the feeling that if they disclosed their concerns they would not be able to contain them or to deal with the associated emotions.

The belief that distress is an inevitable part of cancer disease and its treatments and consequently is understandable by everyone may explain also the reluctance. Finally, the belief or experience that nothing can be done about disclosed concerns is another factor that negatively affects communication.

Use of Denial and Avoidance

Particular reactions of patients to their diagnosis, treatment, or prognosis may limit the opportunity for open communication. Some people use denial when facing a threat; others may repress or suppress their affects. A third group will use active avoidance of expected threat and discomfort.

Denial, repression, and avoidance of threatening situations partially or totally prevents realistic, and thus painful, awareness of the situation and its implications. In a laboratory study, increased anxiety was observed in personalities labeled as repressors when relevant information concerning the experiment were transmitted to them and a decrease in anxiety when irrelevant information was given. The opposite process was seen in individuals described as sensitive: they were hypervigilant to anxiety-producing stimuli, using intellectualization and control as the main defense mechanisms.[14] These findings illustrate the diversity of individual responses to different types of information. In oncological practice, the same variations of behavior can be found in patients who are naturally anxious: frequent dissatisfaction with transmitted information that is considered insufficient, and greater use of alternative medicines, which probably give more global answers despite uncertainties.[15] Nevertheless, certain alternative medicines favor denial rather than control, emphasizing emotional support to the detriment of providing realistic information and/or administering active treatment. Factors influencing communication are summarized in TABLE 1.

TABLE 1. Factors Influencing Communication

Variables inherent to senders	
	What is known?
	What decision has been made about transmitting?
	What is said/unsaid?
	How is it said?
Variables inherent to receivers	
	What is already known?
	What is requested?
	What is heard?
	What is retained?
	What is integrated?
Variables inherent to content	
	Nature of the disease
	Prognosis and evolution
	Treatments/side effects
	Psychosocial consequences

NOTE: Sender and receiver can be either patient or health care professional.

KEY SKILLS FOR BETTER COMMUNICATION

Some abilities are fundamental to good communication, whether it be breaking bad news or eliciting patients' needs and concerns. These skills include listening, empathy, response to cues, and appropriate use of reassurance.

Listening

First of all, listening gives the health professional a reference point to evaluate the problems, perceptions, needs, and personal resources of the patient. Listening is a very difficult task for physicians, who are primarily inclined to action. Moreover, in medical education, the art of listening is not adequately taught. Listening is facilitated by using techniques that encourage the patient to express himself (calm attitude, the possibility of silence, etc.). In can be usefully integrated into the process of evaluating the patient's need for information. This process must include an assessment of what the patient already knows and what he wishes to know. After the transmission of information, listening also allows one to check if the new information has been understood.[16]

Empathy

Listening requires an empathic attitude that makes it possible to create confidence between the patient and his physician, and to obtain information concerning the emotions and perceptions of the patient. Empathy, however, must be conceptually differentiated from sympathy and identification with the patient and, of course, must be used in an appropriate way to suit the numerous clinical situations encountered.[17]

Response to Cues

Precise identification and assessment of the patient's problems are essential and constitute the first phase of active support. It enables health professionals to understand patients' feelings and to anticipate (if possible) their future reactions. The attention given by health professionals to present and future problems helps the patient in his own assessment of the situation. This helps avoid confusion and distress, which are frequent consequences of a loss of control over poorly assessed outside events. A physician-assisted reevaluation of meanings associated with reality often enables the patient to regain control.

Recognition of the patient's experience in a climate of understanding enables the patient to feel less alienated and to consider his experience in a temporal perspective. It is not unusual for patients to see their experience as dissociated from time, giving it a never-ending dimension. Finally, the carers may mention the existence of interventions (medical, psychological, social) that may help the patient deal with problems or adapt to situations, or they may generate alternative solutions that help support patients in their readjustment efforts.

Reassurance

Reassurance is an important component of support. Reassuring patients takes place at two levels: on the one hand, by introducing outside resources—for example, the possibility of responding to an experimental treatment; and on the other hand internal resources—for example, the capacity of controlling anxiety.

The failure of reassurance may also occur in situations arising more and more frequently in preventive and curative medicine, especially because diagnostic and therapeutic techniques have made it possible to recognize and treat patients at an asymptomatic stage. Painful and/or mutilating surgery is often necessary when patients subjectively do not feel ill. Preventive and curative medicine in certain cases can thus be perceived as a source of pain and suffering rather than what it often was before, a source of relief from suffering. The repercussions of this situation for the patient and his relatives have not been studied systematically. A possible consequence of this development is the growing success of "unorthodox" medicine in the last few years, systematically opposed to "scientific" medicine, which is presented as technological and aggressive. Informing and educating patients in these situations must replace too-rapid reassurance.

Reassurance given at other periods can be helpful in avoiding tensions resulting from unjustified fear related to the short-term consequences or evaluation of the disease. Specific phases of the disease determine and require particular reassurance. Reassurance—in the case of long remissions, for example—helps the patient recover physically and psychologically. Information/education about possible symptoms the patient must look out for will help him refrain from dramatizing certain signs not associated with his disease. In the terminal phase of the illness, reassurance plays an essential role, particularly for isolated patients and for those who are understandably distressed. Reassurance in the case of "negative" and "irreversible" disease evolution is not always advised because it does not help prepare the patient to deal with vital, uncontrollable threat.

Another common question in cancer medicine concerns the reassurance of a patient showing hope in the face of a poor prognosis. Hope and optimism, among other reactions, may be a way to cope with the distress caused by cancer and its prognosis. Optimism in these cases is thus either related to denial and/or to a way of living. This optimistic attitude often generates discomfort in families and clinical staff because it contrasts with the distress of other patients who anxiously question their physicians about their uncertain future. If physicians actively and without moderation support this optimism, it is likely to lead to severe distress when evidence of a fatal outcome becomes clear. A certain medical neutrality is, therefore, useful. Hope must be considered as a real "creation" that enables the patient to cope. False reassurances by physicians may lead to the loss of confidence in the medical team, especially when the disease is obviously progressing.

CONCLUSIONS

Can informing a patient be damaging? There are examples of cancer patients who either refused proposed treatments or developed severe psychological reactions (aggressive behavior, anxiety, depression, psychotic state) after having been informed. Some clinicians report that they have never been confronted with these extreme reactions. How can such contradictory experience be reconciled? First of all, such extreme reactions are infrequent in cancer populations. A second explanation is that information may be harmful when given without communication skills and when it is not accompanied by sufficient support.

Good communication is essential in facilitating the best possible adjustment to cancer. For instance, it enables the patient to anticipate problems, assists rehabilitation in patients with curable cancers, and avoids unnecessary distress. For some people, it gives the possibility of preparing for death, which is sometimes more bearable than an uncertain future.

Nowadays medicine in general and oncology in particular are facing an exponential growth of scientific knowledge, generating difficulties in the process of decision making.[18] This context and the changes of attitudes of health professionals in general and physicians in particular in favor of giving patients more complete information require more detailed knowledge of the patient's reaction and need for support. The more information the health care professional gives, the more the patient reacts on a verbal and nonverbal level. These reactions require additional attention from health care professionals with regard to the patient's needs, and increased readiness to offer emotional support.[19] However, it is unrealistic to expect physicians and nurses to give their patients such support and break bad news optimally unless they have been equipped with the necessary skills through training, which is generally still unavailable. There is thus an urgent need to offer training in communication skills.

REFERENCES

1. McIntosh, J. 1974. Processes of communication, information seeking and control associated with cancer: A selective review of the literature. Soc. Sci. Med. **8:** 167–187.
2. Broclain, D., P. Aiach & D. Cebe. 1988. What does "to tell" mean? Doctors' attitudes to informing cancer patients. Cancer J. **2**(2): 53–57.
3. Mount, B. M., A. Jones & A. Patterson. 1974. Death and dying. Attitudes in a teaching hospital. Urology **4:** 27–33.
4. Novack, D. H., R. Plumer, R. L. Smith, H. Ochitill, G. R. Morrow & J. M. Bennett. 1979. Change in physicians' attitudes toward telling the cancer patients. JAMA **241**(9): 897–900.
5. Greenwald, H. P. & M. C. Nevitt. 1982. Physician attitudes toward communication with cancer patients. Soc. Sci. Med. **16:** 591–594.
6. Goldberg, R. J. 1984. Disclosure of information to adult cancer patients: Issues and update. J. Clin. Oncol. **2**(8): 948–955.
7. Manos, N. & J. Christakis. 1980–1981. Attitudes of cancer specialists toward their patients in Greece. Int. J. Psychiatry Med. **10**(4): 305–313.
8. Razavi, D., C. Farvacques & N. Delvaux. 1988. Les soignants face à l'information du patient cancéreux et da sa famille: Une enquête. Rev. Med. Suisse Romande **108:** 127–134.
9. Anderson, J. L. 1982. Evaluation of a practical approach to teaching about communication with terminal cancer patients. J. Med. Educ. **16:** 202–207.
10. Blumenfield, M., N. Levy & D. Kaufman. 1979. Current attitudes of medical

students and house staff toward terminal illness. Gen. Hosp. Psychiatry **1:** 306–310.
11. RAZAVI, D., N. BERGER, S. FRISCH & M. SOURIS. 1982. Les médecins spécialistes hospitaliers et le mourant: Une étude comparative. Psychol. Méd. **14**(6): 895–902.
12. GIVIO (Interdisciplinary Group for Cancer Care Evaluation) Italy. 1986. What doctors tell patients with breast cancer about diagnosis and treatment: Findings from a study in general hospitals. Br. J. Cancer **54:** 319–326.
13. WEISMAN, A. D. & J. W. WORDEN. 1976. The existential plight in cancer: Significance of the first 100 days. Int. J. Psychiatry Med. **7**(1): 1–15.
14. COOK, J. R. 1985. Repression-sensitization and approach-avoidance as predictors of response to a laboratory stressor. J. Pers. Soc. Psychol. **49:** 759–773.
15. PRUYN, J. F. A., R. M. RIJCKMAN, C. J. M. VAN BRUNSCHOT & H. W. VAN DEN BORNE. 1985. Cancer patients' personality characteristics, physician-patient communication and adoption of the moerman diet. Soc. Sci. Med. **20**(8): 841–847.
16. BILLINGS, J. A. 1985. Sharing bad news. *In* Outpatient Management of Advanced Cancer: 236–259. J. B. Lippincott. Philadelphia, PA.
17. BOOK, H. E. 1988. Empathy: Misconceptions and misuses in psychotherapy. Am. J. Psychiatry **145:** 420–424.
18. FORROW, L., S. A. WARTMAN & D. W. BROCK. 1988. Science, ethics, and the making of clinical decisions. JAMA **259**(21): 3161–3167.
19. GOLDBERG, R. & R. M. TULL. 1983. The Psychosocial Dimensions of Cancer. A Practical Guide for Health Care Providers. The Free Press. New York, NY.

The Relationship with the Cancer Patient

ROBERT FLAMANT

Faculty of Medicine
University of Paris-Sud, and
Institute Gustave-Roussy
39-53 Rue Camille-Desmoulins
Hautes-Bruyeres
94800 Villejuif, France

CANCER IS UNLIKE OTHER ILLNESSES

In spite of tremendous progress made in diagnosis and treatment, cancer continues to instill fear. It is closely related to the image of death and the decay of the body. Cardiovascular disorders, relatively more frequent and with a higher mortality rate, are feared less. Everyone accepts that the heart wears out and one day will stop, but no one accepts being the victim of some kind of monstrous parasite, composed of an anarchy of cells that come to interfere with the balanced order of the human body. In other words, having a deficient heart is looked upon as quite natural. Having cancer is considered to be a malediction and unjust. In addition, we regularly use the word cancer to describe a major disturbance in many nonmedical fields, e.g., social, economic, political.

This fear of cancer falls within the realm of the irrational. To deny it by saying it is illogical is pointless. It must be accepted and taken into account in the relationship between the doctor and the patient. Cancer doctors, especially the younger ones, are not always aware of this need. They are oriented wholly towards diagnosis and treatment, which require increasingly complex technical and scientific skills. It is difficult for them to take into consideration this psychological aspect, which is based on communication. Finally, along with diagnosis and treatment, it is communication between the doctor and the patient that leads to a high quality of healing or of survival.

CANCER IN FRANCE

Much greater emphasis is placed on the above considerations in Latin countries than in Anglo-Saxon countries. Education in France does not prepare the individual to confront illness or to accept death. Cancer is still the illness most feared by the French, in spite of the more recent arrival of

AIDS. It is quite symptomatic that a death is never announced as being the result of cancer, but "following a long illness." Cancer has supplanted tuberculosis as the socially unacceptable illness. A person having suffered from cancer, even once cured, is never regarded by others as having every chance of living.

THERE IS COMMUNICATION IN ANY CASE

The patient does receive communication from the doctor, even if the doctor is not aware of this. For example, the patient carefully observes the reactions of the doctor and the nursing staff and interprets them. A silence or hardening of the doctor's face when reading the results of an examination are given a negative interpretation by the patient. The doctor may lack tact without realizing it. There is nothing worse for a hospitalized terminal-phase patient than seeing the doctor making his rounds without stopping to see him because he no longer has anything to say to him.

Therefore, since communication exists even independently of the doctor's volition, it is better that it be controlled. Communication needs to be active, not merely passive.

Communication is based first on listening to the patient. Only too often the doctor talks without heeding the patient, as if he were afraid to hear him. It is psychologically easier for a doctor to repeat a few stereotyped words, identical from one patient to another, than to adapt his words to the patient's needs.

After listening to him, the doctor must consider the information he wishes to convey to the patient. Contrary to what certain doctors believe, the patient does not want a technical description of his illness. He wants most of all to know if it is serious or not, if the treatment will be long or painful, if he can carry on working. All these questions must be answered, without side-stepping any of them but also without adding to the anxiety. It is not essential, for example, to go into all of the discomforts that may arise during chemotherapy; but the most important ones should be discussed, such as the hair falling out and digestive problems, with emphasis on the medication used to reduce these effects. Information should be given gradually and be expanded on at later interviews. It should be remembered that the patient is already worried. He must not be destabilized; this may cause him to give up the fight completely. Every patient has a limit to the amount of information he can absorb at a given time, and this should not be exceeded. Special emphasis should be placed on explaining the current stage of therapy so that he is forewarned of what is going to happen to him. Giving all of the information at once is pointless: it is too sudden, and the patient will not remember it all.

Written and illustrated documents may help when giving information, but again we should make no mistake as to the patient's degree of attentiveness. He will not read them with as open a mind as he would if he were reading a scientific magazine and were in good health. Sometimes, contact with a patient who has already begun treatment may prove more effective than long discussions and the use of audiovisual resources.

The informed consent that is signed by a patient beginning a clinical trial is inspired more by legal than by ethical considerations. A patient who knows he is suffering from cancer is not capable of logical reasoning in order to give a cognizant consent to a clinical trial. He should therefore be informed and his endorsement obtained, but with tact, gradually and without adding to his anxiety.

The impact of the information given should be assessed and, where necessary, the information should be reiterated or corrected. In effect, there are often differences between what the doctor means and what the patient understands and remembers. The doctor and the nursing staff should therefore ensure that the patient has understood what he has been told and, if need be, provide him with the information he is missing.

SHOULD WE TELL THE TRUTH?

The question of whether to tell patients the truth is particularly pertinent in cancer treatment. Many discussions have been held on the subject from various aspects: ethical, philosophical, religious, and, of course, medical. Positions vary, and in certain cases this leads to controversy.

Telling the truth on any subject is a normally accepted necessity. In justice, we are asked to swear to tell the truth. This is the only means of determining the guilty and acquitting the innocent. We can only surmise that the truth must be told whenever necessary. For a patient with cancer, hiding the nature of his illness from him may lead him to neglect treatment. On the other hand, if the patient knows that his doctor always tells him the truth, a relationship of confidence may be established, and he will not suspect the doctor of "hiding something" from him. Cases are known of persons with a phobia about cancer not believing the doctor even after he has established that their cancer tests had proved negative. We should therefore act in order to preserve the patient's confidence in the doctor, and telling the truth is a good way of doing so.

But telling patients the truth is a principle that involves complex practical aspects. Should we tell the whole truth about the type of cancer and its prognosis? Should we tell everything immediately when revealing the diagnosis? We can see that there is a whole range of attitudes from which the doctor has to choose.

Optimally, the doctor should not have a basic attitude that he systematically applies in all cases. On the contrary, he should vary his behavior on the basis of the degree of receptivity of the patient before him. The aim is to avoid increasing the anxiety of the patient excessively when he suspects he has cancer. More often than not, it is preferable to inform him about the type of cancer in stages. For example, the first positive effects of treatment could be awaited before announcing that the cancer is of a serious nature.

This measured attitude, adapted to each patient, is not subscribed to by the dogmatic partisans of truth at all costs. Their reasoning is based on a philosophical principle: respect for human dignity means the patient must be told the truth in all circumstances. This is a noble principle established by healthy persons who are unaware of what their reaction will be the day they themselves suffer from a serious illness. There are numerous examples in which ardent defenders of the truth when fit and healthy cannot face the truth when they fall ill themselves. The mere idea of having cancer deeply alters an individual's personality. He no longer reacts as he used to since what had previously been a subject for intellectual discussion viewed from the outside has become a source of affective reaction experienced from the inside.[1]

Only the doctor with his own human sensitivity can assess the best conditions in terms of time and means in order to gradually conduct the patient towards satisfactory knowledge of his illness. It is for this reason that there is such a variation among doctors, some of whom are manifestly more capable than others of bringing the patient to accepting the truth. This skill is independent of the doctor's technical and scientific skills. It is difficult to teach this skill except within the context of the practical training a student receives in his daily contact with a senior doctor.

COMMUNICATION WITH THE PATIENT'S RELATIVES

Communication with the patient's relatives is important, as they can help him appreciably in enduring his ordeal. This is particularly so, of course, where the patient suffering from cancer is a child. It is through the mother that most of the information is passed on to the child, which nevertheless does not mean the doctor cannot communicate directly with the patient. But the relationship is three cornered: pediatrician, mother, and child; the essential factor is harmony. This is a considerable help to the doctor, as dialogue with the parents, as healthy adults, is sometimes much easier for the practician. Furthermore, the father and mother are in the best position to break any bad news to the child.

When the patient is an adult, communication is more often through the husband or wife. It requires great sensitivity on the part of the doctor to first of all assess the relational situation between the patient and the spouse. The situation in which the anxiety of the spouse adds to that of the patient must be avoided. It is especially when the person close to the patient proves to be of the right caliber that it is to the doctor's advantage to use him or her as an intermediary in order to break any bad news.

In all cases, communication with the relatives is the doctor's duty, and he should not try to have this done by anyone else. He will need to find the time necessary, and this is another of the keys to success along with diagnosis and treatment. Communication with the patient and his relatives is an integral part of the care that a doctor should give his patient.

THE ROLE OF THE NURSING AND SUPPORT STAFF

The role of the nursing staff and auxiliaries, including secretaries and medical auxiliaries, such as physiotherapists, is by no means negligible. Patients often spend more time with them than with the doctors and feel more at ease in asking them questions. It is therefore essential that these personnel know what the doctor has said in order to converse along the same lines. It is very bad when they do not know how to answer or contradict what has previously been said. This adds disorientation and suspicion to the patient's anxiety, damaging his morale. Here again, it is the doctor's duty to work in close cooperation with his medical team and to take the time to keep them informed.

INVOLUNTARY COMMUNICATION

Involuntary communication consists of the attitudes that the doctor or nursing staff may have without taking measure of all their consequences. It often happens that the patient observes the doctor while he is engrossed in a technical matter. This happens, for example, when the doctor receives the results of tests or looks at an X-ray plate. The doctor should control his reactions, as he is being spied upon by the patient. By the same token, he should refrain from making comments of a technical nature to another doctor in the presence of the patient. The patient will interpret the slightest sign, and the degree of error will be proportional to the insufficiency of communication with the doctor.

On the other hand, a strong, relaxed attitude on the part of the surgeon prior to an operation may be perceived as very reassuring by the patient. Here again, this is a lesson in self-control that the doctor should learn. It is practically never taught in medical schools, where everything is restricted to the technical and the scientific. This gap needs to be filled. Improving the results of cancer treatment in terms of healing is not enough. The quality of life of the patients healed or in remission can also be improved at the human level.

CONCLUSION

The more complex the treatment of cancer becomes, leading to better results, the more essential is improved communication between the doctor and patient, as this is the only guarantee of being healed in terms of morale. There is currently a dissociation between improvement in the rate of survival and the increasing feeling of patients' dissatisfaction with doctors. This could even lead to the bringing law suits not founded on the technical quality of care. The only way to overcome this major difficulty is to treat the relationship with the patient with the same degree of importance as the technical aspects of diagnosis and treatment.

First, young doctors should be trained to be not merely good technicians or scientists. Training can be theoretical, but should above all be practical. Second, the relationship with the patient should be incorporated into medical practice and the time necessary for it set aside in the doctor's schedule. This means allowing time not only for technical matters but for communication as well.

Third, the effectiveness of the communication should be assessed with equal attention to that given to assessing the technical effectiveness of treatment. This assessment is accomplished mainly by questioning the patients. Experiments may be used to compare the different methods of communication in order to select the most effective ones.

Finally, cancer doctors need to adopt a new attitude. After the revolution some twenty years ago that brought a scientific dimension into the training and practice of cancer doctors, the new human relationship dimension should be added. This consists of excellent communication between the cancer doctor and his team on the one hand, and the patient and his relatives on the other.

Insofar as cancer treatment is increasingly successful, surviving and healed patients should be helped to achieve a comfortable standard of living. Communication between the doctor and the nursing team with the patient and his relatives is of prime importance, is on the same plane as the technical and scientific aspects of treatment. Its aim must be to tell patients the truth, but gradually, in a manner adapted to each patient, taking care not to exceed the person's capacity to receive it.

REFERENCE

1. FLAMANT, R. 1994. Malade ou cobaye. Plaidoyer pour les essais therapeutiques. (Patient or guinea-pig: The case for clinical trials.) Albin Michel. Paris.

Straight Talking about Cancer

Duty or Danger?

ROLF VERRES

Abteilung Psychotherapie und Medizinische Psychologie
Psychosomatische Klinik
Ruprecht-Karls-Universität Heidelberg
Bergheimer Strasse 20
69115 Heidelberg, Germany

This chapter is about the ways in which we face up to things that threaten our lives. Risks and dangers have the power to make us afraid. But if we see them as a challenge they can also enhance our awareness and represent a source of greater personal courage and self-confidence. By at least making the tentative attempt to face up squarely to some of the risks we run in our everyday lives, we may ultimately achieve a clearer picture of who we are.

Our lives are prone to all kinds of unpredictable illnesses and accidents. Cancer, whether as a risk or a reality, is no more important than the other dangers we are exposed to. But the effect it has on people's lives is particularly well documented. In my fifteen years as a physician and medical psychologist, I have made a special study of the physical and psychological aspects of cancer prevention, cancer detection, cancer conditions and their treatment and have come to the conclusion that we can live our lives more intensively by facing up to the specific threat posed by cancer and actively improving our knowledge of what it implies, rather than closing our eyes to it. Squaring up to the antithesis of life can teach us a great deal about life itself.

The cancer phenomenon is a paradoxical one. Unlike normal cells in the body, cancer cells proliferate wildly, their growth is rampant, uncontrolled, seemingly unstoppable and it is precisely this that makes them potentially so deadly. They threaten the very order of the human organism and with it the entire person whose body they are assailing.

In my experience of people forced to come to terms with the existential threat that cancer represents, I have witnessed a great deal of fear and despair, but also hope and courage, not only in cancer patients themselves but in their families, their loved ones and also in the doctors and medical staff taking care of them. When I myself have been affected by these feelings in all their intensity, I have frequently asked myself: "Why have I concentrated my research as a doctor and psychologist on cancer and the fear it causes, rather than on something more positive and life-affirming?" It took me a long time to realize how much awareness of the value of life and the art of living can be derived from the personal encounter with cancer sufferers by allowing the fear of death as much room in one's own personal experience as the will to live, and by consciously withstanding the collision between these two extreme perspectives on life, wherever and however they may present themselves.

Many people have a marked instinctive resistance to thinking about what it would be like if cancer were to break into their lives. They feel they know for sure what the consequences would be—despair, suffering, death.

Thinking about this eventuality does indeed require courage. It is probable that a multitude of cancer cells form in our bodies every day. Some cancer experts believe that, within hitherto undefined limits, our immune system can deal with them without our noticing anything at all.

Thus it may be a salutary experience for each of us to reflect on the need for medical guidance on personal health questions that we have in the present stages of our lives. This will make us better able—in the event of such a doctor-patient exchange—to codetermine the course that such an exchange should take. Anyone seeking guidance on how to come to terms with a potentially fatal illness may be well advised to reflect on his own attitude towards death and to bear in mind that the people he talks to on this subject (e.g., his physician) will themselves be bringing their own (preconceived) notions into that encounter.

A reliable guide in this connection is Philippe Aries. In his *Studies on the History of Death in the West* he distinguishes four phases in the development of our attitudes towards death[1]:

Familiarity, or the "taming" of death: In the first thousand years A.D., Aries detects a widespread familiarity, not to say companionability, in human attitudes towards death. Apart from wars and accidents, it was part and parcel of the dying process to prepare oneself consciously for it. In death scenes in the literature of this period, we frequently find death being anticipated by a species of existential premonition. Wolfram von Eschenbach speaks of this "clairvoyance about our own end" as an important prerequisite enabling the dying to make their final arrangements and give themselves over to a death ritual where they were both the focus of interest and "master of ceremonies." In almost all cases children were allowed to approach the deathbed. This ritualization made dying a relatively straightforward affair, providing a species of emotional neutralization (what Aries calls "taming") and incorporating it, by virtue of a relatively public leave taking, into the familiar routines of everyday life.

Personalization: From about the 11th/12th century onwards, the significance of taking stock, of looking back over one's life became more marked, not least in connection with an altered view of the "Last Judgment." Received religious thinking now taught that the salvation of the soul was not decided at the end of time but immediately after a person's death. The unsparing, uncompromising deathbed retrospective on life was seen as the way of achieving the highest possible awareness of one's own self.

Spectatorship: Between the 16th and the early 18th centuries, Aries detects an increasing dramatization of death. There is a desire to experience death as something impressive and hence to "have a part" in it. This increasing dramatization is accompanied by a greater tendency to experience death as "happening to other people." Death is now interpreted more as a "curtailment," and acceptance of it becomes correspondingly more resentful.

Banishment: With the onset of the 20th century human attitudes towards death change in an almost revolutionary manner. In the course of a few decades familiarity turns into banishment. This goes hand in hand with a new tendency to "spare" the dying, which is synonymous with keeping the truth away from both the dying person and his immediate family. This increasing trend towards declaring death "out of bounds" is mirrored in the conviction that children should be "spared" the sight of the dying.

Today, at least two further widespread attitudes towards death have established themselves:

Abstraction: As the 20th century comes to an end, death and dying—as Wolfram Eberbach puts it—have been "dis-emotionalized and divested of their taboo status."[2] With the increasing impact of the mass media, death is constantly being scrutinized and scientifically analyzed from all points of view. Much attention is given to controversies revolving around decisions of fundamental importance such as whether mercy covenants (interventionist or noninterventionist) can ever be justified, whether—given the increasing sophistication of medical technology—life must invariably be prolonged at all costs. etc.

The "pornography" of death: To my mind, it cannot be seriously maintained that in our society death is still a taboo subject. I would prefer to speak of *alienation*. The action and horror films shown in cinemas and lent out by video shops dwell with gloating, pornographic insistence on scenes of killing and death, while the so-called news sections of newspapers, magazines, and television programs display scenes of violent death in such minute and horrifying detail that readers and viewers are first sickened and then, after continuing overexposure, finally lapse into a state of apathy and stupor. Fears that this will have a lasting effect on the way people experience, think, and talk about death are only too justified. I am convinced that this widespread pornography of death makes it more difficult for people to come to appropriate terms with the fact of their own mortality.

However simplistic and black-and-white the above classification of attitudes towards death may appear, there is surely no denying the subliminal effect they will have on the way people talk about fatal illness. This applies equally to doctor-patient encounters. In such situations, the doctor is unfortunately conceded a greater degree of control over the proceedings than the patient. For the latter this means that the doctor's own personal attitude towards existential risks, dying, and death will be the operative factor determining the extent to which a sincere and helpful exchange can take place. Only a doctor willing to accept death in all its consequences will be in a position to talk credibly about the possibilities of prolonging the patient's life and the limits imposed on them. A doctor who is unable to accept death and goes on fighting with all the means at his disposal even when the fatal illness has clearly triumphed runs the risk of tormenting his patients rather than helping them.

At this point I should like to introduce a term that will be central to my argument: health education. In Germany, where I come from, the word generally used for this is *Aufklärung*, which literally means "enlightenment."

The late 17th century in Europe saw the first flowerings of an epoch in the age of ideas which we refer to today as the Age of Enlightenment. In the literature and philosophy of that period much thought was devoted to the question of how, by the exercise of his powers of reason, Man could be "liberated from his own self-inflicted lack of autonomy," as Immanuel Kant put it.

The optimistic faith in Reason and Progress made great strides, and many highly sophisticated ideas were put forward as to how, via a broad education, each and every individual could have instilled in him a self-determined and genuinely human approach to his dealings with himself, with others, and with Nature. This was tantamount to inquiring how he could best be instructed in a liberal and autonomous use of his faculties of reason and securely provided with a sound fund of knowledge.

I should like to draw upon this concept of "enlightenment"—one which inspired generations of thinkers and writers and, thanks to its universalist claims, had a profound effect on all spheres of social life, including medicine—as a yardstick by which to measure the present conception that we have of *Aufklärung* in terms of the information and (interpersonal) guidance offered to patients in the highly technological world of modern medical care. To put it bluntly, what we encounter in reality is but a shadow of what an "enlightened"—and truly enlightening—approach to patient education could look like. My intention here is not, however, to pillory this state of affairs but rather to analyze the reasons for it and thus, it is hoped, contribute to an improvement.

When we speak of doctor-patient information, interaction, or guidance in modern medicine, what we are usually referring to is the narrow question of to what extent and in what way a doctor should reveal to a person that he is ill and that certain measures are going to be necessary to treat him for his condition. Both in the medical community and in the general public, debate on the principles and informative value of such doctor-patient encounters has on occasion been heated. Legal experts have been called in to further define, standardize, and tighten up the requirements that medical care and the guidelines on medical documentation have to satisfy.

At present, the way we look at this question is far too clinical in its bias, centering almost exclusively around the fundamental question "How much do we tell them?" Thus medical information has gradually come to be looked upon almost exclusively as the "bad news" imparted to a patient about his illness, usually in circumstances placing a considerable strain on all concerned.

What we need here, throughout our entire health system, is a much broader conception of what education on medical matters should be. People should not have to wait until they fall ill to be told how they can best use their faculties of reason to minimize the risks they run by the simple fact of living. This is something that should be conveyed to them throughout their lives by medical experts who are just as concerned to preserve health as they are to cure illnesses. But where does one find such experts?

One of the most striking features of the sources of general information about prevention, detection, treatment, and consequences of cancer is that hardly any effort has been undertaken to make the highly specialized expert knowledge on the subject available in an integrated, easy-to-understand form. There is a need here for initiatives and institutions setting out to provide this kind of integrated information.

For the nonmedical public it is extremely difficult to obtain well-substantiated, ordered information on these questions, although they are obviously of vital importance. There appears to be an invisible but highly effective political lobby putting up resistance to genuinely preventive medicine and the unhindered flow of information on health and sickness.

Although nearly one person in four gets cancer in some form or other and almost everybody is confronted with this topic by contact with cancer sufferers, young people at school are told next to nothing about this phenomenon and most adults have to rely on the mass media for their information. Also, as can be expected in a society like ours, differences in the degree of access to well-presented information on this point are, of course, very much a function of a person's educational status.

Medical psychologists Fritz Muthny and Michael Bechtel have analyzed the coverage of medical issues in major German news magazines.[3] Certain of these magazines (*Stern* and *Spiegel*) tended to associate chronic illnesses such as cancer with factors like aggression, personal troubles, and suspicion on the part of the sufferers. By contrast, a magazine with a different kind of readership *(Neue Illustrierte)* emphasized more positive emotions—relief, happiness and hope. In general, *Spiegel* and *Stern*, both of which cater to an educated audience, were more accurate, critical, and reflective in their reporting. But members of the better-educated classes also frequently succumb to the morbid fascination of the tabloid style when it comes down to questions of life or death. Day in and day out, these papers cater to the lust for sensation in their readers, causing sheer informational havoc in the process.

In the drawer of the bedside table of a clerk who had died from the effects of prostate cancer, his family found a thick wad of carefully collected press cuttings. Here is a selection of the headlines to these articles: The Big Fear of the Cancer Test; Smoking and Alcohol—the Deadly Duo; Beech and Oak Cause Cancer; Blood from Ring Finger Shows Cancer Risk; Merciless Therapeutic Overkill; Magic Marbles Defeat Cancer; Laughter Good For AIDS and Cancer; Sedentary Workers Prone to Colorectal Cancer; Why Sunlight Stymies Colorectal Cancer; Overweight? Watch Out for Ovarian Cancer!; Dieting Encourages Tumors; Poverty Makes Cancer More Likely; Love Prevents Cancer; Marriage Protects You Against Cancer; Psychic Features Indicate Risk of Cancer and Heart Attack; Sawdust Causes Cancer of the Nose; Our Daily Poison; Doctors Fail the Communication Test; Cancer Therapy: Have They Been Cooking the Statistics?; The Sick Become Sicker; Pill Increases Breast Cancer Risk; Breast Cancer Not Caused by Pill; Unhappy Women More Prone to Breast Cancer; Breast Cancer: Cry Your Fears Away!; The Hackethal Case: Feel My Breast—The Cancer's Gone!; Mind Over Cancer!; Does Our Outlook on Life Have an Effect on Cancer?

I have spent hours thinking about what went on in the head of this man as he tried to make sense of this pseudoinformation in a situation full of fear, uncertainty, and hope. In all those weeks he spent in hospital he had plenty of time to think things over. He did not even tell the doctors looking after him that the pain had become unbearable and that even methadone was no longer sufficient to deal with it. Instead he rang me up and although I lived 400 kilometers away and had no part in the treatment he was receiving, it was to me that he turned with his request for higher doses of methadone. He said if he asked the doctor in the hospital, the doctor might see this as a criticism and turn against him. As we all found out when it was too late, he had tried to satisfy his need for information by collecting newspaper articles. But here, as elsewhere, the information purveyed by the tabloids is a farrago of garbled facts.

The confusing and inconsistent information spread by sensationalist journalism has its consequences. What, for example, must an obese person feel like when he opens his newspaper and a headline screams at him: "Fat People More Likely to Get Cancer"? What goes on in the mind of someone fond of the sun (like most of us, presumably) when they read "Sunshine Causes Skin Cancer"; and then get told elsewhere how important ultraviolet light is for vitamin D production; and two days later see the headline "Sun Stops Colorectal Cancer"? These half-truths haunt some people like evil spirits. They cause fear and provide nothing in the way of guidance.

Information from the mass media on dangerous illnesses is felt by most people to be confused, unpleasant, and contradictory. So why do so many people stand for it, considering that such illnesses can strike at any time and that proper information on prevention, at least, can be a life-saver? Do people want to be informed or entertained? Can we really only have one without the other?

At this juncture I should like to go into some detail. The present restrictive view of patient education written into our health systems can be illustrated by the following quote taken from the *Ärzteblatt Baden-Württemberg* (Baden-Württemberg Medical Gazette):

> The responsible adult patient, who is sound in mind and in possession of his faculties of reason, must be given the following 'safety and diagnosis information'. He must be told: the diagnosis (diagnoses) and the results of the medical examination; what is going to happen to him (a) generally, (b) in concrete terms (medication), (c) in terms of the risks (e.g., psychoactive drugs) and consequences (e.g., post-hospital care) involved; what alternatives there are (if any) to the proposed course of action.
>
> Once these questions have been answered, the doctor has satisfied the contractual obligations incumbent upon him vis-à-vis the patient at this stage, and the patient can exercise his right of self-determination.[4]

The doctor tells the patient *what is going to happen to him.* But does he also help him to find out *what the patient himself can do?*

When in 1985 the *Bundesärztekammer* (Federal German Medical Society) and the *Deutsche Krankenhausgesellschaft* (Association of German Hospitals) published their "Recommendations for Guidelines on Informing Hospital Patients about Proposed Medical Care" in the *Deutsches Ärzteblatt* (Federal Medical Gazette),[5] the reason they gave for elaborating these recommendations was that there had been a steep increase in *compensation lawsuits* against hospital authorities for failing to ensure that patients were given the requisite medical information. This phenomenon had thus made it necessary to revise the existing *Instructions for Medical Staff* in their present form and thus achieve a more standardized approach.

Obviously, nobody will deny the necessity of averting compensation lawsuits. But in the wording quoted above we see a definite tendency to reduce the broad, comprehensive view of medical information and education to comply with a legalistic, bureaucratic mentality where the doctor is constantly on the defensive, hemmed in by "instructions," which he ignores at his (legal) peril. The upshot is a minimalist approach to patient information limited to telling him *what is going to happen to him.* "Enlightening" the patient with a view to enabling him to decide what he himself intends to do in the given situation is obviously a minor priority compared with getting him to agree to the course of treatment lined up for him by the doctor.

Medical students at the university are given little or no opportunity to prepare themselves for patient education as one of the tasks awaiting them as doctors. In isolated cases voluntary student groups or individual professors may address the question. But even when the topic is tabled in seminars on medical ethics or occasionally at medical congresses, discussion will almost invariably revolve around the question of cases in which doctors (and patients) are freed from the obligation to inform (and be informed). This is generally felt to be the case when information on the diagnosis would in all probability actually aggravate the patient's condition—i.e., the patient would be unable to come to terms with what the doctor discloses to him. In such cases the courts will usually concede to the doctor the right to a "compassionate lie." The legal criteria governing this decision will, however, differ somewhat in almost all countries of the world.

In our clinical practice both my staff and myself have frequently noted that patients will praise a certain Dr. X. for being frank and honest. On closer inspection we have found that such statements almost always refer to colleagues who have reassured the patients in question in tones of unassailable confidence. "We'll soon have you back on your feet," they say, or "We're in the driving seat on this one, you have no cause for concern." Behind the scenes, however, the doubts sometimes outweigh the credibility.

Only rarely is a doctor commended for his honesty when he says things like "Your life expectancy is not very high." And hardly any patient will have the fortitude to welcome the statement "We have exhausted the medical possibilities of halting the disease" as an indication of laudable integrity on the doctor's part.

Younger doctors are frequently criticized by patients for being vague and nebulous about the further course of the illness in question. It appears that over time older doctors develop more convincing strategies in their dealings with patients. The paternal/maternal aura disseminated by older physicians can frequently convey a sense of security, even when the statements they make to patients are ambivalent. The essential thing for the patient is that there should be recognizable grounds for optimism. In doctor-patient explanation it may thus be that information is not all-important. Feelings obviously play an equally significant role.

Frequently, part of the temptation that physicians may feel to impart the necessary information to patients in terms that are vague, not to say downright euphemistic, derives from the patients themselves. It would thus be entirely erroneous to put the entire blame on the doctors for the unsatisfactory medical information situation that exists. Patients, too, bear a responsibility for what they are told or not told in interviews with their doctors.

This brings us to the question of whether one can have a clear conscience about advising patients to insist that their doctor give them the "whole truth" about their condition, the course it is likely to take, and the chances they have of recovering. Experience suggests that people's desire for complete honesty on this point decreases proportionally to the extent to which they themselves are personally involved. A sensitive physician will perhaps be able to "read" the questions put to him by the patient and decide on that basis whether total frankness on the nature of the malignant disease he has diagnosed is truly desired or not. Almost every physician finds himself in moral conflicts of this kind at one time or another. Some doctor-patient couples develop ambiguity and inference to a fine art. This requires a high degree of sensitivity on both sides if indirectness is not to degenerate into mere nebulosity and consequent misunderstandings.

As the 20th century comes to an end we also encounter some perverted forms of patient guidance. One such is the proposed use of standardized videotapes to lighten the information burden resting on the shoulders of doctors. The scenario is a horrific one. A female patient who has just been told that she has breast cancer has a video recorder wheeled into her room. A film describes the various forms that breast cancer can take, the various kinds of surgery and postsurgical treatment, including side effects and complications (risks), and closing perhaps with a whole series of women reassuring the viewer that they all got over it without too much trouble and that cancer can be an opportunity . . . .

Fortunately the German *Ärztekammer* has clearly signaled its rejection of this kind of mechanization. This rejection is squarely based on the realization that any kind of "counseling" that does not take into account the specifics of the individual case and the personality of the patient is by definition highly dubious. True, surveys have revealed that most patients desire "unambiguous information on the diagnosis in the case of an incurable condition." But it is doubtful whether such methods can reliably reflect the needs of patients in a situation that cuts so deeply into their lives and personalities. Of course, as a preparation for certain kinds of therapy (say the insertion of an artificial anus) a video film may indeed represent an acceptable aid for some patients, always provided that it is used as a supplement to the personal exchange between doctor and patient and that the patient is given the opportunity to ask questions.

It is by no means rare for persons who—as long as they are healthy—insist that they want to be told the whole truth if they should fall ill to change their minds on this point *after* the onset of illness. When faced with a dangerous disease, doctors themselves are not necessarily an exception. It may indeed be inhuman to force a person to face up to the knowledge of his own inevitable death, thus plunging him into a state of despair. Information and guidance, properly understood, should be a gradual process, taking full account of the needs and fears of the patient and also his level of education and his ability to cope with what he is being told. The question of the right way of going about this is bound to differ from case to case.

In clinical terms, medical information for patients is designed ultimately to assure the ongoing principle of self-determination subsequent to the onset of illness. A patient must not only be advised about *what is going to happen to him,* he must also receive counseling about *what he himself can do.* Before initiating therapeutic measures it is incumbent upon the physician to provide the patient with information of three different kinds. Ernst Wolf, one of the judges at the Regional Appeal Court in Munich, summarizes the present legal situation in Germany in connection with obligatory information for cancer patients as follows[6]:

Information on the diagnosis: Here a certain degree of vagueness is permissible. Words like "cancer" or "carcinoma" do not have to be uttered by the physician. If the condition diagnosed is terminal beyond all doubt and not even palliative measures are available to alleviate the symptoms, the doctor may either clothe the diagnosis in more indirect terms or even keep it from the patient altogether.

Information on the course of the illness: This is a description of the probable course that the illness will take without treatment and with the proposed treatment.

Information on risks: This aspect of patient orientation has to do with the dangers and the temporary or permanent effects of the course of treatment proposed by the physician, even though the greatest possible care is exercised in administering it. In the treatment of cancer, in particular, the side effects and subsequent impairments can be so substantial that the patient must be informed of them before deciding whether to consent to the treatment.

Drawing upon years of experience at the Regional Court of Appeal in Munich, Ernst Wolf paints a "discouraging picture" of what doctor-patient communication looks like in reality:

> Is it because patients frequently do not understand the language used by doctors? Is it because such interviews have a statistical average length of 3.5 minutes? Do doctors really have too little time to inform their patients properly? Or do the nature and duration of such exchanges genuinely reflect the attitude of doctors and their annoyance at having to do something that they consider to be the domain of the courts, compounded with discomfiture at having to admit that there are limits to what medical science can do? Is it because doctors are unshakably convinced that whatever they do will by definition be for the good of the patient? Is it perhaps the fears of the patient that make it so difficult for him to understand what he is being told?[6]

In a study of almost 500 surgery patients, Höfer and Streicher came up with findings verging on the devastating. After doctor-patient information sessions, only 18% of the patients had correctly understood the risks and dangers of their condition and the operation they would be undergoing; only 49% could remember that this topic had been talked about and had understood that the operation was "necessary and involved risks"; the other third either had no memory at all of what they had been told or a completely inaccurate one.

Today, it is not only physicians and law experts who take an intensive interest in information and guidance for cancer patients. Medical psychologists are equally concerned. However, according to the 7th *Approbationsordnung* (Regulations on Medical Training) for physicians, only 4.5% of the obligatory classes in the preclinical stage of medical studies are devoted to medical psychology, while in the clinical curriculum psychology disappears almost totally except in connection with the genesis of psychosomatic and psychiatric disorders. Thus budding doctors obviously have too little opportunity to acquire skills in patient care of the psychological variety.

Clinical counseling of this kind should not be regarded in all-or-nothing terms. What is needed is a gradual concerted attempt on the part of doctor and patient to find common ground in terms of language and a basis for mutual sincerity. Hans-Jörg Senn is a specialist in internal medicine treating cancer patients at the Canton Hospital in St. Gallen (Switzerland). He has made a study of those cases where sincerity does *not* take place.[7] On the medical side a number of reasons are typically advanced for *not* being frank and sincere to tumor patients. Unflinching honesty, it is said, will have detrimental effects. The patient must be protected by concealment of the facts or compassionate lies. Another factor felt by physicians to play an important role is the level of education and maturity of the patients involved. They fear that young, "uneducated," and elderly patients will have particular difficulty coming to terms with matter-of-fact disclosures about a dangerous or fatal condition. Many doctors are also apprehensive about the likelihood of suicide among informed cancer patients, feeling that it is sufficient to put the immediate family in the picture and leave it at that. This, of course, has the added advantage of being less difficult.

The important thing is that the doctor should be self-critical enough to ask himself who it is that he is protecting by holding back unpleasant information. Is it really because he thinks the patient may not be able to take it? Or is he perhaps protecting himself as well? In-depth studies on tumor patients aware of their condition have demonstrated that on average the percentage of suicide candidates is no higher here than it is in the rest of the population.

The following arguments can be adduced *in favor of* frankness and sincerity vis-à-vis patients with so-called malignant disorders. Disinformation and half-truths can isolate the patient. If nobody knows what the patient has been told, everyone involved with him will tend to avoid further discussion of the case, thus depriving themselves of the opportunity of learning more about it. Evasion becomes the order of the day. It becomes more difficult for doctors and nursing staff looking after that patient to concert their efforts. Insincerity leads to a loss of credibility and ultimately forfeits the trust between patient and doctor that is so essential to a therapeutic alliance. Patients are cheated of valuable living time. They are deprived of the opportunity of putting their affairs in order, retaining full autonomy via comprehensive information, and coming to terms with the new demands made on them in terms of personal maturity and the ability to "let go." Only an "enlightened" patient in possession of the requisite information appropriately imparted and acting on a true understanding of his condition can assume his rightful share of the responsibility for the decisions to be made in such a situation.

Hans-Jörg Senn has collected statements made retrospectively by tumor patients who had been poorly advised on their condition (if at all).[7] Here are some examples:

> I think my doctor was afraid of me. He never let me get a word in the whole time I was in his office, and after that he avoided me.
>
> I felt like some kind of leper or pariah. There was a lot of whispering with my family, and people were generally evasive.
>
> My G.P. thinks I don't know I have cancer. I don't want to bother him with that as well; that's why I prefer to talk to you about it, here in the hospital.
>
> Why wasn't I told much earlier? I've been done out of an important part of my life.

According to Karl Jaspers,

> Ideally the relationship between doctor and patient is a relationship between two sensible human beings . . . . Given information by an expert, a sensible person is able and willing to understand, and to act on the basis of what he has understood . . . . The patient is instructed about his condition, knows what is at stake and is prepared to play a constructive role in the conduct of therapy."

Patients should therefore be given a much greater opportunity than before to assume partial responsibility for the degree of "enlightenment" they are to be given. If a new culture of medical information and guidance is to evolve, the responsibility for it cannot rest with the doctors alone. Wolfram Eberbach, a specialist in legal aspects of medical care, sees little need for any further *theorizing* about doctor-patient relations, except perhaps in the "finer points."[2] By contrast he bewails the almost total neglect of the actual situation in which these theories are supposed to be transformed into reality—i.e., the interaction between doctor and patient and the factors operative within that interaction.

In my experience, too many people today give themselves up entirely to the decisions of their doctors, waiting almost humbly for the doctor to dictate what kind of tone the encounter is going to be conducted in—a tone largely determined by the personal convictions and attitudes of the physician involved.

Painstaking and detailed though the thoughts expended by physicians and legal experts may be on how best to "spare" the patient, one extremely important aspect frequently goes by the board. Doctors are often heard to say that they avoid straight talking in their encounters with cancer patients because they would not be able to face up to the truth. With this attitude they are ultimately cementing a far-reaching "dis-enlightenment" of the people placed in their charge, a disinformation that has political dimensions. The real reason why most people cannot take truthful information in this situation is that in their previous experiences of life nobody has ever given them any guidance in facing up to the nature of potentially fatal disease, let alone encouraged them to envisage the likelihood of contracting such a disease themselves. Then, when it happens, the reaction is shock and panic in the patient and the corresponding evasions and euphemisms on the part of the doctor. Looking back on the detection phase after undergoing breast amputation surgery, a 48-year-old woman had this to say:

> I suspected it myself. I thought it was bound to be malignant because it was so big. It was terrible, as if the ground was giving way beneath me, as if I was blacking out—it was awful, that moment.

It is imperative that doctors not wait for this kind of situation to occur before they start being supportive. So-called compassionate lies would in most cases be unnecessary if people in general were given a greater degree of enlightenment about the nature of the risks they run simply by being alive. As things stand at the moment, however, this is a very remote prospect indeed.

REFERENCES

1. Aries, P. 1975. Essais sur l'histoire de la mort du moyen âge à nos jours. Editions du Seuil. Paris.
2. Eberbach, W. H. 1984. Die Aufklärung des Patienten vor dem Hintergrund der Einstellung zum Tod. Medizinrecht **6:** 201–240.
3. Muthny, F. & M. Bechtel. 1988. Chronische körperliche Erkrankungen in der Sicht der Medien. Medizin-Mensch-Gesellschaft **13:** 188–197.
4. Diehl, L. W. 1985. Aufklärung des Patienten. Einge Stellungnahme zur Rechtssprechung aus ärztlicher Sicht. Ärzteblatt Baden-Württemberg Heft 6/1986: 433–434.

5. BUNDESÄRZTEKAMMER. 1985. Empfehlungen für Richtlinien zur Aufklärung der Krankenhauspatienten über vorgesehene ärztliche Maßnahmen. Deutsches Ärzteblatt B, 26 April 1985 (82. Jahrgang): 1272–1274.
6. WOLF, E. 1987. Die Aufklärungspflicht des onkologisch tätigen Arztes: Rechtliche Beurteilung unter besonderer Berücksichtigung der klinischen Prüfung. Onkologischer Service Lederle, 7. Ausgabe. Wolfratshausen.
7. SENN, H. J. 1985. Wahrhaftigkeit am Krankenbett. *In* Einführung in die Psycho-Onkologie. F. Meerwein, Ed.: 59–74. Huber. Bern.

SUPPLEMENTARY BIBLIOGRAPHY

LAMSZUS, K., R. VERRES & K. H. HÜBENER. 1994. Wie erleben Patienten die Strahlentherapie? Strahlentherapie Onkologie **170:** 162–168.

OLSCHEWSKI, M,. R. VERRES, H. SCHEURLEN & H. RAUSCHECKER. 1988. Evaluation of psychosocial aspects in a breast preservation trial. Recent Results Cancer Res. **111:** 258–269.

VERRES, R. 1977. Psychosoziale Faktoren der mangelnden Inanspruchnahme von Krebs-Früherkennungsuntersuchungen. Eine Interviewstudie mit 115 männlichen Patienten einer allgemeinärztlichen Praxis. Lang-Verlag. Frankfurt.

VERRES, R. 1978. Wie beeinflusst Angst vor Krebs die Motivation zur Krebsvorsorge? Medizin—Mensch—Gesellschaft **3:** 153–160.

VERRES, R. 1982. Psychological problems in early-diagnosis cancer screening. *In* Public Education about Cancer: Recent Research and Current Programs. UICC Technical Report Series, Vol.67. P. Hobbs, Ed.: 51–63. International Union Against Cancer. Geneva.

VERRES, R. 1986. : Krebs und Angst. Subjektive Theorien von Laien über Entstehung, Vorsorge, Früherkennung, Behandlung und die psychosozialen Folgen von Krebserkrankungen. Unter Mitarbeit von S. Schilling, H. Faller, U. Michel, R. Daniel, A. Völcker. Geleitwort von Th. v. Uexküll. Springer-Verlag. Berlin.

VERRES, R. 1986. Cancer and fear: Laymen's theories about early detection and therapy of cancer. J. Cancer Res. Clin. Oncol. **111**(Suppl.): 61.

VERRES, R. 1987. Zur Bedeutung kollektiver Umgangsweisen mit Krebsängsten für die Rehabilitation Krebskranker. *In* Psychotherapie in der psychosomatischen Medizin. H. Quint & P. L. Janssen, Eds.: 100–106. Springer-Verlag. Berlin.

VERRES, R. 1987. Ethische Probleme bei der Krebsvorsorge und der Krebsfrüherkennung im Lichte von Diskrepanzen zwischen Laientheorien und professionellen Theorien zur Krebsbekämpfung. *In* Ethik in der Behandlung Krebskranker. D. Schmähl & H. Erhart, Eds. Zuckschwerdt. Munich.

VERRES, R. 1988. Subjective theories on etiology and treatment of cancer. Recent Results Cancer Res. **111:** 179–184.

VERRES, R. 1989. Zur Kontextabhängigkeit subjektiver Krankheitstheorien. *In* Patientenkonzepte von Körper und Krankheit. C. Bischoff & H. Zenz, Eds.: 18–24. Huber. Bern.

VERRES, R. 1990. Wechselwirkungen zwischen Rehabilitation und Prävention: Implikationen für die künftige Forschung zur Rehabilitation bei Krebserkrankungen. *In* Krebsrehabilitation und Psychoonkologie. U. Koch & F. Potreck-Rose, Eds.: 134–140. Springer. Berlin.

VERRES, R. 1994. Die Kunst zu leben—Krebsrisiko und Psyche. 3d edit. Piper. Munich.

VERRES, R. 1991. Gesundheitsforschung und Verantwortung—Gedanken zur Differenzierung und Vertiefung der Rekonstruktion subjektiver Gesundheits- und Krankheitstheorien. *In* Alltagswissen über Gesundheit und Krankheit—Subjektive Theorien und Soziale Repräsentationen. U. Flick, Ed.: 305–317. Asanger Verlag. Heidelberg.

VERRES, R. 1993. Responsabilité et recherche sur la santé. De la facon de différencier et d'approfondir la reconstruction de théories subjectives de la maladie et de la santé. *In* La Perception Quotidienne de la Santé et de la Maladie. Théories Subjectives et Représentations Sociales. U. Flick, Ed.: 360–375. L'Harmattan. Paris.

VERRES, R. 1995. Vom Handlungsdruck zur Begleitung in die innere Ruhe. Deutsches Ärzteblatt **92:** A-3615–3618.

VERRES, R. & M. HASENBRING, Eds. 1989. Psychosoziale Onkologie. Jahrbuch der medizinischen Psychologie, Vol. 3. Springer. Berlin.

VERRES, R., I. LOPAU, K. LAMSZUS & H. SCHAAF. 1994. Subkapsuläre Orchiektomie versus LHRH-Analogon: Therapiepräferenz und psychische Befindlichkeit von Patienten mit fortgeschrittenem Prostatakarzinom. Urologe B **34:** 214–218.

VERRES, R., M. ROSER & M. WEICHENTHAL. 1991. Medizinpsychologische Aspekte der Früherkennung und Prävention des malignen Melanoms. *In* Diagnostik und Therapie maligner Melanome. W. Meigel, W. Lengen & G. Schwenzer, Eds.: 110–122. Diesbach. Berlin.

Cancer and Truth-telling in Greece

Historical, Statistical, and Clinical Data

GERASSIMOS A. RIGATOS

1st Department of Medical Oncology
St. Savvas Cancer Hospital
171, Alexandras Avenue
115 22 Athens, Greece;
Athens University Medical School; and
Hellenic Society of Psychosocial Oncology

HISTORICAL AND PHILOSOPHICAL ASPECTS

Aletheia (Truth) was, according to ancient Greek tradition as it has been preserved by the poet Pindar (518–438 B.C.), the daughter of Zeus, who was the father of gods and men. According to the Roman tradition Truth (Veritas) was the daughter of the god Saturn (Cronus), who was also the father of Jupiter (Zeus). Thus, one can see that, according to the conceptions of the peoples who created contemporary Western culture, Truth holds an honorary place in the pantheon of ancient gods and goddesses. Very early, also, Truth was connected to Medicine. Plutarch mentioned that she was the wetnurse of the god Apollo—the god of light, poetry, and music—but also of Medicine; one must recall here that the Oath of Hippocrates starts with an invocation to "Apollo the physician." Besides this, according to Philostratus, Truth is always depicted by the side of Oneirus (Dream) and the mythical healer and magician Amphiaraos, dressed in a plain long white gown.

Etymologically the word *aletheia* (αλήθεια) comes from the privative prefix *a-* and the word *lethos* or (in the Doric dialect) *lathos* that means error, mistake. According to another interpretation the word is composed of the privative *a-* and the word *lethe,* oblivion. Thus, the original meaning of the word is the unmistaken, the correct, or, that which, being truth, cannot be forgotten.

From a philosophical point of view many theories about truth have been developed. The *theory of correspondence* goes back to Plato (427–347 B.C.) and mainly Aristotle and maintains that truth is the agreement of knowledge with the object, the correspondence of what we think or maintain and what exists. In the Middle Ages the Aristotelean theory predominated, and truth was believed to be the agreement of intellect and object or, as expressed in Latin, *adequatio intellectus et rei.* Subsequent philosophers holding the same opinion are Thomas Aquinas and, more recently, B. Russell , G. E. Moore, and early Wittgenstein. Other theories to be mentioned are: (a) the *semantic theory* of A. Tarski; (b) the *pragmatic theory* of W. James; (c) the *theory of common consent* of W. Kamlah and P. Lorenzen; (d) the *theory of coherence* with roots in Hegel; (e) the *sociological theory* of K. Mannheim, M. Scheler and others; (f) the *Marxist theory* as maintained by Marx (correspondence or agreement of knowledge with objective reality, as in Aristotle) and Lenin (dynamic social function connected to the whole of scientific applications and political actions).[1,2]

HISTORICAL DATA ON TRUTH–TELLING IN MEDICINE

Concerning the problem of truth-telling to the patient, the conflict between the protection of the patient from psychotraumatic information and the right of a person to know the truth and to maintain his autonomy has long been recognized. Various authors[3–5] mention that the Greeks and Romans ignored the ethical dilemma between the announcement or the concealment of truth, adopting a more pragmatic attitude: physicians simply had to do their best for the patient with their best skills and interventions. But even if one supports this opinion, it was, of course, not the general attitude. Hippocrates himself, the "father of medicine," expresses at various points in his work a completely different attitude.[6] He wrote: "I think the best physician is the one who has the providence to tell to the patients according to his knowledge the present situation, what has happened before, and what is going to happen in the future". (*Τον ιατρόν δοκέει μοι άριστον είναι πρόνοιαν επιτηδεύειν, προγιγνώσκει γάρ και προλέγειν πάρα τοίσι νοσέουσι τά τέ παρεόντα καί τά προγεγονότα καί τά μέλλοντα έσεσθαι.*) At another point he wrote: "Whatever absurd is happening, it has to be told." (*Ό, τι αν παράλογον γένηται λέγειν χρή.*).

Rufus of Ephessos (1st–2nd centuries A.D.), in agreement with the physician Xenophon of Kos (c. 280 A.D.) and Oribase (c. 360 A.D.), wrote: "It is useful, according to what Xenophon has written and to what occurs to us when we have gained experience, to foretell the evolution [of diseases] and to treat these diseases carefully."[7] According to medieval moralists, Galen—the physician who wrote more books than any other—was the first who advised physicians to tell white lies in order to comfort their patients and diminish their suffering.[3,8] It is not known why this great epigone of Hippocrates changed his opinions from those of his teacher. Perhaps the appearance of Christianity and the allied philosophy of love and going beyond human logic and knowledge are connected with this important change in Galen's opinions. Galen lived in the second century (128–200 A.D.). A century later and during the following centuries of the Byzantine empire (330–1453 A.D.) the great church fathers supported similar opinions.

Gregorius, Bishop of Nyssa (335–394 A.D.), maintains that "real truth" goes beyond the boundaries of human knowledge. Thus, what is asked for is not simple truth, such as in diagnosis, but going beyond truth to holistic—somatic, psychological, and mental—support, and good communication between the physician and the patient.[9,10] John (344?–407 A.D.), one of the great fathers of the Eastern Orthodox Church, who was called Chryssostomos (the golden mouth) because of his appealing speeches, supports similar opinions. He compares lies to drugs and knives, whose use is permitted for the overall good of the patient, although they may cause pain."[11] Basil (330–379 A.D.), who has been called the Great and who founded the first big hospital during the Byzantine empire, recommends the use of truth with prudence: "The reasoning of the mind has been given to us to use truth with prudence." (*Δέδοται ημίν το του νου κριτήριον εις της αληθείας σύνεσιν.*) So one can see that for this great father of the church, with his humanistic studies, classic medical education, deep theological and philosophical knowledge, but also practicing social care, truth was not an end in itself but a means toward the welfare of the patient.[12]

Other church fathers, mainly those from the western part of the Roman Empire, maintained other opinions. Saint Augustine (354–430 A.D.) condemned lies no matter what their cause in his work *Contra mendacium*.[5] Centuries later Saint Thomas Aquinas (1225–1274 A.D.) condemned lies in the manner of St. Augustine, but admitted the possibility of careful dissimulation.[13] During the same century the official Catholic Church intervened in this ethical and deontological problem. Of course, one can notice that throughout the centuries these Catholic positions have changed from time to time.

Many such regressions occurred in the West during the Renaissance. During the same period in the eastern part of the Roman Empire, the Byzantine Empire, dark times were to come, because the famous empire was subjected to a new dynamic, but barbarian, people—the Turks. These dark ages lasted four centuries. A small part of Greece was liberated in 1821 after a painful revolution. Throughout this period, education was not encouraged; often it was forbidden. So physicians of this period studied in Italy, France, Germany, Austria and Hungary; and the opinions they espoused were those of the scientists of the countries where they were educated. The first modern Greek university was founded in Athens in 1837 with Bavarian professors and Greek professors who had studied abroad. Although some types of cancer are mentioned in the medical books of that time, the need for communication with the patient or informing him is not mentioned, nor is the problem of telling the diagnosis. The only subject is treatment with the poor means of the time.

TRUTH-TELLING IN CONTEMPORARY GREECE

In modern and contemporary Greece, under the influence of European authorities of the first half of the twentieth century, medicine—the whole structure of medical services, perceptions, and the attitudes of physicians— was paternalistic. The diagnosis of cancer was not communicated to the patient, only to his relatives. The only ethical and practical obligation of the physician was to provide therapy. The choice of the method of treatment, the decision about its application, and the evaluation of its efficacy were the entire concern of the physician. No participation by the patient in the decision making was needed. Very often the patient was misled by a false or naive diagnosis, always with the consent and often under the pressure of the family. One has to mention here that in Greece, even today, there are still strong family bonds; in most cases the family is still the strongest support system. The education of medical students, at least through the 1960s, has not included subjects like psychology, ethics, and deontology, communication, etc. As a rule even now these subjects are not included in the educational program of medical schools. This gap, has been partly filled during the last two decades by continuing medical education, which has been taken over mainly by scientific societies. A number of very interesting discussions and scientific events have taken place on the subject of physician-patient communication. Also special publications and patients' associations have taken up this subject.[14]

The first extensive public discussion on the subject of informing the cancer patient took place in Athens in April 1974.[15] It is interesting that internists as well as surgeons engaged in oncology firmly supported the opinion of not telling the truth. On the contrary, psychiatrists, theologians, and lawyers were in favor of telling the truth.

By the late seventies, the attitude of physicians in the United States concerning telling the truth had already changed. According to a study from Philadelphia in 1953, among 442 physicians only 31% always or almost always told the truth.[16] At the beginning of the sixties 90% of 219 doctors did not inform the patients about serious truths.[17] Another study in 1970 among 178 physicians showed that 66% sometimes told the truth, 25% always did, and 9% never did.[18] In 1974 this subject is still a matter of study and reflection, with the tendency of telling the truth constantly becoming stronger.[19] Five years later a study by Novack *et al.*[20] among 264 physicians showed the complete reversal of the negative attitude towards truth: 97% preferred to tell the patients the exact diagnosis (TABLE 1). During the same period the attitude of European physicians was not uniform. It seems that in Finland[21] and England the percentages of patients informed about their diagnosis of cancer were greater than in Germany—

TABLE 1. Comparison of Data on Truth-telling to Cancer Patients Showing the Great Differences between 1953 and 1979[a]

Study			Truth-telling by Physicians		
Author(s)[b]	Year	No. of Physicians Queried	Always or Almost Always	Sometimes	Very Rarely or Never
Fitts and Ravdin[16]	1953	442	31%	–	69%
Oken[17]	1961	219	10%	–	90%
Friedman[18]	1970	178	25%	66%	9%
Novack *et al.*[20]	1979	264	97%	–	–

[a]See, for comparison, Achte *et al.*,[21] who report that 30% of cancer patients ignore their diagnosis; of the 70% who know it, only 30% asked for it. See also Reference 15 for a discussion on the subject of truth-telling.
[b]All papers are from the United States.

where paternalistic attitudes still prevailed, the former Soviet Union (personal data), and France.[22]

STUDIES OF ATTITUDES OF PHYSICIANS AND THE HEALTHY POPULATION IN GREECE

In the 1970s the Hellenic Anticancer Society performed a study of the beliefs and attitudes of the public concerning cancer.[23] The sample consisted of 3,154 healthy persons living throughout Greece. One of the questions people were asked was whether they would want to be informed about the true diagnosis if they had cancer. The results are shown in TABLE 2.

One can see that at the beginning of the seventies at least 71.5% of the unselected healthy Greek population did not want to know the truth

TABLE 2. Results of the Study by the Hellenic Anticancer Society of an Unselected Healthy Greek Population[23]

Would you like to be told the truth if you were a cancer patient?	Urban Areas		Rural Areas		Total	
	n	%	*n*	%	*n*	%
Yes	639	27.1	108	13.5	747	23.7
No	1652	70.2	603	75.5	2255	71.5
Don't know	64	2.7	88	11.0	152	4.8
Total	2355	100	799	100	3154	100

TABLE 3. Physician Truth-telling to Cancer Patients[a]

	Never	Very Rarely	Occasionally	Often	Total
How often do physicians tell the cancer patient the truth about the diagnosis?	52 (Never + Very Rarely)				
	37 (52%)	15 (21%)	14 (20%)	5 (7%)	71 (100%)
	(73%) (Never + Very Rarely)				
How often do physicians inform their patients that their death is imminent?	67 (Never + Very Rarely)				
	58 (82%)	9 (13%)	4 (5%)	– –	71 (100%)
	(95%) (Never + Very Rarely)				

[a]Detailed results of the research by Manos and Christakis,[22] modified.

about cancer. Corresponding beliefs and attitudes of physicians in Greece were first measured in 1980 and were presented at a domestic congress and also published during the same year in an international journal. A questionnaire was distributed to 110 physicians working in anticancer and university hospitals. Seventy-one of the physicians responded, half of whom were medical and hematological oncologists. The results of the study showed that 73% never or rarely announced the diagnosis of cancer. The percentage reached 95% about not informing the patient of imminent death (TABLE 3). Although the physicians queried ascribed this attitude to reasons concerning the patient (protection from psychological breakdown, lack of willingness to be informed, etc.), I believe the main problem is the physicians' relative inability and lack of appropriate education.

In the meantime, in the context of social and economic progress, improvement of public education, better information through the mass media, and general changes that have occurred, public opinion and attitudes have begun to change. Thus, also, the ways the public faces the announcement of the truth have changed. While in 1971 only 23.7% declared that they wanted to know the truth about cancer, in 1977 45% did, and in 1987 51.9%.[24] The changes in attitudes of different parts of the population are shown in detail in TABLE 4.

Let us compare the percentage of the population that wants to know the truth in two different countries during the same time period. While in Greece only 45% wanted to know the truth according to the study men-

TABLE 4. Changes in Greek Population of Attitudes concerning Truth-telling to Cancer Patients[a]

Population Sample	Want to Be Told the Truth		Do Not Want to Be Told the Truth		No Response	
	n	%	*n*	%	*n*	%
Entire country						
1971	747	23.7	2255	71.5	152	4.8
1977	1457	45.0	1570	48.5	213	65.5
1987	1766	51.9	1143	33.6	491	14.4
Urban areas						
1971	639	27.1	1652	70.2	64	2.7
1977	1121	46.0	1190	48.7	129	5.3
1987	1171	41.7	1143	40.8	491	17.5
Suburban areas						
1971	–	–	–	–	–	–
1977	–	–	–	–	–	–
1987	440	44.0	399	39.9	161	16.1
Rural areas						
1971	108	13.5	603	75.5	88	11.0
1977	336	41.6	380	47.8	84	10.6
1987	155	48.0	134	41.5	34	10.5

[a]Data from successive population studies by the Hellenic Anticancer Society.

tioned above, in 1978 the percentage was much higher in the United States. According to a study by Blumenfield *et al.*,[25] among 1,518 healthy persons interviewed, the percentage who wanted to know the truth about cancer ranged from 82% to 92% in various groups of the population. We can also see that even in 1987 the percentage of Greek people who wanted to know whether they had cancer (51.9%) was much lower than the percentage in the 1978 American study.

But although the percentage of those who favored the announcement of the truth seems to have more than doubled, the attitude of physicians does not seem to have changed. In the most recent study, 120 physicians were interviewed in 1986.[26] Of the physicians interviewed 110 (91.6%) were men; 98 (81.7%) were between the ages of 31 and 50; 75(62.5%) were surgeons, and 40 (33.3%) were internists. We also noticed that 109 of the physicians interviewed were practicing in the capital (90.8%), and 78 (65%) had studied only in Greece.

Fifteen out of 120 (12.5%) stated that they usually tell the truth to cancer patients, while 105 (87.5%) usually not. Out of these 105 physicians 32 (26.6% of all interviewed) did not reveal the truth to any patient, while the rest followed a more differentiated policy. The physicians over 50 years of age (6.7% of the sample) never told the truth, and the same was true for all the female physicians (8.4% of the sample). All 120 physicians reported that they informed the patients' relatives of the diagnosis. In their discussion of their results the investigators point out that physicians do not have well defined opinions on the subject, that they have not been taught during their medical studies ways of communication with patients, and that a number of physicians do not accept or are not informed about the internationally recognized "rights of the patient."[27] Although in general many physicians and other scientists refer to a specific personality type and cultural background in Greece and other Mediterranean countries, it seems that the problem concerns the physician and his lack of relevant communication rather than the personality of the patient.

My own opinion about the problem of truth-telling is that our attitude should not be dogmatic. I support that the truth must be told to a great percentage of patients, if they ask for and want to know the truth. But because truth is not an end in itself but a means contibuting to the well-being of the patient, we have to respect those who do not want to know or who could not endure the burden of truth. Of course, revealing the truth carries with it more responsibilities for the physician: he has to learn the ways through which he will succeed in approaching his patient; he has to learn details of his personality and precancerous psychological situation before he begins to discuss the diagnosis and the prognosis of the disease with his patient. In telling the truth, the doctor has also to take on responsibility for the holistic support of the patient, including his biological, psychological, and social needs, until the end.

I also think that concealing the truth as a rule results in worsening communication with the patient, which is disadvantageous to both patient and physician. The development of this disturbance is shown in FIGURE 1.

CONCLUSIONS AND PROPOSALS

From the data presented here the following observations become evident:

1. Physicians in contemporary Greece tell the truth to only a small percentage of cancer patients, and they almost never inform them about imminent death.
2. The percentage of the population who would want to know the truth in the case of cancer is growing little by little; during the 16 years between 1971 and 1987 it has more than doubled.
3. On the contrary, the attitudes of physicians seem to have remained stagnant, not having changed between 1980 and 1987.
4. Among possible causes of physicians' attitudes is their lack of education about communication techniques and psychology at med-

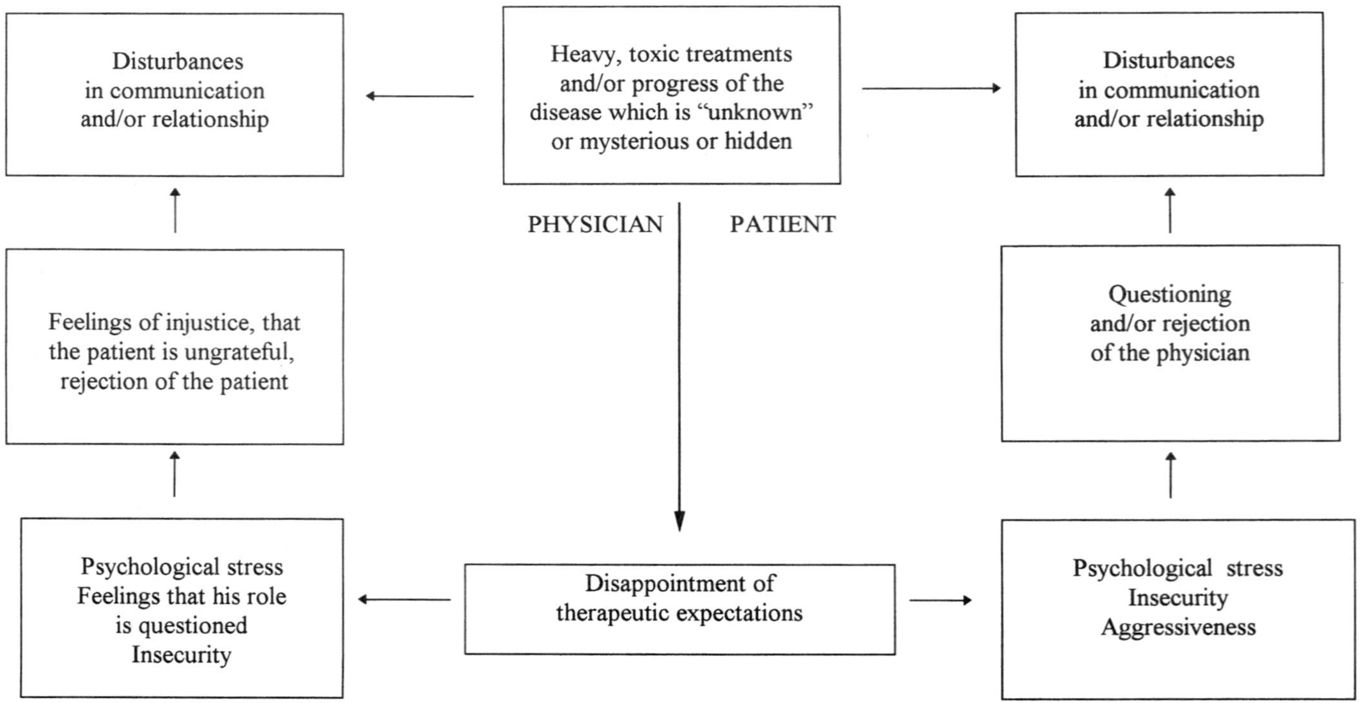

FIGURE 1. Model showing the disturbances in the relationship between doctor and patient that might result when the truth is not told.

ical schools, perceptions about a specific Greek personality, and lack of information among a large part of physicians about the rights of the patients.

Although these conclusions were drawn in one country, they may be valid in other countries, too.

Greece is now in a state of mobility concerning social changes. Rights are being claimed, communication about therapeutic achievements and attitudes is rapid, education and public information concerning medical and other subjects are broad. Certainly the accelerating movement toward a common perspective among the countries of the European Union will bring about changes in the way of practicing medicine. All the above will favorably influence truth-telling to cancer patients, especially if these proposals are carried out:

1. A new study must be carried out among a representative sample of physicians concerning present-day attitudes towards truth-telling to cancer patients.
2. A greater number of psychiatrists must be appointed to cancer hospitals and, of course, also to general hospitals, where a great number of cancer patients are also treated.
3. Psychologists must be appointed to cancer hospitals.
4. Medical schools should include the subject of communication with the patient in their educational curricula.
5. The subject of clinical psychology should be taught more systematically and extensively.
6. The subject of medical ethics should also be introduced, with emphasis on patient's rights, the ethics of clinical trials, etc.
7. Medical oncology should become a specialty in Greece, and it should include at least half a year's training in psychosocial oncology.

If all the above does not happen, the disagreement between public perceptions and attitudes and those of physicians will become greater, as will the disturbance of the patient-doctor relationship.

REFERENCES

1. HOSPERS, J. 1967. An Introduction to Philosophical Analysis. Prentice Hall. Englewood Cliffs, NJ.
2. SKIRBEKK, G., Ed. 1977. Warheitstheorien. Frankfurt am Main.
3. MOLL, A. 1902. Aerzliche Ethik. Enke. Stuttgart.
4. GRMEK, M. D. 1964. Le pieux mensonge du medecin et le droit du malade a la verité. Concours Med. **86:** 2855–3858, 4021–4030.
5. WEIL, M., M. SMITH & D. KHAYAT. 1994. Truth-telling to cancer patients in the Western European context. PsychoOncology **3:** 21–26.

6. POURNAROPOULOS, G. 1967–1970. Introduction to Hippocrates. Vols. 1–6. Publ. Martinos. Athens. (In Greek.)
7. BUSSENMAKER, C. 1851–1876. Oeuvres d'Oribase. 6 Vols. (Vol. 4, 1854). Paris. (Reprint: Amsterdam, 1962.)
8. KUHN, K. G. 1821–1833. Claudii Galeni Opera Omnia. 22 Vols. Medicorum Grecorum opera quae exstant. Leipzig. (Reprint: Hildesheim, 1964-65; in Greek and Latin.)
9. CHEMISS, H. F. 1930. The Platonism of Gregor of Nyssa. University of California Press. Berkley, CA.
10. DANIELOU, J. 1940. Gregoir de Nysse. Paris.
11. MIGNE, J. P. 1858–1860. Johannes Chrysostomos: Opera Omnia. Patrologia Greca. Vols. 47–64. Paris.
12. PASCHOS, A. 1994. Vassileios the Great, Educated General Practitioner. Ioannina. Athens. (In Greek.)
13. DIEPPEN, P. 1958. Ueber den Eingluss der autorisativen Theologie auf die Medizin des Mittelalters. Steiner. Wiesbaden.
14. RIGATOS, G. 1985. Introduction to Psychosocial Oncology. Zeta Medical Publishers. Athens. (In Greek.)
15. NOUSSIAS, M., K. ATHITAKES, I. GARAS, I. DASKALOPOULOS, G. LYKETSOS, X. BETSIDES, N. BRATSIOTES & N. SAKKAS. 1975. Roundtable Discussion: Should cancer patients be informed? Bull. Sci. Union Athens Municipal Hosp. **6:** 7–51.
16. FITTS, W. T., JR. & I. S. RAVDIN. 1953. What Philadelphia physicians tell patients with cancer. JAMA **153:** 901–904.
17. OKEN, D. 1961. What to tell cancer patients: A study of medical attitudes. JAMA **175:** 1120–1128.
18. FRIEDMAN, H. S. 1970. Physician management of dying patients: An exploration. Psychiatry Med. **1:** 295–305.
19. ROSNER, F. 1974. Emotional care of cancer patient: To tell or not to tell? NY State J. Med. **74:** 1467.
20. NOVACK, D. H., R. PLUMER, R. L. SMITH, I. T. OCHITILL, G. R. MORROW & J. M. BENNET. 1979. Changes in physician's attitude toward telling the cancer patient. JAMA **241:** 897–900.
21. ACHTE, K. A., M. C. VAUKHONEN, R. O. VIITAMAKI & L. SONKIN. 1970. Cancer and Psyche. Monogr. Psychiatr. Clin. Helsinki Univ. Cent. Hosp. Helsinki.
22. MANOS, N. & J. CHRISTAKIS. 1980–1981. Attitudes of cancer patients in Greece. Int. J. Psychiatry Med. **10:** 305–313.
23. SARFATIS, D. & G. PAPACHRISTODOULOU. 1972. Research on attitudes and behaviour of the public towards cancer. Publ. Hellenic Anticancer Soc. Athens.
24. HELLENIC ANTICANCER SOCIETY. 1988. Sampling research on public attitude and behaviour towards cancer (1987). Hellenic Anticancer Society. Athens.
25. BLUMENFIELD, M., N. B. LEVY & D. KAUFMAN. 1978. Do patients want to be told? N. Engl. J. Med. **299:** 1138.
26. DOSSIOS, TH., CH. MARKOPOULOS, I. VLAKHOS & P. LIATSOS. 1986. Aspects of Greek doctors on the subject if the cancer patient should know his disease. Hellenic Armed Forces Med. Rev. **20:** 309–315. (In Greek.)
27. RIGATOS, G. A. 1990. Revelation or concealment of cancer diagnosis? *In* The Truth and the Patient with Neoplasia. N. Kordiolis & G. A. Rigatos, Eds.: 89–96. Hellenic Anticancer Society. Athens. (In Greek.)

Being Honest with the Patient and Ourselves: Do We Give Our Patients Accurate Insight into Anticipated Results of Treatment?

An Irish Perspective

JAMES J. FENNELLY

St. Vincent's Hospital
Elm Park
Dublin 4, Ireland

In Ireland there are about 15,000 new cancer cases per year. With these the specialist staff is indeed quite limited, with five medical oncologists in the public service, two pediatric oncologists, four hematologist/oncologists, and seven radiotherapists—giving a total of 18 people. There are two radiation centers and three public hospitals with staff dedicated to dealing with cancer cases,—i.e., with full staff including medical oncologists, attending radiation oncologists, and a trained oncology nursing staff.

One has to ask the question of why patients find the information that they have cancer so drastic and frightening? Most patients' interpretation of the word *cancer* as mediated by attitudes portrayed by the press, television, and radio. In the Irish scene, attitudes in general tend to be negative rather than positive. Most patients accept the diagnosis of cancer as if it means they are being condemned to death, a death associated with major symptoms, particularly pain that may not be subject to control. Such factors tend to influence our attitude in informing patients.

To overcome these very negative attitudes in patients in our communications it is vitally important to have as much time as possible to devote to informing them of the implications of their illness, the implications regarding symptoms, the radical or nonradical nature of treatment, and the fact that palliative care of the highest quality is now available. If all patients who have been cured of cancer had been told they had cancer at the start, and were prepared to let this be known generally, then the negative aspects of cancer diagnosis would be reduced.

HOW DO WE INFORM THE PATIENT?

From my experience of many years, in interviewing cancer patients I am aware that first of all over 80% make a particular request that any important information relating to their diagnosis be imparted by the consultant in charge. Certainly this is not the type of information to be given by a young intern; perhaps a good senior registrar with adequate training would be more appropriate, with the information being followed up by specialist oncology nurses.[1]

It is informative to review a difficult problem with which I have dealt over the last year.

> A 50-year-old lady came came to me for management of an advanced primary breast carcinoma with adjacent supraclavicular nodes. (Unfortunately she, as well as her husband, was also known to me as a friend for many years.) The cold facts were given: "You have cancer in your right breast, and it has advanced; but it can be removed, and the nodes in your neck will shrink after radiation. We will give you chemotherapy to prevent the cancer from coming back both locally and elsewhere."

Here is my first mistake. I gave the cold facts without including the prognosis—i.e., the reality in my own mind as to the limitations of the efficacy of surgery, radiotherapy, and chemotherapy to control the disease locally and to prevent systemic recurrence. It is difficult to give the patients such negative news if one is starting with radical surgery, radiation, and chemotherapy.

> She completed her chemotherapy, and unfortunately had many side effects, as she was on ACMF, a program devised by Bonadonna[2] that is used for high-risk breast cancer.
>
> Sixteen-and-a-half months later she came in with what looked like a rash on her chest wall at the incision site. It looked nonspecific, but I did suspect it might be a malignant recurrence. I said I would keep an eye on it and referred her to a surgeon for a further biopsy of the axilla, where there was a palpable node that did, indeed, turn out to be positive. By the time she got to the radiotherapist the rash had cleared and become a confluent atypical type of recurrence on her chest wall. Having had radiation before, the only hope was that electron beam therapy might give some benefit. She was extremely upset at this time, feeling that if the recurrence had been diagnosed earlier, there might have been a radical difference in her outlook. Naturally I found it difficult to explain that it really did not matter that much if I had diagnosed this recurrence earlier.

Obviously in this situation if we had been absolutely truthful from the start, perhaps the patient might have found it difficult to accept the treatment with all its side effects; hence the tendency to be evasive in the initial presentation.

It is often said that if we start by telling lies, then we must have a terrific memory for all future communications. Communication with patients must be taken in stages after the diagnosis. Initially I would have seen patients as they are getting over an operation, and perhaps 24–48 hours after an anesthetic. They are not at that stage ready for information, and we still do not know the full pathology results. Therefore, we just inform them that they have had a good operation and await finer results

Once these are available ideally we should have a senior relative with the patient at the time of our discussion. This should be very much a question-and-answer type of conversation, in which we give the patient plenty of time for questions and try to deal with him or her as honestly as possible. Regarding the prognosis, it is best to answer questions rather than making very negative statements.

On the following day, when I meet the patients again, the relatives are much better able to assimilate the facts and ask pertinent questions. It is imperative that when we feel there is a life-threatening illness and that we impart this to the patient in some way, to avoid his or her getting involved in major financial commitments or serious domestic commitments that could create major problems later.

In my experience there are situations in which the patient demands to know information that is not to be imparted to his or her relatives. This may occur when one partner is involved in major business and wants to keep this confidential from the other.

PERCEIVED KNOWLEDGE OF THE DIAGNOSIS

Many communications stress the lack of knowledge imparted to patients, saying that they know very little by the time they leave the hospital. I find that if one is prepared to take time with question-and-answer type communication, one will in most cases find that the patient really does know that he or she has a tumor or cancer. This often arises following the first question, when I ask what is wrong and the patient answers, "I know absolutely nothing." Many patients with breast cancer who have had a mastectomy will initially say they know nothing about their illness. When they are questioned fully as to why they are in the hospital, they admit that, yes, they had a lump in the breast; when asked why the mastectomy was carried out, they say because the lump was suspicious. Further questioning on this will bring out the information that they realize that there were malignant cells in the tumor.

Therefore, we have moved from the initial stage in which the patient has said "I know absolutely nothing" to her telling me she has a malignancy in the breast. When this information comes from the patient, further communication becomes much easier.

INFORMATION ON BREAST CANCER: HOW TRUTHFUL ARE WE REALLY REGARDING THE OUTLOOK?

We may tell the patient that she has a 2-cm breast tumor and that three axillary nodes are involved; but after a very good operation, all are perfectly clear, and we are going to give treatment to prevent any recurrence. In reality we know that 60 to 70% of such patients will have recurrence and probably die of their disease. If we are embarking on chemotherapy to prevent recurrence and realize we have failed in a lot of cases, we do like to be optimistic with our patients. This attempt to be optimistic often does, indeed, mean that we are not being fully truthful. But one has to ask whether we need to focus on the negative aspects at this stage. I do not think so. To be treated with an intensive adriamycin-containing program for high-risk tumors, where she will loose all her hair, develop oral ulcers, diarrhea, and many other problems, does not make sense to a patient who is being told that her disease is very early and the outlook is very good.

One of the major questions in breast cancer at present is the role of high-dose therapy and bone marrow transplantation in high-risk cases or early metastatic disease. Certainly in the United States the information on consent forms in these cases is so extremely detailed that it is doubtful that patients could be in any real doubt of the truth of their diagnosis before they sign such documents. Perhaps such forms, however, are too daunting for patients. Many of these forms are designed to avoid major medical/legal problems that may subsequently arise because of lack of confidence in patients and truthfulness in doctors; therefore, they really are used for the protection of the doctor in the end.

CONTROLLED CLINICAL TRIALS

I personally find it difficult to encourage patients with a very bad outlook—say, advanced non–small cell lung cancer or gastric or pancreatic cancer with metastases–to participate in a controlled trial, since the anticipated results are so bad; usually the results are in the order of a 20% response, and one is looking for about a 5% difference. In these cases we may be able to show marginal benefit for the patients versus the best supportive therapy, but do we need to do further major studies to prove this point with such poor results? In my opinion we need to go back to the laboratory to get more effective agents.

THE TRUTH RELATED TO THE DIAGNOSIS

Patients with localized Hodgkin's disease are usually in their teens, 20s or 30s. For them the future is very good, and the cure rate is high, in the order of 75%. We can indeed be absolutely truthful, very optimistic, and very detailed in speaking with them regarding their tests and treatments. We must, however, cover our statements by saying that we cannot guarantee 100% results. But are all of our patients told about the possibility of infertility, which may occur in about 90% of males treated with MOPP and in about 50% of females?

Are patients told that there is an increased incidence of second malignancies in Hodgkin's disease, particularly in those treated with radiation and chemotherapy?[3] It is understandable that if we are trying to cure a patient of one malignancy, we want to encourage them as much as possible to return to normal living. Since in any population there is a one-in-four chance of getting cancer anyway, it is debatable whether we contribute anything by telling patients that they have an increased risk of another cancer because of their treatment.

LUNG CANCER

It is tragic that, in a situation in which disease is so preventable, in most cases once lung cancer is diagnosed, the outlook is very bad, with 80–90% of patients dying within one year.[4] There is an editorial in the National Cancer Institute Journal headed "Hope for Non Small Cell Lung Cancer."[5] In the summary regarding chemotherapy of advanced disease the statement is made that survival for one year following chemotherapy is now tripled; that really does sound fantastic. This is then further spelled out as 5–10% survival at one year and as a real increase of from 4 to 10 weeks.[6] At this stage one must say that how one interprets these statistics depends very much on one's own philosophy. But it is the latter statement—increase of survival from 4 to 10 weeks—that is of real importance. Usually in lung cancer we are dealing with older patients, who have chronic lung disease, and perhaps heart disease from their long-term smoking or other vascular disease as well.

Even at this bad stage, however, it is essential to get across the truth regarding the future, particularly regarding the limitation of life. I start by informing the patient that there is a tumor pressing on the lungs that may cause collapse of the lungs and cause very serious problems. He may have had a good operation, but with residual disease.

I try to get patients to ask about the future, and if they do, I say it is like pneumonia: if there is no response, we could be talking in very short terms; and if there is a good response, we might have a survival of many months or a year or so.

At present with chemotherapy available to us it is my opinion that non–small cell lung cancer is grossly overtreated with chemotherapy, particularly in the case of advanced disease. Coming to a difficult decision regarding treatment, it is important to discuss seriously with the patient as well as with relatives the advantages and disadvantages of chemotherapy, how the side effects may outweigh any benefit in terms of improvement in the size of the tumor, and possible increase in survival.

It is imperative that we always make our decision according to the patient's wishes, since there are regrettably cases where family members may make a decision that is not in agreement with that of the patient.

Having said the above, it must also be said that there are encouraging reports from newer combinations of platinum with drugs such as taxene (docetaxel and pacltaxel), but it is going to take another few years of rigidly controlled trials to tell us exactly what progress they may lead to.

GASTROINTESTINAL CANCER

There are many vogues that persist in cancer treatment. One such is the use of eponyms such as FAM (5 flurouracil, adriamycin, and mitomycin), which has been used for many years in the treatment of gastric or pancreatic cancer. When FAM is compared to single-agent 5 flurouracil, the very good results shown by the former are not really significant.[7] In spite of this, FAM still retains the top place in most textbook recommendations on treatment for cancer of the upper gastrointestinal tract. A radical educational report should be adopted to eliminate treatments that initially looked encouraging but have not stood the test of time.

Adjuvant chemotherapy in Duke's C colon carcinoma, using 5 flurouracil with levamisole or folinic acid, no doubt has a place in reducing recurrence and does increase survival,[8,9] but the impact in metastatic disease is significant in only a few studies. Regarding upper gastrointestinal malignancy, Klein used a biochemical modulation of 5 flurouracil with high-dose methotrexate (FAMTX), and reported a response rate of 59% with mortality of 3%.[10] Subsequently Wils *et al.*[7] did an extended study, which found the response rate to be 41%, with a 4% toxic death rate. In both studies most patients did not survive 2 years, and with a mortality rate in the order of 3–4% one must question whether such a toxic program is valid. It is interesting that Kelsen commented that at this time "no combination regimen has clearly demonstrated its superiority over single-agent chemotherapy for gastric cancer."[11]

In pancreatic cancer, Kelson again commented that no combination chemotherapy regimens have demonstrated superiority over 5 flurouracil alone. In the largest of the studies on pancreatic cancer, the median survival of patients on chemotherapy was 3 months on 5 flurouracil and lomastine versus 3.9 months for those on observation alone.[12] There is no doubt that newer, more effective drugs are required for gastrointestinal cancer. Having said that, most patients who go to specific cancer units will nonetheless end up getting active treatment where major results may not be anticipated, such as with advanced colon, gastric, pancreatic, or esophageal cancer.

The answer to these problems is that a complete audit of the results of our treatments for the various malignancies is required, and it is vitally important that patients be aware of such results before embarking on such toxic programs.

There are many other areas where treatments may work extremely effectively, such as with testicular tumors, bone tumors, osteogenic sarcoma, and Ewing's tumor; imparting knowledge in these situations is, indeed, quite easy. Regretably the major areas—lung, gastrointestinal, breast, and prostate cancers when in the advanced stage, remain resistant to effective treatments.

CONCLUSIONS

It is the author's impression from 30 years of experience that most patients still do not know the implications of their illness, and they do not know the prognosis. In the 1990s many more patients are aware of their specific named diagnosis, as compared to 20 or 30 years ago; but continuing with their various treatments, many are unaware of how really bad the outlook is.

REFERENCES

1. HERITY, B, N. HILLIARD, M. MORIARTY, J. J. FENNELLY & R. CONROY. 1987. Ir. J. Med. Sci. **156**(6): 172–181.
2. BUZZONI, R., G. BONNADONNA & P. VALAGUSSAUSSA. 1991. J. Clin. Oncol. **9:** 2134–2140.
3. TUCKER, M. A., C. N. COLEMAN *et al.* 1988. N. Engl. J. Med. **318:** 76–81.
4. STEWART, L. A. & J. P. PIGNON. 1995. Br. Med. J. **311:** 899–909.
5. 1995. Editorial News. J. Nat. Cancer Inst. **87:** 1661.
6. MYERS, M. H. & L. A. RIES. 1989. CA Cancer J. Clin. **39**(1): 21–32.
7. WILS, J. A., H. O. KLEIN, J. WAGENER *et al.* 1991. J. Clin. Oncol. **9:** 827–883.
8. ERLICHMAN, C., S. FINN, A. WANG *et al.* 1988. J. Clin. Oncol. **6:** 469–475.
9. POON, M. A., M. J. O'CONNELL, C. J. MOERTEL *et al.* 1989. J. Clin. Oncol. **7:** 1419–1426.
10. KLEIN, D., O. T. ATIGO, L. SALZ *et al.* 1992. J. Clin. Oncol **10:** 541–548.
11. KELSON, D. 1994. Semin. Oncol. **21**(4, Suppl. 7): 58–60.
12. FREY, C. P. TWOMEY & R. KEEHAN, D. ELLIOTT & G. HIGGINS. 1981. Report of the Veterans Administration Surgical Adjuvant Chemotherapy Study Group. Cancer **47**(1): 27–31.

Ethics of Relationship

From Communication to Conversation

M. A. ANNUNZIATA

Centro di Riferimento Oncologico
Istituto Nazionale Tumori Centroeuropeo
Via Pedemontana Occidentale, 12
33081 Aviano, Italy

INTRODUCTION

The first part of this chapter describes the present situation in Italy as to whether physicians should inform cancer patients of their diagnosis. Italy seems to have reached a middle ground between two opposite models—the paternalistic view of the past and the American or Northern European approach. The second part of the chapter deals with an analysis of the communication process, with the aim of demonstrating the impossibility of controlling information, and therefore the necessity of finding new guidelines. The assumption is that no direct correlation exists between what the doctor tells and what the patient knows, and therefore the "to tell/not to tell" dilemma is true more in theory than in reality. In fact, the patient who has received no "official" communication often knows more than the patient who has been given detailed information.

Daily clinical practice is definitely too complex and dramatic to be reduced to such a simplistic quandary. A more appropriate question, then, may be "does or doesn't the patient know?" It is the patient's awareness, not (or at least not only) the information given that allows an individual space for personal choices, autonomy, and self–determination.

The awareness of disease is not only a *dynamic* process influenced by a number of factors, such as a patient's personal characteristics, the clinical situation, and the adequacy of the information provided; it is also an *interactive* process through which doctor and patient communicate.

A more educated population, scientific progress, and the various difficulties encountered in clinical practice are just some of the reasons behind the need, felt by many physicians, for a theoretical solution of the dilemma of what to tell the cancer patient. General guidelines may, in a sense, free doctors from the emotional burden of a more personal approach.

In the author's opinion, the solution is multifaceted, requiring a better patient/physician relationship, a careful assessment of the needs and expectations within the relationship, and the physician's specific preparation for effective communication.

The term "ethics of relationship" indicates respect for definite guidelines in the relationship, which are nevertheless subject to modifications and adjustments, depending on the constantly changing aspects of the relationship itself, its requirements and goals.

The internal guidelines are determined by the patient's emotions, his needs, values, and hopes, which the doctor must comprehend, discuss, and respect. The resulting relationship is therefore based on the complete recognition of the patient as a person and the establishment of a balanced form of communication (conversation), which stems from the doctor's equally complete recognition of his own personal history, feelings, and needs as separate and distinct from those of his patient.

In this relationship, the foremost right of the patient is to receive correct and adequate information about his disease—as is the current indication in clinical practice—but according to rules and times determined within the relationship itself. What we have termed "ethics of relationship" simply indicates the doctor's ability to *be,* to face his patients as a human being.

The Italian Situation

The question "Should patients be told they have cancer?" has been addressed for a long time. Whether or not to withhold information regarding the diagnosis of cancer is the most studied aspect in the literature,[1–10] and this has led to a more constructive philosophy toward this disease. An interesting survey carried out in 1984 by J. Holland and colleagues[9] in order to determine the number of oncologists who tell the truth to their patient, showed a much lower percentage in Italy (40%) compared to Northern Europe and the United States (80%). There are a number of considerations, both professional and personal, that contribute to the doctor's decision, and many of them depend on the effects of the rules of behavior shared by doctor and patient.

Cancer is often associated with suffering and death; other diseases may be equally fatal, but cancer is regarded generally—not only by the layman, but often by counselors and physicians as well—as a horrible, incurable, disfiguring disease. It is therefore not surprising that today many cancer centers in Italy have adopted a different approach, more common in the United States and in Northern Europe. In Italy, the current approach may be placed somewhere between the paternalistic view of the past and the modern trend, which considers patients as autonomous individuals. It is undoubtedly attractive to contemplate the idea of a patient/doctor team confronting the disease together, thanks to an open line of communication that allows each individual to tap his own physical and emotional resources in order to meet the challenge he is facing and to be aware of his alternatives and choices.

Spinsanti[11] has described two different aspects of the behavioral spectrum: on the one hand, doctors feel an "a priori hostility," preferring a leading, fatherly role toward their patients, whose behavior remains dependent and passive; the other approach is what Spinsanti describes as "acritical acceptance," in which a doctor merely relays information in an impersonal, often brusque, manner, with little or no consideration for the patient's emotional needs.

In Italy the patient/doctor relationship is undergoing a deep change. Often the doctor is no longer considered infallible, and his diagnoses unquestionable. Patients are more informed and less passive about their decisions and options. The balance of the relationship, however, is based on a number of specific aspects, such as social and cultural background, personal expectations and attitudes. It is unwise to overestimate the vulnerability of the patients to distressing information, but it would be equally unwise to proceed in the opposite direction and simply conclude that each patient is now perfectly able to deal with the right to know and the decision–making process.

La Bianca[12] has stated that in Italy and other Latin countries it is commonplace for many patients, in particular cancer patients, to avoid all responsibility and to assume that the right to choose and decide remains solely with the doctor. Such an attitude often fails to distinguish blind trust from realistic faith, but it is still quite common in Catholic countries. Nevertheless, it would be wrong to believe that only geographical or religious limitations determine a patient's attitude.[13]

A recent non–Italian study[14] showed that the majority of the patients polled (54%), when asked to choose among five different options, decided not to get involved in the decision making and to relinquish it to their physicians. Conversely, a larger percentage (64%) of the healthy control group chose to participate fully in all medical decisions. It would be interesting to find out what triggers a dependent type of trust in a sick individual, and whether this may be based on cultural characteristics. Santosuosso[15] has reported on the institution of a National Committee on Bioethics and the recent laws on blood transfusions (1990 and 1991) and on the prevention of AIDS (1990), which have confirmed the need for informed consent, and the introduction in 1992 of the European Guidelines for Good Medical Practice for the experimentation and use of new drugs. The new attitude toward the medical profession is, therefore, emphasized by a growing interest in the legal aspects of delicate matters such as patients' rights and therapeutic privilege.

In the Italian medical community, some claim that it is entirely possible to adopt the "open" approach currently used in the United States and elsewhere in Europe; however, it is important to remember that differences in cultures, attitudes, and behaviors may modify, sometimes radically, the results sought.[16] If, for example, the concept of benefit is the same in both Italy and the United States, the concept of autonomy may differ.[12]

Many doctors have reservations about a more "transparent" physician/patient relationship because of their "a priori hostility"[17] and "semantic rigidity,"[18] deriving from their own unconscious phobia of death, which they share with their patients, and a feeling of frustration in their professional role.

The crisis of the paternalistic approach and the subsequent question "to tell or not to tell?" are spurred not only by the increasing interest in the patient as a person, but also by recent medical advances, which have produced more aggressive and effective treatments extending survival, and a culture that seemingly denies the fear of death.

I believe that the real question here is not whether or not to inform the patient, but, rather, the search for the optimal approach. Evidently, those who support the view of denying the patient information about his own disease will continue to believe in the patient's need to be protected from unnecessary misery, painful decisions, and emotional burdens; those who choose to discuss the disease openly with their patients will just as surely continue to sustain the importance of self-determination, compliance, coping, and mutual trust.

These two modalities, if considered alone, separated from each specific doctor/patient relationship, with its own unique implications, may indeed bring negative results. There is no general answer for every case. Too often we forget that providing information to a patient is as important as what happens *before* and *after* the dreaded to tell/not to tell dilemma. There is no approach ethically valid for everyone, above and beyond the personal characteristics and limitations of each patient and doctor, in their respective roles. What we call "ethics of relationship" should be the ideal approach that satisfies the patient's needs within specific rules of behavior shared by doctor and patient.

INFORMATION AND TRUTH IN THE PATIENT-PHYSICIAN RELATIONSHIP

In the patient/physician relationship, information is mediated by communication; through it, the patient learns about his diagnosis, prognosis, and treatments, which refer to data (symptoms, test results) about his own disease. Information may be given orally or in written form, or it may be somehow *perceived* by the patient; finally, information may be gathered autonomously by the patient from several different sources. Therefore, it is important to make a distinction between information and the mere transmission or verbal communication of data:[15] in other words, the patient may already know much about his disease *before* the communication of his diagnosis.

The to tell/not to tell dilemma arises from the assumption[19] that information can be controlled by the doctor alone. Thus, we have two diametrically opposite views:

Information

- Doctor and patient are equal (two individuals with equal dignity and capacities)
- The patient is the master of his or her person and well–being (self–determination)
- No one can decide for someone else (except in the case of mental incompetence)
- In the doctor/patient relationship there is no contradiction between trust and truthful information

Noninformation

- Doctor and patient are not equal
- The relationship between them is characterized by help, either requested or given
- The management of disease does not need active participation by the patient
- The rules of the medical profession control the doctor/patient relationship

These two approaches seem to imply that communication causes an almost automatic transformation of the patient into an individual able to think and decide for himself. But communicating information is often one–sided, as it consists mainly of the doctor's input, not the patient's; and inadequate, since the "informed" patient and his doctor do not ultimately have the same knowledge. This model of information is, therefore, based on rules of behavior inherent to the medical profession that are predetermined and restraining, not necessarily appropriate to every patient/physician relationship.

This type of "informative communication" does not promote the possibility of the patient questioning or verifying the information received, nor does it recognize a relationship between equals. What makes a difference is a doctor's willingness to reexamine himself (self–reference)[20] and his ability to recognize his position within the relationship and to enrich it with a different type of communication—conversation, during which both doctor and patient contribute their own experiences, emotions, and specific knowledge.

Another aspect of the physician/patient relationship is help. The patient is "not only physically, but also emotionally sick; he has many fears: fear of the disease, of recurrence and death, of losing his job, of depending on others."[21] As with any other major disease, cancer exacts an enormous price, both physical and psychological; upon knowledge of the diagnosis, a cancer patient must face head–on his own mortal fragility. He needs solutions; often he has precious little time to learn more about his disease, in order to come to a decision that is in his best interest. He does not need input alone: he needs reassurance, information about his symptoms, and trust. He needs his doctor's human touch and compassion. From a systemic evaluation of the communication process,[22–25] we will attempt to answer some common questions of interest to anyone working with cancer patients.

Is the Information Provided Understood Correctly?

It is important to remember that—whatever the doctor's decision about what to tell the patient—the person he is facing may already have had contact with other physicians and patients, and he may already have gathered data from several different sources. All this knowledge not only plays a role in his own definition of the disease, in his hopes and expectations, but it may also hinder the comprehension of the information he is receiving. Consequently, the most important consideration for the doctor is not the decision of what information to disclose, but, rather, how to do it.

He may opt for *partial information,* to be completed later on in the relationship; *overinformation,* providing more input than requested and/or necessary; *contrainformation,* withholding facts and actually lying to the patient; or *"right" information,* providing correct data that is adequate for that particular patient.

The individual providing verbal information shares—or presumes to share—a common code with the receiver. If, however, the information is perceived but not verbally expressed, it does not require a code in order to be received. Verbal communication, to put it quite simply, means *to tell something to someone;*[22] it requires a sender, a receiver, and a common code. The terms "information," which we have used above, and "transmission of data"[15] are not as specific as the term "informative communication," which includes different types of information: "direct" (what the speaker actually means); "inverse" (what he may "involuntarily" say), and "indirect" (what is received by the listener, by adding direct, inverse and "perceived" information gathered from one or more sources). The receiver makes all these connections, depending on the information he already possesses or is able to infer. Mediated information is so complex that it frequently causes misunderstandings: what the doctor transmits, or means, is often not what the patient receives, or understands. Other limitations may make matters worse: doctor and patient may not even share the same code; the nonverbal aspects of the communication process may be ambiguous; the message may be missent or too difficult to comprehend. Patients often feel that doctors hide behind the barrier of their technical language in order to withhold information; this type of communication is unidirectional and leaves the patient confused and frustrated.

In conclusion, mediated information may be misdirected (purposefully or not) by the sender, by either the use of a highly specialized language or a number of other factors (professional and/or personal experiences, cultural background), even when sender and receiver share the same code. We have seen how the message may be poorly transmitted and/or received. It is therefore crucial for patient and doctor to have an equal relationship, in which information can be constantly and freely checked and verified, thanks to mutual trust and common rules of behavior.

What Do Doctors Inform Their Patients About?

Doctors inform their patients about the diagnosis, treatment, and prognosis of a disease—cancer—that in our culture is synonymous with death. There is obviously a deep personal involvement when a doctor speaks of a patient's pain, of his life and death. To tell the truth to a patient is clearly an easier task in the initial stages of the disease, when treatment options and strategies are possible and the patient feels motivated to fight the disease rather than surrender to it. But when doctors are bearers of not–so–good news (recurrence, progression, lack of adequate therapeutic prospects), then communication becomes more complex, and scientific information is insufficient. The emotional well–being and personal gratification of both doctor and patient must be found in a more meaningful rapport. In addition, the concept of information varies, depending on a number of factors: the patient's age and his personality traits, the type and stage of the disease, the doctor's age, experience, and attitudes. Given all the variables and all the possible combinations, the solution can be found only within an ethical relationship.

What Does Noninformation Mean?

We know that it is virtually impossible for an adult who is newly diagnosed as having cancer to know nothing about his disease. Any patient can gather sufficient information from symptoms, diagnostic procedures, surgical interventions, and/or medical treatments to understand that he is indeed sick, and at least to suspect the nature of his disease. And yet, the debate goes on about disclosing or withholding information. Why? Probably because we still equate communication with words—either spoken or written—and therefore feel that we can somehow control them (by saying or not saying them). It is, therefore, difficult to define noninformation exactly or to find a link between information, in the commonly accepted sense of the term, and a patient's autonomy and self–determination.

Is noninformation the failure to openly inform a patient that he has cancer, to tell him his disease is not cancer, or to tell him he is not sick at all? If so, how may treatments be justified?

Partial information may mean not telling the patient the exact name of the disease, while nevertheless acknowledging the seriousness of his situation and discussing his therapeutic options. We may attribute noninformation to the doctor's deep understanding and respect for the unstated decision of his patient to be kept in the dark about his real situation. But giving the patient a false diagnosis or even reassuring him of his perfect health is certainly not noninformation, but contrainformation, which lacks the respect for the patient's rights as a person and cannot be the basis for a good doctor/patient relationship. "In order to preserve patients' autonomy in their best interest, doctors must know them well and understand their deepest needs."[26]

Is the Communication of Information Always Accurate and Definite?

Information on diagnosis and prognosis usually differ because the first is usually quite accurate, while the second is frequently indefinite and uncertain. But it is important to assure the patient that, as precise as the diagnosis may be, it is not a "sentence."

Tamburini[27] has written that "the communication of a diagnosis should not be information that is provided only once, but it must be repeatedly adjusted, questioned and verified . . . it is ultimately the continuing updating on the course of the disease."

Taking into consideration all the factors that play a role in this crucial moment of the patient's life—his diagnosis and prognosis, treatment plans, emotional needs, family and social role—information on his disease is never definite; it does not begin and end at a specific time but continues throughout the course of the disease, in a process that requires honesty, confidence, and compassion. However, the flow of information does not stop even when doctor and patient meet impersonally, with little or no verbal exchange.

Does Information Equal Truth?

As commonly accepted, the term "truth" indicates the objective reporting of facts, the realistic recounting of data, the veritable version of events. But in reality there may be many "truths" about the same fact, data, or event. Inevitably, what we see is filtered through our own experiences. The uniqueness of our point of view depends on a number of factors, such as cultural background, beliefs, and education, to name just a few. The concept of truth is, therefore, neither absolute nor individual. In dealing with cancer, it seems that the only possible reference to the word "truth" is death. In our culture, death is rarely acknowledged and often denied; the task of disclosing the truth (death) is usually delegated to physicians.

In the field of oncology, scientific truth and psychological truth merge into a cultural truth, shared by doctor and patient. The answer to the question "Does information equal truth?" is consequently "No." In fact, the question is more complex than it appears.

Saunders[28] has stated that "physicians must not modify or betray truth, but choose from it the aspects more useful or less traumatizing for the patient. They must instinctively make a distinction between 'truth' and 'all the truth.'" The author here uses the term "truth" as a synonym for objective datum when he says it must not be modified or betrayed, and for information, when he says that it must be adapted for each patient, admitting, therefore, the existence of two truths (the doctor's and the patient's) according to a hierarchic type of relationship totally controlled by the doctor.

We provide information *of* facts, and we tell the truth *about* facts. This difference is not trivial; by *talking about* the truth physicians are able to expand bare facts into a conversation more naturally and spontaneously. Information does not equal truth because it implies a certain behavior on the part of the doctor beyond the mere reporting of data, the patient's verification of the received message, and a type of ethical relationship that is made possible only in a conversation. The truth–telling process is more than just the factual notification of the patient's disease; the doctor's task includes his ability to humanize sterile data and adapt them to a more personal context. He must take into consideration his patient's (and his own) needs and emotions, which cannot, however, interfere with his diagnostic and therapeutic decisions. Truth cannot be separated from the patient's need to be informed, his hopes and expectations; it may cause changes and adjustments; it is a precious commodity within the relationship, merging the individual values and truths of patient and doctor. "To tell the truth is much more than just to provide information; it is not exactly the opposite of lying, nor the sum of correct facts, but a situation of mutual interchange in the doctor/patient relationship. This correlation is established on the basis of mutual responsibilities"[16] and roles.

CONCLUSIONS

What we have termed "ethics of relationship" is not restricted to a predetermined model of medical behavior, but it strengthens the autonomy of the doctor/patient relationship through open discussion and conversation. It establishes, within the relationship, a set of rules mediated by ethics—the doctor's (professional and personal convictions) and the patient's (experience based on personal principles and values). It provides emotional gratification of both doctor and patient, in the fulfillment of their respective roles.

REFERENCES

1. Fitts, W. T. & I. S. Ravdin. 1953. What Philadelphia physicians tell patients with cancer. JAMA **153:** 901–904.
2. Rennick, D., Ed. 1961. What should physicians tell cancer patients? N. Med. Materia **2:** 1120–1129.
3. Oken, D. 1961. What to tell cancer patients: A study of medical attitudes. JAMA **175:** 1120–1128.
4. Friedman, H. S. 1970. Physicians' management of dying patients: An exploration. Psychiatr. Med. **1:** 295–305.
5. Novak, D. H., R. Plumer, R. L. Smith *et al.* 1979. Changes in physicians' attitudes toward telling the cancer patient. JAMA **241:** 897–900.
6. Hardy, R. E., D. R. Green, H. W. Jordan *et al.* 1980. Communication between cancer patients and physicians. South. Med. **73:** 755–757.
7. Greenwald, H. P. & M. C. Nevitt. 1982. Physicians' attitudes toward communication with cancer patients. Soc. Sci. Med. **16:** 591–594.
8. Golberg, R. J. 1984. Disclosure of information to adult cancer patients: Issue and update. J. Clin. Oncol. **8:** 948–955.
9. Holland, J. C., N. Geary, A. Marchini & S. Tross. 1987. An international survey of physicians' attitudes and practice in regard to revealing the diagnosis of cancer. Cancer Invest. **5**(2): 151–154.
10. Mosconi, P., B. E. Meyerowitz, M. C. Liberati & A. Liberati (on behalf of G.I.V.I.O.). 1991. Disclosure of breast cancer diagnosis: Patient and physician reports. Ann. Oncol. **2:** 273–280.
11. Spinsanti, S. 1993. Orizzonte Medico, anno XLVIII–n.3(4) Marzo 1993.
12. Labianca, R. 1993. Un'alleanza terapeutica per condividere le decisioni. Quad. Cure Palliative **3:** 225–227.
13. Santosuosso, A. 1993. Modelli ideali e situazioni reali. Quad. Cure Palliative **3:** 233–235.
14. Degner, L. F. & J. A. Sloan. 1992. Decision making during serious illness: What role do patients really want to play? J. Clin. Epidemiol. **45:** 941–950.
15. Santosuosso, A. & M. Tamburini. 1990. Dire la verità al paziente. Alcuni motivi psicologici e giuridici. Fed. Med. **43:** 503–507.
16. Surbone, A. 1993. Dire la verità ai pazienti. JAMA (Ital. Edit.) **5**(1): 33–35.
17. Amir, R. 1987. Considerations guiding physicians when informing cancer patients. Soc. Sci. Med. **9:** 741–748.
18. Annunziata, M. A. 1993. Dalla comunicazione diagnostica alla conversazione. *In* Il disagio psichico in oncologia. L. Grassi, Ed.: 283–288. Spazio Libri Editori. Ferrara.

19. NESPOR, S., A. SANTOSUOSSO & R. SATOLLI. 1992. Vita morte e miracoli. Medicina, genetica, diritto: Conflitti e prospettive: 113–117. Feltrinelli Editore. Milan.
20. TELFENER, U. 1991. Il rapporto terapeuta–paziente, ovvero il sistema osservante. *In* Dall'individuo al sistema. M. Malagoli Togliatti & U. Telfener, Eds.: 21–30. Boringhieri. Turin.
21. SCANNI, A. & G. FARINA. 1993. Il gruppo come modello di lavoro. Quad. Cure Palliative **3:** 229–230.
22. WATZLAWICK, P. 1971. Pragmatica della comunicazione umana. Astrolabio. Rome.
23. WIENER, M., S. DEVOE, S. RUBINOW & J. GELLER. 1972. Non verbal behavior and non verbal communication. Psychol. Rev. **79:** 185–214.
24. RUESCH, J. & G. BATESON. 1968. Communication. The social matrix of psychiatry. Norton. New York, NY.
25. VIARO, M. & P. LEONARDI. 1990. Conversazione e terapia. L'intervista circolare: 47–54. Raffaello Cortina Editore. Turin.
26. PELLEGRINO, E. D. 1993. Dire la verità al paziente è un artefatto culturale? JAMA (Ital. Edit.) **5**(1): 36–37.
27. TAMBURINI, M. 1990. Tumore al seno: Meglio informare per meglio curare. Psichiat. Med. **4:** 18–19.
28. SAUNDERS, D. C. 1982. Principles of symptom control in terminal care. Med. Clin. North. Am. **66:** 1169–1983.

Telling the Truth to the Patient with Cancer

A Cross-Cultural Dialogue

ERCOLE BRUSAMOLINO[a] AND ANTONELLA SURBONE[b]

[a]*Istituto di Ematologia*
Università di Pavia, and
Divisione di Ematologia
Policlinico San Matteo IRCCS
Pavia 27100, Italy

[b]*Department of Medicine*
Memorial Sloan-Kettering Cancer Center
1275 York Avenue
New York, New York 10021

INTRODUCTION

And you shall know the truth and the truth shall make you free.
—JOHN 8: 32

The issue of truth-telling to the cancer patient is much like a pendulum, which can swing from a cold, nontherapeutic truth-telling to a paternalistic, unjustified truth-withholding. Several different attitudes and policies are in between; each of them stems from cultural differences in different societies and are the result of the complex interaction among patient, physician, and society.

Complete, accurate, continuous information to the patient with cancer is a requirement of deontology in the United States,[1] while it is far less imperative in Italy and most of the European countries. On one side, truth-withholding is deemed a limit to the patient's freedom; on the other side, it is considered protection from an unbearable, shattering reality.

What lies behind these different approaches has been discussed in previous articles.[2–4] Briefly, in the cultures more strongly bound to the Hippocratic tradition of medicine, even though information is the basis for the covenant between patient and physician, the first aim is not information but what is good for the patient (beneficence). At the root of this approach is substantial distrust of the possibility of effectively communicating knowledge; the layman (the patient) is not believed to be able to make informed decisions, and the doctor becomes a powerful, distant figure exercising unilateral power on the basis of incommunicable knowledge.[5] Even today the essence of what the Roman Emperor Hadrian said in the second century holds true: "It is difficult to remain Imperator in the presence of a physician."[6]

On the other hand, in the United States the importance of the learning process is valued much more highly, and thorough information is considered the prerequisite for a therapeutic relationship between patient and doctor.[7] The balance between the two principles of beneficence and autonomy dictates practical directions in bioethics.[8] In patriarchal or hierarchical societies, beneficence is the preeminent organizing principle, taking precedence over justice and personal rights; while in liberal democratic systems, personal rights and liberty are purportedly the organizing principles of society. Truth-telling to the patient is possible and beneficial where autonomy is synonymous with freedom, while it is much more complex where the principle of beneficence has absolute priority over that of autonomy.[9]

The metaphorical implications of the word *cancer* (which are still very strong) are not equally perceived in different cultural contexts; even the comprehension of the words we use to disclose the diagnosis and the prognosis to the patient is emotion and culture related and may vary widely among different persons and social groups.

Furthermore, the nature of suffering and the goals of medicine in this respect,[10] and the issue of dying are subjects of open discussion and confrontation in some cultures, whereas they are timidly or never approached elsewhere.

Despite these differences, a thorough, honest disclosure to the patient of his or her cancer diagnosis and prognosis should be considered morally mandatory in our modern multiethnic societies; incomplete information and the consequent web of half-truths can be even worse than truth-withholding itself. But what is really thorough information? How is it to be handled with the patients? And what are the ultimate goals of truth-telling?

Thorough information must not be a fetish or an obsession; and the information provided must be nondogmatic and fully understandable by the patient.[11] As such, it must be adjusted according to his or her cultural background, educational level, and willingness to hear a truth that can be severely disrupting and even defeating.

Thorough information to the patient with neoplasia concerns not only the diagnosis but also the therapeutical program and the prognosis. We shall try to approach each of these different steps, with reference to our direct experiences in clinical practice.

TRUTH-TELLING ABOUT DIAGNOSIS

Thoughtful disclosure of the diagnosis of cancer is probably the most arduous part of our task. The word *cancer* has a mighty and dismaying metaphoric meaning; for this reason, we should from the outset dismantle the all-or-nothing concept of uniform clinical behavior of cancer and of an invariably fatal outcome. We can try to oppose discouragement and fear by conveying the idea of the great heterogeneity of neoplasia and outlining to the patient appropriate, rational medical strategies to deal with this kind of disease.

The technical knowledge inherent in the medical diagnosis must be translated with layman's words in a plain—and as much as possible serene—conversation adjusted to the cultural level of the patient and attuned to the patient's emotional state. Along with the direct conversation with the patient, the diagnosis of cancer should be supported by further ad hoc informative material such as booklets compiled by trained oncologists and psycho-oncologists at major institutions. National Cancer Institute educational material, for instance, is available worldwide and could be translated and adapted to each cultural situation, and given to the patient for reading. The oncologist should then encourage questions and comments.

Comparison of patients' individual experiences with others affected by the same disease is inevitable, as patients wait together for long periods and exchange their impressions and experiences. However, this does not generally help and may even be detrimental. The oncologist should be well aware of this reality and be available to openly confront this issue; indeed, every personal situation is unique, and any individual is also unique in facing cancer physically and emotionally. While being accurate in presenting the published data and the results to patients, the oncologist should always also instill this sense of the uniqueness of each individual case, so as to allow the patient to make good and full use of his or her own personal resources.

Consulting of encyclopedias or medical dictionaries by the patient is strongly to be discouraged; indeed, the accuracy and correctness of these publications are generally very poor, and the room for misinterpretation is very large. The role of the mass media is also often questionable and open to misinterpretation.

However, patients will look for such sources of information and will rely on them if their doctor is reluctant to make the necessary medical knowledge available to them.

One of us (E.B.) is a hematology attending physician at a large university center in Italy: The diagnosis of acute leukemia can strike the patient very strongly, with a feeling of impending, unavoidable death. The disclosure of such a diagnosis must be handled with particular sensitivity because of the state of the patient, who is often very sick due to anemia and other severe complications such as infections or bleeding. In this situation, the patient needs to be immediately assured of the availability of prompt, effective supportive therapy (transfusions, antibiotics). Informed consent for blood transfusions is mostly a formal procedure and does not take the place of more detailed, personal communication when clinical conditions improve and the initial contact with the hospital is over. I do not usually go into many details about the numerous varieties of acute leukemia; instead, I emphasize that acute leukemia is a chemosensitive disease (responsive to chemotherapy) and that a complete remission can be achieved in a substantial proportion of patients. The patient must be assured that all the urgent procedures the situation requires will be promptly carried out and that he will be properly informed of any new developments; often there is a need for reassurance of other family members about the nonhereditary or nontransmissible quality of the disease.

A quite different example is provided by chronic leukemias, which at onset may progress slowly and may well be picked up by chance. A large cohort of patients with chronic lymphocytic leukemia do not need treatment at all. Even though these cases are much less demanding than those of acute leukemia, we are faced with the twofold difficulty of disclosing the diagnosis of leukemia while at the same time withholding treatment. This can be difficult to accept by the patient; it may generate skepticism and apprehension and may prompt the patient to seek another opinion.

The diagnosis of chronic myeloid leukemia implies that after a period of almost normal well-being the patient will experience an acceleration of his disease, which in all features will come to resemble acute leukemia. When the quality of his life is good, it may be very hard for the patient to accept burdensome therapeutic measures such as bone marrow transplantation to prevent transformation to the acute phase. The disparity between present well-being and eventual problems adds to the difficulty of judicious medical counseling in the stable phase of chronic myeloid leukemia.

One of us (A.S.) is a solid tumor attending physician at a large teaching hospital in New York City: When I see a patient for an initial consultation, I spend at least one hour discussing in great detail the pathologic findings and their meaning. Patients come to me already aware of their diagnosis of cancer. However, it is only when they discuss it with the medical oncologist that the reality of it hits them completely. Patients do not generally discuss the details of their prognosis and treatment with their surgeons; it is the task of the medical oncologist to inform them. Often I draw a picture of the cancer, not unlike what I used to do during my training in pediatric oncology; this helps patients see their disease, and it provides a very good start for a detailed conversation. In my practice, too, I try to listen a lot to my patients, and I let them lead the conversation with me. Issues come up regarding diagnosis, prognosis, and treatment in a very haphazard way initially, following the patients' questions, rather than through a fixed approach. Later on in the first encounter I summarize what we have said, put it in a precise order, and fill in all the missing information.

TRUTH-TELLING ABOUT THE THERAPEUTIC PROGRAM

A.S.: Due to the cultural and legal requirements of medicine in the United States, most of the time I give patients further detailed information, including data and statistics on their prognosis with different treatment options, at the time of our first encounter. Often, details on the side effects of the proposed therapy are also discussed. As I do not find my first conversation with a patient an ideal situation (the patient is generally overwhelmed), I arrange to see patients at least once more before they actually start therapy, for a conversation only, and I provide them with educational material that they can read before seeing me again. In this time-consuming enterprise I am supported by the excellent work of the nurse collaborating with me, who also dedicates long sessions with the patients and their loved ones. The role of the nurse is essential, indeed, in that patients can hear the same information from two different voices (at least). Also, they can phrase their concerns in different ways and express some particular concerns either to the doctor or to the nurse, at their preference.

E.B.: The whole body of our experience must be offered to illustrate to the patient the rationale and outline of the therapeutic program. In combined modality programs, each phase must be presented as part of an integrated approach, whose prospective efficacy and toxicity should be discussed in as much detail as possible.

Some forms of therapy, such as severely impairing surgery, intensive chemotherapy, or bone marrow transplantation, can be particularly disruptive; the patient needs to know to what extent the therapy will affect his or her present and future life. In this respect, it is of the utmost importance to know from the beginning the duration of the whole therapeutic program and its acute and chronic toxicity; when the patient can weigh present hardships against future benefits, he usually becomes more calm and cooperative. Because scientific medical words often have different meanings to the patient and to the physician, great attention should be paid not to use medical jargon or confusing technicalities.

When in the early 1970s I was the responsible investigator of one of the first studies on breast cancer adjuvant chemotherapy,[12] the practice of randomized studies in Italy was at its very beginning, and informed consent was optional. Even though the rationale for adjuvant treatment was sound, its efficacy was still to be proved, and its long-term toxicity was still to be evaluated. Proposing year-long chemotherapy on a randomized basis after impairing surgery was not an easy task, as it was not easy to decide what to tell the women who, after the randomization, were not offered treatment. After the positive results obtained in the last 20 years,[13] adjuvant or primary chemotherapy in breast cancer is now standard and no longer poses problems. There remain difficulties, on both the patient's and the physician's side, for the vast majority of current adjuvant chemotherapy, including that for brain tumors, head and neck squamous carcinomas, non–small-cell lung cancer, and cervix and colorectal cancers. Indeed, the results in these areas have yet to be proved as unequivocally beneficial; adjuvant therapy can still be viewed as "experimental."

TRUTH-TELLING ABOUT EXPERIMENTAL TREATMENTS AND TRIALS

A recent study illustrates the standard of informed consent in European multicenter randomized clinical trials.[14] Not surprisingly, this study confirms that the amount of information given varied largely between Mediterranean and non-Mediterranean clinicians. Altogether, 38% of clinicians did not always tell patients that they had been assigned to their treatment at random; 42% used verbal consent only; and 5% did not seek consent at all. A commentary from the United Kingdom[15] raises important issues on how to handle information in randomized studies. Indeed, presenting randomized treatment options can be particularly difficult if consent is sought before randomization; one has to explain to all patients the potential advantages and disadvantages of a new treatment even though only half of them will eventually receive it. As previously suggested by Zelen,[16] commentators suggest that randomization should be done before consent, and they support its ethical (although paternalistic) use; this argument is still open to debate and controversy. One of us (A.S.) is very hesitant in accepting prerandomization: it seems to invalidate the essence of honesty toward the patient, which should lead to sharing the responsibility for his or her medical treatment. If doctors are reluctant to explain the nature of a randomized trial to their patients, why are they? Should we proceed with prerandomization, or should we refrain from enrolling patients in a trial if we cannot justify its nature to the patient? (This is a comment from a United States perspective and might not apply to other cultures.)

In nonrandomized studies using new therapeutic agents, the "experimental" nature of the therapy must be clearly explained to the patient and consent sought for using the new drug, which is viewed as a workable alternative to ineffective standard therapies. In the case of random allocation, the patient should be assured that if he refuses to adhere to the prospective study, he will be offered treatment according to the highest conventional standards. In any case, informed consent should not be regarded as a fixed object that has only to be verbalized in a one-way process (the culture of informed consent); on the contrary, informed consent should belong in a culture of communication, which is by definition a two-way process between the doctor and the patient that develops over

time and correlates with other variables, such as the outside society.

Illustrating the risk of long-term toxicity inherent to therapy may be particularly distressing to patients; they are confronted with not only their present difficult situation but also the looming of troubles to come.

E.B.: The risk of infertility is perceived as severely impairing normal life and, in men, is somehow connected with apprehensions about sexual potency. The leukemogenic risk of radiotherapy and chemotherapy should be properly weighed against their efficacy and curative potential. In clinical situations such as Hodgkin's disease[17] and breast cancer adjuvant chemotherapy[13] rather conclusive data are available; these data should be used to put the problem of secondary neoplasms into perspective and to assess its real magnitude. Accordingly, patients with Hodgkin's disease, for example, who have been treated with radiotherapy only or with chemotherapy without alkylating agents can be reassured because their risk of leukemia is very small, if any. On the other hand, patients who have for the past been treated with combined radio- and chemotherapy with alkylating agents have a definite risk of leukemia; the duration of this risk time is, however, limited to the first 10 years after therapy, and that can be alleviating for long-term survivors.

A.S.: The risk of infertility is a main subject of discussion with my patients, most of whom are young women of child-bearing age, who would like to have children after adjuvant chemotherapy for breast cancer. Data from the literature are limited to experience with two drug regimens used in an adjuvant setting—namely, CMF and CAF; but many young women are now receiving more intensive adjuvant programs. Therefore, we face a lot of uncertainties, about how successful a new treatment might be, and also about long-term toxicity, with its important symbolic elements. I always discuss the issue of infertility after chemotherapy with my patients, and I do take it into consideration when offering a particular regimen. At times, it seems to be the most distressful part of the conversation with a young woman, which is easily understandable as children are a projection into the future, and taking the possibility away can have tremendous metaphoric implications.

Inevitably, the discussion of long-term side effects of treatments is particularly demanding, since we ask patients to weigh immediate benefit against potential future damage. It is indeed at this point that most patients, even in the United States context, ask for the doctor's help in making the decision. I remain convinced that doctors should not merely present options, but that they should, on the contrary, be willing to assume full responsibility when requested to do so by an informed patient. I shall never forget a young patient with leukemia, sitting on her bed with her two-month-old son and being told she could choose between experimental treatment, in-hospital support therapy alone, or immediate discharge home. After presenting the options, the team left her alone in her room; I found this most unethical, and still do.

TRUTH-TELLING ABOUT PROGNOSIS

Telling about prognosis means indicating how long the patient is likely to survive and the probable quality of life with and without treatment.[18] The approach to the disclosure of prognosis can obviously vary widely according to a number of factors, including the stage of the neoplastic disease, the age of the patient, the type and the prospective efficacy of the therapy.

One delicate aspect of truth-telling regarding prognosis is our limited ability to accurately prognosticate—something we often forget. When we both worked at the same institution in Milan, we were often told that what makes a doctor is the ability to prognosticate. This was an important incentive to be very accurate with each patient. Young oncologists must be trained to judge the patient's most likely course of disease and life expectancy, which are relevant not only to truth-telling, but also to the proper medical management of patients, so that excessive treatment as well as all forms of undertreatment may be avoided. However, over years of clinical experience the ability to prognosticate becomes stronger on the one hand and yet on the other becomes questionable. There are in each oncologist's personal experience a multitude of different cases, and experience teaches us not to behave as prophets but to be humble before patients and their families. Discussing prognosis should help the patient rather than being a way for the doctor to affirm his or her power.

If cancer is in an early clinical stage and is well manageable by therapy with high cure rates, giving a good prognosis can be very encouraging for the patient and rewarding for the physician. On the other hand, if cancer is advanced and therapy less likely to be effective, problems may ensue. There is a tendency to confuse telling of prognosis with the mere disclosing of statistical life-expectancy data; while providing more response rates or survival percentages does not in itself increase the quality of the information. The thrusting of bare percentages and statistics onto a patient who may have difficulties in properly interpreting them or, as has been suggested, may even expect "to be buffered against news of impending death is a gratuitous and harmful misinterpretation of the moral foundations for respect for autonomy."[9] The increasing knowledge of response rates and survival derived from controlled clinical studies should obviously help in decision making; but, as in the case of informed consent, it should not be viewed in a rigid, absolute way. A good example is provided by the perception of risk of recurrence after surgery or after achieving complete remission. A 30% risk of recurrence after surgery for early breast cancer does not have the same meaning to all patients at all times; women's perception of their risk may vary greatly depending on how the risk is presented by their doctors, as well as on their own individual values, beliefs, and goals. The same holds true when we inform the patient of the risk of recurrence in other cancers, such as Hodgkin's disease, aggressive lymphomas, or testicular carcinoma, that can be expected to be cured in a high percentage of cases.

E.B.: Some forms of acute leukemia do require immediate intensive therapy because of the risk of early death due to acute complications such as severe hemorrhage or sepsis with endotoxic shock. As suggested by others,[19] I do not think that in such a dramatic situation all the available prognostic information should be given at once: the patient is usually very sick and frightened; he may find himself unable or unwilling to know and may prefer instead to have his physician or family doctor informed about his immediate prognosis. Achieving complete remission sheds new light on prognosis and revives the patient's hope. Postremission therapy may include allogeneic bone marrow transplantation; while telling of long-term prognosis, we should clearly illustrate the potential acute and chronic toxicity of such an intensive approach and its effect on the quality of life. Indeed, acute mortality related to this procedure is still unacceptably high (about 15–20%); life-threatening complications can develop in the first three months after transplantation and chronic graft-versus-host disease developing after this period may be severely disabling.

CONCLUSIONS

One's personal attitude toward suffering and dying strongly influences one's medical approach to patients with refractory disease and terminally ill. In our Western culture there is a tendency "to deny death altogether and celebrate new forms of medical technology designed to forestall death"[18]; on the other hand, there is a debate over the "sheer futility"[20] of such experimental interventions in fully refractory diseases. Some have coined the term "bearable truth"[21] to refer to the information to be offered not to lie and "not to put too much pressure" on the patient. In these situations, the most important things are not withholding the ultimate hope and preventing despair; for a physician, the maximum effort toward these goals is an ethical mandate. Hope can be sustained and despair prevented by assuring our patients that they will not be denied any form of treatment (supportive therapy or even chemotherapy) and also that they absolutely will not suffer from unproved or futile therapies. Also, hope will be sustained by assuring patients that they will not be left alone by the doctors.

In writing these pages we have put together our thoughts and experiences as longstanding friends, having been colleagues at the same institution in Milan, sharing a common cultural background and common ideals in life and medicine. We now find ourselves practicing in two different countries, with different medical deontologies: the physician in Italy still protecting patients from painful truths, the physician in the

United States requesting complete written disclosure of all medical information to the patients in order to respect their autonomy. These differences are the result of a different perception of the concept of self-determination, viewed as the leading ethical principle in the United States but not in Italy. Although there is a trend towards more active participation of Italian patients in their health care decisions, it is unlikely that these two situations in medicine will ever be comparable. Also, this is not necessarily to be advocated, since each country is and should remain different.

It has been remarkably important, though, for the two of us to find that we share the same ethical principles and values, although we express them according to our present cultural contexts. It also has been reassuring to verify that after many years of different experiences and working styles we still believe that autonomy and beneficence do not exist without each other. They are interrelated principles, and they demand to be respected simultaneously. When there is conflict between autonomy and beneficence, it is either because we have not strived hard enough in our communication efforts, or because we have given absolute priority to one or the other, rather than aiming at a balance. Neither of us ever forgets that truth-telling, however best expressed, is a fundamental part of the medical act and of the patient-doctor relationship. But also, we do not forget that the medical responsibility rests with the physician, who is consulted for being an expert in his or her profession, that the patient is in a uniquely dependent state because of the nature of disease itself,[22] and that the patient-doctor relationship should see the doctor in the position of an educator. Finally we do not forget that we may be patients one day.

REFERENCES

1. AD HOC COMMITTEE ON MEDICAL ETHICS. 1984. American College of Physicians ethics manual. Part I. History of medical ethics, the physician and the patient, the physician's relationship to other physicians, the physician and society. Ann. Intern. Med. **101:** 129–137.
2. SURBONE, A. 1993. The information to cancer patient: Psychosocial and spiritual implications. Support. Care Cancer **1:** 89–91.
3. SURBONE, A. 1992. Truth telling to the patient. JAMA **268:** 1661–1662.
4. SURBONE, A. 1994. Informed consent and truth in medicine. Eur. J. Cancer **30A:** 2189.
5. ZITTOUN, R. 1990. Patient information and participation. *In* Psychosocial Aspects of Oncology. J. C. Holland & R. Zittoun, Eds.: 27–44. Springer. Berlin.
6. YOURCENAR, M. 1974. Memoires d'Hadrien suivi de Carnets de notes de memories d'Hadrien. Gallimard. Paris.
7. SUCHMAN, A. L. & D. A. MATTHEWS. 1988. What makes the patient-doctor relationship therapeutic? Exploring the connexional dimension of medical care. Ann. Intern. Med. **108:** 125–130.
8. THOMPSON, I. E. 1987. Fundamental ethical principles in health care. Br. Med.

J. **295:** 1461–1465.
9. PELLEGRINO, E. D. 1992. Is truth-telling to patients a cultural artifact? (Editorial.) JAMA **268:** 1734–1735.
10. CASSEL, E. J. 1982. The nature of suffering and the goals of medicine. N. Engl. J. Med. **306:** 639–645.
11. SURBONE, A. 1992. L'informazione al paziente. Il medico d'Italia. Organo Ufficiale della Federazione Nazionale dell'Ordine dei Medici Chirurghi **199:** 8
12. BONADONNA, G., E. BRUSAMOLINO, P. VALAGUSSA *et al.* 1976. Combination chemotherapy as an adjuvant treatment in operable breast cancer. N. Engl. J. Med. **294:** 405–410.
13. BONADONNA, G., P. VALAGUSSA, A. MOLITERNI *et al.* 1995. Adjuvant cyclophosphamide, methotrexate, and fluorouracil in node-positive breast cancer. The results of 20 years of follow-up. N. Engl. J. Med. **332:** 901–906.
14. WILLIAMS, C. J.& M. ZWITTER. 1994. Informed consent in European multicentre randomized clinical trials. Are patients really informed? Eur. J. Cancer **30A:** 907–910.
15. TOBIAS, J. S. & J. HOUGHTON. 1994. Is informed consent essential for all chemotherapy studies. Eur. J. Cancer **30A:** 897–899.
16. ZELEN, M. 1979. A new design for randomized clinical trials. N. Engl. J. Med. **300:** 1242–1245.
17. BRUSAMOLINO, E., G. PAGNUCCO, G. CASTELLI *et al.* 1992. The risk of secondary myelodysplasia and acute leukemia in Hodgkin's disease is related to the combined modality therapy and to the use of nitrosourea derivatives. Proc. Am. Soc. Clin. Oncol **11:** 329.
18. ANNAS, G. J. 1994. Informed consent, cancer, and truth in prognosis. N. Engl. J. Med. **330:** 223–225.
19. VARIOUS AUTHORS. 1994. Informed consent, cancer, and truth in prognosis. (Correspondence.) N. Engl. J. Med. **331:** 810–812.
20. MOERTEL, C. G. 1991. Off-label drug use for cancer therapy and national health care priorities. JAMA **266:** 3031–3032.
21. ESPINOSA, E., M. GONZÁLES BARÓN, J. ORDOÑEZ & P. ZAMONA. 1993. The information given to the terminal patient with cancer. Eur. J. Cancer **29A:** 1795–1796.
22. PELLEGRINO, E. D. 1987. Altruism, self-interest and medical ethics. JAMA **258:** 1939–1940.

Communication in Cancer Care

The Dutch Situation

JOLANDA SCHOUWSTRA AND JOEP W. VAN DEN BLINK

Dr. Daniel den Hoed Cancer Center
P.O. Box 5201
3008 AE Rotterdam, The Netherlands

Responsibility *to* the patient as an autonomous, self-determining individual, instead of responsibility *for* the patient as a paternalized dehumanized person, implies telling the truth instead of lying and deceiving; this is a professional ability that needs to be further developed.

This chapter starts with an outline of how the truth is to be told according to Dutch legislation. Then this legal formula is translated into everyday practice, followed by an example of truth-telling in a cancer center. Finally, we will comment on the ethical question "Is it right to tell the patient the truth?"

THE LEGAL CONTEXT

Until recently, a Dutch medical practitioner more or less followed his own guidance in informing or not (fully) informing the patient. This situation has changed, however. On April 1, 1995 a new law was enacted in the Netherlands—"The Law concerning Agreement on Medical Treatment." The term "agreement" in this law carries the same meaning as it does in commercial law, such as an agreement between a client and a building contractor concerning the conversion of a house. The law is a result of the need to bridge the "paradox of medical aid." "Being a patient places people in a vulnerable position, and he is therefore to be protected against a system which was, on the one hand, created in order to help him but, on the other hand, is justified only by the patient's need for help." The law also reflects recent developments in the doctor/patient relationship and the individual's right to autonomy and self-determination. The medical practitioner is no longer responsible *for* the patient (paternalism), he bears responsibility *with regard to* the patient in a horizontal relationship. The law stipulates the rights and obligations of both parties towards each other, aiming at an *equal* cooperative relationship between medical practitioner and patient. The law is based on:

- the obligation to supply adequate information either way;
- the obligation to receive the patient's prior consent for treatment;
- the obligation to respect the privacy of all parties concerned.

Informed Consent

The patient's right to information, the medical practitioner's obligation to inform the patient, and the obligation to obtain the patient's consent prior to treatment or examination have now, in the Netherlands, been laid down in law. The law obliges medical practitioners to inform the patient in understandable language about:

- his disease or disorder;
- the nature of the suggested treatment or examination;
- possible alternative treatments;
- the consequences and possible risks connected with the suggested treatment or examination;
- medications and their possible side effects.

The medical practitioner is to inform the patient clearly about exactly what is the matter with him, what is going to happen to him, and why. The patient needs this information in order to come to a considered decision about his treatment (informed consent).

It is not easy, however, to decide on the extent of the information the patient must receive. On the one hand, he must have adequate information to come to a considered decision; on the other hand, he should not suffer any unnecessary anxiety or be burdened with information he cannot cope with. Recent research on the psychological effects of the level of information on head and neck cancer patients showed that the highly informed were better adjusted in interpersonal relations and were more intimate with relatives. On the other hand, they experienced more fears, anxiety, changes in their lives, worries about their health, and physical symptoms of their cancer.[1] The patient's ability to understand all the relevant medical-technical considerations depends on his intelligence and emotional condition as well as on other factors, which may be difficult to assess. With these considerations in mind, the obligation to inform the patient consists of more than just providing relevant medical data. The greater the importance of the information, the greater the obligation on the part of the medical practitioner to soothe the patient and to present the information in such a way to achieve maximal results under the circumstances—*to optimally inform the patient*.[2] If the patient cannot cope with all the information in one session, the medical practitioner is obliged to divide the information into more than one session. He is responsible for the patient's understanding of the information given, and he is to check if the patient has, indeed, understood the information and if he is aware of the consequences of his consent to a certain treatment or examination. The way in which the medical practitioner presents the information may, therefore, vary from patient to patient.

Thus, the transmission of information is a reciprocal process between doctor and patient, for which no fixed set of rules can be given. In any case, the information will have to be attuned to the patient's personality. Some patients need more extensive explanations than others. One patient wants his doctor to come straight to the point, the other does not. There is also the possibility of providing the patient with written information to study, as a supplement to prior oral information. However, according to the new Dutch law, written information by itself can never be considered adequate.

Will the Patient Always Be (Fully) Informed?

If, in the medical practitioner's opinion, a patient does not want to know, or will not be able to cope with, certain information, this may not be adequate reason for him not to give this information. Not informing the patient, according to the law, is allowed only in those very rare cases, known as "therapeutic exceptions," when, in the medical practitioner's opinion, the information might be harmful to the patient. In order to be able to refer to this therapeutic exception clause, the medical practitioner has to consult a fellow practitioner. A slower rate of recovery or insecurity about the prognosis is not in itself a reason for withholding information on the grounds of therapeutic exception. Only when an actual harmful effect on the patient, like a possible suicide attempt, is to be expected, does the law allow the practitioner to refer to the therapeutic exception clause. In such cases he informs a third party, such as the patient's partner, if he considers this to be in the patient's interest. As soon as the patient is considered to be able to cope with it, the practitioner is obliged to give him the information he has withheld.[3]

Another exception to the medical practitioner's obligation to inform is the patient's right not to receive unwanted information. The practitioner has to respect the patient's decision, unless the lack of information is considered extremely harmful to the patient or to third parties. In this case he has to inform the patient anyway. Even if the patient does not want to know about the side effects of his medication, for instance, he has to be informed if, for instance, they will affect his ability to drive a car. Another example: a patient is to be operated on for a mammary tumor. She has tated that she does not want to be given detailed information. She requires only information about the anesthetic and her prognosis. Therefore, only this information will be given by her doctor; she will not be informed about the actual surgery, frozen sections, etc.

Right of Access to and Transcript of Medical Files

Apart from the right of information the patient also has a legal right of access to his or her medical file. The medical practitioner is obliged to keep a medical file, in which all information concerning the patient's treatment is included. The patient has a direct right of access to this file, with the exception of any information not concerning his person. Information that may infringe on the privacy of third parties is also excluded from the right of access. Letters of referral and other information given by other practitioners are not available to the patient. He may, however, obtain this information directly from the practitioner in question, who, because of his "agreement on medical treatment" with the patient, is obliged to give it. Thus, the agreement on medical treatment is a personal agreement between two parties.

The patient does not have just a right of access, he also has a right of transcription. This means he is entitled to a photocopy of his file, which right he may, if necessary, enforce by means of a legal procedure. He can also assign this right to a third party. Thus, he may authorize a lawyer to obtain a copy of his file. In civil procedures this is of increasing importance, as the file may be used as evidence. A positive side effect of this right of access to one's medical file and to copy it is the improvement of the quality of reporting.

The Patient's Obligations

The patient is obliged to clearly and fully inform the medical practitioner, in order to enable the practitioner to diagnose and treat the patient correctly. He is also obliged, within reasonable limits, to follow the practitioner's advice. In practice, this means that the patient must fully answer any relevant and specific questions and that he must, of his own accord, give any information that may be important for diagnosis or treatment. The patient's legal obligations are limited insofar as he may not be expected to be fully aware of the relevance of the information he may have to offer. These obligations of the patient may be of great importance in legal procedures in case adverse results of medical treatment are caused by the patient's actions, such as deliberately withholding or distorting information or not complying with the doctor's advice.

The Medical Practitioner's Obligations

A medical practitioner has the right to make his own decisions. He is not obliged to blindly fulfill the demands of a patient or his representative. His own expertise and convictions play a part in this decision. If a doctor is convinced a treatment is medically unnecessary or useless, he may refuse to perform it. This is laid down in the law. Moreover, according to current medical-ethical beliefs, it is a medical practitioner's duty not to perform useless treatments. The law and the ethical code thus form a basis for the medical policy of abstinence: no resuscitation in cancer patients in an advanced stage of the disease, cutting off life-support treatment in comatose patients with no chance of recovery, etc. These are examples of decisions that, as long as they are well-founded, may be made and executed by practitioners without the possibility of a judge revoking them.

Representation of Patients Who Are Incapable of Autonomous Decisions

If an adult patient is unable to act in his own interest, the practitioner's obligation towards the patient concerning information and consent must be fulfilled with a representative who is appointed by the judge or by the patient himself by written authorization; or, if no such authorization has been given, with the (married or cohabitating) partner; or, if there is no partner, with a parent, child, brother, or sister of the patient. The practitioner is obliged to comply with their wishes only in so far as they are in the patient's best interest. The responsibility for medical decisions will always lie with the practitioner. He is, therefore, obliged at all times to test his decision against the criterion of the patient's best interest.

For patients up to the age of 16, the parents or guardians are the legal representatives. However, if a minor, irrespective of his age, is considered adequately capable of assessing his interest in the matter and does not want to be represented by his parents or guardian, he must be able to count on his doctor to give weight to his opinion.

Informing a Third Party

The set legal rule for informing a third party is that the patient's explicit permission is always required. The only exception is a situation in which the patient is unable to give permission and the practitioner considers informing a third party to be necessary for the patient's treatment. If, for instance, a married couple is involved in a car crash, the man is comatose, and the woman is compos mentis, the woman should be informed and may consent to her husband's treatment.

Information to a third party can be given *only* (a) after the patient has given permission; (b) if informing a third party is essential in view of the necessary care and treatment. In his contacts with patients' partners, relatives, and friends, the medical practitioner is bound by his professional oath of secrecy. He can inform relatives only with the patient's permission, except in case of an emergency or "therapeutic exception." No strict rules can be given for this last situation, as it always involves conflicting obligations (professional secrecy against the obligation to inform). The practitioner must consider each case very carefully and, if necessary, consult a fellow practitioner. He should be very prudent and consider informing relatives only as an exception. Unless authorized to do so by the patient, relatives can never give the practitioner permission on the patient's behalf to inform a third party; this responsibility always lies with the practitioner. After the patient's death, this may lead to problems for the next of kin. As professional secrecy is not lifted after death and few patients authorize anyone to request information after their death, the next of kin cannot have access to the medical file of the deceased unless the practitioner feels obliged to violate his professional secrecy. This decision is to be made only if the practitioner is fully convinced that he is serving the deceased patient's best interest and acting on his implicit request.

In this section we have described the legal obligation of medical practitioners in the Netherlands to give information, to obtain the patient's permission (informed consent), to give access to the patient's medical file, and to inform a third party if the patient is not considered capable of making a well-founded decision. The next section will deal with giving information, with particular regard to telling the "truth".

THE TRUTH: TO TELL OR NOT TO TELL, THAT IS THE QUESTION

The description of the role of the doctor in the doctor-patient relationship has been summarized by Dr. John Brown (1810–1882) as follows:

> It is the duty of the doctor in the first place, to cure us; in the second, to be kind to us; in the third, to be true to us; in the fourth, to keep our secrets; in the fifth, to warn us; and best of all, to forewarn us; in the sixth, to be grateful to us; and, in the last, to keep his time and temper.

If an unfavorable diagnosis is made, the inevitable question arises to what extent the patient should be informed. The doctor often worries about whether the patient will be able to face the truth. But a more important factor is the fact that many doctors are afraid to tell the truth and do not know/have not been trained to handle this situation. With the introduction of the new law, this question arises less and less often, as the doctor is legally obliged to inform the patient. If he does not, the patient can demand access to his file and read the truth anyway. This way of receiving information is a much greater shock for the patient than being told by the doctor, and the patient's trust in the doctor is damaged.

It might be advisable to assess right from the beginning of a doctor/patient relationship what information the patient will or will not receive in certain circumstances. In this way the question of which information, given to which patients, in which circumstances will have a positive effect, and why, may be answered with more accuracy. Scientific research in the field of informing the patient usually studies the perception and appreciation of the information supplied and hardly ever includes the question how much and what kind of information a patient can cope with and what would be the best way to communicate it.

The rare studies concerned with the question, what do patients themselves want to know? clearly show that most patients want to know more than doctors, until now, have been willing to tell. According to a number of researchers, doctors tend to assume too often and too quickly that patients would suffer adverse effects from receiving information.[4–8]

Another reason doctors give for only sparingly informing the patient is their fear of the patient's emotional reaction, and of the possibility the patient might lose his trust in their expertise if they voice their insecurity about certain aspects of the disease or the treatment.

The main issue in telling the truth is, What can the patient cope with, and what is the best way to communicate it? The patient's reaction is closely linked to his personal attitude and way of life. Patients who have not avoided difficult situations in the past, are less likely to do so now. Therefore, the doctor should get to know the patient better, in order to gain insight into his weak and strong points.[9] How has the patient dealt with loss and change in the past—the death of relatives or friends, changing working conditions, moving house, children getting married, etc.? The patient's way of dealing with such situations reveals much about his personality. A doctor who also pays attention to the patient's conversation during an examination usually finds a way to address the issue of previous experiences and the patient's perception of loss and change. Listening is an important talent—one that tends to be underestimated and underdeveloped by medical practitioners.

Another aspect of telling the patient the truth is the meaning of the word "truth." If a patient is told that he has cancer, does this mean the same to him as to the doctor who supplies the information? In a questionnaire a doctor said he meant "a tumor localized in a certain area, which can be surgically removed and which may leave a surgical scar." When the patient was asked what cancer meant to him, he answered, "Cancer means dying, being left by everybody, utter desolation, lying alone in a room, spreading an unpleasant odor, having no future whatsoever." This proves that the discrepancy between what the doctor is trying to say and what it implies for the patient may be very great, indeed.

Effect of the Truth on the Patient

The little truth is clad in clear wording;
the big truth is embedded in deep silence.
—R. TAGORE

When a patient proves to have cancer, a Dutch doctor practically always informs him of this fact at once. Then they discuss what steps are to be undertaken. The patient and his relatives often turn out to be unable to adequately take in the information, as a diagnosis of cancer evokes strong emotions. If they absorb any information, the process is usually very selective. The patient now knows what is wrong with him and goes home in a highly emotional state of mind.

A study by Keirse[5] shows that the following problems may occur:

- The patient feels crushed, does not want anything, is no longer capable of anything; he is not coping at all.
- The patient denies that there is anything wrong with him. He does not want to talk about it. He is incapable of making the necessary arrangements to say good-bye.
- The patient acknowledges his disease. He wants to talk about it, but his spouse cannot.
- Good friends are afraid to visit him, because they do not know how to behave. The patient wants to talk with them, but dare not take the initiative. He experiences isolation.
- Acquaintances suddenly impose on the patient out of interest or sheer fascination with his suffering and want to support him or see him suffer. The patient does not need or want this attention, but dares not ask them to leave him be.
- The patient is in pain and/or short of breath, but does not consult the doctor, as he is unable to cure him anyway.[10]

The "Bad News Interview"

Based on the above-mentioned facts, the Daniel den Hoed Cancer Center (DHCC) has developed the following procedure. The "bad news interview" takes place after examining the patient in the presence of the doctor, the nurse, and the patient's close relatives or friends. This interview leaves room for emotions. It is not restricted to information about the patient's condition, but also includes possibilities and strategies for treatment; if possible, the patient is given written information as well. At the end of the interview one must check whether the information has been understood and whether the patient and relatives have any further questions. An appointment for a second interview is always made. During this second interview the patient's understanding of the information given in the first interview is checked. The reason for splitting up the bad news interview into at least two sessions is the fact that a long, detailed conversation is seldom possible because of the patient's and relatives' emotions. Moreover, the patient has to consent to the treatment he is to receive. He can give his consent only once he has fully understood and accepted the information. It is impossible to actively involve the patient in decisions about treatment during a first interview. We know from experience that the patient and his relatives tend to be either very quiet or very angry. In either of these state of mind they will not be able to pose any technical questions.

During the second interview, which is held a week or so afterwards, the patient has come to realize what is wrong with him and is able to discuss the possible treatments and come to an agreement with the doctor, unless the doctor considers a third interview to be necessary. The patient tends to ask many questions during this second interview: is the treatment curative, hopeful, or palliative? are there any side effects? how long will it take? etc.

The doctor always informs the patient where he can get nonmedical aid and counseling. He mentions the possibility of an interview with a social worker; and if there is a patients' association, contacts with fellow patients are encouraged.

If the doctor does not clearly state his diagnosis right at the beginning of the bad news interview, this may have an adverse effect on the patient's absorbing the information: the initial warning may scare the patient so much, that he does not hear the actual diagnosis and, consequently, is not able to come to terms with it. A good method to use is to tell the important news briefly, in a neutral manner, using simple words—the so-called KISS principle, (keep it short and simple). An example: "The examinations show you have intestinal cancer." This gives the patient an opportunity to react to the news. By repeating the diagnosis and discussing the patient's emotions with him, the doctor may be able to help the patient face the news. Studies prove that patients can handle bad news very well when told it in this way, and that they do not think their doctor's approach heartless.[11] A patient's experience:

> First, he very carefully told me I had breast cancer, and I reacted to that. During the rest of the conversation he reacted to me, and not the other way round. His composure was very encouraging.

This patient said she felt that the doctor focused completely on her and reacted to the questions she posed.

> He took his lead from me, gave me the information I asked for. He did not tell me things I was not interested in at that moment, but dealt with my questions very calmly and in great detail. He paid close attention to me, checking whether I had understood his answer, whether the information had been clear enough and he had given enough information.

The patient considered the silences that the doctor allowed to fall very important.

> When he had just given some information, he gave ample time for me to think it over. He would wait patiently until I was ready to hear more or to demand further explanation.[12]

However, it is essential not to give just the bad news, but, in the same session, to point at possible treatments. All too often the patient is told, "I am sorry, but there is nothing I can do for you" when no curative or life-prolonging treatment can be given. When we have no further options to cure the patient, we can still help him in a number of ways. Palliative medicine is an additional art that a doctor can and must master. Telling the truth is an integral part of this art. The effect of telling the truth in the last stage of a patient's life may be very great. A recent example from the DHCC palliative care unit:

> One never gets used to it, but, I get very good counseling. They pay attention to me and ask me how I feel. When I am worse, they do not hush it up; they are very open. Moreover, you see, they have told the truth about not having to be in pain when the end comes. That is a thought I find very comforting.

This patient found composure in her relationship with her doctor, which made it easier for her to discuss her illness and enabled her to face the end of her life with less fear.

POLICY IN ACUTE SITUATIONS: A PRACTICAL EXAMPLE

The new Law concerning Agreement on Medical Treatment has made the demand for agreement on medical treatment more explicit and given it a legal status. From an ethical point of view, the patient's consent had been obligatory for quite some time, especially in cases of major medical treatment, which seriously compromises the patient's autonomy.

Resuscitation definitely falls in this category. However, this kind of urgent treatment is hardly ever performed with the patient's prior consent. Still, in some cases, there might be good grounds for wanting this consent. Resuscitation became a subject of interest with the introduction of CPR (cardiopulmonary resuscitation) as an adequate treatment for cardiac arrest, especially in myocardial infarction.[13] Before its introduction resuscitation was restricted to victims of drowning and suffocation. Modern-day television daily proves the total moral acceptance, even admiration, for this technique, in soap operas like "Bay Watch." In oncology, however, the situation is completely different. Major studies on the value of CPR with oncology patients show that only a small percentage of all clinically resuscitated cancer patients leave the hospital alive.[14] Therefore, the patient may expect the hospital to have a good, detailed DNR (do not resuscitate) policy to protect him against unnecessary exposure to medically useless treatment. Such a policy must also deal with the patient's right to participate and receive information concerning the decision process whenever possible. In acute situations this is usually impossible, which means that the subject has to be discussed before the situation occurs. As this is a difficult subject to discuss with the patient, we describe a method that is used in the Daniel den Hoed Cancer Center.

During hospitalization in the DHCC all patients are classified as Policy I, II or III patients:

Policy I: resuscitate; no limit to interventions.
Policy II: no resuscitation; agreements about:
- admission to intensive care
- artificial respiration
- treatment of infections, loss of blood, cardiac failure.

Policy III: treatment directed solely at counteracting complaints such as pain, nausea, constipation, thirst, fear, dyspnea, etc.[15]

These codes are used to inform doctors and nurses about the desired treatment during an acute situation. Discussion about directions for a "nonmaximal policy" started in 1990. This discussion was based on nurses' experience that uncertainty about what action to take in acute situations led to problems:

- There was no uniform policy for all patients.
- There were no guidelines describing the procedures and the conditions to be met.

Principles

Acute situations are divided into two types: (a) acute failure of vital functions (breathing and/or circulation) that will cause death within minutes if no action is taken; (b) complications (fever, bleeding, etc.) that may prove fatal if not treated immediately. The classification of clinical patients into categories is meant to enable the medical staff to act instantly and adequately, when there is no time for consultation with the patient and getting his consent for treatment. Therefore, it makes sense to outline a policy beforehand, especially as it can be anticipated that, in some cases, resuscitation and/or other interventions in acute situations will be of no avail. Moreover, the patient himself must also be able to demand certain restrictions to treatment.

One must realize that classification in category I, II, or III is based only partially on the phase of the patient's disease. The patient's wishes, the proposed treatment, and the risks involved in the treatment are important additional factors taken into account in classifying a patient.

An example: a patient with metastasized melanoma, who, because of the stage of his disease, would not normally be classified in category I, may nevertheless be classified as such if he is currently receiving immunotherapy. Immunotherapy may cause serious cardiovascular complications, which, however, are treatable and (quickly) reversible. It would be incorrect to let a patient who has given permission for immunotherapy as well as for treatment for its possible complications die of the direct consequences of the treatment.

Assessing and Modifying the Policy in Acute Situations

In the out-patient clinic, the doctor who makes the decision to hospitalize a patient discusses with the patient his reasons for hospitalization, the treatment, its direct and indirect risks, and the possibility of treating these complications, and informs him about his right to express his wishes concerning restrictions on treatment. The doctor asks in particular whether the patient has drawn up a do-not-resuscitate or euthanasia statement. Such written statements are widely known and socially accepted, and the patient usually regards the question as perfectly normal and is not unduly bothered by it, especially if it is one question among a number of others. The doctor makes note of the patient's wishes in the file, including the policy in case of acute situations.

Once the patient is hospitalized, the attending physician discusses and explains the treatment policy as suggested by the doctor of the outpatient department, including the policy in acute situations. On the basis of this consultation and his own assessment of the patient's interest, the attending doctor classifies the patient for the policy in acute situations. This policy is included in the file on a special, easily accessible form. *The policy may be amended* at the patient's request or following changes in the medical situation. It is advisable to have a nurse present during the doctor's conversation with the patient concerning such subjects as amending the policy in acute situations.

Informing the Patient about the Policy in Acute Situations

It is obvious that such sensitive subjects as the policy in acute situations should preferably be discussed *personally*, at the right moment, and, if necessary, in more than one session. Written information about the patient's right to state his own wishes concerning restrictions on treatment is included in the information leaflets the patient receives on admission. The advantage of this leaflet is that the subject has already been brought to the patient's attention by the time the patient and doctor discuss it, and this probably makes their discussion easier.

Information under All Circumstances?

Basically, the decision not to be informed lies with the patient (see WILL THE PATIENT ALWAYS BE FULLY INFORMED? above). Naturally, this also applies to resuscitation policy. Here, too, the doctor may withhold information from the patient (therapeutic exception) only if it can reasonably be assumed that providing the information would cause serious harm to the patient (see above-mentioned section). Therapeutic exception is a exceptional situation; the circumstances must be verifiable, or the scale will tip to the side of paternalism.

Bottlenecks

Of course, the patient does not always have the expertise necessary to fully judge the choice of policy I, II, and III. Moreover, the patient's problems are often complex, changing with time and dependent on many factors. This causes a lot of uncertainty, also concerning policy I, II, and III decisions, which the patient preferably should not be burdened with. Doctors do consider it important, however, that the patient be informed about the phase and prognosis of the disease. The main problem in this respect is how to tell the patient. Many doctors have stated that they find it difficult to tell a patient that resuscitation is pointless and will therefore not be performed. During their training, doctors are not taught social skills and conversational techniques. This may cause a lot of problems when the doctor has to have a bad news interview or when the choice of policy in acute situations is discussed. Doctors who have not had this training as a student should therefore receive it in the institution at which he works. This training may include videotapes and role playing. In the DHCC the training is based on the excellent material provided by Maguire[16] and Buderman[17], as well as on video-tapes in which a psychiatrist conducts interviews with patients, showing all the pitfalls and how to avoid them.

ETHICAL ASPECTS

The issue is not that truth has to be told per se, but that patients have to be properly informed; this means that the issue is how, when, and by whom the truth is to be told.

In the weekly journal of the Royal Dutch Medical Association of 20 October 1995 the following case history appeared under the headline "Eerlijkheid duurt het langst" (honesty is the best policy):

> A woman chose to give birth at a polyclinic with the assistance of a obstetrician. In partu the contractions spontaneously stopped. Without the patient being consulted, the wrong medication was injected (probably the shot of ermetrine that had been prepared beforehand). There were no more contractions; all labor activity stopped. The gynecologist on duty panicked and manually delivered the child. The staff "fought" for the baby's life for an hour and a half. The result was a physically and mentally severely disabled baby. The medical staff did not disclose the full facts of the case, in spite of the parents' insistently repeated requests. The parents remained unaware of the cause of the child's handicap and had all kinds of tests performed, including genetic screening! Employees of the clinic who were aware of the malpractice and asked that the parents be informed were threatened with dismissal. The reaction of the gynecologist responsible, when confronted with the parents' knowledge of the actual course of events five(!) years afterwards, was, *"You should never have known any of this."*

This case history is a true story, which happened in 1982. The mere fact that the editorial board of the journal deemed it necessary to publish this article in 1995 as a warning to Dutch physicians indicates their doubt about truth-telling by doctors and supports the present legislation.

Health legislation and medical ethics partially overlap, especially in those cases where the law represents the average morale and ethics of present-day society. The law lays down standards and general rules, which create certain restrictions but which also establish individual freedom and autonomy. Ethical standards are, by nature, multiform and should be used as a measure of one's behavior and actions. Cultural, religious, historical, and other perspectives are of great importance and may lead to opposing views. In Japan and various other countries, a doctor usually does not tell a patient he has cancer. In many occidental countries, such medical conduct is nowadays considered medically unacceptable. But within one country, too, fierce ethical discussions may take place, like the national discussion about euthanasia in the Netherlands. Ethical values and standards have been kept within certain legal bounds, in spite of the continuing process of law and precedents defining the common judicial (that is, democratically, socially established) bounds. Legally established rules take precedence over ethically accepted values and are usually a few steps behind. This also applies to the law discussed in this chapter. The law follows the ethical consensus and provides the opportunity to legally enforce regulations that have been ethically accepted but have not always been lived up to.

Ethical views on providing information, too, are subject to differences of opinion, which are often defended by the way in which they are described: lying, cheating, not telling the truth, misleading, telling a little white lie, withholding information, telling half truths, providing incorrect information, etc. Some of these forms of not telling the truth are considered acceptable, some are not. In the literature, however, there is a growing consensus that can be paraphrased "to tell the truth or not to tell the truth—that is the question." Whatever the word or expression used, it all comes down to this one question. The prevailing opinion is that hardly any situation can be imagined, let alone encountered, in which not telling the truth might be justified.[18–21] Except in very special circumstances, to mislead patients is to deny them due respect; it implies that they are incapable of understanding, accepting, and controlling their situation. Lying or deception is, therefore, an abuse of power that infringes on the patient's right of self-determination and self-knowledge. It is, in short, an affront to the patient's dignity and autonomy.[22] Consequently, there is practically no ethical defence for not telling the truth; it flatly opposes the patient's right of autonomy and the basic rule, *primum non nocere*.

The legal basis for this right, too, stems from ancient times. As early as Roman times we find legislation based on *alterum non laedere* (doing no damage to others). Medical history, too, shows that quite early on the basic rule, when informing the patient, the truth is to be told, was accepted.[23] In medieval times, for instance, the truth about a fatal diagnosis was to be told to allow the patient to receive the holy sacrament and to prepare for his demise.

This practice, based on Christian theology, was not always followed, however. As time went by and people became less religious, the practice declined, and the acceptance of "white lies" took root. Not telling the truth was even proclaimed as part of the art of medicine: *qui enim nescit simulare, nescit curare* (he who can not dissimulate can not cure).[24] The doctor would urge the patient to have faith in him and lay his fate in his hands; because of this doctor-patient relationship, the doctor would consider white lies acceptable.

These little white lies survived for a long time. Oken's survey of 1961, based on questionnaires and personal interviews, showed that out of 219 physicians at Michel Reese Hospital (in the United States), 90% generally did not inform cancer patients of their diagnoses.[25] The situation in the United States has drastically changed. In a comparable survey, using the same questionnaire, held in 1979 by Novack *et al.*, 97% of all physicians declared that they preferred to inform their patients of the diagnosis.[26] One of the most important reasons for this drastic change, out of a great many possible causes, is probably the dramatic change in the malpractice situation that encourages physicians to minimize liability by transferring knowledge to the patient.[27] In 1991, Jennifer Jackson wrote, "Doctors and nurses, like everyone else, have a prima facie duty not to lie—but again like everyone else, they are not duty-bound to avoid intentional deception, lying apart; except where it would involve a breach of trust."

Nowadays, the patient's trust in the physician and vice versa still form the basis of their relationship. If the physician does not fully inform the patient, or does not tell the truth, this can only lead to an ultimate breach of trust, which means that the basic rule of *primum non nocere* will be violated. It is no coincidence that the main ground the medical disciplinary council has for condemning a physician's conduct is "undermining the public's trust in the medical profession."

So far, medical practitioners have been the focal point of the discussions about informing and truth-telling. The equal partner in this respect, the patient, has been given far less attention. Hardly any research has been done to establish the effect of informing the patient and to learn the patient's own perception of the truth. In Greece, the motherland of Hippocrates, it is very rare for a cancer patient to know what he is suffering from. Hippocratic tradition prevails there even today: "The doctor must not harm, and to inform is to harm." The attitude of Greeks towards truth-telling has recently been studied.[28] The answer to the question, Do the Greeks wish to be informed of the nature of their illness? is, "It depends." It depends on their age, education, family status, occupation, place of birth and residence, and religion. Lo[29] studied a great number of patients ($n = 152$), not excluding anyone. He asked them about their experiences concerning truth-telling. Seventy-one percent of the patients expressed a feeling of "having more grip on the situation," 53 % were relieved, and 53% considered it an example of proper care. Not all patients were positive, however: 22% became nervous, and 16% felt sad; 6% felt the physician had given up on him. Other researchers have reported positive reactions to the truth from a majority of patients.[30]

Bedell[31] points out another reason why physicians do not tend to discuss matters with their patients: they assume they know what the patient wants. Her study shows that physicians know far less about their patients' views than they assumed. Loewy, too, points out that, "Even when doctors have known their patients quite well, their ability to predict the wishes of these patients [with regard to end-of-life decisions] has had virtually no more accuracy than random chance."[32]

In conclusion, we may state that physicians should learn not only to adequately inform their patients, but also to do so in interaction with the patient in his evolving place in the doctor-patient relationship. It is only by shared decision making, not by leaving patients alone with the decision, that mutual trust between patient and physician, which is the basis for their relationship, is strengthened.

FINAL REMARK

While we were writing this chapter, an article from the local newspaper *Haarlems Dagblad* of 20 October 1995 happened to find its way to our desks. The caption read: "Specialists consider information unnecessary. Cancer patient may be involuntary guinea pig." The introduction of the article begins: "Some cancer patients do not know they are guinea pigs in scientific research programs. Medical specialists sometimes do not inform their patients, because they think that these—often desperately ill—people will not be able to cope with the pros and cons of the experiments. But sometimes it is just a question of lack of time."

The Netherlands, too, have a long way to go.

REFERENCES

1. KREITLER, S. *et al.* 1995. Psychosocial effects of level of information and severity of disease on head-and-neck cancer patients. J. Cancer Educ. **10**(3): 144–145.
2. HOUTEPEN, E. & A. MOSSHAMMER. 1995. WGBO: De meest gestelde vragen. EHAM Consultancy. Almere.
3. KNMG CONSULT. 1995. Arts en patiëntenrechten. Bijlage bij Medisch Contact nr. 8.
4. FADEN, R. R., C. BECKER, C. LEWIS, J. FREEMAN & A. I. FADEN. 1981. Disclosure of information to patients in medical care. Med. Care **19:** 718–733.
5. LEY, P. 1982. Satisfaction, compliance and communication. Br. J. Clin. Psychol. **21:** 241–254.
6. MCINTOSH, J. 1974. Processes of communication, information seeking and control associated with cancer. A selective review of the literature. Soc. Sci. Med. **8:** 167–187.
7. WARMENHOVEN, N. E. 1985. De rechten van de patiënt: Opvattingen van huisartsen en patiënten. Stichting Nivel. Utrecht.
8. VAN ZUUREN, F. & J. DE BOER. 1988. Het recht op informatie. De Psycholoog. **23**(11): 623–628.
9. KEIRSE, M. 1987. Psychosociale aspecten van patiëntenzorg, deel 1. ACCO. Leuven/Amersfoort.
10. VISSER, F. J. 1992. Diagnose kanker, hoe vertel ik het mijn patiënt. Medisch Contact **22:** 693–694.
11. SCHOUTEN, J. A. M. 1985. Anamnese und advies. Samson Stafleu. Alphen aan den Rijn.
12. BRAND, E. 1995. Hoe vertel je iemand dat ze kanker heeft. Nieuwsbrief LCBB.
13. KOUWENHOVEN, W. B. *et al.* 1960. Closed chest cardiac massage of the heart. JAMA **173:** 1064.

14. VITELLI, C. E., K. COOPER, A. ROGATKO & M. F. BRENNAN. 1991. Cardiopulmonary resuscitation and the patient with cancer. J. Clin. Oncol. **9:** 111–115.
15. GEVERS, J. M. K. 1991. Beslissen over wel of niet reanimeren. Tijdschrift voor Gezondheidsrecht: 410–418.
16. FAULKNER, A., P. MAGUIRE & C. REGNARD. 1994. Breaking bad news—A flow diagram. Palliative Med. **8:** 145–151.
17. BUDERMAN, R. 1992. How to break bad news: A guide for health care professionals. Papermac. London.
18. RYAN, C. J. *et al.* 1995. Becoming none but tradesman: Lies, deception and psychotic patients. J. Med. Ethics **21:** 72–76.
19. GILLON, R. 1990. Deceit, principles and philosophical medical ethics. J. Med. Ethics **16:** 59–60.
20. GILLON, R. 1993. Is there an important moral distinction for medical ethics between lying and other forms of deception? J. Med. Ethics **19:** 131–132.
21. DUNBAR, S. 1990. An obstructed death and medical ethics. J. Med. Ethics **16:** 83–87.
22. BAKHURST, D. 1992. On lying and deceiving. J. Med. Ethics **18:** 63–66.
23. GRMEK, M. 1964. Le pieux message du medecin et le droit du malade à la vérité. Concours Medicale.
24. HOFFMAN, F. 1749. Medicus Politicus, vol. 5, part 3, ch. 4: 24. Geneva.
25. OKEN, D. 1961. What to tell cancer patients: A study of medical attitudes. JAMA **175:** 1120–1128.
26. NOVACK, D. H. 1979. Changes in physicians' attitudes toward telling the cancer patient. JAMA **241:** 897–900.
27. FREIREICH, E. J. 1979. Editorial. JAMA **241:** 928.
28. DALLA-VORGIA, P. *et al.* 1992. Attitudes of a Mediterranean population to the truth-telling issue. J. Med. Ethics **18:** 67–74.
29. LO, B., G. A. MCCLEOD & G. SAIKA. 1986. Patients' attitudes towards discussing life-sustaining treatment. Arch. Intern. Med. **146:** 113–115.
30. VAN DELDEN, J. J. M. 1993. Beslissen om niet te reanimeren. Een medisch en ethisch vraagstuk. van Gorcum. Assen.
31. BEDELL, S. E. *et al.* 1983. Survival after CPR in the hospital. N. Engl. J. Med. **309:** 569–576.
32. LOEWY, E. H. 1991. Debate. J. Med. Ethics **17:** 156–160.

Communication, Autonomy, and Hope

How Can We Treat Seriously Ill Patients with Respect?

STEIN HUSEBO

Anästhesiologische Abteilung
Malteser-Krankenhaus Bonn-Hardtberg e.V.
Von-Hompesch-Strasse 1
53123 Bonn, Germany

> *What I say isn't necessarily true,*
> *but it explains, just by the fact*
> *that I say it, my existence.*
> —CESARE PAVESE

For patients and their next of kin our manner of communication can determine how successful the rest of their lives are. What significance do autonomy, integrity, and hope have in this communication process? What do we understand by these concepts? How should we put this understanding into practice on a daily basis?

As doctors we face innumerable situations daily where our ability to communicate is set to the test. Our ability to present information and questions; the extent to which we allow patients to ask questions; our choice of what we speak about and what we omit speaking about; the way in which we listen or fail to listen—all these things influence the patient's opportunity to make choices.

PATIENT 1: SHOULD I TELEPHONE HER DAUGHTER?

Marie is a 63-year-old woman with cancer of the large intestine. She is a widow with a daughter of 29. When I meet her in the hospital she is exhausted and bedridden. I realize that she has only a few days to live. She has intense abdominal pain which radiates to her back and pelvis. We deal with her pain first, as a matter of course. This can be relieved by increasing her dose of morphine, and when she is told this, she becomes calmer. We subsequently have the following conversation:

"Do you have children?"

"Yes, I have a daughter. She's an actress. She's got the opening night of her first big role next week."

"Presumably you've told her that you are seriously ill?"

"Yes, I feel that my strength is coming to an end. I really hope the end comes soon—I am looking forward to it all being over . . . ."

"May I call your daughter? She'd obviously want to know how things stand."

"No! You mustn't call! My daughter is more important to me than anything else. This premiere means so much to her."

Marie tells me clearly and lucidly that I should not call her daughter. In order to respect her autonomy, should I call or not? Does she really not want me to call? Is it in her and her daughter's best interests for me to call? Should I call her regardless?

Already we encounter one of the many challenges of a normal working day. When we decide to respect the patient's choices and what the patient wishes or does not wish us to do, how can we be quite sure that they see their options or mean what they say?

Does She See Her Options?

What are her options? Marie has a large number of important choices to make in the last days and weeks of her life. Which of these choices she regards as important is dependent, among other things, on the way in which she herself perceives her situation and possibilities. The choices may include the type of treatment she might request, or accept, and how the treatment should be administered. The choices she makes can also—directly or indirectly—give her the chance of maintaining optimum integrity and autonomy, or not.

What is possibly of equal importance is that in such situations it is our own prioritizing of important choices that is emphasized. This can be seen to be true in Marie's case. My understanding is that Marie's daughter is the most important person in her life, and I choose to emphasize the choice of whether to call her or not. Whether or not this is a correct issue to focus upon depends on my own ability to "read" Marie's situation, and to ask Marie those questions that are most important to her. If Marie is to see and understand her choices she must, above all, see what consequences these individual choices will have.

So, back to the question—should I call her daughter or not? Marie is seriously ill. She will probably die sometime in the next few days. If I do not call her daughter, they will not be given the opportunity to say goodbye. Marie, who has brought her daughter up single-handedly, will die alone. Her motive is to protect her daughter. But what about the daughter? Is she being given the chance to choose? Should it be the mother who makes this decision, or the daughter? Does the mother understand what the consequences will be for her and her daughter if I do not call?

Does She Mean What She Says?

Many would say she does. People mean what they say. But exactly what is she saying?

"No, you mustn't call! My daughter is more important to me than anything else. This premiere means so much to her." She is saying more than that I should not call. She is confirming something I already realize: "My daughter is more important to me than anything else." Maybe she means what she says about not ringing at that exact point in time. However, at the same time she is expressing an intense loneliness and a longing for the person who means more than anything else in the world to her. This intense longing is clear in her face, in the manner in which she is speaking, the manner in which she breathes, in the very pauses between her words—in her entire expression.

My impression is that she is being extremely open in what she says to me concerning the extremely difficult questions she faces. She wants to discuss matters so that she can see precisely what her choices are and make her answers clear to me. The manner in which our discussion progresses shows the difficulties that arise when we fail to see and understand in context the expressions and words of an individual with a particular background.

> "Do you think your daughter loves you?"
>
> Marie fights to hold back the tears. Then she cries for a while. The silence helps us both. I continue to emphasize the relationship between the mother and daughter and say, "Marie, I must call your daughter. You are the only mother she has. If you die in the next few days, your daughter won't have the opportunity to be with you when you need each other most. She has to be able to choose for herself what she feels she wants to do in this situation."
>
> She did not argue.

I took her expression to imply that she was grateful that I had taken upon myself the responsibility for a decision she found difficult to make for herself. But could I know what was right for her? Surely she knew best? Does it not create dangerous and unnecessary pitfalls when doctors and professional caretakers take control of patients' choices in complex situations?

> The reaction of Marie's daughter when I called revealed the complexity of the problem.
>
> In the end she said, "Unfortunately I can't come. I have a big first night next week."
>
> "Only you can decide what is the right thing for you to do. But I think it would mean an awful lot to your mother if you were to visit her."

"It would cause an impossible situation for the theater if I drop out now. I can't leave my son either —he's only three. I really can't speak any longer now. Good-bye."

It was an awkward conversation. Did I go too far? Did I make the situation harder for both mother and daughter? Actors have unique working conditions. If it were impossible for the daughter to come, had I not created unnecessary expectations and feelings of guilt for them both?

The daughter came the next day. Her visit to her mother was deeply intense. She left the same afternoon, but before she did she asked if she could talk to me without her mother present:

"How long is she likely to live?"

"It's always difficult to say. But since it means a lot to you in your situation, I would say it's a question of no more than a few days—at most a week or so."

"What do you think I should do?"

"I understand that it is difficult for you. It's wonderful that you could come today, regardless of what you decide. What do you yourself feel you should do?"

"I don't know. The theater manager will murder me if I say that I can't go ahead with the performance. And I don't know what to do with my son Steffen . . . ."

"Well, perhaps the theater manager has a mother of his own, too; maybe he will also face a similar situation one day. Steffen has a mother, who presumably means more than anyone else to him. What would you want him to do if he were in the same situation as you are now?"

She left for her first night downcast. Two days later she returned with Steffen. They stayed until her mother died. However, there arose an unexpected—but not unusual—problem: her mother did not keep to my well-intended timetable. She did not die after a few days, or even a few weeks, but lived for a further two months.

PATIENT II: SHOULD WE USE THE KIDNEYS OF A BRAIN-DEAD CHILD?

Kristin and Frode's children were three and seven years old. The three year old knocked over a saucepan of boiling water. The consequence was a minor third degree burn. During his first days at the hospital the situation was completely under control. Then one morning he was found in his bed, pale, unconscious, and without a palpable pulse. His condition was rapidly perceived to be septic shock (acute blood poisoning), a sudden and unexpected complication. Despite intensive and exhaustive treatment, he was declared brain dead three days later.

The parents were informed that their son was brain dead. Additionally they were told that we considered it appropriate to switch off the artificial respirator. The parents were in a state of deep shock. The situation was not made any easier by the fact that on their initial arrival at the hospital they had been told that the burns were not life threathening.

At this stage the question arose as to whether organ donation should be suggested as a possibility. Should one make such suggestions, or is it too great a burden on parents already in a state of severe shock to pose such a difficult question? Would it present a significant additional burden that, in this particular situation, the boy's life could perhaps have been saved?

Before I discuss the various ethical, human, and professional perspectives of this and the previous case studies, a few definitions might clarify the issues involved.

AUTONOMY OR PATERNALISM: WHICH IS IN THE PATIENT'S INTERESTS?

Autonomy = respect for the patient's integrity and choices.

Paternalism = we understand better than the patient what is most in their interest, and make the choices on their behalf.

"Gentle" paternalism = respect for the patient's integrity and choices while protecting them from having to make impossible decisions.

Integrity = self-respect, self-value, freedom, responsibility.

How can these concepts, and our understanding of them, shed light on the ethical and professional problems we meet with regard to serious illness? Should we always respect the patient's choices and integrity? Are there some situations where we place unnecessary anxiety and suffering on people by the questions we raise? Are there situations in which the patient has no choice?

Kristin and Frode were in a state of acute shock. The personnel in the intensive care unit are used to relating to relatives at a time of crisis. They have considerable experience in conveying difficult information and raising the question of organ donation. But how do relatives feel at being asked about this? How does it feel to have to make such a difficult decision? Should we, out of consideration for the prospective recipient of the child's kidneys, ask anyway?

After some discussion we chose not to ask Kristin and Frode. We felt that it would place too great a burden on them. For quite a while afterwards there was disagreement about this decision among the professionals involved. I have met Kristin and Frode on a regular basis in the three years following these events. They say now that they are glad the question was not raised, but that such a request would have been acceptable. They did, however, stipulate a number of criteria:

1. That the person making the request be someone they know, and for whom they have respect.
2. That this person demonstrate genuine interest and respect for them and their situation.
3. That he/she have the ability to listen.
4. That their answer or uncertainties be respected, whatever the result.

Even if these criteria had been met, they both say categorically that they would have considered such a request intrusive. They would have said no at the time and would say no now.

Kristin and Frode's situation was unique. We can, however, conclude that in clinical practice there are often situations in which we should refrain from posing particular questions, or from giving information that presents patients, or relatives, with impossible choices. We should also recognize that, to a large extent, the choices we give the patient are often not real choices, because the patients are completely at the mercy of our expertise and evaluation of the situation.

It is common to encounter situations in which this is so. If the options for treatment are complicated or have considerable risk attached to them, the process of giving information presupposes that we employ a high degree of tact and consideration. The person presenting the information must allow for the possibility that the patient's or relatives' choices may represent a distressing "last straw"—one that may well contribute to delay and aggravate a major crisis. Such a process is painful for all those involved—the patient, the relatives, and the informant. "Giving bad news" is an extremely demanding task. The result can often be disheartening—the bad new may simply not be conveyed, or it may be presented bluntly to the patient and relatives. The giver of bad news often cannot manage to show sufficient emotional and human involvement to enable him/her to present the information in as constructive a way as possible.

Perhaps some would disagree with this conclusion. Such decisions will be greatly influenced by the information we have and our own understanding of the people and situation involved, but to an even greater degree they are influenced by our own values and emotions. In different countries, different doctors in different hospitals handle these questions in different ways. In many countries this type of decision is characterized by the fear of doing something wrong. Often we neglect to make unpleasant decisions or delay making them in the hope that conditions may change. Frequently patients and relatives are exposed to considerable suffering because our fear of doing something wrong prevents us from doing something right.

If we concentrate on the information regarding bringing treatment to an end, it is perhaps easier to demonstrate that a paternalistic approach is often necessary to protect the patient or relatives from impossible choices. When the information that a child is brain dead arises, is it appropriate to ask the parent's permission to terminate intensive care? Of course not. This approach would lead to a lasting burden on the parents. They may well suffer for the rest of their lives from the thought that they bear the responsibility for their child's death. Ultimately it is the doctors who must decide which treatment an individual patient should be offered. Autonomy for patients means that they at all times have the right to reject a particular course of treatment. Autonomy does not mean that patients can demand treatment that we consider medically or ethically indefensible—for example, active euthanasia.

I gave the parents much of this information.

> When I explained that unforeseen complications had led to the child's becoming brain dead, and that we could say with certainty that there was no possibility of the brain functioning again, their reaction came as a shock to me. After a few minutes the mother said, "You know that I have money. I will hire the best lawyer in the world. I will pursue you to hell and back if you attempt to shut down the respirator."

I was shattered. To start with, I was tired out because of the way we had battled for the last few days to save the child's life. It was not only extremely difficult to relate such news; it was also almost impossible to comprehend the mother's pain. I now had a complex disagreement to deal with. Those who remark condescendingly about doctors' inability to communicate should attempt to understand how difficult it often can be.

What did the mother really mean? Did she really want to pursue me to hell and back? Or was she actually saying something else? When I had gathered my wits about me again, I heard something that was not said aloud—but that was nonetheless clearly stated: "You are trying to tell me that my child is no longer alive. You are threatening to take him away from me. I cannot bear to hear that news from anybody. At this moment what I need most is someone to shout at. I hope you don't mind bearing the brunt. I need it more than ever."

> I remained sitting there. She gave me a dressing down that I will never forget. After several hours (lasting about 10 minutes) I said cautiously,"It's not a question of turning the respirator off now. You can stay with your child as long as you like. But I would just like to ask you to think about one thing until we see each other again tomorrow: what do you think is best for your child?"

> They sat with their child for three days. In this time they did not want to speak to me. Then I was told that the mother had broken down during the night. The next day they came to see me and said, "Thank you for giving us time. You can turn the respirator off now."

To many people it may seem tragic that we sometimes have to give up. It can be hard to accept that we sometimes stop active intensive care, as this can hasten the patient's death. But experience shows that it is far worse for all involved to draw out the end of life when death is unavoidable. This is perhaps most true when the death concerned is that of a child.

The mother's aggression towards me was difficult to handle. At first I wanted to run out of the room, or to scream. I found it somewhat easier when I realized after a moment or so, from the context, that she was telling me more than what the mere bones of her words conveyed. She was in need. She needed someone to scream at. It was a sign of trust that she chose me.

Is it so that we show emotions, confusion, and anger only to those in whom we have confidence? Why do we tend not to understand exactly what it is that lies behind someone's verbal abuse? If anger and aggression are normal reactions in such situations, why do we not learn more about how we can make it easier for patients and their relatives to shout at us?

SHOUTING IS GOOD THERAPY FOR ONE WHO IS SUFFERING

We should learn to be able to see outbursts of emotion as therapeutic possibilities, and learn how we can deal with them without making a counterattack. Perhaps most of all we must learn to deal with our own reactions when we experience aggression and fatigue. Next time someone shouts at you, sit back. Listen patiently and without becoming unfriendly. When the outburst is over, continue listening for 12 seconds or so. Then say with heartfelt friendliness: "Are you sure you have said everything you want to say?"

Let us move our attention back to Marie for a moment: did I show her respect for her autonomy? My own impression was that I put pressure on both Marie and her daughter. Would I have been showing them greater respect if I had accepted Marie's express wish that I not telephone her daughter? Did I manipulate them both to accept my solution?

If I reflect on these questions and possible answers, it strikes me just how different the answers are depending on the questions that are raised and the people concerned. Operating within the confines of watertight ethical limits in connection with serious illness is problematic. It sets huge demands on the person with the task of giving "bad news." We should understand which choices the individual patient and relative are struggling with, and also those choices they do not see, but which may have a considerable impact on whether or not they make a success of their lives. Normally we all have time on our side: we can try and fail, we can take the chance that the path we have chosen is right for us, and we can change our minds later if we reach another point of view. But the unique thing in both the situations I have described is that time was of the essence. The choices had huge significance for the individuals involved. And this is often the case with serious illness.

How can we cope when we realize that the information and choices are so difficult? What can we do to ensure that we reach maximum respect for the patient's autonomy and integrity? I catch myself constantly trying to manipulate the individual patient or relative to see, and sometimes choose, those options that I feel are the best in view of the situation. I know that I have sometimes gone too far in my "well-intentioned paternalism". Let me give an example.

PATIENT III: A DYING PATIENT WHO REFUSES TO ADMIT THAT HE WILL SOON DIE

A man in his mid-60s has lung cancer and is facing death. He has from the start been negative, and in a state of denial, about his illness. There has been no indication that he has wanted to acknowledge or talk about the fact that he will never recover. Every day he waits for "a miracle." He begs the doctor to try everything possible, even when there are no more additional treatments which can influence or slow the progression of the disease. When the doctors refuse to give him any more"hope" of recovery, he seeks out one alternative treatment after another. His wife and two children experience growing despair. They realize that he will soon die. They are now prepared to face up to the change in the situation that the man is unable to come to terms with. They ask me repeatedly for help in talking to him about their grief. They wish to say good-bye in a dignified manner. They have a considerable need to comfort—and be comforted by—the dying man.

I make several unsuccessful attempts to make the man open up emotionally, and help him see that "the battle is lost." His refusal leads me to make a last attempt. I take his latest X-ray pictures with me, determined to show them even if he does not want to see them. With his children and wife present, I explain the X-rays to him, which show extensive spreading of his lung cancer.

The desired result fails to materialize. He turns his face towards the wall, pulls his quilt over his head and asks us to leave the room. He dies ten days later, in abject loneliness. His rejection of me as a doctor is total. His relationship to his family becomes considerably worse after my attempt to give him the insight I thought he and his family needed.

For me this experience remains a moving example of just how wrong things can go when I, as a doctor, think I know what is best for the patient and act accordingly. I feel that my problem was not just lack of respect for the man's autonomy and integrity. The problem was to a greater extent inability to communicate, both with him and with his relatives.

What the man communicated to me was that he was not able to cope with the fact that he was about to die. He needed alternative strategies in order to be able to preserve his dignity. He chose denial and repression, and these gave him the necessary defense. I believe that it is sometimes necessary to "break down" a defense that is preventing a patient from seeing his/her possibilities. What I would now criticize in my behavior at the time, however, is that I failed to see how strongly the man signaled:

1. "I can't cope with dealing with death. It is difficult enough for me to deal with life."
2. "You all don't need to keep telling me repeatedly that I am going to die soon. I have already grasped that."
3. "What I need help with is my growing loneliness. It is not easy to die."
4. "Ask me who I am, and you will understand why I react in the way I do."

Why do we continue to ignore the significance of a person's biographical details? This man was a company manager, with responsibility for several hundred employees. For the last three to four years he had shown great strength and enthusiasm in building up his business. He had drawn on unique qualities when the company was threatened with closure and bankruptcy. The motto "never give up" epitomizes his effort and his principles. His eldest child had been killed in a traffic accident. He had dealt with this situation through burying himself in his work. No one had seen him cry following the accident. His solution to the situation was to work longer hours and avoid talking about his child. He was brought up to regard ambition and strength as the most important values; his family seldom showed their emotions.

Today I can see clearly that my methods of dealing with this man were a form of paternalism that clearly contained a gross violation of his autonomy. It is true that crises in life often carry with them the possibility for increased growth and openness. But vulnerability can often lead to regression and denial. Growth and openness can only take place on the individual's own terms. Knowledge of, and respect for, the individual person's life history and value system are decisive for a positive result. We cannot help people cope with a major life crisis unless we know a great deal about who they are. Clearly, we can expect to cause considerable damage if we neglect to trace out their life stories and carefully evaluate the implications of who they are and where they come from for the communication process that, we hope, will have positive results for our patients.

If this patient had received support for the way he was coping with his disease and a great deal of reassurance of how much his family loved him, the end of his life might have been a more meaningful process for both him and his family. He would perhaps have been more able to comfort and receive comfort from his family.

HOW CAN WE INCREASE RESPECT AND UNDERSTANDING FOR PATIENTS AND THEIR CHOICES?

The principle of "informed consent" has been important in the fields of medicine and communication. Informed consent implies that the doctor must always ensure that the patient is well informed and consequently gives his or her agreement to the treatment or treatments the doctor recommends. This principle can easily founder when someone requesting informed consent does not follow good patterns of information-giving and tactfulness. It can be even worse when the giver of information does not show genuine interest in the person being informed and fails to acknowledge the great power the doctor has to gain the answer he/she desires through manipulation. Gaining informed consent is not necessarily synonymous with respect for the patient's integrity and autonomy. At best it can be seen as the basis for such respect. The three examples above can serve to shed some light on these challenges.

> Some months after Marie's death I telephoned her daughter. She said the following: "Thank you for not giving up. It is impossible for relatives to enter into that kind of situation. I was really young when my father died. I was so scared to lose my mother, so scared that I wanted to run away. I really value the time I spent with my mother when she was dying. It has meant a huge amount for both Steffen and myself. Especially the days we took my mother home, just being able to see her eyes light up again. I hope you and your colleagues never give up in situations like these—that you bother to take the time to help us see our choices, and what our true interests are . . . ."

Her comments take us back to the issue we touched upon earlier. Often those of us working with the seriously ill "see what lies in the patients' or relatives' interest": we have a distance from the emotional chaos of the situation that allows us to see and understand in a way those more intimately involved are unable to. Sometimes it is possible to make clear the choices available to the patients or relatives concerned. At other times it is not possible.

Can one therefore not state categorically how the patient's interests can be best protected? What is more important,what is the right thing in a specific situation—respect for autonomy or paternalism?

The true challenge is not to find simple solutions and answers or to avoid difficult questions. The challenge is not to abandon patients or relatives to guesswork and ignorance; this will only increase their anxiety and sense of isolation. Perhaps the worst mistake we can make is to tell "the whole truth" as precisely and briefly as possible. In doing this we may perhaps satisfy our own desire for openness and precision, but we will leave patients and relatives in a bleak desert of anxiety and despair, with their imaginations running riot.

Ethics and communications must constantly be regarded as a continuous process between patients, relatives, and colleagues. This process begins at our first meeting with the patient and continues after the patient has died. Relatives have a considerable need for communication to continue after the death of a family member. The manner in which we prepare them for grief and their sense of isolation can dictate the degree to which they succeed with the remainder of their own lives. On occasion, careful follow-up work can prevent later tragedies. Neglecting to recognize the need for follow-up work can have serious ramifications. It is a fallacy to suggest that this would lead to an increased demand on time and resources.

The ability to communicate with others varies from person to person. I am convinced that the chance of success multiplies significantly if we succeed in listening at the same time as we are giving information, and at the same time realize that communication in this context is a process that occurs over time. To use a cliché, the result depends not on what we do, but on the way we do it. Above all, it is the manner in which we interpret our own value-systems and relate to our own vulnerability that determines the degree to which we succeed in the face of these challenges.

In a recently published work, *The Irreplaceable*, the Danish professor of philosophy Peter Kemp writes that the foremost principle underlying ethics is "the feeling person."[1] Additionally, he underlines that we also find the foundation for ethics in art and history, and especially in tales. His comments give a biting critique of the education and training that health workers are offered at present. Ethical questions are only rarely a central theme of professional meetings—especially among doctors. It is the exception to find that processes and methods of communication are an integral part of teaching and education. Literature and art are visible by their absence in the education of health personnel.

One frequently hears arguments along these lines: "For the patient it is always most important that the doctor is technically able. When given the choice between a doctor who is a skilled communicator and a doctor who knows his medical facts, scientific knowledge will always be preferred." This kind of argument is, to my mind, meaningless. A doctor unable to communicate is useless when it comes to clinical practice. It is not a liver, a kidney, a heart, or a tumor that we are treating. It is a human being—a person. This person will regularly be subjected to appraisals and treatment he/she does not need. Sometimes serious damage or life-threathening complications may occur as a result of unnecessary treatments. Doctors must always possess the ability to communicate. Professional ability carries with it the ability to communicate. In my eyes, nowhere else in modern society do we find such extensive power so often misused as within the health service. The problems may appear irresolvable: one can easily feel unable to effect change. However, there are some signs that things are changing for the better. The strong ties medicine previously had with the arts and humanism, both in theory and practice, are now increasingly reappearing. Communication, the giving of information, and ethics are now being taken more seriously within the various branches of the health service.

Despite this, we still find that demands for "documentation," "facts," and "data" dominate. Frequently these demands are misused in order to hide a lack of ethical commitment and reflection. What our patients regard as "the good life"—their dreams, values and feelings—should, naturally, be uppermost when we set priorities. To a greater extent than before, doctors must be expected to make a clear ethical commitment. This must above all be visible in recruitment to high positions within medicine and among teachers. In day-to-day practice in their contact with patients and relatives, the individual doctor must learn, and gain experience of, what is good treatment: what is it that contributes to make "a good life" for the individual concerned. It is therefore of central importance to have the right professional role models.

Perhaps this should be our top priority. But it is only when we manage to live up to and practice ethical attitudes that we are showing respect for the people we ultimately are serving. A well thought through attitude towards ethics, autonomy, and paternalism is of the utmost importance in all contact with people. When these people because of their situation in life become patients, ethics and courtesy must be the basis of all our practice.

Patients and their relatives also bear some responsibility for this process. They themselves must seek out information and insight that make it possible for them to see their own choices and the consequences individual choices will have. The focus of this article on the responsibility of those involved in treating the seriously ill does not absolve patients and relatives from their own responsibility. But patients and relatives can take charge of their autonomy and integrity only if those of us with power treat them with courtesy, ethical reflection, and respect.

We must also, perhaps, understand that power must be exercised within the health service, that power is a totally necessary part of our clinical day to day life. It is self-evident that someone in the position of giving another person medical treatment possesses a great deal of power. It is important to be able to recognize that patients and relatives are completely at the mercy of the information we provide them and of our manipulation. The question we must ask ourselves daily is how we can increase our sensitivity, "vulnerability," and understanding so that the power, the conflicts, and the ethical challenges are visible. Something visible can be investigated and understood. It is only when we see what choices and power, or lack of power, we are up against that we come close to a fundamental, necessary respect for the patient as a fellow human being. Every single situation in which we come across a patient can teach us endless amounts about ethics and communication, about autonomy and integrity. When a patient becomes seriously ill the possibilities for learning are limitless.

IS THERE HOPE, DOCTOR?

Many patients and a number of relatives say that their doctor has given them the message"There is no more hope." When a life can no longer be saved, both doctor and patient often see this as a defeat. The distressing nature of the feelings this arouses concerns us as well as the patient—we are all future patients somewhere along the line. Most people are quite attached to life. Sometimes we go through difficult phases, we are sad or depressed, or we may see insurmountable obstacles ahead of us. Most people choose to continue living despite everything. For one thing we view the death process as a painful alternative. In addition, death for many of us is something final: a one-way dead-end street without the possibility of continuing or turning back.

History is full of evidence of the ways in which we search for solutions to the problem of death. Practically every religion contains the concept of life after death. Christians believe in the everlasting life of the soul, in a good God, who will help us when needed. The German historian Franz Borkenau has described our own era as "post-Christian." He describes changes that have occurred in the minds of many people. The modern human being tends to regard life as ending at the point of death, without hope of life after death. The conclusion is that we must enjoy life while we have the chance.

There have also been sociological changes. In a review article, Fulton and Owen describe social development in the United States.[2] In 1920 more than half of those who died were under the age of 20, and the average life expectancy was less than 49. Today most people live for closer to 80 years. More than 80% die in institutions—hospitals, old peoples' homes, or nursing homes—and this increases to 95% in cities. In 1920 80% died at home. In 1995 there were seven times as many hospital beds as in 1920. A similar development has taken place in Norway: death takes place outside of the home. It often seems as if it does not take place at all.

The problems become even greater when medical treatment can no longer delay death, or when life ends because of an unexpected accident or illness. In cases such as these the confrontation with death not only releases shock, grief and anger on the part of the dying person and his/her family, but also triggers grief and despair in the patient's doctor and professional carers.

The consequences are significant. The seriously ill are not sufficiently prepared for imminent death. The dying and their relatives are left to deal with their anxiety and emotions on their own. They do not have the opportunity to part as emotionally as possible. They do not have the opportunity to die in the place and conditions in which they would like to die. They are subject to unnecessary treatment with modern techniques and expensive medicines for weeks and months, even in circumstances where the death process has started a long time previously. This is particularly relevant when such treatment merely serves to prolong the final period of suffering.

These problems concern us all. The question is not just how our patients should be treated, or how our relatives will come to die. Above all it is a question of how we ourselves will die. Perhaps alone, isolated in a hospital bed, surrounded by people who do not have it in their power to relate to our despair or loneliness, who often express superficial, groundless optimism until it is too late. What can we do to prevent bewilderment and despair leading to confusion and suppression of necessary emotional reactions?

Perhaps those of us who consider ourselves to be in the prime of our lives should reflect on our attitude to life and death? We are, after all, all going to die—there is no hope of our surviving in this world.

WHEN YOU HAVE VISITED YOUR DOCTOR

Let us do a simple experiment in our heads. Today you have been to your doctor, whom you trust implicitly. She explained the results of your latest tests to you. You have cancer, and it has spread. You asked what can be done. She answered that nothing can be done to halt the development of the disease. You asked how much time you have left. She answered that it is impossible to say for sure. You understood from her answer that it is serious—you probably have no more than six months.

What will you do? What remains of your life? What value, what possibilities, what hope is there for you? Will you nonetheless attempt to clutch at straws—hope to find an undiscovered or unknown miracle cure? Will you go through such a treatment even though you have to sacrifice your last cent to do so? What are your thoughts about your doctor now?

Are you angry with her? Should she have spoken so openly and frankly about your long-term chances? Would you rather she had held back her information, even though this would mean keeping you in the dark?

The reality is that this is the case in many instances. Patients often find they receive incomplete information with regard to the progression of the illness and the possibilities for, and consequences of, treatment. One reason for this might be that the doctor has a well-founded desire to protect the patient. But this information is also difficult to convey. In many cases, the doctor wishes to protect himself/herself because he/she is unprepared, and finds it distressing to deal with his/her own strong, emotional reactions when someone has to receive devastating news.

WHAT WOULD YOU TELL YOUR OWN FAMILY?

Would an open and intimate relationship be important to you? Or would you want to shield those closes to you in such a situation? From experience we know that many of those who are seriously ill need help in order to speak openly with their closest family and friends. It is difficult to establish openness about such personal, existential questions. But we also know that for all those involved, particularly for children, it is best to establish a mutual and intimate understanding of the illness and its consequences.

It is not just the doctor or the patient who holds back information, and who justifies this by saying he/she wishes to protect others from unpleasant news. Relatives commonly react in this way as well. Our urge to hide death from our children is perhaps the clearest sign of how difficult we find it to relate to death. Most children lose close relatives before they leave primary school. Like us, children need to share reactions and feelings with others when they are going through a time of crisis and grief.

Throughout the ages, reflecting on the imminence of our death has been the greatest existential challenge we face as human beings. Death has been a never-ending source of inspiration to artists, thinkers, writers, and philosophers. It has been suggested that a culture's maturity is reflected in the way it relates to the mortality of humans—and that this consciousness more than anything else can help to prevent the inhumanity of man. How, then, can we explain the fact that we, despite this, make such monumental efforts to protect ourselves?

Let us return to the issue of your hope. Did you imagine that you were immortal? Or are you just unprepared for death at this particular moment? When the doctor suggests that you do not have long left to live, what can you look forward to? Is there still hope?

THE EXPERIENCE OF A RELATIVE

Some years ago a woman in her late thirties sat in front of me. Her husband had died some months earlier after a short, traumatic illness. They had gone through an indescribably depressing and difficult experience.

"It was dreadful right from the start. Lars felt unwell for some weeks. We both thought that it was due to his job. At first he didn't even say he had been to the doctor's. But one day he came home early, ashen and reticent. He just spat it out: "I have cancer—there's no hope . . . ."

"We had all the imaginable reactions: shock, despair, anger, grief, loneliness, and the desire to run away. We sought all manner of alternatives. As our doctor could not help, we looked for other doctors who could. When that did not work, we tried alternative medicine. There were arguments, slammed doors, and outbursts of anger daily. The children kept out of the way. Hope? Lars was depressed and bitter. It was hard for him to see our children. Even his religious beliefs, which had always been so important to him, became a problem.

"The way in which the information was relayed to Lars was hopeless—he was alone and unprepared; they didn't even arrange a follow-up appointment for him. He drove home alone afterwards; it's a wonder he didn't crash into the side of the mountain!

"But then, in our everyday lives, we got small things to hope for. Hope for a good night's sleep. Hope for being able to take a boat trip. Hope that the medicines would keep the pain and sickness under control.

"These hopes increased: that the children would be happy; that I would be able to cope financially with the house when Lars was gone; the days we had left together; that Lars not be on his own, that he could stay at home. And love—Lars said that the love we share with other people lives on when we ourselves die.

"He was calm in the final days. It was he who was comforting us. We were all with him when he died in our lounge. Afterwards he lay at rest for two days. We tended to him: it was we who dressed him in the clothes we decided on; and we put him in the coffin.

"After being told there was no longer hope, we cursed you frequently. It is not possible to live without hope! Even if there is no longer hope for survival, there is still hope! It is terrible for patients if you are not capable of treating us in a way that allows us to retain our hope despite developing a tragic illness."

DOES THE DOCTOR LACK HOPE?

Is there more hope for patients than for doctors at times of crisis, or at death? Or, to put it differently, is hope something that can easily disappear in a hospital or nursing home? When everything seems lost, is there actually more hope than ever? Perhaps Lars and his family were an exceptional case. But aren't we all? Isn't there a depth, a tenderness, a contentment, a desire, or a love—something we have succeeded with, or with which we could still achieve success?

To associate with dying patients is a personal burden for doctors—a burden that we as a profession have not taken seriously. Doctors who cannot manage to act with patience, friendliness, and understanding in difficult situations are often themselves physically and mentally exhausted. The consequences of this kind of exhaustion are often significant. A doctor's work and home life can become intertwined in a way that threatens his, and his family's, lives and health. This fact is seldom, if ever, covered in our basic medical training and is given even less emphasis in our daily clinical work. It would go beyond the limit of this article to describe how this serious problem might be resolved. I would, however, like to refer to Bennet's *The Wound and the Doctor.*[3] He writes: "Only the sensitive doctor, who can relate to this sensitivity, can function as a doctor." Each of us possesses the key to this sensitivity. It is not too late to release it.

It is unreasonable to expect our patients to forgive us for not performing well as doctors because of personal problems. It is our task to offer respect, confidence, and alternative hope when the patient is in the throws of a major life crisis. We must beware of making our own "hopeless" day-to-day situation something the patient carries responsibility for.

The confrontation with death is something that concerns our entire culture. This confrontation is often valuable to individuals. I have often heard the bereaved say,"I don't understand why no one said outright to us that there was so little time left. We would have loved to say good-bye before it was too late. I carry so much inside me that I would love to have said . . . ."

It would be of great benefit to patients and relatives if the relatives were more involved in the care of the dying. We should adjust our clinical practice to allow this to occur. For instance, it is quite common for dying patients to be on an intravenous drip the last days or weeks before death. For a long time doctors thought it was wrong to let dying patients suffer thirst when they could no longer manage to drink enough orally. This "final drip" has had a significant role in medical practice for the past 50 years.

But what purpose does the drip serve? Who benefits from it? There is no evidence that shows we can relieve thirst in dying patients by using a drip in this way. On the other hand the experience from hospices shows that dying patients need considerable attention paid to their mouths, and localized moistening of the mouth and throat in order to avert and treat the conditions that arise because of breathing through the mouth. Moistening of the lips with a cloth, small quantities of liquids through a pipette, or small pieces of ice is what the sick person needs.most. Relatives can, with support, carry out these tasks. Delegating such tasks to relatives will encourage them to sit down and spend valuable time with their dying relative.

In addition to depriving the patient of this significant benefit, the drip has a number of other negative effects that should be noted. It can tie the sick person to the hospital and keep him/her unnecessarily reliant on medical personnel. It can also lead to a dying patient's being given too much fluid and suffering from secretions or mucous when pneumonia or heart failure gains a hold. Possibly the greatest problem is that this type of drip prevents communication of the important knowledge that death is approaching.

One of our greatest tasks is to remove the taboo surrounding death in both our and our patients' lives. This is as important for the relatives as for the patient. If death is surrounded by taboo, despite our attempts otherwise, people facing death will experience great loneliness unnecessarily. They can, despite still being alive, feel that they have no significance to those around them. They can thus feel that they, though not yet dead, have already lost their life.

Even though no study has been done regarding the usefulness of intravenous treatment in dying patients, the most crucial argument against this practice is not based in medicine but comes from the field of ethics. The process of dying is a part of life. Neither life nor death is a disease. I want to depart from this life as a living person, not as a patient. I do not want to be dependent on medical treatment or personnel when what I need most is respect for my integrity, a sign that I can now die in peace, surrounded by those who, rather than being concerned with my illness, are concerned with me.

Death in itself is rarely terrible. A dying person becomes weaker, falls back into his dreams, and gradually loses consciousness—if everything proceeds as it should. What is terrible is untreated pain or other insufferable conditions. But a lot can be done about these. What is also terrible is the way in which the living experience the loss of a relative without being properly prepared. What is terrible is the collective and individual images and notions that surround death in our society.

In contact with dying people it is not "illness," "patients," or "prognoses" that are the central issues. Each person has his/her background, experiences, values, and associations. It should be foremost in the doctor's mind to allow each individual to have his/her own personal death. This can happen only if we treat patients and their relatives in a manner that conveys our deep respect for the life of the patient.

Respect for a patient's life bears with it respect for the fact that for many of those with serious illnesses death comes as a release—it is not the "final enemy," to be fought at any price. Performing futile treatments in the final days or weeks is not reconcilable with good medical ethics.

The doctor must with care and empathy be capable of helping the patient comprehend the consequences of diagnosis and treatment. The patient's readiness to receive the truth must be stressed—as must the doctor's own readiness to deliver "bad news" of this kind. Truth does not in this context mean merely blurting out difficult information or predicting the exact time of death. The task is to set in motion a procedure that allows the sick person to understand that time is limited, that death is imminent. It is not our task to desert the sick when cure is no longer possible.

It is crucial for us all that we take this message in and understand how important it is. Clear understanding of the particular situation can give the sick person unimagined mental strength. Most people have within them more courage and vitality than they themselves imagine and than the others expect.

It is also crucial that the doctor do his/her best to help when loneliness, anger, grief, or pain threatens to crush patients and relatives. These reactions are part of the distress experienced in an encounter with grief. When the hope of survival diminishes, when patient and relative seek comfort and a deeper meaning, the doctor's own distress must not be allowed to take over.

IT IS NOT POSSIBLE TO LIVE WITHOUT HOPE

Hope is not just something that is limited to an expectation of the future. Hope is closely connected to a person's life story, position regarding the past and the present, and outlook on life. Although it may seem insignificant, recognition of a life that has been lived, interest in the experiences and values that have given that life meaning can mean an enormous amount to a person. It can stand as an assurance that the patient will not be left to rely on his/her own resources, that in time he or she will be the center of medical and human attention and care.

And what can those of us who imagine ourselves to be in the prime of our lives do? Are we able—before things get serious—to come to terms with our own limitations? We still have the rest of our lives ahead of us. How, and with whom, do we wish to spend it? What are we still able to do for our children, for our partners, for our parents and friends? What can we do for ourselves?

What does life mean to you? What does death mean? Is there hope?

REFERENCES

1. KEMP, P. 1991. Det Uerstattelige. En Teknologi -etikk. Munksgaard. Copenhagen.
2. FULTON, R. & G. OWEN. 1994. Death in contemporary American society. *In* Death and Identity. R. Fulton & R. Benediksen, Eds.: 12–28. The Charles Press. Philadelphia, PA.
3. BENNET, G. 1987. The Wound and the Doctor. Secker and Warburg. London.

To Tell or Not To Tell the Cancer Patient the Truth?

BOGUSŁAW A. MACIEJEWSKI, MARIA MACIEJEWSKA, AND MAGDALENA KRYJ

M. Skłodowska-Curie Memorial Institute and Cancer Center
Wyb. Armii Krajowej 15
44-101 Gliwice, Poland

There are many physicians by title, . . . very few by calling.
—HIPPOCRATES

The physician-patient relationship is a significant component of the treatment strategy. Communication constitutes perhaps the most important process in medicine. Among various aspects of the direct relationship between the physician and the patient, conversation with the patient is among the most important. It is the duty of the physician to supply the patient with full explanations. However, cooperation between the physician and the patient is not merely a question of mutual goodwill and readiness. It also depends on certain other factors, the nature of which may be associated with, for instance, knowledge and competence—i.e., the professional training of the physician for his work with patients. It is increasingly evident that medical knowledge must be supplemented by a basic knowledge of psychology, so that the physician may make fuller use of the therapeutic power of words to enlist the patient's psychological reserves.

The physician-cancer patient relationship constitutes a most complex problem, one of the most difficult aspects of which is sincere communication with the patient. Despite the passage of time this matter still is one of the most controversial questions, and coming to the surface time and again, sometimes evoking heated disputes and arguments. Among the main dilemmas is whether the patient should be told the truth. Most American physicians are willing to inform the patient first of all, who, as they assume, has the right to learn the truth and decide whether the family is also to know. Physicians in Europe, including Poland, are more in favor of telling the family first.

Both attitudes arouse many doubts, uncertainties, and moral dilemmas. Should the cancer patient be told the whole truth even when the disease is advanced and there is no chance of cure? Or should the patient be cheated, should the seriousness of the situation be minimized by explanations that there is still hope, that within days the patient's health is going to improve, while telling the whole truth to the family? Is such an attitude an expression of cowardice, mercy, conformity, or pity? Is withholding the truth about the state of his or her condition from the patient a lie, a choice of a lesser evil, or an act of graciousness? How can we separate truth and honesty with respect to the patient, who trusts us and listens with hope to our every word, from the immeasurable damage of the harsh verdict of fate? According to what criteria should the physician decide which approach is best for the other human being? Where is the boundary between the truth and the patient's good? If someone were to ask whether the truth should always be expressed and never held back, when cancer is at stake, it would seem that the answer should be that in medicine words like "always" and "never" do not fit. And though exceptions may be found, they merely constitute confirmation of this principle.

It is hard to talk about the relationship between the physician and the cancer patient in Poland on merely moral and ethical grounds, without taking into account the political, social, and cultural conditions that have influenced this system for decades. The notion of the *summum bonum*, the highest good, and *primum non nocere* have become fundamental guidelines for Polish physicians, including oncologists. Nowadays and in the past the use of Latin in Polish medical practice (histopathological diagnosis, patient records, prescriptions, and autopsy reports), although it comes from long years of tradition, poses from the beginning a barrier of secrecy before the patient by coding information in an unknown language. Poland has been a predominantly Catholic country, and the conservative church still tries to convince people that it is better to pray and believe than to ask for more information. This, indeed, also has an impact upon the physician-patient relationship, and is the source of uncertainty, apprehension, fear, and suspicion. It is very seldom that a patient asks a physician to interpret and to explain the Latin expressions.

The first years of the 20th century mark the beginning of Polish oncology. In 1906 the Committee for the Fight Against Cancer was established, and over the following years polyclinics for outpatients with cancer were opened. Maria Skłodowska-Curie established the Foundation for the Radium Institute in Warsaw, which began operation in 1932. Also, Maria Skłodowska-Curie donated the first gram of radium for treating cancer patients. The Radium Institute was the first comprehensive cancer center in Poland, where the fundamentals of modern oncology, based on close cooperation between pathologist, surgeon, radiotherapist, and medical oncologist were practiced.

After World War II, the Institutes of Oncology in Gliwice (1947) and Cracow (1951) were established. In 1951 all three Institutes were combined to form the single M. Skłodowska-Curie Memorial Institute and Cancer Center. Over the next years a network of polyclinics and oncological centers developed in numerous Polish cities. All of them adopted the professional and organizational concept of comprehensive cancer treatment as the basis for their operation. During the midseventies a Comprehensive Governmental Program was drafted concerning the Fight

Against Cancer. This centralized approach toward organizing the professional components of the cancer treatmentent program contributed to the unified education and training of radiation and medical oncologists and comprehensive therapy for cancer patients all over the county.

During the post-War period, with the entrance of Communism into the political stage in Poland, the good of the individual was replaced by the good of the general society, and the slogan "each one receives relative to his needs," introduced by Communism, became empty words, not only as far as medical care was concerned. A free health system in general and free oncology services in particular were declared; however, this only apparently made medical assistance easily accessible, pretending to bring it close to the patient.

Centrally managed administation, financing, and organization of health care with generally low-budget expenditures for these purposes led over a period of 40 years to a decay that has been hard to rebuild. . The patient frequently was treated mechanically and, although receiving treatment and medicines free of charge, had practically no possibility of expressing his or her needs in spite of the fact that in theory this was legally guaranteed. Within the Communist system physicians were produced en masse, at first with assigned employment. During the first decades after the War their contact with world medicine was almost nonexistent. Low wages, generally low even today, and difficult living conditions for both physicians and patients had their negative impact on the relationship between the two. A Physician's Ethical Code did, in fact, exist, but it was far from perfect; and significant gaps in the legal regulations seriously compromised the modest possibilities of patients' rights being respected. Physicians and lawyers, similarly to the other members of the intelligentsia, were pushed by the political system to the lowest levels of the social hierarchy, although the society continued to praise them very highly. This may to a large extent be ascribed to the authority, knowledge, and ethical standing of the old professors who lived though the War and tried to pass on the highest moral and humanistic values to the next generations of physicians. In view of such serious restrictions, it is surprising that the high educational level of physicians was maintained, so that their practical professional ability and knowledge did not differ from those of their colleagues from Western Europe, as it turned out when the frequency of contacts between them increased. In such a social situation and with health care generally available, although of low quality, ethnic, cultural, and social differences generally vanished, and their impact on the physician-patient relationship disappeared.

Disease became a shameful matter. Cancer has been, and frequently still is, thought of as a death sentence. But a slow evolution of such opinions may be observed over the last few years. Limited access to the physician, in spite of Communist propaganda suggesting the opposite, bad hospital conditions, and shortages of medicines all resulted in a decrease in the patient's trust in the efficacy of the therapy proposed by the doctor. A sociological survey conducted during the eighties[1,2] indicated that as many as 42% of those investigated declared that they "would go to the doctor as the last resort," 63% used their own or their friends' experience, and as many as 29% just waited for their symptoms to disappear. One fifth of the persons investigated used the suggestions of homeopaths and chiropractors. A strange exception to this picture was the inhabitants of Warsaw, the capital of Poland, who almost without exception consulted a doctor whenever they noticed any alarming symptoms. It seems that the needs of the patients were better realized in the capital than in the rest of the country. Communist propaganda sought to use the capital to promote a false image of the country by establishing a number of excellently equipped government hospitals, science and research institutes, and academic clinical hospitals. Workers were generally treated as simply a labor force, although they had various privileges granted by the workers' and farmers' political system. They learned to think of their bodies as something undergoing wear and tear, not worthy of recovery. Prophylactic and rehabilitation activities were neglected. Environmental pollution got continually worse, although the nation was persuaded that the people lived in safe conditions. A dramatic case of this situation and policy was Silesia, where the progressive ecological degradation was concealed from public opinion.

Research conducted at the turn of the eighties[3] indicated that as few as one patient in five evaluated his or her contact with the physician as "good." More than half considered the information obtained to be "insufficient and incomprehensible." Another sociological survey[4] suggests that the most effective psychological influence on the patient proved to be the so-called egocentric communication style. This consists in the physicians' ascribing more autonomy for themselves than for others, thus imposing upon their patients the decision concerning their treatment. Not having much of a choice and worried about possible loss of the available treatment, the patient often would consent to the suggested treatment without futher discussion or full information about it.

The physician-patient relationship has been evolving over the few years since Poland has become a democratic country. This is ensured by the revised physicians' Code of Ethics,[5] as well as by the mandatory principle of informed consent. The empty slogans of "social care" and "Communist health services," inherited from the 40 years of Communism are slowly being filled with meaning with the prevailing care for the health of the individual, although an obsolete and unreformable social insurance system is causing delay in this field.

Although the Chamber of Physicians was recently reconstituted and malpractice regulations are in force, the health policy has not changed very much, and the system is still free. There are still many discrepancies between the declared and real-life accessibility of the health system.

Prices of medicines increase every year. The list of drugs available with full reimbursement is very short; patients generally have to pay 100% or 30% of the cost of drugs. Although hospital treatments for in- and outpatients are declared free, the budget given by the central Ministry of Health is too low to cover all costs, and patients are often asked or even pressured to contribute toward the costs. Many hospitals have long waiting lists, and for the last few years the number of patients admitted to hospitals is increasing. For example, at the Institute of Oncology in Gliwice 9,000 patients were treated in 1990, and more than 12,000 patients were treated and 150,000 consultations provided in 1995. The budget of the Institute did not increase during this period. This may look like a miracle, but it is not. We have to find private sponsors, foundations, and charities to cover the difference between the given budget and actual expenditures. This situation, with its many paradoxes, is making the transition period very difficult. Fundamental changes in the social insurance system are promised by the government every year; however, people do not belive that these will be realized soon.

The political, historical, social, and cultural circumstances of the physician-patient relationship presented have influenced and are still influencing the answer to the question of whether the cancer patient should be told the truth. Some journalists report that patients in the United States are always told the truth and that it would be good to do the same thing in Poland. Our impression from a number of visits to the United States, however, is that this is not always the case, that the principle is not always followed. Also, we doubt whether it would be proper to simply transfer this practice or legal principle onto Polish soil. There is little probability that Americans are different from Poles and do not fear cancer. The scope and justification of the aim of telling the truth may differ—i.e., legal, economic, property matters, etc. may be at stake—but I believe psychological questions are rarely, if ever, considered.

There is a lot of work to be done in Poland before people start to talk openly about cancer and discuss the disease with family, friends, and specialists. For the last few years we have popularized knowledge about cancer more widely and actively by the mass media. There are regular programs on television and radio concerning cancer prevention and prophylaxis, screening for early detection, etc. Besides the financial and organizational problems that have to be solved, there are many psychological and sociological customs that have to be changed, and all these activities need a long time. It can be observed that physicians by themselves carry out more initiatives than the Ministry of Health or politicians in this difficult process of sincere patient-doctor communication.

In Poland as in other countries there are philosophical and ethical aspects of the doctor-cancer patient realtionship that cannot be easily related to doctors' unwillingness to start time-consuming, open communication with patients. Everyday life again and again demonstrates to us that the cancer patient who asks about his or her condition and demands the truth, stating that he or she is strong and capable of withstanding anything, is in fact expecting the denial, not the confirmation, of his or her apprehensions.

Should we, then, tell the truth concerning the diagnosis? What verbal arguments does the physician have to aid him or her? In oncology many words like "if," "maybe," and "probably" are still used; the patient's cure is simply expressed in probabilistic terms. What is the physician's position with respect to the patient, if the physician may offer only a chance, while homeopaths and chiropractors would freely promise to cure the patient? In what way should the physician behave toward a terminal cancer patient, and how should he or she prepare the sick person for death? Even when given the opportunity of learning about one's approaching death, a human being generally tries to avoid awareness of its inevitable coming. Is the physician to break this natural defense mechanism by telling the truth and depriving the patient of his or her last hopes? Who needs patients to be aware of the existence of their illness? *Qui bono?*

The patient may die within a few months, but there are vastly different ways of living through this last period: depressed and in black despair, expecting day after day the final stroke; or living in a rather quiet mood until the end. Seneca has said "it is not death that we fear, but the thought of it." Oftentimes the escape from the consciousness of death is a result of anxiety about the physical suffering associated with it. Many persons seek comfort and relief in religious help, others prefer a psychologist to a priest. Yet, the dominant role in ensuring the patient's proper physical and psychological condition is that of the physician. Everyone feels safer and more certain knowing that he or she has someone who will help until the very end. We have had over 10,000 patients in our oncological practice, and only a few of them quietly and rationally prepared for death. I have witnessed very many psychological breakdowns and have had a number of suicidal cases. And at the opposite end, there is a group of cancer patients who were permanently cured. They passed through the hell of doubt and despair, and only a few took up a conscious fight. We have many doubts, and we are not certain what the truth is in the end. The question of telling the patient the truth is becoming more and more frequently and commonly a subject for discussion, and physicians have many times been accused of usurping for themselves the right not to explain to patients where the truth is.

The regulations of the Polish Physicians' Professional Code of Ethics[5] formulate the principles of the physician-patient relationship by stipulating that the physician should impart to the patient understandable information concerning his or her condition, diagnosis, diagnostic and therapeutic procedures employed, alternative methods, side effects, and the consequences of neglecting treatment. The stipulation is formulated as a suggestion rather than an obligation. The truth, seemingly so expected, only rarely brings about peace. Therefore, although lies are ignoble according to any ethical system, an "optimistic lie" or rather a "misstatement" employed for the benefit of the patient may not be considered to be so.

Such a tentative opinion concerning the physician-patient relationship, perhaps thought of by some as waiving responsibility, has been influenced by the many years of neglect of prophylaxis and promotion of cancer knowledge in Poland. The intense activities of the medical profession and of social circles in Poland in this field in recent years cannot fill the gap. Doubtless, the popular knowledge of the cancer diseases among Americans is incomparably greater than that in Poland. Thus, the plane of the physician-patient relationship is different, too.

Yet, irrespective of continent, country, circumstances, or economic conditions, the question of telling the truth to the cancer patient should also be taken account of from the point of view of the present situation in the cancer research, which is decisively different from the advancements in, say, nuclear physics or space research. In the latter two cases the knowledge available is sufficient for the achievement of the solutions sought—e.g., space flights. What is now known about cancer cannot, however, constitute a basis for the establishment of a program that would offer a solution to the problems of the prevention and treatment of this disease. Although research is being earned out and progress is notable in, for instance, tumor biology, exceeding the practical feasibility of employing this knowledge, at the present stage of development the prospect of success as far as time is concerned is hard to determine. The complex nature of this disease constitutes an extremely difficult obstacle. Cancer is not a single disease, but it is found in many diverse forms, the nature of which are not yet precisely known. This, particularly, makes any planning complex. Thus, one cannot foresee to what degree progress achieved with respect to one type of cancer can be helpful in fighting another. Only full control of this disease would, in my view, give the physician the right to tell the patient the full truth about it.

We still have a long way to go in fighting prejudices, preconceptions, uncertainties, and stereotyped convictions. Thus, no single answer exists to the question about the form the physician-patient relationship should take, nor is there a simple answer to the question of whether or not to tell the cancer patient the truth. There are no racial or religious prejudices among physicians in our country. We do not consider the patient on the basis of what he or she represents or where he or she comes from. Whether he or she is a VIP or a simple farmer, the patient's condition is decisive for the physician's actions. The problems of telling the truth or withholding it and of legal responsibility depend on the patient's good and still have to be solved by the physician in his or her own conscience.

REFERENCES

1. KIELANOWSKI, T. 1980. Ethics and Medical Deontology. PZWL. Warsaw.
2. SOKOŁOWSKA, M. 1986. Sociology in Medicine. PZWL. Warsaw.
3. WIREFIELD, N. R. & M. Y. PEAY. 1980. Behavioural Science in Medicine. G. Allen & Unwin. London. Copyright for the Polish Edition by PZWL, Warsaw,1986.
4. KHOURY, S. & C. JASMIN, Eds. 1979. Cancer, Dr Grands specialistes respondent. Hachette. Paris. Copyright for the Polish Edition by PZWL, Warsaw, 1983.
5. 1992. Medical Profession Law. Journal of Law No. 25, chaps. 2–5.

Truth-telling, Information, and Communication with Cancer Patients in Poland

JERZY MEYZA

M. Skłodowska-Curie Memorial Cancer Center
ul. Findera 101
02-781 Warsaw, Poland

Communication with patients has improved progressively in the civilized world, including Poland.[1] These changes in relations between patients and physicians have recently been more profound and rapid here. With the collapse of Communism, major socioeconomic changes have occurred, but some of the previous rules remain valid. One of the best examples is the durability of the National Health Service (NHS), which has existed since the beginning of the Communist state, and is still fully dependent on the will or whim of the government. Consequently, physicians, as government employees, are fully subordinated to the rules imposed by an administration interested mainly in the realization of the five-year plans. Physicians, usually insufficiently paid, are treated as professional "guardians" providing medical services not always concordant with the preferences and needs of the patient. Medical confidentiality in the NHS is questionable because it is still shared with administrative and paramedical personnel, and computer databases. Finally, and not exceptionally, the patient remains the only one unaware of the truth about his illness. Due to the decline in the prestige of the medical profession,there is a distrust of the public towards the NHS.

Sick people are emotionally the most vulnerable and tend to experience ambivalent feelings towards medical personnel and anger at any negative behavior of the staff. They expect more than technical competence, looking for social and psychological as well as physical relief.

The Polish Civil Code, in paragraph 19 of Bill Number 408[2] enacted in October 1991, gives the patient the right to information about the condition of his/her health. This short, simple statement does not impose upon the physician delivery of information as to the scope of diagnosis, prognosis, and treatment.

The Chamber of Physicians, closed during the Communist period and reopened in 1989, proclaimed the Code of Medical Ethics in a new version in 1993.[3] The Code states that the patient has the right to be informed clearly and understandably about his/her illness and to decide jointly with the physician on the preferred type of treatment. The same Code prohibits euthanasia but bestows on the physician the right not to introduce, or to postpone, treatment in terminally ill cases.

The majority of the population of Poland is Catholic, and the Church in Poland is rather orthodox. Its attitude against abortion is still rigid. A more flexible approach exists concerning the information level for patients, which should depend on their need and on the physician's understanding of the patient's willingness. Indirectly, the Church demands that the patient should be aware of his fate, because extreme unction before death remains a must in the mind of all Catholics. Some members of the clergy do not permit burial in a Catholic cemetery of one who did not receive the last sacrament.

Communication should be more than the divulgence of a diagnosis or the giving of information. It involves the communication of caring, understanding, respect, support, reassurance, and continuing availability. There is an impediment to communication, a conflict between autonomy and health, between the values of the patient and values of the physician. It is due to the unbalanced nature of the interaction, in which one party is sick and searching for security and in which judgment entails the interpretation of technical information. This impediment shapes the expectations of patients and physicians, and underlies the ethical and legal standards for physicians' duties, informed consent, and medical malpractice.[4]

The first level of communication means talking, listening, tactful explanation, and a sensitive common approach to a particular problem. The next, deeper, level means sharing of emotions and imparting of confidence and trust. Medical staff providing care to cancer patients should help them to "ventilate," to express their emotions, to increase their willingness to work against the disease, to maintain a fighting spirit and overcome the tendency to give up. The ideal role for the physician is to be a friendly teacher. The care must provide comfort to the body, the mind, and the soul. In this model the patient has the opportunity for his values to be preserved.[5]

Mutual understanding between patient and physician in Poland has been restricted to a small number of patients, mainly to the educated population. It is frequently difficult for the physician to adapt his explanation to the cultural and educational level of the patients. Even educated patients cannot always understand the medical vocabulary because the physician may not take enough time to explain the situation in the rush to start treatment immediately.[6]

Patients may find it hard to ask questions because they fear that they will hear the worst news, that they will not be able to cope with the information, or that they will get an evasive answer. They fear that their questions may be interpreted as a lack of trust in the doctor or may cause discomfort. Another reason is the preference to accept a passive role as a subordinate patient and to avoid uncomfortable discussions about uncontrollable illness.

The most important task for a doctor is to listen to the patient, to his personal hopes, desires, and dreams. Hope has an important role in the humanization of technical progress, during which the creation of belief has been lost. However calm they may seem, cancer patients are almost always anxious. It is necessary to remember that they need reassurance to allay their fears, create confidence, and establish a feeling of security and hope. Hope in palliative care is not false optimism but means that a better time can yet come despite a bad diagnosis. Labeling the patient as hopeless means blocking the active help, care, and goodwill of the surrounding friendly people.

Effective communication is important not only to the management of anxiety, depression, and emotional problems but also to the relief of pain and other symptoms. More suffering is caused in the advanced stages of cancer patients by poor communication about their illness than by all other problems except unrelieved pain.

With the advancement of the disease patients become more vulnerable emotionally, and their feelings towards their caregivers become ambivalent. The attitude of those around changes dramatically when a person is known to have cancer. Frequently the cancer patient is completely avoided by family or friends; this is probably due to the discomfort of not knowing how to deal with, or what to say, in this situation. The family is alarmed that cancer implies pain, invalidism, disfigurement, and death. Family and friends, after initially being sympathetic and attentive, may in time drift away to their own lives, inadvertently isolating the cancer patient. Family may be reluctant to attend the bedside of the terminally ill, may fear that cancer could be contagious, and especially dangerous for children.[7]

Some patients do not want to inform the family about their illness; others do not accept a reversed role whereby instead of caring for their children or other family members they receive care from them. Some may wish to control the spread of the news or to spread it in their own way, especially if relationships within the family are strained. Others have feelings of envy towards healthy members of the family. How the patient will cope depends also on the availability of resources on which he can draw, such as family help, and economic and social support.

Social support is an important factor in helping the patient adjust to his problems. How the patient copes depends to a large extent on the availability of an adequate support system. External support involves people from the environment, social services, and hospices. It is important that the patient have at least one person who can listen with understanding and compassion to his fears about illness and death. Usually the strongest support comes from the family or caregivers.

The Anticancer Campaign is one of the voluntary organizations bringing support to cancer patients in Poland. They have organized "Confidence Calls" in many Polish cities, serviced by oncologists and psychologists who reply to each call from a person who suspects he may have cancer or from patients needing help in any form. The number of calls has been growing steadily. More recently fewer people are willing to contact their doctors, or else they prefer this form of intimacy. The response to a discussion on Polish television confirmed the need for continuation of these Confidence Calls. Patients find most useful a social network composed of individuals facing similar diseases and problems. Another form of activity has developed in the "Stoma Club," where help in the management of stoma, instructions about available facilities, and social support for those who feel isolated are provided. The clubs cooperate with surgical units serving patients with permanent and temporary stomas.

In the Rehabilitation Department of the Cancer Center in Warsaw, a club of patients recovering from breast cancer surgery has been organized under the name "Amazon Club." The aim of this club is to offer support by former breast cancer patients, on the basis of their own experience, to new patients, especially those at high risk of psychological risk. The Amazon Club soon gained popularity and has spread to 12 other cities in Poland.

Discussion groups have been formed in which patients and health-care professionals describe to new patients what to expect from the disease, what the possible sequelae of treatment are, and how to prevent the development of disability; and serve as a source of information about available services. Ten years' experience of the clubs was reviewed recently. The 852 members of the clubs were questioned, and it was found that no case of clinically confirmed depression was observed among patients participating in the clubs' activities; 82% stated that their family life did not deteriorate after treatment. In general, 96% of the respondents concluded that the club had an important influence on their lives, helping them communicate with each other, construct a bridge to the healthy population, and return to work.[8]

The goals of the Anticancer Campaign and club activities are rather long-term; shorter-term goals facilitate agreement with the patient's wishes, and appear to be more attainable and realistic, especially for patients whose condition may deteriorate rapidly. A fairly modest goal of caregivers should be individually established and directed at what the patient wishes to do today and tomorrow; most consideration should be devoted to his individual problems. Working toward each goal requires communication and consultation with the patient, and recognition of his self-esteem.

Many people know of their condition but do not speak of it; and if assured of discreet support and assurance from relatives, friends, and caregivers, they experience their disease with quiet courage. Patients with terminal illness who talked openly with medical staff appreciated this, and most criticism is directed at undue reticence. It is erroneous to assume that people either "want to know" or "do not want to know"; they vary continuously in what they want to know, how much they want to know, and from whom. It is necessary to differentiate between the need to give information in an early stage of cancer and its desirability in terminal illness. When a patient is dying, there is less need to inform him about the diagnosis and prognosis. At this stage the patient usually knows what he needs to know; he requires understanding and support, and sometimes an opportunity to unburden himself. The information provided to the patient has a real impact on his ability to cope with the illness and repeated medical procedures, which are sometimes irrational in the patient's opinion. How the patient copes depends to a large extent on the availability of an adequate support system.[9]

Many doctors tell their patients about their prognosis only if asked; others claim that the terminally ill do not really wish to know that they are dying. If the symptoms cannot be relieved, this must be explained to the patient, and the doctor should help him face the situation. As the disease progresses the patient may finally gain awareness that a fatal outcome is likely, but may be able to place this event at some remote time in the future.

COMMUNICATION IN THE HOSPICE

The effectiveness of the help provided in hospices to terminally ill cases is difficult to establish. Hospices began activities in Poland 10 years ago and now include 186 home care and 8 inpatient hospices. The patients in the hospice usually know that they have untreatable cancer; however, very often they request only full understanding of their needs and partial removal of their burden.[10] This is a reflection of improved knowledge about cancer, better general education, and widespread awareness of personal rights. Their anxiety gradually diminishes, and this is followed by adaptation and an acceptance of reality. Patients in the hospice are very receptive to the nonverbal behavior of the staff and look for cues about their condition. Much can be read from the face of a patient not able to communicate verbally. These patients also need eye contact and physical human touch. The doctor and nurses should establish the assurance of support on which the patient will come to rely and should protect the patient from the feeling of isolation and an inability to communicate with the caregivers.[11]

INFORMATION

The idea of Lady Saunders is to maintain open communication with patients; she stresses the need to have their illness explained and interpreted in order to relieve their fears. The commonest cause of complaint by patients about medical services is lack of information about their condition and its management. Generally, patients want to know as much as possible about their illness. Patients' first question is a useful clue to their attitude to disclosure about their illness.[12] The patient needs to know what is happening to him and that the doctor understands his problems. What the patient is really asking is "What is happening to me, and what are you going to do about it?" He requires information he can understand. His main need is to know how his disease will affect him. Withholding information is harmful to the patient's emotional state and lessens the chance of his or her cooperation.

Patients remember the first statement of what they have been told better than later ones, regardless of their relative importance. They more easily remember information given with explicit categorization—e.g., "First I will tell you what is wrong with you, then we will discuss your treatment." Patients who are asked to repeat what they have been told remember it best. It is in the patients' best interest to know the truth, and this becomes for doctors more a question of good medical practice than only the right to know.

The informed patient is better able to cope with the stresses of handling cancer and the traumas that may be involved in its treatment. It is often difficult to determine how much a patient wants to know, and there is fear that he will be told more than he can handle. The decision is frequently made to divulge very little. Some patients feel they have been given too many details initially and that they have been incapable of absorbing them; others would have preferred more information as to what they might expect. The belief that no more information should be given than is required for cooperation in treatment is not supported by acceptable evidence; it is based only on the opinion, conviction and emotional justification of the physician. Patients have an intrinsic need to find explanations about why the cancer happened to them. It is their assumption that cancer is a stigma, a punishment for past offenses. To bolster inner strength, the patient needs to be able to demand information about his illness and to maintain some control over his life.

TRUTH-TELLING

In a recent survey Dr. M. Jokiel asked 976 physicians about their approach to telling the truth to cancer patients. As many as 97% preferred to inform cancer patients of the diagnosis. The chief factors considered in the decision were age, intelligence, emotional stability, and relatives' desire.[13]

A doctor discovering cancer while examining a patient knows that when he says nothing he is saying a lot. But the "telling" often involves the use of vague terms, euphemisms, and circumlocutions or overprecise, incomprehensible technicalities. This type of information teaches patients little more than what they know from the past. Their awareness of their condition will depend not on what they were told, but on what they think they were told. The diagnosis should be free from ambiguity. People tend to dissociate from what they do not understand or do not accept for themselves.[14]

The doctor who wishes to adopt an honest approach and who uses the word "cancer" when initially telling the patient about his illness seldom uses the word subsequently. The doctor must distinguish between making a true statement and telling the truth. He must distinguish between accuracy (insofar as he knows it) and veracity (telling the truth honestly), not withholding or obscuring part of what he believes to be true. The patient needs to understand not only what cancer is, but what it is not. The doctor should not confuse honesty with accuracy. No more is expected of the doctor than to tell the truth as he sees it according to his best knowledge and judgment. While the doctor cannot always be certain of the outcome, or even of the diagnosis, fear of error should not interfere with the giving of information. Many physicians do not give their patients enough information because they think that telling too much may lead to questions they cannot answer or to a demand for a prediction to which they are unwilling to commit themselves. An honest answer of "I don't know" to some questions does not preclude answers to more easily anticipated questions—e.g., about pain, disability, or care. The belief that the doctor will tell the patient the truth in all circumstances creates in a patient a hopeful assurance. This patient does not feel lonely and mistrustful.

Hospital staff is often afraid of upsetting a patient because an open expression of feeling arouses their own anxiety. To avoid personal contact, staff often concentrate on physical and diagnostic tasks. When physicians have difficulty dealing with their failure to cure and with death, they may signal to their patients, sometimes unconsciously, that this topic is to be avoided in further discussions. Medical staff may behave in a way that inhibits patients from asking questions; they may maintain a social distance and in this way create a deterrent to communication. A doctor's refusal to tell the truth is quite often based on nothing more than a wish to avoid emotion-laden confrontation.[15]

In case the patient declares that he does not want to know the diagnosis if it is cancer, his wish should be respected, and further management should proceed in the most sympathetic way. Those who are not "ready to hear," who cannot cope with the information, will not be harmed. They will find a way to handle the situation by denial; knowing does not impede denying. In due course denial is usually replaced by constructive behaviors. Information needs vary over time. Attitudes are not fixed and can be expected to change.[16,17]

In general hospitals in Poland, telling the truth to cancer patients is rarely practiced. As a rule, the physician informs the family about the diagnosis. Usually it is a paternalistic statement, without the quality of counseling. For the hospital staff cancer remains a taboo, not to be discussed openly. The incurable patient is often not treated for associated ailments, but is sent home as soon as possible. Nobody is willing to talk to these patients. Not rarely, the first information about the diagnosis comes to the patient from the staff of a hospice.[18]

Until lately a common practice in Poland was to hide the diagnosis and prognosis of cancer, except in the case of patients who are reluctant to accept the proposed treatment. Even then, the information was restricted to naming the treatment modalities. The doctor plays a paternalistic role and informs his patients about the necessity of the treatment selected by him. In some general hospitals the patient may be discharged if he rejects the surgical option chosen by the doctor, and may be referred to the Oncological Service.

With the change in the Polish economy, some physicians have started their own private practice, which usually obliges them to inform the patient and his/her family about the diagnosis, to explain or even interpret the relevant choices of effective medical intervention, and to suggest the treatment most suitable for the patient.

In an analysis of the scope of information provided and the communication between physician and patient in the Gynecological-Oncological Department an important finding was that the patients admitted and treated in the oncological ward were not informed about the diagnosis of cancer and were given misleading answers with euphemistic explanations. Replying to a questionnaire about awareness of the cancer diagnosis, patients revealed that, despite the lack of information from the doctors, 48% of 285 patients knew the true character of their illness. The main source of information was other patients or, unintentionally, the nurses.

Until the 1950s hospital patients were tended by nuns, who prepared them daily during prayers to be ready to meet their Lord. Thus, in a depersonalized way information about death was brought to mind. Since the nuns were relieved of their duties in the hospitals in 1955 and replaced by professional nurses, nobody has been authorized to inform cancer patients that their treatment might not always be successful.

The institution of general practitioner (home physician, GP) is under development in Poland. I am not sure that our GPs will be competent to inform their cancer patients, willing to communicate with the patients and their families, or provide palliative care for terminal patients.

The frequency of truth-telling to patients depends also on the specialization of the physician. In Poland approximately every third patient of 120,000 new cancer cases per year is treated in oncological clinics or hospitals.[19] Presumably admission to or treatment in oncological units would enlighten most of the patients as to the nature of their illness and inform them about what radio- or chemotherapy means. This assumption was only partially confirmed in the results of two surveys conducted in oncological units.

The results of the first survey performed in the Gyne-Oncological Department of Oncological Hospital confirmed that the majority (78.5%) of 192 patients knew they had cancer, but as many as 81.7% were not conscious of the treatment they were receiving or what would happen if a cure was not attained. Most of them (86%) predicted a high probability of cure and constructed optimistic prognoses.

In a second survey, conducted in another oncological department, 88% of 210 patients wanted to know the diagnosis, but only 72% did on the condition that it was not cancer. Less than half of the patients of the same sample, who had no chance of cure, wanted to be aware of the diagnosis but not the prognosis.

In recent years healthy people in Poland have changed their opinion about the need of informing cancer patients. Twenty years ago half of the 878 randomly selected inhabitants of a big city replied "no" when asked about truth-telling to the cancer patient. A survey performed 10 years later indicated that 82% of 923 asked agreed on the need of providing full information to cancer patients with good prognosis, but only 21% wished the truth to be told to incurable patients. Less than 15% of villagers, members of the older generation, and the uneducated accept the need for information about cancer when the prognosis is bad. They say that the word "cancer" is so ominous and hopeless that it would be inhuman to announce the verdict of death to anybody. These successive investigations show that better information published through the mass media has helped promote an understanding of the nature of cancer and of the growing chances of cure and better care for the terminally ill. The public is starting to accept that cancer is not an anathema or a punishment but, even if not curable, is one of the ways that life ends.

Only 8% of 936 healthy people recently surveyed doubt if imparting full information about a prognosis is always the proper approach in communication between physician and cancer patient. Almost all agree that the patient has the right to know the truth, but nevertheless 15% of those older than 65 years do not wish to be told an the unfavorable diagnosis.[20]

A pilot study examining satisfaction with care in an oncological hospital was performed on a group of 52 cervical cancer patients discharged after completion of irradiation who replied to a 60-item questionnaire. All patients were aware that they had cancer, but 40 respondents did not know the possible consequences. The prognosis was not explained in 46 cases, and as many as 42 patients asked for more detailed information about their future. Despite the full confidence in doctors' expertise expressed by 48 patients, 38 felt intimidated in communication with their physician, except on very important subjects. Communication with nurses was easier for housewives (half of the group), and even educated women (8/52) preferred to ask nurses rather than doctors certain intimate questions—e.g., about sex after radiotherapy. The analysis of data indicate that the medical staff, mainly physicians in the specialist Oncological Hospital, did not provide satisfactory information to the cancer patients concerning treatment and prognosis. This result needs comparison with the scope and quality of information given to patients in the wards of general hospitals.

Patients with little education are significantly more likely to underestimate the seriousness of their condition. Inaccurate views of their disease were probably due to inefficient communication with their doctors as well as denial of the seriousness of their illness. Doctors do not always communicate as well as they think they do. Patient perception of the probability of cure or prolongation of life is more optimistic than the physicians' estimation.

The "sick person" is a social role that is seen as governed by the doctor who is in charge of the patient. When people are ill, they often welcome a dependent position in which responsibility is removed from their shoulders. The majority do not wish to assume full responsibility, but would rather share it with the physician and rely on his expertise. Some patients deny information because they do not like to accept the truth. The phenomenon of denial represents a normal adaptive process that permits the patient to cope with an otherwise unacceptable situation. In the early stage of cancer it is common for the patient to exhibit denial. This is a protective mechanism in the face of threatening events. The denial of diagnosis may be due to panic, resulting in failure to understand what has been said. To some extent this can be avoided by careful, unhurried explanation. Denial of a serious illness may be more common in those with strong personalities who have led successful lives. In the course of time denial is resorted to less.[21]

No treatment should be undertaken without full explanation and discussion with the patient. Decisions should be shared in a collaborative process in which both the patient and the physician make active and essential contributions. The physician brings medical training and expertise, understanding the available treatment alternatives to the diagnosis and management of the patient's condition. Mutual participation must replace paternalism as the basis of the doctor-patient relationship. The burden of decision making cannot be left to the patient. Some patients experience difficulties in accepting randomization and believe that their physicians will decide what is best for them. Before 1972 informed consent standards were required by the physicians; subsequently they have been oriented toward the patients and are therefore easier for them to accept.

The passive sick role of a patient can be successively replaced by mutual participation in the medical decisionmaking. The paternalistic role of the physician is replaced in modern patient-doctor relationships by open, perfect communication with the patient. The patient brings the knowledge of his own subjective aims and values, through which his wishes and the benefits of various treatment options can be evaluated. There is a tendency nowadays among medical personnel to discard the image of authority and encourage the patient to speak more freely. It appears that there is now more effective communication with cancer patients, less fear that it will result in loss of hope, greater understanding of the patient's desire for information, and increased sensitivity to their emotional needs; there is also a greater commitment on the part of the doctor to be constantly available when needed. Though more doctors are being open with their patients, it still seems highly unlikely that the vast majority of physicians tell their patients about their illness. This reflects the actual position in most of the world, and unfortunately it is true also in Poland. All the changes that have occurred recently in this country bring hope for improvement in the standards of the health care and communication between patient and doctor.

REFERENCES

1. NOVACK, D. H., R. PLUMER, R. L. SMITH, H. OCHITILL, G. R. MORROW & J. M. BENNET. 1979. Changes in physicians' attitudes toward telling the cancer patients. JAMA **267**(9): 897–900.
2. DZIENNIK USTAW RZECZYPOSPOLITEJ POLSKIEJ. 1991. Ustawa Nr. 408 z dnia 31 sierpnia 1991 O zakladach opieki z zdrowotnej. Art. 19 paragraf 3 str 1245.
3. NACZELNA RADA LEKARSKA. KOMISJA ETYKI LEKARSKIEJ. 1993. Kodeks Etyki Lekarskief. Projekt nowelizacji. Gazeta Lekarska **6**(Wkladka 1): 3–6.
4. LICHTER, I. 1987. Communication in Cancer Care. Churchill Livingstone. Edinburgh.
5. MCKILLOP, W. J., W. E. STEWARD, A. D. GIMBURG & S. S. STEWARD. 1988. Cancer patients' perception of their care and its treatment. Br. J. Cancer **58:** 355–358.
6. JOKIEL, M. 1987. Zmiany w uświadomieniu społeczeństwa polskiego w zakresie chorób nowotworowych na przestrzeni 10 lat (1976–1986). Nowotwory **37**(3): 190–194.
7. EZEKIEL, J. E. & L. E. LINDA. 1992. Four models of the physician-patient relationship. Special communication. JAMA **267**(16): 2221–2226.
8. ADAMCZAK, M. 1988. Wybrane procesy poznawcze i emocjonalne u kobiet po mastektomii. Wyd. Nauk. UAM. Poznań.
9. CASSILETH, B. R., R. V. ZUPKIS, K. SUTTON-SMITH & V. MARCH. 1980. Information and participation preferences among cancer patients. Ann. Intern. Med. **92:** 832–836.
10. SAUNDERS, C. & N. SYKES. 1993. The Management of Terminal Malignant Disease. 3d edit. Edward Arnold. London.
11. HUGGINSON, I. 1995. Clinical Audit in Palliative Care. Radcliffe Medical Press. Oxford.
12. WEIL, M. M. SMITH & D. KHAYAT. 1994. Truth telling to cancer patients in Western European context. Psychooncology **3:** 21–26.
13. JOKIEL, M. & E. SIKORSKA. 1990. Opinia publiczna o informowaniu pacjentów o rozpoznawaniu choroby nowotworowej. Nowotwory **40**(1): 60–64.

14. ŁUCZAK, J. & A. ROSZAK. 1990. Co wiedza o swojej chorobie pacjenci leczeni w szpitalu onkologicznum. Nowotwory **40**(1): 65–68.
15. JAREMA, M. & A. JAREMA. 1975. Psychiczne aspekty choroby nowotworowej. Pol. Tyg. Lek. **30**(49): 2049–2052.
16. ESTAPE, J. H. PALOMBO, E. HERNANDEZ, M. DANIELS, T. ESTAPE, J. J. GRAN, N. VINOLAS & J. M. MANE. 1992. Cancer diagnosis disclosure in a Spanish hospital. Ann. Oncol. **3:** 451–452.
17. SURBONE, A. 1992. Truth telling to the patient. Letter from Italy. JAMA **268**(13): 1661–1662.
18. SIEDLECKI, P. 1987. Czy mówić prawdę chorym na nowotwory? Nowotwory **37**(2): 185–187.
19. ZATOŃSKI, W. A. 1993. Nowotwory złośliwe w Polsce. Centrum Onkologii. Warsaw.
20. JOKIEL, M. 1995. Opinia publiczna o informowaniu pacjentów o rozpoznaniu choroby nowotworowej w latach 1984–1994. Nowotwory. Submitted for publication.
21. BROCK, D. W. & S. A. WARTMAN. 1990. When competent patients make irrational choices. Sounding Board. N. Engl. J. Med. **332**(22): 1595–1599.

Characteristics of Physician–Cancer Patient Relationships in Russia

N. N. BLINOV AND K. P. HANSON

Professor N. N. Petrov Research Institute of Oncology
Pesochny-2
68 Leningradskaya str.
189646 St. Petersburg, Russia

INTRODUCTION

Malignant tumors are the second most frequently reported causes of death among the population of Russia. According to statistics, in 1994. 411,800 cancer patients were registered for the first time, and 300,600 patients died from cancer—i.e., 28.5% and 34.7% higher than the similar indices in 1980, respectively.

Direct and indirect relationships of cancer patients with physicians, relatives, and society are among the complicated unsolved problems in clinical oncology. This is explained by both the annual increase in the number of cancer patients and the growth of the number of patients in society who have already received radical treatment and are considered to be cured of this serious disease. Thus, each year we meet more patients who have cancer or have been cured of it. These people remain an inalienable part of our society, and many of them, after returning to their activities after treatment, encounter numerous social, medical, and psychological problems. All these problems are closely intertwined, and their solution requires a complex approach.

SURVEY OF PATIENTS' ATTITUDES

The first complication of relationships among physician, cancer patient, and relatives is the problem of the diagnosis—whether one should tell the patient about the character of his disease. According to psychological questionnaires[1] the diagnosis of cancer is still a synonym for agony and death for most of the population. Two main groups of patients can be distinguished as far as their relation to the diagnosis of cancer is concerned. Patients of the first group know or suspect their diagnosis and want it made more precise. The second group consists of persons not wanting to know the diagnosis of their disease or trying to deny it ("physician error," or " I cannot have it," and so on). It may be suggested that this motivation is often a reason for refusal to undergo preventive examination, to visit an oncologist, which can result in late diagnosis of the disease and a mournful outcome. But similar complications occurring in the first group as well sometimes bring about refusal to be treated and may cause passive suicide. The medical deontological aspect of disagnosis is whether one should tell the patient the truth, how to tell it, how to cause a minimum of mental disturbance and to mobilize the patient's mind for active treatment and to fight against the disease. It seems to us there can be no common prescription in these cases except the principle of an individual approach to each patient. Psychologists can help oncologists cope with this problem; their presence in oncological institutions is essential. Probably the time is coming to change our ideas about physician–cancer patient relationships, and this may have positive results in the prevention, detection, and treatment of cancer.

The successful development of diagnostic and treatment methods for some malignant tumors allows us to expect the long-term, reliable cure of a vast number of patients; and owing to scientific achievements there is now the possibility of predicting the prognosis of the disease with high probality. In cases with a favorable prognosis it is reasonable, from our point of view, to inform the patient of his diagnosis. Then his recovery and prolonged life after cure will be an excellent confirmation of the achievements of modern oncology. Such outcomes will help change the erroneous opinion of the population as to the fatality of malignant tumors.

In Russia some patients who survive cancer after treatment continue to believe that they did not have cancer, as they had previously been told by physicians. Their relatives are silent about the true diagnosis because they are afraid of the negative attitude of the people around them to cancer patients. This can be explained by the fact that, unfortunately, not knowing the etiology of cancer gives rise to the idea that the cancer patient can infect healthy people. In consequence a "leper" complex arises, and the patient may fall into an atmosphere of social-psychological isolation. Weakening family relationships and disruption of relationships with co-workers and friends bring about painful experiences for the patient. Another complication is the erroneous idea that all cancer patients will soon die even after treatment and that people treated at oncological institutions who survived for a long time did not have this fatal disease ("They were lucky."), and therefore the patient was treated ("tormented") for nothing. These problems are one of the main causes of fear of cancer—sometimes not fear of death, but fear of suffering unbearably and for no purpose.

Nowadays in different countries there are several points of view on the question of whether the cancer patient should be informed about the diagnosis of his disease or not. Many of our authors keep to the principle of sparing the patient's psyche by creating a "deontological legend" (concealment of the true diagnosis from cancer patient).[2] Authors of many other countries consider it necessary to inform the patient completely about his health, arguing that the patient's ignorance causes feelings of loneliness and isolation, keeps the patient more and more distant from the physician, and produces rupture of relationships instead of the unity needed.[3] Many clinicians report their refusal to conceal the diagnosis from the cancer patient, emphasizing the need for emotional support in the critical situation of the meeting of cancer patent with the cruel truth.[4]

Some are of the opinion that it is reasonable to inform the patient of his diagnosis only at the early stages of cancer, but to conceal the diagnosis when the disease has become widespread because of the fatal prognosis. Some authors recommend the following rules of physician–cancer patient relationships: (a) to inform the patient about disease and its consequences by using terms that are clear to the patient both intellectually and emotionally; (b) to give information to those patients who really want it by authoritatively providing the true nature of complications and lethal risks in a psychologically spare form of conversation; (c) to explain the information given about the disease to the extent needed by the patient.[5–7] The diversity of judgments on the type of information about their disease permissible for oncological patients in various countries and in Russia made us turn our interest to the analysis of patients' opinions on the subject, which are still not understood.

In the present investigation we tried to examine to what extent cancer patients are informed about their disease and to estimate their own psychological readiness to receive true data about their diagnosis. Information was gathered anonymously from 280 patients (200 women and 80 men, with mean ages of 55.5 and 54, respectively) by means of questionnaires consisting of 22 items. In addition clinical and psychological conversations took place with all the patients. External tumors (breast cancer) were detected in 65 patients, 194 patients suffered from diseases of internal organs (lung cancer, stomach cancer, gynecological cancer), and in 21 cases diagnosis needed to be defined more accurately.

Analysis of the mood of the patients under observation showed that a third had a pronounced level of alarm, half demonstrated a moderate degree of anxiety, and a fifth were neither anxious nor uneasy about the situation. Pronounced alarm was most characteristic of the women with internal tumors.

Knowledge of their disease, including the true diagnosis, mode of treatment, and prognosis proved indefinite for most of the patients studied. Only 12.5 % of the patients were fully informed about their disease; 31.1% had only a partial notion of it. These data demonstrate that the general notion about the disease among the patients observed was fragmentary.

Only one-fourth of the patients were satisfied with the quality of information about the disease and the diagnosis obtained from a district oncologist; one-third of the patients remained unsatisfied; and almost half gave uncertain answers. These data reflect a definite degree of psychological stress—confusion, disorientation, and emotional shock—as a result of the suggested oncological diagnosis and fear of their future. This is confirmed by the fact that uncertainty was most evident among the patients with internal tumors, where there is higher degree of obscurity and menace to life.

A desire for additional information about cancer, its nature and prognosis, was expressed in only half of the cases (140 patients). Of them, 59 were interested in learning about the disease in detail by reading literature on medicine (reference books, encyclopedias, scientific literature, etc.); 25 obtained their ideas about the disease by sharing their experiences with their relatives and friends. These facts can be explained by peculiarities of individual character (active, passive, tolerant of stress, and so on) and by certain psychological attitudes of the patient toward informative interaction with a physician, consisting either in a desire to know his situation, to remain in ignorance, "playing at silence," or to remain within the limits of the "deontological legend" about the origin and nature of the disease detected Certainly the education and intelligence of the patient play important roles.

Several patients (49.6%) demonstrated a desire to become informed about the situation and have a confidential conversation with a qualified specialist; the desire for such contact was indicated in 39.4% of the cases, with only 10.8% of the patients not wanting such a conversation.

The opinion of the cancer patient about informative interaction with an oncologist is of great, even of primary, importance, as there are still a large number of patients who, not knowing the situation with the disease, miss the opportunity for timely examination and radical treatment and turn instead to nontraditional medicine and put their hope in "popular" remedies.

Most of the respondents noted that full frankness and truth were desirable in their conversation with the physician; one-seventh of the patients wanted to have only suitable (convenient), acceptable information about the diagnosis and the disease, preferring not to know all the unpleasant, frightening facts and details. The information considered by the physician as necessary for the patients was sufficient for most of them; 15.3% of the patients were inclined to inquire after peculiarities of the disease and to have unclear things explained; only 6.4% stressed their unwillingness to know any details of their disease.

Most of the patients agreed with the statement that knowledge of the true diagnosis helps to fight the disease. Only 10% disagreed, and one-fifth of the patients were uncertain of their reply.

Thus, the data obtained in this research show the desire or need of most cancer patients to learn the nature of the disease and details of treatment already at the stage of examination. This data throws doubt on the necessity of keeping to one of the main deontological principles—to conceal the diagnosis from the patient. The opinions of the respondents demonstrate their desire to know the details of the disease and the possibility of their being able to return to work after treatment—i.e., they want to take active part in deciding their fate, of bearing some of the responsibility for their situation, of being allies of the physician in the struggle against the disease. Furthermore, the patients who know about the diagnosis and treatment may be excellent propagandists among the general population of advances in oncology.

CONCLUSIONS

Taking into account the opinion of most cancer patients, the physician can avoid stereotyped relationships with the patient. When a patient with a favorable prognosis is not reacting constructively to his disease and the physician believes that information will contribute to a more constructive attitude on the part of the patient, he should provide that information. From our point of view the moral right to inform the cancer patient about his diagnosis should belong only to the physician competent in oncological diseases—only to the oncologist. Undoubtedly, when the patient is experiencing emotional difficulties or is behaving inappropriately, consultation with a psychologist is necessary.

REFERENCES

1. Gnezdilov, A. V., N. N. Simonov & N. B. Shipovnikov. 1979. Psychogenic disorders in cancer patients and possibility of their correction in oncological clinic. Vopr. Onkol. **25**(5): 106–107. (In Russian.)
2. Peterson, B. E. 1981. On treatment of stage IV tumor patients. Vopr. Onkol. **27**(10): 72–77. (In Russian.)
3. Tristram, E. H. 1986. Suicide and the cancer patient. Cancer **36**(2): 105–109.
4. Holland, J. 1975. Psychological aspects of cancer. Klin. Med. **6:** 140–145. (In Russian.)
5. Henrichs, M. & A. Schmale. 1983. Principles of Psychosocial Oncology. Clinical Oncology for Medical Students and Physicians. P. Rubin, Ed. American Cancer Society. New York, NY.
6. Foulder, C. 1983. The patient's right to choose. Clin. Oncol. **3:** 189–191.
7. Holland, J. C. & R. Mastrovito. 1980. Psychologic adaptation to breast cancer. Cancer (Phila.) **46:** 1045–1052.

Communication with the Breast-Cancer Patient

An Opinion from Russia

EUGENY DEMIN

Petrov Research Institute of Oncology
68, Leningradskaya str.
Pesochny-2
St. Petersburg, 189646, Russia

INTRODUCTION

Nobody can disagree that communication is the basis for all aspects of a relationship between two people. By communicating with one another we learn and we receive information, both correct and incorrect. Knowledge is power. Every human being has the right to be informed as much as is necessary to be in charge of his life. A healthy person may be able to respond adequately to the unexpected. It is another matter when the ill, already living under the abnormal conditions imposed by their illness, receive unexpected news.

In this respect the status of cancer patients is very demonstrative. I will base my comments on breast cancer patients, having devoted many years to studying them and their possibilities of having the quality of life they deserve. In Russia breast cancer is the most prevalent form of malignancy in the female population. In St. Petersburg breast cancer is one of the most frequent tumors in women: about 2000 new cases are registered annually. Improved methods of treatment and increased early detection of breast cancer has brought about an increase in the five-year survival rate to 60%. Of course, this result is not good enough. Greater success would depend in part on communicating to the general population the meaning and consequences of cancer.

It is a pity that in Russia cancer has for a long time been covered by a curtain of mystery and dread, both of which derive from a deficiency or absence of communication. The lack of information is not a consequence of our health policy, which continues to promote optimal service despite changes in socioeconomic conditions. Historically and culturally the practical availability of proper, timely health care in our country is quite adequate. Traditionally patients were not given much information about their condition. The transition to openness has involved some general issues and has affected some sides of life that had not been apparent. It has also affected cancer, which is now seen as not only a medical problem.

At present we cannot reduce the incidence of many of the forms of cancer, but the lessening of the mortality of some forms of cancer, among them breast cancer, might be possible. Late diagnosis is still an obstacle to survival of the majority of women with this disease, some of whom fear seeking medical attention even if they have a lump in the breast. Reasonable communication might be one key for correcting this sorrowful situation.

On the one hand the fact that breast cancer is not completely curable inspires apathy and hopelessness; on the other hand the low level of awareness among people makes them so frightened by malignancy that they do not dare visit a doctor at the first suspicious signs. As far as preventive steps that might avoid cancer are concerned, these involve aspects of human behavior and attitudes to health that are difficult to change. Therefore, a vicious circle develops, and one of our tasks as health professionals is to break it. This has to be done by determinedly providing the public with relevant, accurate information.

It is possible that the hoped-for early detection of cancer depends not only on the establishment scientific programs, but on the knowledge and trust that each person would remain a deserving human being after undergoing medical treatment.[1,2] In my opinion adequate communication in this regard is a great catalyst in assisting people, including those already with cancer, to have a proper orientation with respect to the different points of view that surround this disease.

Healthy people subconsciously follow medical progress with cancer, receiving information, verbal and nonverbal, from a variety of sources. If up to now we have communicated chiefly with people with cancer, I would suggest that we communicate as well with other professionals, the mass media, close relatives of patients, and medical support personnel and volunteers. All of these objects of communication function together, in their separate ways, to influence patients' quality of life. I will describe and discuss such communication in the following section. My remarks reflect the reality of the situation today with regard to communication; they do not merely present my own opinions.

COMMUNICATION WITH CANCER PATIENTS: GENERAL CONSIDERATIONS

Giving information in oncology is one aspect of using every possible method to achieve the best possible result.[3,4] For example, in breast cancer it is not absolutely necessary to tell women that their disease is curable or incurable. What they are told depends on the extent of their participation in treatment. When the process is effective, no one is permitted to shock them with the diagnosis. They know about their tumor's existence anyway. If the situation requires that the truth be told—e.g., if the patient unexpectedly refuses therapy, or if the doctor is confident in the possibility of treatment—then it is indispensable to tell the patient about her disease. I can offer no advice as to how this should be told, except that the information must be given by professionals; it is better to communicate first with the patient's close relatives and to wait for the outcome; the final decision concerning what to do belongs to the patient.

Communication with cancer patients is not only a matter of telling or not telling the truth about their illness. Communication is a very wide and rather relative concept; nobody is ever completely outside of it.[5]

COMMUNICATION WITH PROFESSIONALS

The medical team does not pay much attention to communicating with cancer patients. Only when a patient understands what she has a right to expect in the way of prevention, treatment, and care will she know what to ask for and be able to make sure that she gets it.[6,7] Doctors often do not bother to keep their other patients—those who do not ask—informed. There are two reasons for this:

(1) Doctors' inability and unwillingness to contact patients informally and talk to them openly, using an intelligible language. This must be corrected by training doctors to overcome the barrier between them and the ill and their own psychological barriers and to become more available.

(2) The lack of enough time for communication with the cancer patient. This is not an adequate explanation. Of course, doctors performing surgery, chemotherapy, irradiation, and other aspects of treatment like a routine job rarely ponder the need of patients to be not merely passive recipients of, but active participants in, their treatment and their destiny. Patients who are not given adequate information by their doctors seek it out from other sources and often get information that is incorrect.

This attitude to communication in oncology is the result of the difficult, eternal question of whether to tell or not tell the cancer patient the truth. To my mind this is not a problem as long as patients are given sufficient truth to enable them to participate fully in the treatment process and to help the medical team in combating the disease and its consequences. The only philosophic problem in this regard is how to measure the sufficiency of this truth. Nobody knows the answer to this, and, indeed, there is no single answer; it depends. Nobody wants to hurt the cancer patient who survives.

Telling or not telling the truth is a matter that involves skill (or lack of skill) in communicating with cancer patients, and it involves ethical standards. I believe that ethical standards are not culturally related, but absolute. My long-term research and experience in breast cancer have convinced me that truth-telling benefits the individual doctor and patient, as well as the relationship between them.

COMMUNICATING WITH THE MASS MEDIA

It is no secret that cancer patients in Russia suffer from public misunderstanding and ignorance. Unfortunately the mass media contribute to this. Of course, there is much news in the mass media about the possibility of prevention of tobacco-related cancers and the benefits of screening for breast and cervical cancer. Moreover, we can sometimes read, hear, and watch about rather high cure rates for a number of malignancies that can be detected early and are sensitive to modern therapy. This is good, but it is not quite enough for healthy people and patients because this important information comes from specialists in their professional language, which is not clear to everyone.

It is necessary to use all available methods of communication, but even with such methods, how can men and women be convinced to stop smoking or drinking if these products are advertised and are available even to teenagers? Unfortunately television, especially commercial television, often presents stories about new "miracle" drugs that cannot be immediately disproved by cancer investigators. It is a fault of the mass media that they rarely give adequate, up-to-date comments on news relating to cancer control. Former cancer patients are hardly ever presented on the media to share their experience of the disease and offer positive examples of recovery.

The reasons for this are not clear. It is possible that the long-standing closed nature of our society is one of the causes. Another may be the tradition of not speaking openly about cancer. Despite its social importance cancer is still regarded by the mass media as a matter of fatal suffering that may not be mentioned openly, calmly, or confidently. It would be nice if specialists and cancer patients could take part together in popular broadcasts. Such communication would be invaluable, but at present we may only dream of it.

As a medical oncologist and specialist in the rehabilitation of breast cancer patients, I frequently enjoy and envy the approach that can be seen in Western television programs about a healthy lifestyle. At present here almost everything that concerns cancer and its sufferers deals with such matters as pain and terrible death. This is a significant oversight in truthful public education on the problem of cancer, and one of the psychological consequences of this oversight can be late diagnosis.

Fortunately positive changes in life here have made the mass media gradually begin to change its own and the people's attitudes toward malignant tumor and cancer patients. There has also been a gradual change in attitudes regarding the right of the cancer patient to adequate information from the medical establishment. Cancer is a difficult matter in itself, and it places great demands on people's ability to communicate. The mass media must assist this process.

COMMUNICATION WITH CLOSE RELATIVES

Cancer is a very special disease. Its detection not only brings about new problems in health but sometimes changes and even overturns the social relations of cancer patients as well. It is well known that social relations are one of the most significant human values and that life without them loses its normal quality. Therefore, the family's ability to communicate with the cancer patient is of great importance: communication with family members can be interactive, supportive, and loving; if inadequate, it can destroy everything that has been built up over the years.[8,9]

We investigated this matter in families in which a woman had breast cancer. It was not easy to determine the verbal and nonverbal reactions to the diagnosis among family members. The process of adapting to the new circumstances between the affected woman and her relatives, especially her husband, is not very visible. But everyone takes part in this adaptation, whether they want to or not. We were assisted in this study by volunteers who were former breast cancer patients who had had their own experiences with family communication. The families' quite different responses were grouped into six patterns and may be summarized as follows:

(1) The affected woman hides her illness from friends and distant relatives, particularly if they have daughters (to shield them from the fear of getting cancer). The family maintains the same supportive relations as before and prepares itself psychologically for the treatment. The patient's absence from home during her hospitalization is explained as a vacation. Everybody mobilizes the strength and spirit to be attentive to each other. The husband takes care of everything at home. After the patient returns home, nobody can notice anything different from before.

(2) The affected woman hides her disease only from her friends, but her relatives are fully aware of everything. The illness and its circumstances remind them that life is unpredictable and may be short. A warm attitude helps the patient survive the shock. If the family is not friendly, a relative speaks about the husband's unhappiness, that he is sorry for his destiny. The patient suffers doubly—from her illness and her husband's reaction to it; this does not help her recovery.

(3) The affected woman does not hide her disease, hoping desperately that the diagnosis is wrong. The family supports her in any way possible, letting her know that in spite of her cancer she is needed by everybody. The great thing for her is to be alive. The family members believe that her illness is no worse than others, and the patient is urged to undergo the necessary treatment.

(4) The affected woman is aware not only of her disease but also that it was found rather late for management. She undergoes a very stressful period and is ready to refuse treatment. The family submits to these circumstances, does not try to do anything or to make her accept treatment. Not having adequate support, the patient suffers much more and has no hope, despite positive relations in her family.

(5) The situation is rather difficult when another member of the family has or has had cancer. Even if the family members and the patient do everything they can to arrange treatment and promote recovery, recollection of the previous experience, especially if it did not have a good outcome, complicates relationships and diminishes hope and supportiveness. Positive willpower is needed from everybody.

(6) The affected woman shares her troubles with her husband. He is very attentive and compassionate; he accompanies her to the hospital. But after the confirmation of her diagnosis, he leaves her, with various reasons for doing so: e.g., he fears he will be infected by his wife; he does not want to have a wife who has lost her feminine image.

These six patterns of reaction to the diagnosis of breast cancer were viewed and analyzed as though from within the family and the patient. We professionals often forget that we are dealing with live persons with their own psychology, habits, and relationships. We must confess that at least here doctors think that only they have the right to decide what is appropriate for cancer patients and their close relatives, to specify what contact should take place and what to tell or not tell. This view from without is not correct. We know very well that the majority of cancer patients suspect that they have cancer. Some of them try to deny it; others wait, along with their relatives, for an honest conversation. Doctors must take this into consideration. Before making up their minds about the disease, its treatment, and its consequences, they should learn the point of view of the patient and her close relatives. Only by being aware of the patterns of response to disease, such as those presented above, may professionals effectively discuss this very difficult matter with the cancer patient and her close relatives. They have to be told as much as is required for the overall benefit of both effective therapy and successful relationships with others. It is sometimes possible to bring the different stages of cancer into the conversation, but they are more useful for clinicians than for the patients' psychoemotional needs.

No patient should be deprived of the opportunity of communication, least of all the woman with breast cancer and her husband. Only after having been given adequate information are they able to decide how to proceed. No detailed prescription for this communication can be provided to doctors beforehand. Involving patients and their close relatives in a treatment program depends on the doctors' education, skill, and compassion.

It follows that communication—verbal and nonverbal—with the cancer patient is a very important part of general human relationships. Its quality and efficacy depend on several interacting factors. It is necessary to do everything possible to help patients avoid thinking of their exceptionality and exclusiveness so that they not feel isolated from society. It is important to help them live deserving lives, participating in all events within the capacity of their strength and spirit. This can be accomplished through regular, respectful communication with one's patients. Invaluable assistance can be given by voluntary support personnel.

SUPPORTIVE NONMEDICAL CARE AND VOLUNTEERS: REACH TO RECOVERY IN RUSSIA

Relationships with nonmedical persons can be an important part of providing the breast cancer patient with communication that gives her an opportunity to see herself from another point of view and to gain confidence. When an affected woman sees her "colleague," who has gone through "it" and has a chance to speak with her, her attitude become smuch more optimistic and trustful. Former patients, specially selected and trained in accordance with the Reach to Recovery Program—a worldwide program for the improvement of understanding, treatment, and care of breast cancer patients—serve as a bridge between isolation and normality for the cancer sufferer.

This nonmedical program[10] has been designed to help women with breast cancer return to everyday life after treatment by providing person-to-person support. It is based on the premise that women who have had their own experience with this disease and are now physically and emotionally healthy can relate in a positive way to newly diagnosed persons. It is essential in carrying out this noble work that volunteers ascend to a higher level, where they become more listeners and assistants than former patients and advisors. Their power to communicate and to present correct information generally meets with the appreciation of everyone involved in nonmedical support care. However, sometimes it is regarded with more of a haughty than a cooperative attitude; this can be explained by the difficulty some doctors have in sharing their privileges with others.

Naturally there are many difficulties in overcoming routine professional habits. It is well known that Mrs. Terese Lasser,[11] the initiator of rehabilitation and nonmedical care for breast cancer patients in 1952, has had many problems in developing her idea. The same situation was met by Mrs. Francine Timothy,[12] who was responsible for the International Reach to Recovery Program as its president and who retired at the end of 1994 after 20 years of pioneering work. They both managed to make surgeons allies in achieving their mutual goal.

We have witnessed and felt the effect of this program for almost eight years, since the first Russian Reach to Recovery program was established in St. Petersburg by me and medical psychologist Valentina Chulkova.[13] Many women are active in this association, called Hope (Nadezhda), devoting their morale, knowledge, and experience to effective communication with present-day patients despite the very strained sociopolitical and financial conditions here. Since 1992 Hope/Nadezhda has had the status of an affiliated member of Reach to Recovery International. Since 1995 our association has been a member of another rather new project, Europa Donna, a coalition of organizations and individuals concerned with breast cancer that aims to raise public awareness of the disease and to mobilize the support of women throughout Europe in pressing for better physical and psychological care and treatment and more resources for breast cancer research.

One of the main problems is to persuade professionals of the necessity of volunteer assistance, so that the professionals will accept their support as an important part of the complete program for treatment of and communication with patients. Our association is carefully following all the traditions that have been designed for the sake of breast cancer patients in the West and adapting them to our situation.[5] Our volunteers provide different kinds of help, free of charge: visits, psychosocial support for patients and their families, rehabilitation, help in coping, a telephone hot line, etc. All of these activities are in essence communication—the most important object of the entire program of recovery.

Ours is the first group in Russia to host annual city conferences—Open Door Days—for cancer patients, particularly for women with breast cancer and their relatives. This is helpful because here it is not the rule that cancer patients talk openly to anybody except doctors about their disease. Also, they do not have regular opportunities to see people like themselves and listen to professionals in informal settings, because these people are usually separate from the outside world. It should be stressed that these events have a positive influence on the volunteers as well as on the patients. The former patients who volunteer with the association do not conceal their names and illness during such conferences, held under the motto "Together against Breast Cancer." They speak from the stage and in private conversations with members of the audience. This is a beneficial psychological victory for the volunteers, and they are a good example for present breast cancer patients to follow in not remaining isolated. We are very excited and happy to welcome to these conferences many doctors, who begin to overcome barriers created by themselves and decide to make contact with patients outside of the hospital. They gradually begin to understand that only together is it possible to reach recovery. It is important for cancer patients to become convinced that health is not merely the state of nondisease; it means a deserved quality of life. Mass media participating in these optimistic conferences begin to change their own and the public's attitude to cancer patients from one of ignorance and fear of death to one of respect and correct information, which encourages survivors of cancer to remain members of society. It is good to hear some women speak words of great appreciation for the concrete support that they have had from our volunteers and specialists. Each year we invite lecturers to speak on various subjects and give up-to-date news about the latest achievements in cancer research and management of breast cancer patients through therapy to the giving of psychosocial aid. Together with the audience we try to discuss issues of the day. Many problems exist around us: fund-raising, providing affected women with prostheses and convenient underwear, social questions, etc. The majority of these problems are shared during roundtable time, and it is very interesting to watch people helping others by helping themselves. Once we arranged a fashion show in which our volunteers served as models. The volunteers experience being seen on television and heard on radio. Almost everyone becomes united in the whole process, and the benefits of such communication are obvious. Many in the audience enroll in our association. This is a very serious step, and it tells much about the progress of our Reach to Recovery.

Our movement is spreading to other parts of Russia. Regrettably, such nonmedical activity does not have adequate financial support here; perhaps this might be obtained from the West. Meanwhile, step by step the extraordinary activities of the St. Petersburg Reach to Recovery Association Hope/Nadezhda is helping professionals carry out their recovery programs.

CONCLUSION

We have described and discussed four ingredients of communication with breast cancer patients that are applicable to almost every person who suffers from malignant tumor. Other aspects of relationships with people affected by cancer have been shown as well.

It is a pity that until now cancer survivors in our country have sometimes felt an unfriendly or hostile attitude toward them. This has had a negative effect on their recovery and has impeded the process of their resocialization. This attitude comes from the low level of education and of awareness of the importance of communication in the general public and the mass media. Specialists are still rather closed in their communication with cancer patients. This "mist" is not good for the overall program of early detection and treatment of cancer, and the rehabilitation of cancer patients. The greater the openness of communication, the better the results with this social problem. There are some projects on public education in oncology, and undoubtedly this will gradually improve the whole situation.

It is well known that improving medical results in cancer patients is not the same thing as improving their quality of life. Certainly it is necessary to continue the search for the causes of cancer and to work toward early diagnosis and effective therapy. But no one can predict when advances in these matters will take place. What we can do now is apply all our knowledge, skill, compassion, and will to be as supportive of cancer patients as possible. Everyone who communicates with cancer patients should help them find their individual, independent self.

Communication in oncology must convince people of the possibility and necessity of being examined when they need it; must explain to them the correct meaning of "malignancy" as determined by current research; and must help cancer patients understand that they are no less worthy as human beings than others, no less deserving of the best possible quality of life.

REFERENCES

1. DEMIN, E. V. & V. A. CHULKOVA. 1992. Possibilities of improvement of quality of life of cancer patient. Probl. Oncol. (Rus.) **38:** 84–89.
2. BECK, L. E. GRUNDMANN & W. SCHNEIDER, Eds. 1985. The Cancer Patient: Illness and Recovery. Gustav Fischer Verlag. Stuttgart.
3. DEWING, W. J. A., K. DUFFY, R. SCIANDRA & S. KARLINS. 1988. What the public wants to know about cancer: The cancer information service. Cancer Bull. **40:** 384–389.
4. SHEVCHENKO, I. T. 1979. Thoughts on oncological deontology. Clin. Surg. (Ukraine) **5:** 34–37.
5. VILLEJO, L., V. FLYNN, S. KLUCHARICH & A. PLUMMER. 1988. Strategies for cancer patient education: Overcoming barriers. Cancer Bull. **40:** 365–369.
6. PETERSON, B. E. 1974. Physician and oncological patient. Probl. Oncol (Rus.) **20:** 118–121.
7. MOHRING, P. 1988. Krebs Leben: Maligne Erkrankungen aus therapeutischer und personlicher Perspektive. Springer-Verlag. Berlin.
8. DORRIS, W. L. & K. F. KENNEDY. 1986. Family involvement in the treatment process: Implications for the health care professionals. Cancer Bull. **38:** 248–250.
9. GOODWIN, J. S., W. C. HUNT, C. R. KEY & J. M. SAMET. 1987. The effect of marital status on stage, treatment, and survival of cancer patients. JAMA **258:** 3125–3130.
10. WIESENTHAL, M. 1984. Reach-to-Recovery program of the American Cancer Society. Cancer (Phila.) **53:** 825–827.

11. LASSER, T. 1953. Reach to Recovery: A Manual for Women Who Have Had Radical Breast Surgery. Reach to Recovery Foundation. New York, NY.
12. TIMOTHY, F. 1980. Back to normal life after breast cancer: The success story of the Reach-to-Recovery Programme. Bull. Cancer **18:** 1–3.
13. DEMIN, E. V. 1994. Reach to recovery: The effective way of psychosocial support in breast cancer (The first experience in Russia). *In* Psychological and Social Issues in Supportive Care: An Update. Abstract No. 7. International Psycho-Oncology Society and Indian Psycho-Oncology Society. New Delhi.

Telling the Truth—Yes? Maybe? No?

Yes!

STEFAN KOREC AND M. ANDRASIOVA

National Cancer Institute
Klenova 1
833 10 Bratislava, Slovakia

COMING OUT OF THE DARK AGES

When recalling the era of shamans and tribal healers, one can not avoid the sensation of a physical barrier between the help-seeking object (the patient) and the healer. The defenseless object with no knowledge of his disease, and even less informed about treatment options, is left at the mercy of the powerful, unknown character who uses obscure methods and often connected to divine forces.

Even today, this cliché is still in patients' subconsciousness at the time of their first contact with their physicians. And this atavistic reaction is unfortunately all too often at play (subconsciously) in the heads of some physicians. The situation has changed dramatically in the last couple of centuries, and in the field of oncology in the last couple of decades. The general knowledge and medical education of the general public have reached an unprecedented level.

The rapid development of medical technology and the pharmaceutical industry, the rapid spread of information, and the need for team work have stripped the healer of special powers and have shed light on obscurity. At the same time, readily available information has given the patient the chance to become an active participant in the treatment process. The environment has changed. It is time for us physicians to transform our minds and act accordingly.

CULTURAL BACKGROUND

Cultural traditions, written and unwritten laws, and customs all form the stage for physician-patient interaction and jointly determine the quality of communication. The closer the society is to the open society model the more the patient-physician relationship resembles a partnership and vice versa. In Slovakia, for instance, until very recently, according to the law physicians were not permitted to tell the patient with cancer the truth about his diagnosis, much less discuss the prognosis. The patient was excluded from the decision-making process. Not very differently from in the dark ages, the ailing individual had to trust his healer blindly. The relatives were informed; often the colleagues at work or the neighbors were informed, too. This practice was accepted by the society and was considered normal, moral, and culturally sanctioned.

Moreover, patients, though frustrated, accepted these rules as part of the game, with only minimal resentment. The first ones to break the tradition were young physicians exposed to the practice of medicine abroad. And surprisingly enough, the first ones to object were the unprepared patients. This point is important and must be remembered for future considerations of changing long-standing, deeply rooted rules. The next opponent to better informing the patient was the generation of almighty, all-knowing physicians. The idea of losing their special powers and status was threatening. And the suggestion of having to involve someone else without any medical education was unacceptable. Similarly, the first reaction of relatives to the notion of a better informed patient was a negative one. Here, the most important argument was the protection of the patient.

The three partners (patient, physician, and relatives) in the countries with a long-standing tradition of open communication and respect for individual rights hold completely different views. The patient as an individual has the right to learn all that is known about his health status. The patient-physician relationship has another meaning as well. The patient is a customer purchasing a service from the physician; the physician, who is to provide it, has to inform the patient as thoroughly as possible—that is the first step. For the physician not to inform the patient to the patient's satisfaction amounts to low-quality service, which will result in loss of business. This is because the patient bases his business and private life plans on the purchased information. The third party, the relatives, are usually informed to the same extent as the patient, but can be completely left out if the patient wishes.

The hierarchy just described, in which it is the patient who is in the driver's seat at the time of crucial decisions, is the reverse of the Central European tradition. The arrangement is considered natural, and all the parties involved feel comfortable with it. Any attempt to restrict the flow of information or change the position of the patient in the decision-making process would be opposed and considered unacceptable by the whole society. A developed society does not accept changes out of step with its cultural orientation.

Quite a different thing happened recently in several Central European countries where the laws have changed drastically. The patient who would not have been told his diagnosis before now, under the new law, has the right to see his medical records whenever he wants. At first the process of easing restrictions had opponents from all three of the involved parties (patient, physician, and relatives); all rejected the changing scenario, mostly because of the fear of the unknown. This opposition was only transitory and, after the first experiences, changed to whole-hearted support. This is further proof that providing the patient with complete information about his diagnosis and prognosis, to the extent he can comprehend it, is fully compatible with human nature.

BUILDING ALLIANCES

Cancer is a chronic disease. Caring for cancer patients means a long-lasting relationship. Effective treatment of the cancer patient requires close cooperation between the patient and his physician. The cooperation is close to impossible without trust and mutual information. An appropriately informed patient can become an ally, a partner assuming part of the responsibility and also assuming part of the "ownership" of the treatment.

Therefore, his tolerance for treatment-related complications or treatment failure is substantially higher. This means not only easier communication and possibly shared responsibility, but, most importantly, improved life for the patient. The same principle of informing the patient to the extent that he can comprehend his disease has to apply to the entire health care team caring for the patient.

PRACTICAL CONSIDERATIONS

What

Telling the truth is an act that initiates a higher-quality relationship between the patient and his physician. Before anything happens the physician should understand that the information he is to give the patient will confront him with several facts: that the disease is serious and may not be curable; that the treatment may not bring the expected effect; that the disease has become part of his life and will change it; and, most importantly, that the time he has left is limited.

Therefore, the physician should be clear in his mind about: the nature of the disease, its expected course, and the general prognosis; whether or not the patient himself wants to know the truth and to what extent; and, very importantly, to what extent is he able to comprehend the truth; the reactivity and emotional stability of the patient.

When

With the progression of the disease the patient is repeatedly confronted with thoughts of incurability. At a certain point he suffers his way through to the truth. If at this point the physician is still trying to keep him under an illusion, it is more painful than well-timed, full information.

How

All too often patients complain about the way they were given crucial information. More than at any time during this important conversation, the patient has to feel an alliance with and the deep involvement of his physician in his particular case. He should have the definite feeling of not being left alone, of being given full support by the physician. We have to remember that it is here that bonds are built or lost. And besides possible loss of the patient's confidence, the physician may run the risk of losing self-confidence, which may in turn result in worsened communication with the patient.

The Psychologist

During the whole process of sharing information, easing its impact on the patient, and building a support system the role of the psychologist is becoming more and more pronounced, though not in all cases and at every visit. It is part of the art of the clinician to recognize the need for and the value of real team work. The less the physician can offer medically, the more he should rely on the help of the psychologist, who should be an inherent part of any oncology team that has the well-being of the patient as its highest priority. We should not let the patient die mentally while he is still alive physically.

To Tell or Not To Tell?

Communication with Cancer Patients

BRANKO ZAKOTNIK

Institute of Oncology
Zaloska 2
61000 Ljubljana, Slovenia

INTRODUCTION

Slovenia is a small new country, a former Yugoslav republic, situated between Italy, Austria, Hungary, and Croatia. More than 90% of the population consists of Slovenes; the main religion is Roman Catholic. About three-quarters of the population lives in small towns.

After cardiovascular events, cancer is the second most common cause of death. We see about 6,000 new cancer cases per year in a population of two million. About half of these patients come to the hospital (Institute of Oncology, Ljubljana) where I have worked for almost 15 years. The other half of the cancer patients are diagnosed and treated (surgery) in regional hospitals. We are the only cancer center in the country.

The perception of reality in the human being is mediated mainly through the cultural environment where the individual has grown up. Culture provides a person with models for understanding and responding to experiences of all sorts.[1] In all human societies there are specific beliefs and practices related to health and illness. In the following lines I would like to point out some observations concerning the influences in our cultural environment on communication with cancer patients.

DOCTOR-PATIENT COMMUNICATION: CANCER DIAGNOSIS

Although some books have been published on cancer in the past years in our country, the average inhabitant is very little informed about cancer from the sources of information that most people are susceptible to, such as television, newspapers, and magazines. The best information one might pick up is, for instance, that a tumor of 5 kg or so was removed from someone; one hears more about alternative than about official treatments. So the patients I see know little about cancer, and even less about the possibilities of treating it. Doctors (nononcologists) are also not educated enough about cancer during their medical studies, and as a consequence it is extremely difficult for them to tell their patients the truth.

They are afraid to hurt the patient, because with their words "You have cancer" they think that they are telling him "You are going to die." From an overview of Slovene medical literature I could find only one paper[2] that deals exclusively with how a doctor should behave with cancer patients. Although the title is "How should a doctor behave with patients with malignant disease," the authors start the paper with a citation[3]: "It is our duty to prolong life, but it is not our duty to prolong the act of dying"; and in the paper they mainly discuss the rights of the dying (= cancer) patient from different points of view. This hopeless equation is anchored deeply in the heads of our people (patients and doctors). In Slovene medical literature there were until only recently few reports about the survival of patients with malignant disease. These are probably the reasons that communication between our doctors and their cancer patients is regarded mainly as communication between doctors and dying patients, while the rest of the story is nonexistent. This leads to such standard situations as the following. A patient with diagnosis of cancer established elsewhere comes to me accompanied by his spouse or relatives, who get to me before the patient and beg me not to tell him that he has cancer. Then the patient comes to me, frightened, not informed about his disease, very suspicious from the way his nearest relatives and doctors have handled him and because he had come through an entrance where he could read "Institute of Oncology." Maybe the logic of this process is just to get the patient to the oncologist so that he will give him the information in the best possible way. I think that the best judge of this is the patient, and most of them say that they would prefer to be informed of what was going on from the beginning. The laws in our country actually take all this into account—the right to be informed, the right to decide who else can be informed, etc. Although the laws exist, I have never heard that a patient went to court because he was not informed that he had cancer. But even for other things regarding their relationship with health personnel, people rarely go to court in our country.

Should we change this situation? I see a lot of arguments that say yes. Only exceptionally have patients not asked me, "Doctor do I have cancer?" Beside the right of the patient to be informed, sincere communication from the start is also a very good basis for better cooperation of the patient in the treatment process, which in oncology at this time is not always very pleasant. If communicated with sincerely, patients tolerate the treatments better, and then even the outcome may be better. Even in cases when we fail with our treatment (too often!) the patients may then cope better with the terminal stage of their illness.

Of course these lines are obsolete for readers in countries where patients come to oncologists with a bag of recently published papers on their disease asking which treatment would be the best. But with us in many cases it is still a matter of to tell or not to tell?

In Western countries the moral issue of whether to tell the truth has shifted from disclosure of diagnosis to disclosure of prognosis.[3,4] In other countries[5] the disclosure of diagnosis still seems to be an issue for debate. Although we know that lack of information can increase uncertainty, anxiety, distress, and dissatisfaction,[6] orthodox medical education (at least in our country) does not equip doctors with the necessary communication skills or give them the opportunity to learn how to deal with their own emotional reactions when giving difficult information. Therefore, every doctor has his own way of communicating with his cancer patients, which is "valid" for the environment where he works. When it comes to the moment of truth, everybody is balancing hope with honest disclosure. *Dum spiramus, speramus!* is very true for every human being.

How do I communicate with my patients? Disclosure of diagnosis: to all patients I treat with specific treatments, and to all others who ask me. Disclosure of prognosis: only recently have data on survival of cancer patients in Slovenia been published;[7] since then I can talk with patients of their prognosis much more easily. Actually, disclosure of diagnosis does not seem easier than the disclosure of prognosis; they are complementary. I tell the patient, "You have cancer." (The patient understands the words as, "You are going to die!") Then I tell him that the prognosis (which is never 0%) is, for example, 50% five-year survival, or I even show him the data in the book that is valid for the Slovene population, and the patient understands, "Yes I have cancer, but I can be cured!" He has hope! Many times patients ask, "Doctor, how many months or weeks do I have left?" I never answer them, because I know how wrong I can be. This scheme of communication varies from patient to patient; it is not a cliché. Its aims are honesty and hope.

PATIENT-DOCTOR COMMUNICATION

Insincerity can exist on both sides of the doctor-patient relationship. Patients do not always tell doctors everything. I do not mean only the relevant facts about their illness, but about other treatments they are undergoing. Often patients take treatments that they think will help them (e.g., diets, drugs), but even more often they visit people who practice alternative medicine. Although alternative medicine is quite popular in our country, patients are embarrassed to admit that they are visiting these voodoo people. Usually they take both the official and the alternative treatments, just in case. Sometimes I am informed about this from their relatives.

There are two kinds of alternative healers. The smart ones do not charge anything (give as much as you want); they are very happy if the patients are treated concomitantly by an oncologist (if they are not, they advise them to do so); they usually drive a BMW or Mercedes. Then there are the orthodox, who deny any treatment except their own and have a fixed price, which is not small for our society (two examples: $8000 for five two-hour manipulations; $2000 for 100 ml of "Onco syrup"). They spend most of the money for "research." This second kind of alternative healer drives me crazy sometimes, but I really cannot do much about it in our circumstances.

Much more information is devoted in the mass media to alternative methods for cancer treatment than to official oncology—perhaps this sells more newspapers. But as the only cancer center in the country, we have not done enough to confront this issue.

PATIENT-PATIENT COMMUNICATION

In a small country like ours, where most patients are treated at one place, people with similar diagnoses meet when they are waiting at the outpatient clinic or in the ward for radiotherapy or chemotherapy. And when people meet, they usually talk, exchanging experiences and information. This communication works very quickly, which I found out some years ago. When I was a fellow, I saw a lot of patients with advanced disease, where only symptomatic treatment was indicated. One woman, on her first visit at our institute, came in crying. She was a retarded women of 40, and she had spent most of her life in closed (psychiatric) institutions. She had stage II breast cancer (it is difficult for me to treat psychiatric patients with cancer, for many reasons: the treatments are often interrupted due to their psychiatric disease; sometimes the patients do not cooperate; their reactions are unpredictable). I asked her why was she crying, and she answered, "Only the worst patients come to you, and I am going to die." Sometimes patients ask me why their treatment was different from the treatment her/his friend is getting. Of course, as a doctor you can make up a reason, but this patient-to-patient communication seems to me another very strong argument for complete sincerity with your patients regarding diagnosis, treatments, randomization, etc.

COMMUNICATION WITH PATIENTS: SPECIFIC TREATMENTS

Standard Treatment

As we are all aware, most patients are not included in clinical trials.[8] These patients get the so-called standard treatment. Usually these standard treatments have acute side effects that are unpleasant for the patient, such as nausea, vomiting, mucositis, alopecia, etc. With better antiemetic therapy alopecia is perhaps the side effect that bothers us and the patients the most in our environment. Of course, all patients are informed about these side effects, but alopecia is usually accepted more readily by the patients than by society (and the treating doctors). My discussions with patients (mainly women) who have had this side effect have indicated that for most of them this was not a great concern: their real concern was always about their disease. Only in rare cases, when the information about alopecia was not given in an understandable manner so the patient was surprised when she lost her hair, was this an important issue. So it is very important that side effects are clearly and thoroughly explained to the patients. Communication between patient and health care personnel is an important aspect of the treatment process.

In talks with friends, colleagues, and neighbors I often hear, "If I had cancer, I would refuse treatment." But in 15 years it has rarely happened to me that a patient refused treatment. Is this inadequate communication?

Experimental Treatment: Clinical Trials

There are numerous papers, books, letters, and newspaper and magazine articles all over the world about experimental treatments in medicine. In our country the words "clinical trial" have a negative implication. No one likes to be an experimental rabbit, as they say in Slovenia; but of course everyone wants to be treated in the best possible way. Nevertheless, we do conduct clinical trials. There are no phase I trials, some phase II trials, and mostly phase III trials (some our own: IBCS, EORTC, etc.) in Slovenia. With clinical trials some problems arise regarding the information given to the patients, the informed consent, etc.

All clinical trials performed at the Institute of Oncology in Ljubljana are presented to the Institutional Ethical Committee. Since 1993 this committee has included members from outside the Institute (lawyer, philosopher, journalist, priest, biologist, nurse, and six medical doctors). Regarding informed consent, the recommendation of the committee is that a written, signed informed consent is needed for phase I and II trials. Somehow it was agreed among members that oral informed consent would be satisfactory for phase III trials; but it became apparent in the last sessions of the committee that a written and signed informed consent will be required here, too.

An interesting debate is going on regarding the information about randomization that should be given to the patient. Some committee members are for the postrandomization concept,[9] while others are for the classical timing, with information being given before randomization. One who conducts clinical trials can imagine how many practical problems this dilemma may present, but I think that local cultural and ethical maturity (here more mature does not necessarily mean better; perhaps the situation is like that with grapes) must be respected. So how does the information process with the patients look in practice. It is impossible to answer questions like this in an exact, scientific way. So I speak only for myself. After I have spoken thoroughly with the patient about his disease, the treatment, and his participating in the trial, most of my patients say, "Doctor, I completely trust you; do whatever you think is best for me." If they are asked, they sign the informed consent, usually without questions. But I, some of my colleagues, and our research nurse have noticed that some of the patients who get more attention because they are included in a clinical trial are not used to it. This is something new in our environment. They begin to complicate matters, report problems that do not exist (now that they know what can happen to them!), and feel unusual because they know so much about their treatment and side effects. This may also be a reason why only a small percent of cancer patients are included in clinical trials. I know that exact, written, signed information is necessary for legal reasons in countries where the legal system functions (hyperfunctions?). But I am not sure what the main goal of these procedures is. Is it to protect the patient or somebody else? Is this the job of a doctor or a lawyer?

COMMUNICATION WITH PATIENTS: SYMPTOMATIC TREATMENT

From data of our cancer registry the five-year relative survival of all cancer patients (skin cancer included) in Slovenia is about 40%.[7] This means that at present about 60% of patients will die from cancer and will need medical and psychological support (communication) in the last months of their life. Euthanasia is not legal and is not practiced in Slovenia. Only in recent years has there been some debate on this issue in the *Slovene Medical Journal*.[10] In this phase of the illness everything must, of course, be done for pain control, but equally important is communication with these patients. Patients who are cared for by their relatives with the help of their general practitioner and nurses are satisfied when I talk with them. Although they do not receive specific treatment, they come to a visit at my outpatient clinic if they can. From my experience this really means a lot to them. When they leave, their biggest concern is, "Has he given me a date for the next visit?" Again we can speak here of hope, which is probably one of the essential feelings of human beings. What would we be without love, hope, and faith? To see these patients is time and energy consuming, especially at the outpatient clinic, where I see an average of 25–30 patients per day. But some are not so lucky to have relatives who take care of them There are no hospices in Slovenia; we have homes for the elderly, which are usually fully occupied.

COMMUNICATION WITH RELATIVES

As I said in the beginning, the relatives of our cancer patients are usually more informed about the disease that the patient. They know the diagnosis before the patient, often also the prognosis (usually the patient lives longer than they were told they would; I see surprises both ways). Although the rights of patients on this issue are very clearly spelled out by our laws, I think that much more time will have to pass before this situation changes. Doctors will still for some time give more detailed information to the relatives than to the patient. Traditionally our people have been protected from the truth if it was not good news, and I think that in a warm family this is what one would expect and be proud of in our country.

EXPENSIVE TREATMENTS AND THEIR IMPACT ON INFORMATION AND TRUTH

It is not my intent to discuss prices, but I want to point out situations that emerge in a country where expensive treatments are not available because of limited resources and technology (for example, very expensive drugs, procedures like bone marrow transplants). People—usually relatives and friends of the patient—hear very quickly about these "miraculous" treatments from newspapers and television, but rarely are our patients treated outside our country (a few per year). If the expenses are covered by an insurance company, a positive opinion from a team of oncologists must be given. If the decision is made that profit from the treatment is not expected, it is very important that the relationship between treating oncologist and patient was sincere and based on truth from the beginning. In such cases patients are treated with whatever is proposed to them. Otherwise the expenses must be paid by the family; if that is not possible, the money is collected from the company where the patient was employed, and relatives. Sometimes—usually when children are involved—public collections are made with the help of mass media.

CONCLUSION

A doctor stands on two legs. One of his legs represents medical knowledge and all the information and intelligence necessary for diagnosis and treatment. The other leg represents the ethical and moral principles he applies through communication with his patients, colleagues, friends, and the society. Both legs must be in optimal condition and are equally important if we want to reach our goal, which is not easy when dealing with cancer patients.

REFERENCES

1. DONNELLY, E. 1995. Culture and the meaning of cancer. Semin. Oncol. Nursing **11**(1): 3–8.
2. DOLENC, A. & J. BALAZIC. 1990. Zdravnikovo ravnanje in dolznosti pri bolnikih z maligno boleznijo. Med. Razgledi **29**(Suppl. 3): 15–24.
3. JENSEN, P. J. 1968. Criteria of Brain Death: 91–105. Munksgaard. Copenhagen.
4. KODISH, E. & S. G. POST. 1995. Oncology and hope. J. Clin. Oncol. **13**(7): 1817–1822.
5. VERONESI, A., C. BUSATO, M. A. ANNUNZIATA, M. D. MAGRI, S. FOLADORE, M. ZANO, S. TUMOLO & S. MONFARDINI. 1995. Prospective analysis of the information level of Italian cancer patients. Eur. J. Cancer **31A**(3): 425–426.
6. FALLOWFIELD, L., S. FORD & S. LEWIS. 1994. Information preferences of patients with cancer. The Lancet **344:** 1576.
7. POMPE-KIRN, V., B. ZAKOTNIK, N. VOLK, T. BENULIC & J. SKRK. 1995. Cancer Patients' Survival in Slovenia. The Institute of Oncology. Ljubljana.
8. MARTIN, J. F., W. G. HENDERSON & L. R. ZACHARSKI. 1984. Accrual of patients into a multihospital cancer clinical trial and its implications on planning future studies. Am. J. Clin. Oncol. **7:** 173–182.
9. ZELEN, M. 1979. A new design for randomized clinical trials. N. Engl. J. Med. **300:** 1242–1245.
10. DRINOVEC, J., M. CEVC & Z. FRAS. 1995. Oregon initiative—the liberation, agreement and action. Zdrav. Vestn. **64**(3): 133–193

Informing Cancer Patients: Whose Truth Matters?

MARZIO E. E. SABBIONI

Medical Division
C. L. Lory-Haus
Inselspital
3010 Bern, Switzerland

Mr. M. suffers from cancer and has been informed of the diagnosis, prognosis, and treatment options. He has been offered the opportunity to discuss these issues in the presence of his wife. He does not want us to speak with his wife, preferring to tell her himself. Months later, the wife and the patient tell us that she had been aware of the diagnosis but that they had spent many weeks in silence, neither knowing whether the other knew.

Mrs. S., a gypsy queen, was hospitalized, and her disease was progressive. She seemed not to be aware of the diagnosis and poor prognosis. A member of the tribe was always in her room; she was never left alone. Thus, the tribe knew of our attempts to understand what information the patient had about her situation and whether she wanted to know more. The husband and leader of the tribe requested a private appointment with us and explained to us that the tribe would not tolerate our giving bad news to Mrs. S. If we insisted on informing the patient, they would have her removed from the hospital, so that she could be treated by the rules of the tribe.

These cases are neither unique nor, scientifically speaking, particularly interesting. Every physician experiences such situations. However, they do reflect some of the difficulties that arise in dealing with sick people who are looking for medical help. Physicians see patients who have a personal story to tell in their specific sociocultural context. On the other hand, physicians have been trained to use scientific methods in understanding and treating health problems in their specific sociocultural health system. As the cases illustrate, there may be a number of factors contradictory to everyday practice. Migration, social mobility, social welfare have reduced the sociocultural parallels between patient and doctor. This is why, since implicit rules of behavior for physicians and patients do not seem to work any more, it is not surprising that physicians and society in general are struggling to find explicit ones.

In the following paragraphs I attempt to analyze, from a clinical point of view, some of the sociocultural factors influencing patient information and patient-doctor interaction. In a second part I will address some common difficulties in patient information and shared decision making. I have trained as an internist and in psychotherapy. Our medical department works according to a biopsychosocial model of medicine.[1] We offer rehabilitation, treatment of psychosomatic disorders and palliative care for in- and outpatients, and a consultation service for a 1000-bed teaching hospital.

In many Western industrial countries there has been a notable change in the manner of informing cancer patients on the nature of their disease and their prognosis. Although the doctrine of "informed consent" governs the way information must be given in these countries, the question has shifted from "whether to tell" to "how to tell."[2,3] However, this major change has taken place only with people suffering from cancer, not from other diseases.[4] In Great Britain in 1969, 29% of persons suffering from terminal cancer knew their diagnosis; 16% knew certainly and 21% probably that they were likely to die. In 1987, 73% knew their diagnosis, 44% knew certainly and 20% knew probably that they were likely to die of their disease. In contrast, in 1969 57% of persons dying from causes other than cancer knew their diagnosis, 18% knew certainly and 20% probably that they were likely to die. In 1987, the situation was unchanged, 60% knew their diagnosis, 22% knew certainly and 20% probably that they were likely to die. Another interesting finding is that, whether the person who died was informed or not, most relatives felt that information had been handled in the best manner. Of those people who were said to know they were dying, respondents (relatives, friends, or doctors) in only 11% of the cases thought it would have been better not to know, 60% felt that knowing had been best. Of those who were said not to know they were dying, respondents in only 3% of the cases felt it would have been better for the person to have known; 79% found that not knowing had been best. The results may be biased by the method of collection. The dying person's relatives, friends, and doctors were asked, by not the dying person him-/herself. As expected, information was provided mostly by the general practitioner and hospital doctor, whereas support was given by relatives.[4] The attitude towards cancer continues to differ from that towards other similarly critical diseases. The changes in information practice are probably due in part to the recruitment of a greater number of cancer patients in clinical studies with higher information requirements. Furthermore, educational efforts on the part of oncologists in improving patient information have induced a change especially in younger physicians.[4] Does this change also indicate that it is easier today for cancer patients to talk about their illness?

In a recent study differences were found in the attitudes of elderly subjects from different ethnic groups in Los Angeles County toward disclosure of the diagnosis and prognosis of a terminal illness. Korean Americans and Mexican Americans were less likely than African

Americans and European Americans to believe that a patient should be informed of a metastatic cancer diagnosis or a terminal prognosis. However, they were more likely to favor a family-centered model of medical decision making rather than the patient autonomy model.[5]

In an international survey of physicians' attitudes and practices with regard to revealing a cancer diagnosis, a high percentage of disclosure was estimated for the northern part of Europe, including Switzerland. A low percentage of disclosure was estimated for the Mediterranean countries.[6] The practice of informing patients in Switzerland has evolved over the last 20 years towards telling the truth and involving patients in decision making.[7] However, there is no data available to analyze this process or to help understand possible sociocultural differences—e.g., between the German-speaking part of the country and the French- or Italian-speaking part, or between rural and urban parts of Switzerland.

The situation is different in Mediterranean European countries. In a recent study in Spain, 68% of terminal cancer patients had not been informed of the diagnosis.[8] However, of the noninformed, 42% did not want more information, whereas 30% wanted it. In another study in Spain, 15% of 167 cancer patients were correctly informed of their diagnosis.[9] In the same hospital, 71% of 380 health workers would want to know their own diagnosis if they had cancer. However, only 19% would want a cancer diagnosis revealed to their relatives.[9]

In Italy, only 38 of 100 patients with incurable advanced cancer knew their diagnosis.[10] Sixty-eight patients said that they were satisfied with the information given. However, 83 patients stated that they wanted to know the truth about their health situation. In another study in Italy, 47% of breast cancer patients reported having been told of their cancer.[11] In these countries patient information on diagnosis and treatment options follows other rules.[12] The patient-doctor relationship can be described as paternalistic, and patient information and participation in decisions follow the patient-assent model. However, these countries seem to be progressing towards the model of informed consent.[13]

Due to increased mobility and migration, it becomes more and more likely that patients and physicians from different sociocultural backgrounds may meet, thus increasing the basic problems in patient-doctor interaction. Patients view their ill health in terms of "illness," physicians describe it in terms of "disease." The physician's perspective is based on scientific rationality, with the emphasis on objective measurement and physicochemical data. "Diseases" are viewed as entities, using a reductionistic approach based on a mind-body dualism, with the emphasis on the individual patient rather than on the family or community. The patient's perspective is based upon his experience of ill health and the meaning he gives to that experience.[14] For example, the patient may ask the following questions: What has happened? Why has it happened? Why has it happened to me? Why now? What would happen to me if nothing were done about it? What are the likely effects on other people (family, friends employers, workmates) if nothing were done about it? What should I do about it? To whom should I turn for further help?[14] Lay theories on the causes of illness play an important role in helping patients make sense of what has happened to them. These lay theories may often be scientifically incorrect, but they have internal logic and consistency and are socioculturally determined.[14]

Physicians must present their information in probabilistic terms and expect their patient to understand the meaning of probability. However, it is difficult even for a physician to make decisions based on probability.[15] Common errors, apart from a lack of knowledge in decision and probability theory, have been described, such as thinking in terms of magic or morality, and biased considerations.[15] From the subjective perspective of the individual patient, probabilistic information makes little sense. The patient usually has only two possibilities: either cure or progression, either life or death. The patient cannot be 30% cured or 30% alive.

Information has to be tailored to the specific patient and can be effective only within a workable patient-doctor relationship. Physicians require communicative skills in order to assess the "illness" perspective of the patient. Information and decisions are two-way processes and not discrete events. From a clinical point of view, information must be helpful and not merely a legal medical requirement. A process of shared decision making seems to better fit these requirements than a single instance of informed consent.[16] First, patient and doctor must determine the focus of treatment. Second, they must agree upon treatment goals. Third, they have to choose ways to achieve them. Clinical experience teaches us that these steps cannot all be taken at the same time and that they must be continuously updated.[17]

In patients suffering from hypertension, physicians seem to underestimate the patients' desire for information but to overestimate their desire to make decisions.[18] Cancer patients, too, seem to have a greater desire for information than for making decisions. Sixty-three percent of patients felt the physician should take the primary responsibility in decision making, 27% felt it should be an equally shared process, and 10% felt they themselves should play a major role.[19] Patient satisfaction with information seems to be relatively high as it is.[4] However, informed patients seem to have a higher degree of satisfaction, with the highest being found in patients who agree with their physician on the information conveyed.[11]

The disclosure of a cancer diagnosis is a major stressor.[20] Therefore, the aim in informing cancer patients must be not merely to include them in decision making, but also to provide the necessary help in coping with this event. Social support has been recognized as one of the most important helps to a cancer patient.[21] Personal coping resources must be sustained.[22] Family members and other significant persons are most likely to provide social support.[4] However, they are often excluded from doctor-patient interaction in Western industrial countries. Some oncological services include a psychooncological service or offer other support, such as self-help groups, in order to help patients and their families cope with their disease.

Principles of medical ethics such as "beneficence," "autonomy," and "justice" are discussed elsewhere in this book.[23] The basic requirements for informed consent are "competence" (of the patient), "adequate information," "voluntariness."[16] As mentioned earlier, a model of shared decision making fits clinical reality better than an event model of informed consent. However, it is impossible to inform patients without communicative skills. Unfortunately, these are not taught in most medical schools. It is imperative to provide the clinician with adequate training and supervision in communication.[24–26]

Let us consider again the examples at the beginning of this chapter. What communicative skills could have improved the care of the patients? In both examples it would have been helpful to consider the patient not only as an individual but also as part of a social system (partnership, family, or tribe) and to better integrate these aspects into patient care. We should have tried to understand with the patient the importance and role of his social system. We should have looked for adequate means to allow his social system to provide social support.

A biopsychosocial model of medicine[1] that considers the individual reality of each patient and his family, together with specific communication skills, is a basic requirement for discussing treatment options, decisions, or ethical conflicts with the patient. In patient-doctor interaction ethical conflicts can arise from communication failure. An ethical approach in clinical practice must be based on improving the clinicians' communication skills and their awareness of sociocultural factors.

REFERENCES

1. ENGEL, G. L. 1977. The need for a new medical model: A challenge for biomedicine. Science **196:** 129–136.
2. NOVACK, D. H., R. PLUMMER, R. L. SMITH, H. OCHITILL, G. R. MORROW & J. M. BENNETT. 1979. Changes in physicians' attitudes toward telling the cancer patient. JAMA **241:** 897–900.
3. OKEN, D. 1961. What to tell cancer patients: A study of medical attitudes. JAMA **175:** 1120–1128.
4. SEALE, C. 1991. Communication and awareness about death: A study of a random sample of dying people. Soc. Sci. Med. **32**(8): 943–952.
5. BLACKHALL, L. J., S. T. MURPHY, G. FRANK, V. MICHEL & S. AZEN. 1995. Ethnicity and attitudes toward patient autonomy. JAMA **274:** 820–825.
6. HOLLAND, J. C., N. GEARY, A. MARCHINI & S. TROSS. 1987. An international survey of physician attitudes and practice in regard to revealing the diagnosis of cancer. Cancer Invest. **5**(2): 151–154.
7. SENN, H. J. & A. GLAUS. 1991. Wahrhaftigkeit am Krankenbett—auch bei Tumorpatienten? Schweiz. Rundsch. Med. Prax. **80**(9): 200–205.

8. CENTEÑO-CORTES, C. & J. M. NUÑEZ-OLARTE. 1994. Questioning diagnosis disclosure in terminal cancer patients. A prospective study evaluating patients' responses. Palliative Med. **8:** 39–44.
9. ESTAPE, J., H. PALOMBO, E. HERNANDEZ, M. DANIELS, T. ESTAPE, J. J. GRAU, N. VINOLAS & J. M. MANE. 1992. Cancer diagnosis disclosure in a Spanish hospital. Ann. Oncol. **3:** 451–454.
10. PRONZATO, P., G. BERTELLI, P. LOSARDO & M. LANDUCCI. 1994. What do advanced cancer patients know of their disease? Support Care Cancer **2:** 242–244.
11. MOSCONI, P., B. E. MEYEROWITZ, M. C. LIBERATI & A. LIBERATI. 1991. Disclosure of breast cancer diagnosis: Patients and physician reports. Ann. Oncol. **2:** 273–280.
12. SURBONE, A. 1993. The information of the cancer patient: Psychosocial and spiritual implications. Support Care Cancer **1:** 89–91.
13. SABBIONI, M. E. E. 1991. Speech is silver, silence is gold? Ann. Oncol. **2:** 244.
14. HELMAN, C. G. 1994. Culture, Health and Illness. 3d edit. Butterworth-Heinemann. Oxford.
15. GILLICK, M. R. 1988. Talking with patients about risk. J. Gen. Intern. Med. **3:** 166–170.
16. ARNOLD, R., L. FORROW & L. R. BARKER. 1995. Medical ethics and doctor/patient communication. *In* The medical Interview. M. Lipkin, S. M. Putnam & A. Lazare, Eds.: 345–367. Springer-Verlag. New York, NY.
17. APPELBAUM, P. S., C. W. LIDZ & A. MEISEL. 1987. Informed Consent: Legal Theory and Clinical Practice. Oxford University Press. New York, NY.
18. STRULL, W. M., B. LO & G. CHARLES. 1984. Do patients want to participate in medical decision making? JAMA **252:** 2990–2994.
19. SUTHERLAND, H. J., H. A. LLEWELLYN-THOMAS, G. A. LOCKWOOD, D. L. TRITCHLER & J. E. TILL. 1989. Cancer patients: Their desire for information and participation in treatment decisions. J. R. Soc. Med. **82**(5): 260–263.
20. JACOBSEN, P. B. & J. C. HOLLAND. 1991. The stress of cancer: Psychological responses to diagnosis and treatment. *In* Cancer and Stress: Psychological, Biological and Coping Studies. C. L. Cooper & M. Watson, Eds.: 147–171. John Wiley & Sons. Chichester.
21. BLOOM, J. R., S. H. KANG & P. ROMANO. 1991. Cancer and Stress: The effect of social support as a resource. *In* Cancer and Stress: Psychological, Biological and Coping Studies. C. L. Cooper & M. Watson, Eds.: 95–124. John Wiley & Sons. Chichester.
22. HEIM, E. 1991. Coping and adaptation in cancer. *In* Cancer and Stress: Psychological, Biological and Coping Studies. C. L. Cooper & M. Watson, Eds.: 197–237. John Wiley & Sons. Chichester.
23. SURBONE, A. 1996. Information, truth, and communication: For an interpretation of truth-telling practices throughout the world. Ann. N.Y. Acad. Sci. This volume.
24. ZITTOUN, R. 1990. Patient information and participation. *In* Psychosocial Aspects of Oncology. J. C. Holland & R. Zittoun, Eds.: 27–44. Springer-Verlag. Berlin.
25. HÜRNY, C. 1990. Patient information: Practical guidelines. *In* Psychosocial Aspects of Oncology. J. C. Holland & R. Zittoun, Eds.: 45–47. Springer-Verlag. Berlin.
26. ADLER, R. & W. HEMMELER. 1992. Anamnese und Körperuntersuchung. 3. Auflage. Gustav Fischer Verlag. Stuttgart.

Communication with Cancer Patients

The Influence of Age, Gender, Education, and Health Insurance Status

MEHMET ŞEN[a]

Department of Radiation Oncology
Dokuz Eylül University Medical School
İnciraltı-İzmir, Turkey 35340

INTRODUCTION

Effective and clear communication is essential to the physician-patient relationship.[1] It is particularly important in the care of cancer patients because of their wish to be informed and involved in medical decision making[2–4] and the legal requirements now in place for informed consent for recommended investigatory procedures and treatments. A diagnosis of cancer goes against common sense and often evokes emotions that can be difficult to deal with. Interactions between cancer patients and their doctors generally concern issues of vital importance to the patient which may be emotionally charged and can lead to psychiatric disturbance in a certain proportion of patients.[5,6] The possible costs of poor communication include increased anxiety, distress, coping difficulties,[7] noncompliance with treatment,[8] loss of confidence in medical staff, and dissatisfaction with medical care.

The object of doctor-patient communication is to relate correct and useful information to the patient in a way in which patient recollection will be accurate and consistent. Improvement of this communication process, particularly within the cultural context of the patient population, requires a degree of sensitivity concerning the various communication styles of physicians, and the various coping styles of patients. A hypothetical model of this issue, and various methods of improving communication, are published in the literature.[9,10]

The information and statistics presented in this study were gathered in İzmir, Turkey from questionnaires administered to Turkish cancer patients. While there are great differences between the Turkish patient population and the European patient population in terms of culture and religion, mass communication media appear to have "leveled the playing

[a]Present address: Christie Hospital, Department of Clinical Radiology, Wilmslow Road, Manchester M20 9BX, England.

field" in terms of general awareness of the disease. However, in Turkey the general ability to squarely face the prognosis in severe cases is very limited when compared to that of the patient population in Europe.

Despite increasing recognition of the need for effective doctor-patient communication, there are still big differences in communication with cancer patients. In the Western world there is no argument regarding disclosure of diagnosis and the possible treatment strategies, but there is still a debate regarding disclosure of the prognosis. Ninety percent of all United States physicians reveal a diagnosis of cancer to their patients.[11] But in many countries nondisclosure is still common.[12] In Turkey, as in some European and many Middle Eastern countries, the public regards the diagnosis of cancer as a death sentence. In such situations physicians are reluctant to pronounce the diagnosis, and even more reluctant to reveal the exact prognosis to the patient directly. Written informed consent for recommended investigatory procedures and treatments is not a routine procedure throughout the country. Experienced oncologists realize that most of their patients know their diagnosis, even if it is not discussed openly between patient and physician. Through increasing availability of information on cancer in the media, even patients with minimal general education have become aware of many facts about the disease. A high percentage of patients now know that if, after a certain surgical intervention, their physicians advise "electrical polishing" or limited dosages of slightly toxic drugs so that "the disease should not recur," this actually means that they are undergoing radiotherapy or chemotherapy. Of 45 cancer patients investigated in the chemotherapy day clinic in İstanbul, no significant differences were found between groups of different educational levels in awareness of disease or in patient satisfaction with the available medical services. High educational level patients had significantly different patient-physician dialogue: these more educated patients asked significantly more questions, and more pointed questions, which resulted in a better communicative relationship between the patient and physician.[13]

In this study the percentage of patients who were given information about diagnosis, the degree of accuracy of their recollection of this information, information about treatment methods and results, the patients' role in therapeutic decision making, satisfaction of the patients with the given information, and patients' expectations of their physicians were assessed by a questionnaire. The influence of age, education, gender, and health insurance status on these parameters was analyzed.

SUBJECTS AND METHODS

The subjects included 120 cancer patients receiving treatment at the radiation oncology department of Dokuz Eylül University in İzmir,

TABLE 1. İzmir Questionnaire for Assessment of Influence of Age, Gender, Education, and Health Insurance Status on Communication with Cancer Patients

Age:		
Gender:		
Education:		
Health insurance status:		
1) Have you been informed about your diagnosis?		
	Yes	No
2) Your diagnosis:		
3) Have you been informed about treatment methods and results?		
	Yes	No
4) Have you played a role in choosing your treatment?		
	Yes	No
5) Have you been satisfied with the given information about your diagnosis and treatments?		
	Yes	No
6) What would you request from your physician?		

Turkey. They were given a questionnaire as in TABLE 1. Of the 120 questionnaires distributed, 108 were returned, and an assessment was done by the author. TABLE 2 shows the demographic and disease characteristics of the subjects.

RESULTS

Ninety-six of 108 (88%) patients were informed about their diagnosis; 89 of 108 (83%) were informed about treatment methods and results; 53 of 108 (49%) played a role in the making the therapeutic decision; 68 of 108 (63%) were satisfied with the given information; 43 of 108 (40%) requested more information from their physician. TABLES 3–8 show comparisons of age, education, gender, and health insurance status on these parameters.

High-educational level patients and females were informed more often than patients of low educational levels and males ($p < 0.05$). Age and expense coverage status were found to be of no influence on the patients' perception with regard to physician-provided diagnosis information (TABLE 3).

Females were more aware of their exact diagnosis than males ($p < 0.05$). Age, education level, and expense coverage status were not found to be significant (TABLE 4).

Females were more accurately informed about their treatment methods and results than males ($p < 0.05$). Age, education level, and expense coverage status were not found to be significant (TABLE 5). The accuracy of this information is a result of several factors, including physician-pro-

TABLE 2. Demographic and Disease Characteristics of Subjects (n = 108)

	Number	Percentage
Gender		
Male	52	48
Female	56	52
Education level		
Elementary	78	72
Higher	30	28
Health insurance status		
With	90	83
Without	18	17
Age		
< 50 years	54	50
> 50 years	54	50
Type of cancer		
Lung	28	26
Gynecological	10	9
Breast	22	20
Head and neck	35	32
CNS	7	7
Lymphoma	4	4
Genitourinary	2	2

vided information, intuition, and information from other sources. Further study will be needed to quantify more carefully the effects of each of these sources.

Younger patients (age < 50 years) played more of a role in their therapeutic decision-making process than did elderly patients ($p < 0.05$). Patients who cover their own health expenses also played a greater role in the therapeutic decision-making process. Age and education level have no influence on this parameter (TABLE 6).

The patients who were most satisfied with the diagnostic and treatment information they were provided were patients who covered their own health expenses ($p < 0.05$). There was no satisfaction difference among the other parameters (TABLE 7). It should be explained that in Turkey there is no private health insurance program. Almost all of the population has governmental health coverage. This system is used almost exclusively by people of limited economic means, but it offers little opportunity for patient choices. Patients of greater economic means often opt to pay for their own medical treatment, which allows maximum freedom to explore alternative options.

It can be seen in TABLE 8 that females' expectations were for more information to be provided, while males' expectations were for more care to be provided ($p < 0.05$).

TABLE 3. Percentage of Patients Who Were Informed of Their Diagnosis According to the Variables under Study

Variable	% Informed	% Not Informed	χ^2
Age			
< 50	85	15	1.43
≥50	75	25	
Education			
Elementary	73	27	6.05[a]
Higher	96	4	
Gender			
Male	62	38	18.14[b]
Female	96	4	
Expense			
With insurance	77	23	1.93
Without insurance	94	6	

[a] $p = 0.0139074$.

[b] $p = 0.0000205$.

TABLE 4. Percentage of Degree of Patient Awareness of Diagnosis According to the Variables under Study

Variable	% with Suspicion	% with Certainty	χ^2
Age			
<50	30	70	1.27
≥50	19	81	
Education			
Elementary	28	72	1.87
Higher	13	87	
Gender			
Male	38	62	9.89[a]
Female	11	89	
Expense coverage			
With insurance	27	73	1.23
Without insurance	11	88	

[a] $p = 0.0016620$.

TABLE 5. Percentage of Patients Informed about Treatment Methods and Results According to the Variables under Study

Variable	% Informed	% Not informed	χ^2
Age			
< 50	89	11	2.30
≥50	76	24	
Education			
Elementary	83	17	0.02
Higher	80	20	
Gender			
Male	69	31	10.32[a]
Female	95	5	
Expense coverage			
With insurance	81	19	0.20
Without insurance	89	11	

[a]$p = 0.0013150$.

DISCUSSION

Though it is not a routine procedure to pronounce the exact diagnosis to the patients in Turkey, the results of this study showed that at this institution 88% of the patients were informed about their diagnosis; this level compares favorably with the levels to be expected in Western Europe and the United States. In another study done in the same town 67% of patients who were referred from a radiation oncology treatment to psychiatric treatment were aware of their diagnosis, and 46% of these used the word "cancer." An additional 17% of these patients used similar words such as "bad illness, tumor," etc.; and the rest of the group used neither "cancer" nor any similar word. However, in the control group of this same (those not referred for psychiatric treatment) study the percentage of patients knowing their diagnosis was very low (23%).[14] We have no data to draw conclusions regarding the necessity for psychiatric treatment of the patients in our study who were informed of their condition. This very interesting relationship to a previous study will be a subject of future investigation. In our study, however, highly educated patients and females were given more information than others ($p < 0.05$). In our study the fact that females tended to be more informed might be due to the fact that their disease (e.g., breast and genitourinary cancers) results in a high percentage of body-altering surgery, and is by its very nature more difficult to avoid recognizing. In another study of patients with breast cancer the patient-related characteristics of age, education, and stage of disease

TABLE 6. Percentage of Patients Who Played a Role in Decision Making on Their Therapy

Variable	% with Role	% with No Role	χ^2
Age			
<50	61.1	38.8	
			5.34[a]
≥50	37.0	62.9	
Education			
Elementary	51.2	48.7	
			0.28
Higher	43.3	56.6	
Gender			
Male	51.9	48.0	
			0.14
Female	46.4	53.5	
Expense coverage			
With insurance	44.4	55.5	3.59
Without insurance	72.2	27.7	

[a] $p = 0.0208994$.

were independent predictors of accuracy of information.[15]

In our study 80% of patients correctly identified their diagnosis. Females were more often accurate in their awareness of the diagnosis than males ($p < 0.05$). In Mackillop's study 98% of patients recognized that they had cancer, and 87% correctly identified the tumor type. Local and regional disease patients were also aware of this, but one-third of the patients with metastatic disease incorrectly believed that the cancer was localized.[16] This indicates that the accuracy of information concerning the status of the disease tends to deteriorate as the disease progresses.

Females were given more information about treatment methods and results ($p < 0.05$). This is likely due to the nature of their disease as innumerated above; and mostly the aim of the treatment was curative.

Published studies indicate that it is the wish of most cancer patients to be informed and involved in medical decision making concerning their disease.[2–4]

In our study younger patients and patients who covered their own health expenses played a greater role in their therapeutic decisions. Young early-diagnosed patients wanted to keep their body image as intact as possible, and patients who covered their own medical expenses sought medical advice that agreed with their own desires to limit the invasiveness of recommended procedures. Patients who desired an active role in treatment decision making also desired detailed information.[17]

Two-thirds of the patients in our study were satisfied with the information provided, and overall satisfaction levels were generally high. The

TABLE 7. Percentage of Patients Who Were Satisfied with the Information Provided According to the Variables under Study

Variable	% Satisfied	% Dissatisfied	χ^2
Age			
<50	59.2	40.7	0.36
≥50	66.6	33.3	
Education			
Elementary	61.5	38.4	0.07
Higher	66.6	33.3	
Gender			
Male	61.5	38.4	0.01
Female	64.2	35.7	
Expense coverage			
With insurance	57.7	42.2	4.96[a]
Without insurance	88.8	11.1	

[a]$p = 0.0258917$.

patients most satisfied with the information provided were patients who covered their own health expenses, as indicated earlier ($p < 0.05$). In Brooks's study, on the other hand, factual knowledge about cancer was greater among patients who were less satisfied with communication. Patients reporting the highest level of satisfaction with the information provided tended to want to avoid the harsh truth of their condition, and, at the same time tended to be less anxious about their prognosis.[18] General satisfaction also depended not just upon communication with physicians, but also upon communication with other staff members in the department.[19]

As mentioned earlier female expectations were for more information to be provided, while male expectations were for more care to be provided ($p < 0.05$). Males in this study mostly had inoperable and incurable disease. The prognosis of their disease generally was not provided to them because their health condition offered little hope of improvement, and they generally were not interested in learning the prognosis. Their interests generally centered on treatment that resulted in greater comfort levels.

While these findings should be interpreted cautiously, the results of this study done in the radiation oncology department of Dokuz Eylül University give some indications as to the expectations of cancer patients in their communication with their physicians.

The problems associated with physician-patient education on the subject of cancer are greatly aided by printed information of a specific nature

TABLE 8. Percentage of Patients' Expectations from Their Physicians According to the Variables under Study

Variable	% More Information	% More Care	χ^2
Age			
<50	48	52	2.47
≥50	31	69	
Education			
Elementary	35	65	2.43
Higher	53	47	
Gender			
Male	27	73.0	5.96[a]
Female	51.7	48.2	
Expense coverage			
With insurance	41.1	58.8	0.12
Without insurance	33.3	66.6	

[a] $p = 0.0146621$.

on the subject of the various forms of this disease. Unfortunately these materials are not readily available, and it is hoped that this situation will improve.

It should be pointed out that the oncology department at Dokuz Eylül University has made a concerted effort to increase the level of physician-patient communication about diagnosis and prognosis, and this effort is reflected in this high percentage. The staff at Dokuz Eylül University is largely European trained, and this certainly has influenced this effort, but very likely does not represent a general trend in the Turkish medical population.

The larger and more far-reaching question, however, is to define the situations within which more information is useful to the patient, and those within which more information is, indeed, to the patient's detriment. Some data explored in this chapter indicate that for some patients forcing acceptance of the reality of their disease results only in a deterioration of the quality of life for their remaining time. In other circumstances, and with other patients, more information is an absolute necessity. Some indications are that if the disease is treatable, and if the prognosis offers hope for remission or recovery, more information is useful. If, on the other hand, as shown in male lung cancer patients in our study, the prognosis offers essentially no hope, indications are, at least in the Turkish environment, that the patient would prefer to avoid confrontation with this harsh reality. How this interplays with the legal requirements for disclosure and informed consent for diagnostic procedures and treatment is a very complicated issue, and beyond the scope of this chapter; but it should certainly be addressed in detail at some point. Further, how this set of data influences the overall physician-patient communication process also requires considerably more research, both in Turkey and in other cultural contexts.

ACKNOWLEDGMENTS

I wish to thank Professor Gazanfer Aksakoğlu and Dr. Özlem Ataman Uruk for their kind help in the statistical analysis of this data; and all members of the Department for their great effort to improve communication with cancer patients. Also I wish to thank Dr. John Logue for his review and Mr. James Rimer for his kind assistance in straightening out the prose of this chapter.

REFERENCES

1. MORROW, G. R., A. C. HOAGLAND & P. J. CARPENTER. 1983. Improving physician-patient communications in cancer treatment. Psychosoc. Oncol. **1**(2): 93–101.
2. CASSILETH, B. R., R. V. ZUPKIS, K. SUTTON-SMITH & V. MARCH. 1980. Information and participation preferences among cancer patients. Ann. Intern. Med. **92:** 832–936.
3. SUTHERLAND, H. J., H. A. LLEWELLYN-THOMAS, O. LOCKWOOD, D. L. TRITCHLER & J. E. TILL. 1989. Cancer patients: Their desire for information and participation in treatment decisions. R. Soc. Med. **82:** 260–263.
4. TATTERSALL, M. H. N., P. N. BUTOW, A-M. GRIFFIN & S. DUNN. 1994. The take home message after a cancer consultation: Randomized trial of consultation audiotapes and individualized letters to patients. J. Clin. Oncol. **12:** 1305–1311.
5. CHIATCHIK, S., S. KREITLER, S. SHAKED, I. SCHWARTZ & R. ROSSIN. 1992. Doctor-patient communication in a cancer ward. J. Cancer Educ. **7:** 41–54.
6. DEROGATIS, L. R., G. R. MORROW, J. FETTING, D. PENMAN, S. PIASETSKY, A. M. SCHMALE, M. HENRICHS & C. L. CARNICKE. 1983. The prevalence of psychiatric disorders among cancer patients. JAMA **249**(6): 751–757.
7. COHEN, F. & R. S. LAZARUS. 1979. Coping with the stress of illness. *In* Health Psychology. G. C. Stone, F. Cohen & N. E. Adler, Eds.: 217–254. Jossey-Bass. San Francisco, CA.
8. CARTWRIGHT, A. 1964. Human Relations and Hospital Care. Routledge and Kegan Paul. London.
9. HUMPHREY, G. B., J. L. LITTLEWOOD & W. A. KAMPS. 1992. Physician-patient communication: A model considering the interaction physicians therapeutic strategy and patients' coping style. J. Cancer Educ. **7**(2): 147–152.
10. DAMIAN, D. & M. H. N. TATTERSALL. 1991. Letters to patients: Improving communication in cancer care. Lancet **338:** 923–926.
11. NOVACK, D. H., R. PLUMER, R. SMITH *et al.* 1979. Changes in physicians' attitudes toward telling the cancer patient. JAMA **241:** 897–900.
12. HOLLAND, J. C., N. GEARY, A. MARCHINI *et al.* 1987. An international survey of

physician attitudes and practice in regard to revealing the diagnosis of cancer. Cancer Invest. **5**(2): 151–154.
13. DERMAN, U. & P. SERBEST. 1993. Cancer patients' awareness of disease and satisfaction with services: The influence of their general education level. J. Cancer Educ. **8**(2): 141–144.
14. ELB, H. & A. HAYDAROĞLU. 1992. The recognition of psychiatric morbidity and risk groups on radiation oncology department. Ann. Oncol. **3**(Suppl. 5): 178.
15. 1986. What doctors tell patients with breast cancer about diagnosis and treatment. Br. J. Cancer **54**(2): 319–326.
16. MACKILLOP, W. J., W. E. STEWART, A. D. GINSBURG & S. S. STEWART. 1988. Cancer patients' perceptions of their disease and its treatment. Br. J. Cancer **58**(3): 355–359.
17. HACK, T. F., D. F. LESLEY & G. D. DENNIS. 1994. Relationship between preferences for decisional control and illness information among women with breast cancer: A quantitative and qualitative analysis. Soc. Sci. Med. **39**(2): 279–289.
18. STEPTOE, A., I. SUTCLIFFE, B. ALLEN & C. COOMBES. 1991. Satisfaction with communication, medical knowledge, and coping style in patients with metastatic cancer. Soc. Sci. Med. **32**(6): 627–632.
19. BROOKS, C. 1989. Idealism and realism in patient care during radiotherapy treatment. Radiogr. Today **55**(627): 16–21.

Truth Sometimes Hurts but Deceit Hurts More

LESLEY FALLOWFIELD

CRC Communication & Counselling Research Centre
Department of Oncology
University College London Medical School
London W1P 7PL, United Kingdom

What tormented Ivan Ilyich most was the pretense, the lie—which for some reason they all kept up . . . that he was merely ill and not dying, and that he only need stay quiet and carry out the doctor's orders and then some great change for the better would result.

—TOLSTOY

INTRODUCTION

Many doctors unwittingly hurt their patients by trying to protect them from the truth. This situation usually occurs because of a variety of misguided assumptions doctors may have about human behavior, including a notion that what you do not know does not harm you.[1] This supposition is particularly apparent in the field of cancer medicine and can be seen at all stages of the disease trajectory from the time that a patient reports a sinister symptom, through diagnosis and discussions about the therapeutic benefits of different treatments, to the confirmation of disease relapse and terminal illness. In their desire to shield patients from reality, clinicians often create further difficulties for patients, their relatives, and other members of the health care team. A conspiracy of silence usually produces the opposite effect to the one intended, creating a heightened state of fear and anxiety instead of calm and equanimity. Ambiguous, deliberately misleading, or overly optimistic information can achieve short-term benefits while things go well; however, such misinformation precludes opportunities for patients to receive honest reassurance and, worse still, prevents them from restructuring their lives around more achievable, realistic hopes and aspirations.

Contrast the two following quotations from women with breast cancer, both of whom had been told about their metastases by clinicians with very different attitudes towards truth-telling.

My immediate reaction was to see it as life threatening, but when I asked how long it would be, the doctor said , "I don't know, it could be

> two months, or you could live till you're 80 . . . it depends . . . it might even stay as it is.
>
> I am realistic . . . . I know it has shortened my life, but of course I accept that no one knows at this point [the exact prognosis]. As long as they carry on telling me the truth and will give me warning when time is getting short, so I can sort out practical details.[2]

Doubtless the intention of the clinician who saw the first woman was to stop her worrying about her imminent death, but the result of the doctor's evasion and dishonesty was confusion. Cancer is an enigmatic disease, and it is never easy or prudent to give patients a precise answer to questions about prognosis, but one can always provide cautious estimates in terms of weeks rather than months or months rather than years in a supportive, honest manner that will enable patients to plan ahead and have confidence in their clinicians. The quotation from the second patient is a good example of how much this approach is valued. A patient who is aware enough, and brave enough, to pose the question about diagnosis and prognosis cannot be fobbed off with false reassurances, incomprehensible jargon, or prevarication. Such a patient needs and deserves the truth; and, if it is delivered sensitively, all the evidence shows that it relieves rather than adds to distress.[3]

In this chapter I will outline some of the problems encountered when doctors fail to disclose sufficient truthful information about diagnosis, treatment, and prognosis. I will draw mainly on the data from studies conducted in the United Kingdom.

FAILURE TO DISCLOSE THE DIAGNOSIS

Few doctors in the United Kingdom or the United States admit that they actively withhold the diagnosis of cancer from patients.[4,5] In a study comparing senior hospital doctors' attitudes with those of family practitioners in the United Kingdom, 44% of the hospital doctors said that they "normally" told patients with cancer the real diagnosis, compared with 25% of the primary care doctors.[6] This seems a rather low figure, and, as what people think they say often differs from what they actually do say in practice, it is probably an overestimate of honest disclosure. For example, when one observes patient-doctor interactions in clinics or listens to audio- or videotaped recordings, it is clear that clinicians are often "economical with the truth," and some may never actually use the word cancer. As most studies show that lay populations have a universal dread of cancer[7-9] and feel less than optimistic about the likely benefits of treatment, a doctor's failure to employ accurate terminology squanders an opportunity to correct myths and misunderstandings about the disease.

Euphemisms, such as growth or inflammation of the cells, are nothing other than an intentional, albeit subtle, deceit. When patients eventually see through the lie, further distress may be created, as euphemisms serve only to reinforce the idea held by many that cancer is an unspeakably awful disease. In the words of Michael Simpson, "what remains unspoken is unspeakable."[10]

A doctor who deals with euphemisms and who cannot bring him or herself to say the word cancer to a patient does that patient (and those who may become patients in the future) no favor in the long run. For example, it is still common practice in parts of Europe to describe abdominal cancers in euphemistic terms such as an ulcer or a blockage of the bowel.[11] As the real diagnosis would surface only when metastases occurred, a situation could quickly develop among lay populations that gastrointestinal cancers were invariably fatal. Patients with so-called bowel ulcers or blockages, who may have fared well, leading longer lives, would not help promote the concept of successful treatment or cure to the general public.[12] Thus, when a patient first sees a doctor, this pessimistic view of treatment efficacy may overshadow the interview and contribute to some of the difficulties experienced by a newly diagnosed patient. As Smith, the one-time editor of the *British Medical Journal,* once aptly observed, "The malignant reputation of cancer is enhanced by the secrecy surrounding it."[13]

Why do doctors mislead patients about the diagnosis either by what they say, the way they say it, or omitting to say anything at all? Some are plainly unaware of the fact that their words have conveyed a somewhat different meaning to the one intended, whereas others undoubtedly choose phrases or terminology that mislead. There is a great difference between a true statement and the truth. For example, "You have some abnormal cells in the lining of your bowel" is a true statement; however, if the patient actually has colorectal cancer, he or she has not been told the truth. As Lichter and Davidson have pointed out, "It seems likely that the use of words and phrases capable of subtle distinctions of meaning are deliberately used in the expectation that patients will derive from them a meaning that bears little resemblance to the known situation."[14] Hiding behind lame excuses and justifications, such as that it is kinder to use less emotive words, is an untenable position. Such rationalization of intentional deceit often says more about the doctor's desire to avoid emotionally challenging communication and his/her own difficulty in dealing with issues concerned with cancer, dying, and death.

Many doctors fail to disclose information out of a misguided belief that patients do not wish to know. There is no evidence other than personal hunch, anecdote, and intuition to support this view. In fact, several authors have shown that the majority of people do wish to know if they have cancer. For example, Cassileth *et al.*[15] reported that only 2% of their heterogeneous sample of 256 patients did not wish to know. Likewise, in a recently reported British study only 3 of 101 patients with a variety of different cancer sites would rather not know if their diagnosis was cancer.[1] In other work, a week after receiving a diagnosis of lung cancer, 50 patients were interviewed and asked about their reactions to the news. Two patients claimed not to have been told the truth, two would have preferred not to know, two were uncertain, and 46 (92%) felt that honest disclosure had been correct. None of the patients felt that they had been given too much information, but 26% thought that they had received insufficient discussion about prognosis.[16]

Some doctors, especially those with paternalistic attitudes, feel that patients would not be able to cope emotionally with the news, although there is little evidence for this assertion. Despite being given bad news about a diagnosis of lung cancer, 62% of patients in the study previously discussed felt more reassured after their interview with the doctor.[16] In research reported by a psychotherapist[17] most of the patients referred to her for anxiety management, who had failed to adjust to their cancer, had not had an honest disclosure of their disease. Similarly, in a study of 101 patients with inoperable tumors, drug usage, anxiety, and depression were highest in those who had not been told the truth of their condition.[18]

It has been said that "no news is not good news, it is an invitation to fear."[19] An example of this can be seen in the following quotation from a 72-year-old woman with breast cancer who was being treated by a doctor who belonged to the "no news is good news" school of thought. The patient was perfectly aware of the sinister implications of her breast lump, which she discovered after a fall. She felt extremely anxious, resentful, and unhappy about the doctor's unwillingness to discuss with her the results of her mammogram and the cytology report.

> He was rather vague really, looked awfully uncomfortable about it all, which started me off worrying that it might be something even worse. He kept on talking about a few abnormal cells, never said the word cancer at all, but you don't take a breast off for just a few abnormal cells, do you? I'm not sure if he thought he was being kind or something or whether he thought I was too stupid to realize what was going on. The nurse who does the breast clinic was the only one I could get anything sensible out of. I don't know what I'd have thought or done without her.[20]

The failure to discuss cancer and its implications openly with a newly diagnosed patient can be an extremely isolating experience. This is an important period, when patients need honesty, support, and help to express their changing thoughts and feelings. The following quotation is taken from an interview I had with a young man with colorectal cancer. It reveals quite graphically the misery caused by a code of silence and has echoes of the passage from Tolstoy's "Death of Ivan Ilyich,"[21] quoted at the beginning of this chapter.

paternalistic on the part of the doctor, but sometimes it is also a reflection of the expectations and attitudes of the patient population being treated. Charlton and Dovey[32] reported an interesting study of lay population, cancer patients, and their informal carers and medical students in three culturally different settings in New Zealand, the United Kingdom, and Japan. I can only summarize briefly some of their findings, but it was clear that significantly fewer people in Japan (including medical students) would wish to know the truth if they themselves were dying, and more considered that doctors should hide the truth if the prognosis was gloomy. Regardless of culture, most people wanted their relatives to be told about their diagnosis and prognosis truthfully. The family of a patient with cancer will have their own informational and emotional needs, which have to be addressed if the family is going to be able to function adequately and be able to support their relative. This can involve doctors and other care givers in potential conflicts. Obviously the family must have honest information about the diagnosis, likely prognosis, and treatment plans—but there are extremely few situations when a family should receive this information but not the patient. The rights of a competent patient to confidentiality should override the needs of the family, and a delicate balance may have to be struck between these. There are different moral and ethical positions on this issue, but in general families should not be the gatekeepers of information exchange unless the patient has given explicit permission for this.

FAILURE TO DISCUSS DEATH

There is no substantive evidence to support the notion that patients with cancer who have not been told the truth die in blissful ignorance about their disease.[33] Dying patients can usually see for themselves the deterioration of their bodies. Furthermore, the powerful verbal and nonverbal clues given by relatives, friends, and medical and nursing staff make concealment of the truth virtually impossible. The hollow cheerfulness and optimism about unreachable future goals, the stress and anxiety on the faces of loved ones trying to maintain a lie, together with the sudden, inexplicable reappearances of long-lost friends or relatives start to convey a rather obvious message even if things have not been discussed explicitly. As I have argued before,

> misguided evasion or frank dishonesty may add considerably to a dying patient's distress and prolong the adjustment process. Patients not given the chance to reveal their fears about impending death are left in anxiety-

> The fact that you've got the dreaded big C, that you've got to have an operations, wear a bag, and you might die anyway—that's not the worst of it, you know. It's being treated like a changed person and not being able to talk about it. Everyone sort of clammed up, or they were so overly nice it drove me crazy. I just wanted to be me, to cry about it, be angry about it, say how scared I was, and sometimes even be brave about it; but no one wanted to listen. They all just wanted me to be a good patient. I had to listen to them talking about how lucky I had been that they had caught it early, what a good surgeon Mr. X was, and don't forget all those endless conversations about the bloody weather or my nice flowers and cards when they changed the dressing. Did they really think that could make you feel better about it all? Then everyone who visited did the same sort of thing—this great big game of pretense. I just wanted someone to ask me how I felt, I didn't want to pretend this nasty thing hadn't happened. It had, and it was real for the rest of my life, and no one could help. I've never felt so alone.[20]

It is interesting to note that this patient described his cancer in euphemistic terms, which is what his surgeon had done at the outset. The efforts by his doctors, nurses, relatives, and friends to jolly him along and not discuss his fears and concerns openly led to deep depression and major adjustment problems.

FAILURE TO DISCUSS TREATMENT OPTIONS ACCURATELY

Several studies have shown that the overwhelming majority of patients with cancer not only want to know the truth about their diagnosis, they also would like to have as much information as possible about treatments and side effects.[15,22–24]

One of these research projects involved 50 patients with inoperable lung cancer. Among the 32% of patients who said that they would have liked more information, many commented that they had been reluctant to ask for it as they felt they were wasting the doctor's time.[23] This demonstrates the fallacy of thinking that patients who want more information will ask for it. In the United Kingdom, despite a more consumerist climate within our National Health Service, patients still have a somewhat deferential attitude towards their doctor and will not ask unless given very clear opportunities and encouragement to do so. Too many doctors assume that silence on the part of a patient reflects a desire not to have any further information. In work done by myself and colleagues in the United Kingdom 94% of 101 patients with mixed cancer diagnoses expressed a desire for as much information as possible, be it good news or bad. Only 4% wished for extra information provided it was good news, and 2% said that they would rather have as little information as possible and preferred to leave everything up to the doctor.[1,24] In order to protect the very few patients who genuinely wish to have limited information, we potentially harm the majority who wish for much more. Provision of good information is extremely important, as there is evidence that patients who rated the information given them as inadequate at the time of diagnosis, when treatment options were discussed, never adjust properly to their disease. In a study of 269 women with early stage I or II breast cancer, those who perceived the information given as inadequate suffered significantly more anxiety and depression than those who felt the information given had been good.[25,26]

It is important to note that an expressed preference for more information does not mean that patients necessarily wish to become involved in the final decision making about treatment. Some doctors confuse the need for information with a desire for more autonomy regarding medical management. Several studies have shown that fewer patients than one might imagine wish to make decisions about treatment; nevertheless, the vast majority wish to know a great deal more about the rationale behind the decisions.[25,27,28] Work by Degner and her co-workers, for example, showed that the majority of their sample of women with breast cancer wanted a passive or collaborative role in decision making rather than an active one.[29]

Obviously, patients cannot make properly informed choices about anything, including opting to let the doctor make treatment decisions, if they have not been given sufficient truthful information in the first place.

Doctors often minimize the extent of patient's disease and then withhold important information about the true intent of treatment and likely side effects. The following quotation comes from a woman with breast cancer who died from lung metastases nine weeks after her interview:

> The doctors said, "Take the Tamoxifen, that'll hold it.... it's quite simple to have your lung drained." They did say only evidence of secondaries in the lung, so I presume that means it's not too bad hopefully.[2]

Such subterfuge might produce some short-term advantages in that the patient may be less distressed, but this is maintained only while things continue to go well. The patient who has been lied to or misled at this stage is unlikely to have any confidence in assurances that her pain will be controlled or that further treatments are available to hold the disease in check if it fails to respond to initial therapy or when the disease relapses. Furthermore, this sets up a climate of mistrust for other health carers who may come in contact with the patient.

Some doctors are economical with the truth on the grounds that they cannot possibly give accurate information about cancer and the likely outcome of the treatments. This argument is mere sophistry. One can always be honest about one's own uncertainty; e.g., "I cannot say for certain that

this treatment will cure you, but we do have evidence from our research trials that some patients do respond well" is an honest statement that is likely to be of more help to a patient than premature reassurance that treatment will cure them or giving so little information that the patient assumes cure is a real prospect.

Doctors often justify their giving patients misleading information or relatives may ask for patients not to be told the truth on the grounds that patients will give up hope especially those who can cope only through the use of denial. However, this assertion is based on a misunderstanding about denial. Patients who can use such a strategy effectively do so even when told the truth. The maintenance of hope is a strange and futile pursuit if this involves encouraging people to hope against hope that a miracle will occur. If health carers' energies were directed at helping patients redefine their hope to realistic goals, such as freedom from pain or an ability to maintain a good quality of life, much could be achieved. This can be seen in the following quotation from a woman of 34 years with breast cancer who had been encouraged by everyone not to give up hope. This involved her embarking on a variety of diets and other quasi-medical programs.

> I just cracked and told H [her husband] that I couldn't do it anymore. Somehow we seem closer and happier than we've ever been now we've stopped pretending what's going to happen to me. I've got more time to think about all the good things that have happened to us instead of concentrating on cancer cells all the time.[30]

TELLING THE RELATIVE BUT NOT THE PATIENT

Sometimes the doctor tells the relatives the truth but not the patient. Few doctors in the United Kingdom claim that they do this. For exampl only 2 of 106 senior doctors attending communication skills courses r by the author, said that they often told relatives the diagnosis but not t patient, and only 5 said that they often told relatives but not the pati about the prognosis.

Thomsen *et al.*[11] reported differences in attitudes to this issue betw northern European and southern and eastern European clinicians. N in northern European countries claimed to disclose information a diagnosis and prognosis to both patient and spouse, whereas tho southern and eastern Europe usually concealed the diagnosis fror

patient but gave truthful information to the spouse. It is easy for th us brought up in the West to be extremely critical of this lack of hone closure to a patient and question the ethics of telling a relative wi patient's permission. Such behavior appears unethical and unacc

ridden isolation. If, because of the desire by medical staff to avoid distressing disclosures, they fail to make necessary adjustments, such as setting realistic goals and accepting the inevitable, then they are usually unable to enjoy whatever remaining period of life is left.[34]

As Colin Murray Parkes has pointed out,

> if a dying person has the situation revealed to him . . . little by little, at his own pace, and provided he is encouraged to share with others the feelings which these facts evoke, and provided that others are not constantly feeding back to him their own fears, he will move progressively closer to a full realisation of the situation without suffering overwhelming panic and despair.[35]

Concealment of truth means that patients cannot reveal their fantasies about death and their anxious ruminations about what lies ahead. Consequently, unnecessary fears cannot be allayed. Lichter provides a sensitive, succinct description of this:

> Silence may be eloquent [but] . .; . if we do not tell, it is not just the diagnosis we have withheld, we have not told the patient that we understand his illness, understand how he feels; we have not told him that we shall support him and that we shall keep him comfortable—this, at a time when he is dependent upon the emotional support of others. It is when the prognosis is bad that there is a need to belong to family, friends, people.[36]

Death remains a taboo topic in many cultures; thus a failure to discuss the subject sensitively and supportively fuels the misconceptions and misapprehensions that many people have. It is particularly distressing to watch families who have not been helped to confront the reality of the situation locked in communication about trivia or frozen in silence. In Lawrence Goldie's words, "couples instead of drawing closer together wither in each other's arms."[37] Relatives who beg the doctor to withhold information about the prognosis or, worse still, ask for further treatment to be given when it is unlikely to be of any therapeutic benefit, are revealing as much about their own reluctance to discuss death as their anxiety about their loved one.

In an interesting study by Gotay[38] of women with breast cancer and their partners, talking about it to others was found to be the most useful coping strategy. She found that men were more upset about their partner's imminent death than were the women themselves. Doctors and others can help enormously by facilitating more open communication between a dying person and his or her relatives.

WHAT CAN BE DONE?

On balance, it appears that although the need for specific information varies between patients and over time, in general patients with cancer wish to be well informed about their diagnosis, outlook, therapeutic options, and side effects. Some patients prefer to have more limited information, but their number is far smaller than many doctors might assume. At the moment clinicians have few formal means of deciding in advance of an interview what an individual patients needs and information preferences are. There has been some interesting experimental work looking at ways of determining this more formally, prior to an interview, and then getting the clinician to tailor his or her communication with the patient accordingly.[39]

We hear a great deal about patients' rights to accurate information, and it is clear that these are often violated. Blunt, brutal truth-telling is not acceptable either, and patients also have rights to more limited information if they have been given an opportunity to express the preference clearly and are always given the chance to change their mind if the situation changes.[40]

The compromise of offering to tell patients the truth rather than imposing the truth on patients who genuinely would prefer to know less is, of course, open to abuse. Doctors deciding to take this line have to become more adept at interpreting the variety of verbal and nonverbal patterns of communication used by individuals.

True autonomy logically should include patients' preferences for less as well as more information being respected. However, this area remains confused and is not well informed by empirical studies. When information is withheld from patients about prognosis and therapeutic benefits, it is usually the result of an intuitive decision made by the doctor, and this intuition is often faulty.

Lies always beget more lies. They impose stresses and strains on everyone and rarely protect patients from anxiety and despair. One always has to remember what has or has not been said, and everyone involved with the care of a patient has to tell the same story. This rarely works for long, and a patient is left wondering who or what to believe. As Mark Twain once said, "If you tell the truth, you don't have to remember anything." We all need to learn how to become better, more supportive truth-tellers; able to pace and tailor the information that individual patients tell us they want rather than relying on our own, often faulty, patronizing assumptions about what people want. We also need more research efforts directed at identifying ways to train doctors how to impart difficult and challenging information in a way that helps patients and does not compromise the doctor's own emotional survival. It is easy to criticize, but few doctors are given sufficient training in communication or personal management skills to fulfill their roles adequately.

REFERENCES

1. FALLOWFIELD. L. J., S. FORD & S. LEWIS. 1995. No news is not good news: Patient preferences for information. Psycho-Oncology **4:** 197–202.
2. HALL, A, L. J. FALLOWFIELD & R. A'HERN. 1995. When breast cancer recurs: A 3-year prospective study of psychological morbidity. Breast **2**(2): 1–7.
3. STESIN, M. L. 1987. Talking about cancer: How much is too much? Br. J. **40**: 56–59.
4. HOLLAND, J. C., N. GEARY, A. MARCHINI & S. TROSS. 1987. An international survey of physician attitudes and practice in regard to revealing the diagnosis of cancer. Cancer Invest. **5**(2): 151–154.
5. NEWALL, D. J., E. M. GADD & T. J. PRIESTMAN. 1987. Presentation of information to cancer patients. A comparison of two centres in the UK and USA. Br. J. Med. Psychol. **60**: 127-131.
6. WILKES, E. 1984. The "quality of life." *In* Palliative Care: The Management of Far-Advanced Illness. D. Doyle, Ed.: 9–19. The Charles Press. Philadelphia, PA.
7. WYLER, A. R., M. MASUDA & T. H. HOMES. 1968. Seriousness of illness scale. J. Psychosom. Res. **2**: 363–374.
8. JENKINS, C. D. 1966. The semantic differential for health: A technique for measuring beliefs about disease. Public Health Rep. **81**: 549–558.
9. MCINTOSH, J. 1974. Process of communication, information seeking and control associated with cancer. A selective review of the literature. Soc. Sci. Med. **8**: 167–187.
10. SIMPSON, M. A. 1982. Therapeutic uses of truth. *In* The Dying Patient. E. Wilkes, Ed.: 255–262. MYP Press. Lancaster.
11. THOMSEN, O., H. R. WULFF & A. MARTIN. 1993. What do gastroenterologists in Europe tell cancer patients? Lancet **341**: 473–476.
12. FALLOWFIELD, L. J. & A. W. CLARK. 1994. Delivering bad news in gastroenterology. Am. J. Gastroenterol. **89**(4): 473–479.
13. SMITH, A. 1976. Should a doctor tell the truth when a patient has cancer? The Times (London), March 31.
14. LICHTER, I. & G. P. DAVIDSON. 1981. Care of the dying; questions and answers. Part 2: Pain management and communication. New Zealand Family Physician **8**: 56–59.
15. CASSILETH, B. R., R. V. ZUPKIS, K. SUTTON-SMITH & V. MARCH. 1980. Information and participation preferences among cancer patients. Ann. Intern. Med. **92**: 832–836.
16. SELL, L. B., DEVLIN, S. J. BOURKE, N. C. MUNRO, P. A. CORRIS & G. J. GIBSON. 1993. Communicating the diagnosis of lung cancer. Resp. Med. **87**(1): 61–63.
17. STEDEFORD, A. 1984. Facing Death. Heinemann. London.
18. GERLE, B., G. LUNDEN & P. SANDBLOM. 1960. The patient with inoperable cancer from the psychiatric and social standpoints. Cancer **13**: 1206–1217.
19. FLETCHER, C. 1980. Listening and talking to patients. Br. Med. J. **281**: 994.
20. FALLOWFIELD, L. J. 1991. Counselling patients with cancer. *In* Counselling and Communication in Health Care. L. J. Fallowfield & H. Davis, Eds.: 253–269. John Wiley & Sons. Chichester.
21. TOLSTOY, L. 1960. The Death of Ivan Ilyich and Other Stories. Penguin Books. London.
22. BLANCHARD, C. G., M. S. LABREQUE, J. C. BUCKDESCHEL & E. B. BLANCHARD. 1988. Information and decision-making preferences of hospitalised adult

cancer patients. Soc. Sci. Med. **27**(11): 1139–1145.
23. HUGHES, J. 1985. Depressive illness and lung cancer: 11. Follow-up of inoperable patients. Eur. J. Surg. Oncol. **11**: 21–24.
24. FALLOWFIELD, L. J., S. FORD & S. LEWIS. 1994. Information preferences of patients with cancer. Lancet **344**: 1576.
25. FALLOWFIELD, L. J., A. HALL, G. P. MAGUIRE & M. BAUM. 1990. Psychological outcomes of different treatment policies in women with early breast cancer outside a clinical trial. Br. Med. J. **301**: 57S–580.
26. FALLOWFIELD, L. J., A. HALL, P. MAGUIRE, M. BAUM & R. P. A'HERN. 1994. A question of choice: Results of a prospective 3-year follow-up study of women with breast cancer. Breast **3**: 202–208.
27. SUTHERLAND, H. J., H. A. LLEWELLYN-THOMAS, G. A. LOCKWOOD, D. L. TRITCHLER & J. E. TILL. 1989. Cancer patients: Their desire for information and participation in treatment decisions. J. Roy. Soc. Med. **82**(5): 260–263.
28. RICHARDS, M. A., A. J. RAMIREZ, L. F. DEGNER, L. J. FALLOWFIELD, E. J. MAHER & J. NEUBERGER. 1995. Offering choice of treatment to patients with cancers. A review based on a symposium held at the 10th Annual Conference of The British Psychosocial Oncology Group, December 1993. Eur. J. Cancer **31A**(1): 112–116.
29. DEGNER, L. F. & J. A. SLOAN. 1992. Decision making during serious illness: What role do patients really want to play? J. Clin. Epidemiol. **45**(9): 941–950.
30. FALLOWFIELD, L. J. & A. CLARK. 1991. Breast Cancer. The Experience of Illness Series. R. Fitzpatrick & S. Newman, Eds. Routledge. London.
31. FIELDING, R. L. S. F. KO & L. WONG. 1995. Inconsistencies between belief and practice—Assessment of Chinese cancer patients' knowledge of their disease. J. Cancer Care **4**: 11–15.
32. CHARLTON, R. & S. DOVEY. 1995. Attitudes to death and dying in the UK, New Zealand and Japan. J. Palliative Care **11**(1): 42–47.
33. KÜBLER-ROSS, E. 1970. On Death and Dying. Macmillan. New York, NY.
34. FALLOWFIELD, L. J. 1990. The Quality of Life: The Missing Measurement in Health Care. Human Horizons Series. Souvenir Press. London.
35. PARKES, C. M. 1978. Psychological aspects. *In* The Management of Terminal Disease. C. M. Saunders, Ed.: 44–64. Edward Arnold. London.
36. LICHTER, I. 1984. Communication. *In* Palliative Care: The Management of Far Advanced Illness. D. Doyle, Ed.: 444–460. Croom Helm. Beckenham, Kent, U.K.
37. GOLDIE, L. 1982. The ethics of telling the patient. J. Med. Ethics **8**: 128–133..
38. GOTAY, C. C. 1984. The experience of cancer during early and advanced stages: The views of patients and their mates. Soc. Sci. Med. **18**: 605–613.
39. SIMES, R. J., H. H. N. TATTERSALL, A. S. COATES, D. RAGHAVAN, H. J. SOLOMON & H. SMARTT. 1986. Randomised comparison of procedures for obtaining informed consent in clinical trials of treatment for cancer. Br. Med. J. **293**: 1065–1068.
40. TOBIAS, J. S. & R. L. SOUHAMI. 1993. Fully informed consent can be needlessly cruel. Br. Med. J. **307**: 1199–2001.
41. FALLOWFIELD, L. J. 1995. Can we improve the professional and personal fulfilment of doctors in cancer medicine? Br. J. Cancer **71**: 1132–1133.

Afterword

Right now I'm very angry with doctors. I think part of me is—irrationally—blaming them for my illness, or at least for not having an easier, more straightforward way of curing it.

But I'm also angry because not one of them ever asked me how I felt about this or what I wanted. They all made tremendous assumptions about me and galloped forward in their treatments without any consideration of me as an individual. I galloped along with them as best I could until I couldn't stand it any more, and then I had to dig in my heels. I think there's something wrong about this.

—S. K. T.

Not long ago a friend of mine, whose words I have quoted above, invited me to accompany her on a visit to her oncologist. She was going to learn the results of the surgery and chemotherapy she had undergone for ovarian cancer. She had been encouraged to believe that with these treatments she could be cured.

The results were not good. There was significant new cancer growth. When she asked how often this occurred in similar cases, the physician's answer—in about fifty percent of cases—did not accord with what she recalled having been told when she was being encouraged to undergo the treatment.

The physician recommended more surgery and chemotherapy. When my friend asked what would happen if she did nothing, the physician replied—with a marked change in his hitherto friendly tone of voice—that her digestive system would eventually shut down and she would, in effect, puke to death. For readers not familiar with American slang I will explain that "puke" is a crude word for "vomit."

That exchange was a turning point in my friend's life. She was shaken by the bad news she had just heard and felt that she was being manipulated a second time into treatment that might well not be effective, and that she did not think she could go through again. And she felt that she was being censured by the physician for having questioned his recommendation for that treatment.

At that moment she lost trust in her physician and hope in further treatment.

This incident forcefully brought home to me the crucial importance of the subject of this book. In this country there is general agreement that the physician should tell the truth to the cancer patient. My friend's physician is an experienced, highly regarded oncologist, who does not shun but welcomes human contact with his patients. There seemed to be a good rapport between him and my friend. If in such favorable circumstances communication could take such an unfortunate turn, how much more easily might this happen in less favorable circumstances! I hope and believe this book will help make this less likely.

RICHARD STIEFEL
Associate Editor
The New York Academy of Sciences

Index of Contributors